COCAINE: EFFECTS ON THE DEVELOPING BRAIN

ANNALS OF THE NEW YORK ACADEMY OF SCIENCES

Volume 846

COCAINE: EFFECTS ON THE DEVELOPING BRAIN

Edited by John A. Harvey and Barry E. Kosofsky

The New York Academy of Sciences
New York, New York
1998

The photo on the softcover version of this book shows three children born to drug-abusing mothers followed up in the SAEF (Substances of Abuse Exposure Follow-up) Clinic at the Massachusetts General Hospital. The children demonstrate various features of neurodevelopmental compromise seen in the subset of infants exposed in utero *to drugs of abuse. These features include those of fetal alcohol syndrome/hypoxic ischemic encephalopathy (E.C., right); microcephaly (J.M., middle); and selective language delay (R.K., left). The children are in the arms of their adoptive mothers, who collectively have participated in the raising of more than 500 biologic, foster, and adoptive children.*

Library of Congress Cataloging-in-Publication Data

Cocaine : effects on the developing brain / edited by John A. Harvey and Barry E. Kosofsky.

p. cm.—(Annals of the New York Academy of Sciences ; v. 846)

"This volume is the result of a conference entitled Cocaine : effects on the developing brain sponsored jointly by the New York Academy of Sciences and the Allegheny University of the Health Sciences and held in Washington, DC, September 16–19, 1997"—Contents p.

Includes bibliographical references and index.

ISBN 1-57331-127-8 (alk. paper). — ISBN 1-57331-128-6 (pbk. : alk. paper)

1. Cocaine—Toxicology—Congresses. 2. Fetus—Effect of drugs on—Congresses. 3. Brain—Effect of drugs on—Congresses. 4. Children of prenatal substance abuse—Development—Congresses. 5. Drug abuse in pregnancy—Congresses. 6. Developmental neurobiology—Congresses. 7. Toxicology—Congresses. I. Harvey, John A. (John Adriance), 1930– . II. Kosofsky, Barry E. III. New York Academy of Sciences. IV. Allegheny University of the Health Sciences. V. Series.

Q11.N5 vol. 846
[RG627.6.N37]
500 s—dc21
[618.3′268]

98-6824
CIP

ComCom/RRD
Printed in the United States of America
ISBN 1-57331-127-8 (cloth)
ISBN 1-57331-128-6 (paper)
ISSN 0077-8923

ANNALS OF THE NEW YORK ACADEMY OF SCIENCES

Volume 846
June 21, 1998

COCAINE: EFFECTS ON THE DEVELOPING BRAIN[a]

Editors and Conference Organizers
JOHN A. HARVEY AND BARRY E. KOSOFSKY

CONTENTS

[a] This volume is the result of a conference entitled **Cocaine: Effects on the Developing Brain** sponsored jointly by the New York Academy of Sciences and the Allegheny University of the Health Sciences and held in Washington, DC, September 16–19, 1997.

Part 2. Postnatal Effects: Neurobehavioral Models

Part 3. Developmental Mechanisms

Part 4. Functional Deficits

Part 5. Longitudinal Studies in Humans/Public Policy

Part 6. Poster Papers

Financial assistance was received from:

- ALLEGHENY UNIVERSITY OF THE HEALTH SCIENCES
- NATIONAL INSTITUTE ON DRUG ABUSE (NIDA)
- NATIONAL INSTITUTE ON CHILD AND HUMAN DEVELOPMENT (NICHD)
- NATIONAL INSTITUTE OF MENTAL HEALTH (NIMH)
- MARCH OF DIMES
- CULPEPER FOUNDATION

Introduction

JOHN A. HARVEY[a] AND BARRY E. KOSOFSKY[b]

[a]*Department of Pharmacology, MCP ◆ Hahnemann School of Medicine, Allegheny University of the Health Sciences, Philadelphia, Pennsylvania 19129, USA*

[b]*Laboratory of Molecular and Developmental Neuroscience and Department of Neurology, Massachusetts General Hospital and Harvard Medical School, Boston, Massachusetts 02114, USA*

This volume is the result of a meeting dealing with the consequences of cocaine exposure on brain development that was held on September 16–19, 1997. This meeting was attended by approximately 200 scientists and clinicians who spent 3 days presenting, reviewing, comparing, and discussing the latest data from studies in animal models and in humans. As reflected by articles published in *Newsweek, Science,* and the APA monitor as well as by the enthusiastic comments from meeting participants, this was a landmark conference. Two of the key ingredients that contributed to its success included presentations from research groups who have developed improved methods to more clearly identify some of the consequences of prenatal cocaine exposure, and interdigitation of clinical and preclinical presentations and discussion which emphasized the convergence of findings from studies in humans with animal research. The consensus which has emerged from this "second generation" of clinical research is that as some cocaine-exposed children enter school, they have particular difficulty modulating arousal, attention, impulsivity, reactivity, and other components of behavior that are essential for academic success. Parallel behavioral findings have been observed in animal studies, suggesting that particular neurochemical systems which subserve attention and reactivity are permanently altered following prenatal cocaine exposure. The convergence of data and conclusions suggests that some infants and children exposed to cocaine *in utero* will demonstrate selective handicaps in significantly important behaviors.

The importance of identifying the specific behavioral deficits evident in cocaine-exposed offspring was appreciated by all who attended the meeting. Animal researchers realized that the models that they have developed in mice, rats, rabbits, and primates are informative and relevant. These researchers are now able to use their models to identify basic mechanisms underlying cocaine-induced alterations in brain structure and functions which may lead to prevention or amelioration of behavioral deficits. Clinicians realized that the methods that they have developed to control for the multitude of genetic, environmental, prenatal, and postnatal confounders have permitted identification of specific behavioral alterations induced by cocaine. It is clearly not the case that every child exposed to cocaine *in utero* demonstrates brain growth retardation, motor system abnormalities, and behavioral compromise. The clinical expression of *in utero* cocaine exposure is contextual: as with other prenatal insults, the outcome of cocaine-exposed infants is critically dependent on the richness of the postnatal environment. Indeed, this conference demonstrated the subtlety of some of the behavioral effects of *in utero* cocaine exposure that are not always apparent in standard tests but appear only in more complex situations. However, it does appear that children who sustain higher levels of prenatal cocaine exposure are more likely to demonstrate selective impairment in postnatal brain growth, as well as postnatal impairments in attention, reactivity, and impulsivity. By focusing on those particular behaviors that are altered in cocaine-exposed children, clinical studies can now focus on the effectiveness of particular interventions to improve those specific outcomes.

The improved clarity and insight provided by this meeting will stimulate clinicians and scientists to develop new strategies for improved diagnosis and therapy for cocaine-exposed children. With the greater sophistication that was achieved through the presentations and discussions at the meeting, we have gone beyond the polemic of "nature versus nurture"; clearly both are relevant. Cocaine can disrupt programs for brain development in specific ways with unique behavioral consequences. The expression of that insult is critically dependent on the postnatal environment. Exposed children may be at risk for lifelong behavioral handicaps that are biologically induced and environmentally exacerbated and that will put some children at a permanent disadvantage regarding educability, adaptability, and socialization. Having identified these facts, we must now educate the public and in particular educators and individuals who shape public policy to develop strategies for prevention, intervention, and amelioration of one of the most significant preventable causes of developmental disability in our society today.

Foreword

ALAN I. LESHNER

Director, National Institute on Drug Abuse, National Institutes of Health, Rockville, Maryland

Drug use during pregnancy, particularly the use of cocaine, has engendered significant attention in recent years as a serious threat to public health. In fact, few emergent issues of the past decade rival prenatal cocaine exposure in its scientific, clinical, societal, and political complexity. During the mid- to late 1980s, rising trends in cocaine use among pregnant women coupled with reports that appeared in both the scientific and the popular press implicating prenatal cocaine exposure in adverse neonatal outcomes triggered a premature "rush to judgment" with regard to the fate of cocaine-exposed children. But, importantly, these events also aroused heightened research interest in this relatively understudied area and generated increased research efforts to better understand the extent to which cocaine can affect the developing brain. Since that time, despite the unique challenges and barriers that have confronted researchers in this field—from the methodologic limitations they face to the social, legal, and public policy aspects surrounding the topic of prenatal drug exposure—a great deal of scientific progress has been made.

Research on the developmental sequelae of prenatal drug exposure has been challenged by the complexity of multiple possible influences on outcomes, including the direct impact of drug exposure on biologic functioning and the indirect effects on development resulting from ongoing exposure to the many facets of a drug-using environment. And the nature of this complex mix of influences changes with the age and developmental stage of the child. Despite such challenges, researchers have made significant progress in studying sequelae of prenatal drug exposure and in developing improved assessment strategies and enhanced approaches for dealing with confounding factors. Scientists in a variety of disciplines have developed and refined tools and technologies that are helping to identify children who have been exposed to drugs prenatally and to assess the direct and indirect pharmacologic and behavioral effects of drug exposure. Ongoing longitudinal studies have advanced to the point where subjects have reached school age, and hypotheses that once were pure speculation, including the notion that some of the cognitive effects of prenatal cocaine exposure may not show up until these children's cognitive abilities along certain dimensions were challenged, can finally be tested.

Scientists have also been getting far better at asking the most relevant research questions. Obviously, the central issue that needs to be resolved relates to whether or not children are affected by prenatal cocaine exposure at all. If they are, it then becomes critical to know the type and magnitude of the deficits to look for. Are these effects likely to show up in dramatic ways? Or will the effects be subtle and difficult to detect? Knowing where in the developmental process these effects are likely to appear is another important part of the puzzle. Will the effects of prenatal drug exposure be readily evident at birth? Or will they only emerge at those points in the child's life in which they encounter specific cognitive, social, or environmental challenges?

If the science consistently shows that all of those who are exposed to cocaine are affected, then the task to be accomplished, obviously, becomes relatively straightforward—identifying those children who were exposed and intervening early. However, if the preponderance of data suggests instead that only some children are affected, the task then is to find out who they are and to administer interventions that will be beneficial without adding to their burden by labeling or stigmatizing them. This is, in fact, one of the greatest challenges facing those who work in this field, for such labeling could potentially do as much harm as the direct or indirect effects of the drugs themselves.

Intervention is another important issue. What types of interventions are cocaine-exposed children going to need? What is involved in those interventions that will make a measurable difference to the affected child? How will these interventions be administered? And what types of fiscal and practical considerations do each of these entail?

If the findings relating to cocaine-exposed children that have begun to emerge are, in fact, real, how will the relative roles that biologic and environmental factors play be firmly delineated? Are the consequences observed the result of a child's living environment or can they be attributed to the drug to which they were exposed? Research findings obtained to date in this area have helped us to recognize and fully appreciate the extent to which pharmacologic variables are intricately intertwined with co-occurring biologic, genetic, social, and environmental variables. Thus, the challenge becomes to determine not only the impact of each of these domains individually but also the probable outcomes of their interactions.

The 3-day landmark conference jointly sponsored by the New York Academy of Sciences and the Allegheny University of the Health Sciences on which this document is based brought together many of the major basic and clinical researchers in this field to discuss the current state of the science in this area. Chapters contained in this volume report on research that has attempted to identify the molecular, neurochemical, physiologic, and neuropathologic processes that may mediate the toxicity of gestational cocaine exposure and the behavioral and clinical correlates of that exposure. This important meeting served as an extremely valuable forum not only for disseminating the latest findings in this area of research but also for identifying many of the knowledge gaps that still remain, for discussing many of the key policy issues that need to be addressed, and for charting a strategic course of action for the field. So where do we go from here?

As reported by many of the conference participants, to date, animal models have been particularly useful for studying the effects of prenatal exposure and for modeling drug-related effects on brain development at the structural, cellular, and functional levels. Clearly we need to further cultivate this basic strategy of exploiting animal models that are appropriate to the phenomenon being addressed. As our understanding of the subtlety of cocaine's behavioral effects in humans (cognitive functions, neuropsychological processes, etc.) improves, we must have better animal models to predict these outcomes accurately and to aid us in more fully understanding the underlying mechanisms that are at work.

We also need to generate much more information than we currently have about the effects of drugs of abuse on the developing brain. We started with the assumption that all prenatal cocaine effects would be exerted via systemic or cardiovascular effects on the mother and her reproductive system. But with the recent discovery that there are active neurotransmitters and cocaine receptors in the fetal brain, the whole enterprise has changed. So we need to continue to intensify our efforts to learn more about what is happening at the cellular and molecular level.

Beyond the basic science, the problem of prenatal cocaine exposure needs to be addressed from a clinical standpoint. We need to evaluate the need for and then develop and apply the appropriate interventions. The question here becomes what should these interventions be? And for whom? And how will we know who is about to be affected? Or whose effects are about to be expressed? And who has been protected in some way? And how? The fact is that the complexity, subtlety, and nonuniversality of the effects of prenatal exposure pose incredibly complex research questions. We need to develop strategies to address all of these issues.

Then, obviously, we need to study the affected children with greater intensity, more sophisticated methods, and over long periods of time. To do this more emphasis must be placed on longitudinal studies. To get the full picture we must look at the long-term consequences of prenatal drug exposure at least through childhood into late adolescence, examining outcomes in such domains as neurodevelopment, social development, physical development, physical health, and vulnerability to drug abuse.

We must also continue to bring innovative approaches to the study of this area by drawing additional researchers with neighboring expertise into this fray. For example, the additional perspectives of more cognitive scientists, more developmental cognitive scientists, and the like could greatly benefit the field. And, of course, there must be translational research or research bridging animal and human work to assure that generalizations we make are in fact reliable and valid and that we are generating information that will ultimately be useful in clinical practice.

Overall we must intensify research efforts in this area if we are able to fill the gaps that exist and replace the myths that have been conjured up about "crack babies" with scientific data of high quality. And although our scientific pursuits in this area constitute enormous challenges, our efforts must not end here. Research in this field is far from simply an academic or scientific pursuit. It has tremendous implications for both how we treat children and how we frame policy. Thus, public understanding of this issue is another area of concern that urgently needs to be addressed. We have seen the pendulum swing—from public hysteria about crack babies in the mid- to late 1980s to more recent press suggesting no need for worry or alarm. We need to think about a strategy for rolling out to the public—and to health care providers, child welfare workers, teachers, etc.—the truth, including the truth about the complexity of this problem and the unpredictability of who is or who will be affected and who will not. It is also important for the public to realize that there are many kids who will have serious problems. And we need to explain all this without inadvertently stigmatizing large numbers of children, many of whom may be, at most, minimally affected.

In my view there is an imperative to get a more accurate, even if more complex, understanding out there of what is happening, or at least our best guess at what is happening. Educating the public to withhold judgment about children prenatally exposed to cocaine until we have all the facts will best serve these children's interests. Even in a changing knowledge climate it is essential that we roll out the truth about the effects of prenatal cocaine. It is up to us to employ science to set the record straight. This will ultimately be our best strategy for facilitating effective care of vulnerable mothers and children.

Keynote Address

FLOYD E. BLOOM

It's really a great pleasure to be with you tonight. As John already told you, he and I go back a long ways in this science, and Barry Kosofsky, whom I remember from the time he couldn't get his thesis finished before he went to medical school, and John are sort of the core of a cadre of comrades in monoamines. There is no better home for that than in our present considerations of cocaine in the developing brain.

What I will do is start with a brief mention of what we are doing about this substance abuse science in *Science.* Then I'm going to concentrate on what I got out of your program and with the edification of the papers that Barry and John sent me in advance. Finally, I'll speak to what I think is the core question of the Conference, the issue that underlies the Academy's statement on this meeting in their magazine "Cocaine Effects in the Developing Brain: Fact or Fallacy?"

So, first let me start with what we are doing at *Science* with the science of substance abuse. The October 3rd issue (*Science* 278: 45–75, 1997), which was released for the Society for Neuroscience Meeting, will in fact be devoted to the science of substance abuse, portrayed in a more comprehensive manner than we have heretofore done. That special issue includes the molecular, cellular, and behavioral sciences of substance abuse, but edited in a way that allows you the reader to comprehend what's being done regardless of your prior scientific background. The issue also goes into the status of treatment methods for each substance abuse problem we have to exemplify how in an era of managed care it's still possible to spend a dollar more wisely on treatment than it is on other forms of supply control, let us say. It also deals with the systems in the brain that have evolved to allow drugs of abuse to act on the brain and what we can learn not only in understanding the human problems but also in trying to foresee some strategies in dealing with them. A very thoughtful article is presented by Dr. Leshner on why substance abuse as a disease is an important concept to understand. I hope you will write me with your reactions to that issue after you have looked at it.

Substance abuse is a very pervasive issue, and to me the aspect of it that is most poignant is the tragic waste of human resources. The developing brain is certainly deserving of your attention and I applaud all of you for investing your time and your intellectual activity in its study.

When I talk to young scientist wannabe's, what I ask them is, "What do you think are the two most important attributes you need to be a successful scientist?" A lot of people say "grants"; a lot say "patience." For me the two most important things are logical curiosity and the ability to avoid self-delusion. I will first talk to you about a method of logical curiosity, called the method of Zadig. Zadig was a character in a fable written by Voltaire in the middle of the eighteenth century who had marvelous powers of observation and reasoning. Voltaire borrowed this character and his approach from an earlier book written in the sixteenth century about the travels of the three sons of the King of Serendipo. Serendipo (serendipity) is something that all real scientists love, because it means that while you are busy seriously looking for something you think you are going to discover, you discover something even more important. How many times do we hear, "You know what we expected to find, but instead . . . ," and there it was. And that is really the exciting thing. Zadig's logic was also much appreciated by a man named Professor Joseph Bell, a nineteenth century Scottish surgeon who had the ability to recognize what was wrong with someone as they walked in the door of his clinic. Bell was the professor and mentor of Arthur Conan Doyle who refined the characteristics of Professor Bell into the man we all know today as Sherlock Holmes, an ace in the practice of Zadig's logic, sometimes described as retrospective prophecy because the proper analysis of what has happened sometimes allows one to predict likely future developments. Of course, Sherlock Holmes, like Sigmund Freud, was a user of both opium and cocaine. So we return full circle to the problem that concerns us here.

Zadig's logic applies to every problem that a professional scientist will encounter as he/she goes forward in trying to find his/her way through the world of experimental science. It applies every time one faces a new, unexplained phenomenon and says how did this happen. It gets refined into a skill when you learn to ask "If it happened this way and if I do that experiment, then this is the result I should get." It certainly applies when one asks how cocaine use by mothers can affect the developing brain of their children *in utero.* It especially applies when you do the properly framed experiment with all of the right controls and the results reveal themselves to be totally opposite to your predictions. It is then, at least in my experience, that you need your keenest powers of what Zadig's method—retrospective prophecy—can do to move ahead because now you really have something that's worth your time to study.

If you've read any of my editorials in *Science,* you know that one of my favorite intellectual icons is Vannevar Bush. Bush was the one who coined the term, "the endless frontier." He was the person who single-handedly converted the World War II scientific effort into the powers of science for culture and society. He was also the person who predicted computerized information handling, computer networks, hypertext, and desktop computers. In one of his books, called *Science is Not Enough,* he has an essay that runs only about 1,000 words, and is called "The Builders" because it epitomizes the scientific pursuit in a way that I'm sure most of you would agree to be accurate.

> The process by which the boundaries of knowledge are advanced and the structure of organized science is built is a complex process indeed. It corresponds fairly well with the exploitation of a difficult quarry for its building materials, and the fitting of these into an edifice. The edifice, science, itself has a remarkable property, for its form is predestined by the laws of logic and the nature of human reasoning. It is almost as though it had once existed and its building blocks had been scattered, hidden, and buried, each with its unique form retained so that it would fit only into its own peculiar position.

Then he goes on to talk about the people who work in this quarry called science, some of whom he describes as having "even grasped the suggestion of its ultimate meaning . . . (who) sit in the shade and encourage the young workers."

I feel that I'm in that category with you all. This is not a field in which I have participated. But I took Barry and John's invitation to comment with seriousness; having read up on it a bit, perhaps I have a couple of things that will spark some discussions.

Fetal maldevelopment as a result of maternal drug use is not a new or unusual declaration, although it seems to surprise people every time it comes up, as it frequently does. It happened 30 years ago with thalidomide which served to reinvigorate the Federal Drug Administration in a way that the UPS strike did for the Teamsters Union. The same declaration emerged a decade ago with bendectine, a drug once used to treat morning sickness, and in my scientific career time, it has reappeared with the Fetal Alcohol Syndrome, the Fetal Phenobarbitol Syndrome, the Fetal Benzodiazepam Syndrome, and the Fetal Methadone, Dilantin, Aminoptrin, Methyltrexate, Nicotine, Acutane, and THC Fetal Maldevelopment Syndromes.

Crack babies make newsworthy reports says a recent issue (September 17, 1997) of the *Washington Post,* even if it's only pricking open an empathetic thought balloon that may have been filled with somewhat aggressive interpretations. Neuroscientists in the United States have the experimental knowledge of where in the experimental animal and human brain cocaine acts. They have the analytic tools and the animal models to look at the reality of cocaine's actions in the developing brain. They have done so under experimental conditions that can overcome some of the domentable reasons why there are always skeptics for every Fetal Drug X Syndrome that gets reported.

Women who knowingly take substance abuse drugs when they are pregnant are unlikely to have taken only one such drug. And they are unlikely to have been totally healthy before they got pregnant. So, how do we know that cocaine does what cocaine-abusing mothers find in their children? How do we know when in the course of *in utero* development it did it? How much does it take to do it? And why do some people who take cocaine seem to have totally normal babies? You can substitute for the word cocaine any of the other drugs in that list I just summarized.

In getting ready for this presentation, I decided that the thing I know the most about that seems relevant is Fetal Alcohol Syndrome (FAS). I had an Alcohol Research Center for nearly 20 years before my colleague at Scripps, George Koob, relieved me of duty. FAS was one of the things that we looked at quite a lot. Many of the problems that you face with fetal cocaine exposure are problems that were dealt with fairly well in the slowly evolving history of Fetal Alcohol Syndrome: the nature of the toxic effects, the times at which toxicity could occur, the doses required to get it, and its consequences and sequelae. Initially, I assumed there must be many more cases of Fetal Alcohol Syndrome than of Fetal Cocaine Syndrome because of the greater use of alcohol than of cocaine. However, one of the background papers claimed that as many as 10% to 15% of urban newborns have been exposed to cocaine. We are now being presented with the astounding observations that perhaps more than 40% of pregnant mothers in some populations have been exposed to cocaine, an astounding number which makes this problem an enormous challenge.

What is the actual incidence of fetal alcohol-induced problems in infants? The last *Mortality-Morbidity Weekly Report* that I could find on FAS was a 1995 review of the literature collected in the National Birth Defects Monitoring Program from 1979 to 1993, which is a pretty long time. Fetal Alcohol Syndrome in the *Mortality-Morbidity Weekly Report* was based on obstetric hospital discharge diagnoses for children. The physician had to state that the baby met the criteria for the dysmorphology and the maternal use of alcohol that makes it Fetal Alcohol Syndrome, a pretty tough diagnosis to make. When the survey was started in 1979, the incidence of FAS was estimated at 1 of every 10,000 births; by 1993 it had risen to 6.7 per 1,000 births. This assumes that we have sensitized the physician to look for these physical defects, that we've challenged them to ask the mothers about their alcohol use, and that there's a physical dysmorphology involved in the diagnosis of Fetal Alcohol Syndrome. Still this was a nearly sevenfold increase.

Given that we also recognize that the fetal alcohol effect, a diagnosis of maldevelopment cognitively without the dysmorphology, is not too far from some of the working diagnoses of what we call the fetal cocaine effect. Yet I don't have any good feeling from what you all have said as to what the real incidence is. In part, that's because mothers who use cocaine use an awful lot of other things; which of them is the "one" to which we attribute the maldevelopments?

The work that has just been presented covers some of the most remarkable achievements in all of clinical research that I've ever heard in terms of the numbers of mothers and babies diagnosed. The same goes for the preclinical research in experimental animals. I am particularly impressed with the *Trends in Neurosciences* paper that John, Barry, and their colleagues put together and the original research on which it is based.

Their use of reasonable doses of cocaine administered in a consistent way gave rise to many experimental consequences. As I was studying those papers, my initial reaction was to question how they know that these rabbit fetuses have all had the right birth weight or some other variable. But each time their data had indeed measured that: birth weight, weight gain during pregnancy, number of pups per litter, everything seeming to match between control and drug-exposed fetuses. That uniformity wasn't achieved in Fetal Alcohol Syndrome for a very long time.

Dealing with the possible toxic, teratogenic effects of nutritional deprivation is very critical. From all of our work on Fetal Alcohol Syndrome, I can tell you that the healthier, less stressed the mom and her pups, the less toxic the Fetal Alcohol Syndrome. We've been able to give pups pretty potent amounts of alcohol under hands-off, non-controlled conditions in which they are only away from their moms for an hour a day and it's very hard to find anything wrong with them at all. If you stress them a little or compromise their nutrition a little, then all of these things bring out a potential adaptive mechanism that's run its gamut. All those things come to the forefront.

It's therefore very critical for animal researchers to take a leading role in this Fetal Cocaine Syndrome campaign. Earlier, Ted Slotkin called this kind of work, "Cocaine as a Probe of the Developing Animal Brain." Maybe that's a nice way of expressing morbid curiosity about the animal causes of the human problem. But let's assume that there are very specific developmental defects in the human nervous system that we see in the Fetal Cocaine Syndrome, in the rabbit nervous system that we see in the work of Barry, Pat, John, and all their colleagues, and in the work with rats that Linda Spear described.

The question then has to be: Is the site of that maldevelopmental action the same molecular mechanism to which we attribute the reinforcement actions of cocaine, namely, the dopamine transporter? Well, there are problems with that conclusion. One problem is that we don't yet know when in rabbit or rat gestation we must give the intravenous doses of cocaine to cause the effect that unleashes the later neurochemical, cytologic, and behavioral manifestations. As I understand the current protocol extends drug exposure from implantation until 2 days before the end of pregnancy. But we know that the dopamine system develops later and that it certainly doesn't innervate the parts of the brain that Pat Levitt finds to be disturbed cytologically until mid-term or later. In fact, I couldn't find a study on prenatal development of dopamine neurons in the rabbit; therefore, what we think we know about the rabbit we extrapolate from what we think we know about rats and mice. There, dopamine neurons are not born until the middle of gestation. So, if the dopamine transporter is the place where cocaine acts to confuse brain cellular development, you shouldn't have to treat them before day 14 because before then there isn't any dopamine transporter.

On the other hand, a very interesting sidelight to the Levitt, Kosofsky, Harvey, and colleagues' review was the recognition of the recent studies by Lidow this which bring to light certain facts that are in the literature but are not very well known. Lidow points out that there are substantial amounts of catecholamines in the brain long before the central catecholamine neurons are born and long before the blood-brain barrier seals them off, which may have some of the alleged trophic effects that we've always thought we could attribute to catecholamines but could never quite prove.

We all know that in addition to blocking the dopamine transporter, cocaine also blocks the norepinephrine transporter and the serotonin transporter. In digging through this literature, I found an astounding series of observations that in the early embryonic development of the sensory pathways from the thalamus to the cortex, these thalamocortical neuron systems transiently express the 5-HT transporter long before the serotonin neurons actually innervate the cortex. The non-serotonin neurons can use this transporter to accumulate 5-HT into their interior, and because there is no blood-brain barrier at this stage of development, these developing neurons can in principle carry back to their cell bodies serotonin that is present in the blood stream. So if an early dopamine transporter is not the primary site of action for cocaine effects on brain development, then perhaps the serotonin transporter could be. That evidence would change the focus of our experimental spotlight from the dopamine projecting terminal fields to some of the other cortical fields. Moreover, serotonin is much more pervasive in most cortical fields than is the dopamine system.

As I understand, Pat Levitt's work focused on the anterior cingulate cortex because of what we knew about the rodent dopamine innervation being heavy in the prefrontal cortex and heavy in the anterior cingulate cortex. But as several non-human primate neurocytologists have pointed out, when we move from rodents to primates, the picture of the dopamine system changes very significantly to become more intensive throughout many cortical fields than just the tiny area innervated by dopamine in the rodent prefrontal system. So we must then ask: Are all those motor changes that we just heard about—those pyramidal signs of upper motor neuron disorder with spasticity—due to the prefrontal cortex effect that was already described or are there effects of cocaine on the developing dopamine projections to the premotor and motor system that are certainly within the bounds of what could be looked at to pin down where and how cocaine produces fetal maldevelopment. Therefore, a prudent person might well conclude that a lot more work needs to be done before we can conclude whether the learning changes that were so nicely mapped onto what we know so far about the abnormal anatomic pathology are indeed the explicit explanation for the learning changes or whether there are many more things lying beneath the surface.

These are questions that you all can see as well as I can. If I were starting in this field tomorrow and I had to write a grant to the National Institute of Drug Abuse, the question I would like to answer is when during gestation is it necessary to hav cocaine there to do the key disruption? Are there periods when it's safe? Or are there periods when the vascular effects of cocaine on the placenta and uterus are such that the fetus is at risk no matter what part of gestation it is? Are there stress-related effects, such as the ones that Michel Le Moal and his colleague, Piazza, have observed, in which drugs elicit steroid responses and the steroid responses adjust the drug responding systems so that animals become tolerant to the effects of psychostimulants? Some of this has been observed in the field.

Are the dopamine receptor changes that we've heard about, the uncoupling of the GSα subunit from the D_1 receptor, the real critical change? Is it not so much the action of dopamine or of the dopamine transporter, but the post-transductive effects of dopamine that are really the heart of the cocaine-causes-maldevelopment message? If it were, then perhaps some of the therapeutic directions that were hypothesized could be worth pursuing.

Let me say one other thing about the dopamine system that goes to the cortex. The mesolimbic and mesocortical projections are not the same as what we all know about the pharmacology of the nigral-striatal system. In fact, recent work suggests that they lack terminal auto receptors; so if you blocked their ability to perform dopamine reuptake, those terminals would have less chance to adapt to the change in dopamine transmission. The cortically projecting dopamine cell bodies lack the presynaptic dopamine regulatory systems that the striatal-nigral system is. So, if the dopamine transporter is the place where the action occurs, why is it that there aren't changes in the basal ganglia, the main brain region in which neuroscience has built all of what we think we understand about the functional importance of the dopamine transporter?

Recently, David Lewis and Susan Sesack described data that extend other observations in this field and suggest that the mesocortical dopamine axons don't have very much of the dopamine transporter either and that they rely very little on reuptake to achieve their pharmacology. If that's the case, they should be among the least sensitive of the places in the brain to react to cocaine if the dopamine transporter is the place to be.

Well, these are things that my morbid curiosity, my Zadig's logic, would provoke me to study if I had the time and the energy to do some of that exciting work which I am sure all of you will do in a much better way. But the real question is, why are you all here? I think the real question was verbalized at this Conference for the first time. Suppose all this is true? What is the best thing that can happen with all the discoveries that you have made? I would also note that you are here, "here" being in Washington, DC, because establishing the veracity of a cocaine effect on the fetal brain in doses that an unwary, pregnant mother could take is one of the most important public health statements that we could make.

It's important for two reasons: One, pregnant mothers who find themselves using substances should be in treatment immediately. We should find ways to alert them to this fact. If we could alert them to the fact that this is a real syndrome, that not only are they risking their own lives but also the lives of their unborn children, then that knowledge ought to be built into a stepped-up, intensified educational system aimed at the right people, in the right grades of school, to alert them that this is not just playing around with something that momma and daddy don't want you to do. This is really an important issue.

I've been a skeptic of prevention programs. I recall a recent report from the Institute of Medicine of the National Academy of Sciences that examined the prevention of drug abuse problems and that concluded, to paraphrase their summary, that the people who are doing really well with this are the people who sell the programs and the people who are doing really badly are the ones who pay for them and expect something to happen.

The DARE programs implemented for second, third, and fourth graders are really good, the kids feel really splendid, they can come home and say the litany and the catechism of why they shouldn't use drugs, and by the time they get to the seventh grade where their older colleagues are starting to smoke, they have forgotten all about those things. But there was recently a paper in *JAMA* that focused efforts on seventh graders, gave them booster training in the eighth, ninth, and tenth grades, and then did a long-term follow-up 2 years later in the twelfth grade which showed a 66% reduction in polydrug abuse, which is exactly the kind of drug abuse that we're talking about here.

So why isn't it important enough just to have my colleague Gretchen Vogel from *Science* just write this up in *Science* magazine? Because you as scientists have to do more than just do your science. You've got to communicate this pervasive and potentially lethal problem to the communities from which you come and get them to write letters to their Congressmen, to all Congressmen, to make them aware of this. Because like it or not, Congress listens to what was in yesterday's mail. But if it's not in tomorrow's mail, they are going to go on to whatever is.

When Gerald Klerman was Administrator of the now defunct Alcohol, Drug Abuse, and Mental Health Administration, he reported to Congress on the Fetal Alcohol Syndrome in 1978, relying very heavily on preponderant animal data to document the reality of the Fetal Alcohol Syndrome. He began an intensive, nationwide public education aimed at women of childbearing age, employers, women's groups, and schools to train physicians to recognize FAS.

Those suggestions, those findings, and the continued momentum of your science are what's required, and I endorse Alan Leshner to get to the point as to wherein this science we can make such a striking statement.

I am pleased to have been part of your conference and to have heard what you had to say. I look forward to the rest of your meeting. Thank you very much.

Maternal and Transplacental Effects of Cocaine

JAMES R. WOODS, JR.[a]

Department of Obstetrics and Gynecology, University of Rochester School of Medicine and Dentistry, Division of Maternal Fetal Medicine, Rochester, New York 14642, USA

ABSTRACT: Pregnancy is a dynamic process, and maternal as well as fetal risks from cocaine use in pregnancy may differ as pregnancy progresses. Three areas of biology offer opportunities for reevaluating cocaine's effects in pregnancy: (1) Maternal cardiovascular and neurologic responses to cocaine hydrochloride are enhanced when compared with responses in nonpregnant subjects to the same dose per kilogram or to metabolites of crack cocaine. (2) During first trimester placental implantation, oxygen availability to the fetus may normally be limited. Cocaine-induced uterine artery vasoconstriction may lead to reperfusion and oxygen toxicity to the fetus from released reactive oxygen species. (3) Cocaine transport in the first and early second trimester may, in part, be across the placental chorion-amnion. Lacking a skin barrier, the fetus at mid-pregnancy may come in direct contact with high concentrations of cocaine in amniotic fluid, a reservoir that clears cocaine slowly, thereby prolonging exposure during critical periods of fetal neurotransmitter formation. Exploring these three areas of biology may offer new approaches to understanding the ultimate impact of prenatal cocaine exposure on maternal and fetal biology.

Considerable attention has been given to the impact on the developing fetus and newborn when women abuse cocaine during pregnancy. For nearly 15 years, researchers reporting in journals of obstetrics, pediatrics, and the neurosciences have built an enormous knowledge base for a drug that is less used than cigarettes, alcohol, or marijuana, yet is far more provocative.[1–4] For all of the attention that has been directed towards the psychosocial dynamics of the user or towards cocaine's effects on the newborn and child, less effort has been expended to define this drug's actions that are specific to the physiologic adaptations of pregnancy. Are there, in fact, unique biologic characteristics of the pregnant addict, perhaps changes within the maternal cardiovascular system, or vulnerability of the early fetal-placental unit, that place the woman and her developing fetus uniquely at even greater risk from cocaine abuse?

Three theories that I will propose concern excessive risk for compromised health during the first half of pregnancy. Cocaine produces a greater increase in maternal cardiac work and systemic vascular resistance during pregnancy than is seen in the nonpregnant state.[5] This exaggerated cardiovascular response is most marked in the uterine vessels and is evidenced by heightened maternal cardiac and neurotoxicity.[6] The first trimester fetus and placenta, exposed to excessive cocaine-induced vasospasm and subsequent reperfusion within the uterine vasculature, are unprepared to neutralize the tissue-damaging molecules that are released in this ischemic-reoxygenation process.[7] Yet, the first trimester process of placental implantation, once considered a black hole in our understanding of early pregnancy, is known now to occur in a lower oxygen en-

[a] Address for correspondence: James R. Woods, Jr., Department of Obstetrics and Gynecology, Strong Memorial Hospital, 601 Elmwood Ave., Box 668, Rochester, NY 14642.

vironment which may lack defenses for oxygen toxicity.[8,9] Finally, amniotic fluid represents an unappreciated source of cocaine exposure to the developing fetus. Amniotic fluid, until 18–19 weeks' gestation, is principally derived from transudate across the umbilical cord and chorionic plate. The first and second trimester fetus, lacking a keratinized skin layer, is vulnerable to substances that pass into and accumulate within the amniotic fluid.[10] In fact, as understood from premature newborn studies, drug absorption through the skin correlates closely with epidermal maturation. Long after maternal blood drug levels have declined, cocaine accumulating in the amniotic fluid thus may access the young embryo and fetus through the skin freely during critical periods of cardiovascular and neurotransmitter development.

The cardiovascular actions of cocaine have been perceived consistently as fundamental to maternal-fetal risk. After 15 years, it is appropriate to reevaluate our understanding of pregnancy and early fetal-placental development as a unique target for prenatal cocaine abuse. In doing so, the questions that at this point remain unanswered may be far more compelling than those that have already been addressed.

WHY DOES MATERNAL CARDIOVASCULAR ADAPTATION IN PREGNANCY ENHANCE THE HYPERTENSIVE RESPONSE TO PRENATAL COCAINE USE?

Pregnancy is a period of marked cardiovascular change, whose principal purpose is to support nutritionally the growth of the placenta and developing fetus. The first and second trimesters are characterized by a gradual decrease in maternal systolic and diastolic blood pressures until approximately 20 weeks. This phenomenon is attributed mostly to the vaso-relaxing effects of progesterone, rapid growth of the low-resistance vascular bed within the placenta, and the vasodilating properties of nitric oxide.[11] During this period, a progressive expansion in maternal blood volume occurs in response to increasing metabolic needs of the fetal-placental unit, and maternal cardiac output increases 50%. Of note, the effect of increasing blood volume and cardiac output on blood pressure appears to be overshadowed during the first half of pregnancy by dynamic vascular growth by the placenta and uterine artery vasodilation.

The last half of pregnancy presents a different pattern of cardiovascular change. Growth of new placental blood vessels slows, thereby reducing the blood pressure-lowering effect of this low-resistance vascular bed. Blood volume, in contrast, progressively increases, while cardiac output stabilizes. The demands for improved venous return, which are imposed by the expanded blood volume, are met through increased venomotor tone. These physiologic events lead normally to a steady rise in blood pressure throughout the third trimester.[11]

The significance of maternal cardiovascular adaptation in relation to cocaine toxicity was first noted in the heightened hypertensive response to intravenous cocaine observed in late-gestation pregnant sheep.[5] At doses of 1 and 2 mg/kg, intravenous cocaine produced twofold greater increases in blood pressure than that in nonpregnant sheep administered the same dose per kilogram. When these studies were repeated in pregnant and nonpregnant sheep that had been instrumented for cardiac output measurements, the enhanced sensitivity to cocaine in pregnant sheep was seen again.[12] The previously noted heightened blood pressure increases in pregnancy reflected an increase in both systemic vascular resistance and cardiac output. These data indicate that cocaine use during pregnancy produces enhanced vasospasm peripherally and enhanced cardiac effort.

A possible hormonal mechanism for this enhanced cardiovascular sensitivity was evaluated by administering intravenous bolus cocaine to nonpregnant sheep before and after progesterone 10 mg/kg im was administered.[13] This dose was chosen because it produces blood levels of progesterone consistent with those in pregnancy. Enhanced toxicity to Bupivacaine, another member of the "caine" family, previously had been reported *in vivo* in pregnant as compared with nonpregnant sheep and *in vitro* in isolated Purkinje fiber preparations of progesterone-treated nonpregnant rabbits.[14,15] When compared with pre-progesterone responses to cocaine, the blood pressure of progesterone-treated nonpregnant sheep increased twofold, consistent with previously observed differences in cocaine-induced blood pressure responses between pregnant and nonpregnant sheep. In this experiment, norepinephrine was injected before as well as after progesterone treatment, but this produced only the same blood pressure rises at both times in the experiment. These observations suggested that enhanced cardiovascular responses to cocaine in pregnant and nonpregnant progesterone-treated sheep were not due to increased sensitivity of alpha$_1$ receptors. Otherwise, the responses to norepinephrine also would have increased after progesterone administration.

The cardiovascular effects of other derivatives of cocaine offer a different approach to this issue. Crack cocaine now is known to contain, among other compounds, methyl ecgonidine (MEG).[16] Both cocaine and MEG have produced hypertensive responses in sheep. Cocaine-induced hypertension reflects its ability to block norepinephrine's uptake within the synaptic cleft. The blood pressure rise in response to MEG appears to be related to a compensatory hypertension induced by a precipitous hypotension. The blood pressure rise in response to MEG is not influenced by progesterone, however, unlike that observed with cocaine.[17]

Using other species, investigators have witnessed pregnancy's unique ability to alter cocaine's cardiovascular actions.[18] Species differences and method of drug delivery, however, have influenced the patterns of these altered responses. In pregnant rats, intravenously infused cocaine produced decreases in heart rate, cardiac output, and cerebral, myocardial, and placental blood flow that were greater than those responses in nonpregnant rats.[18]

At larger doses, such as 5 mg/kg, late-term pregnant sheep exhibit seizures coupled with cardiac arrhythmias, which are characterized by ventricular tachycardia, atrioventricular dissociation, ventricular fibrillation, and death.[6] Similar electrocardiographic changes in men have been reported.[19–21] Nonpregnant sheep, at this cocaine dose, exhibit only a hypertensive response. Only when given three to four times this cocaine amount (15–20 mg/kg) do they exhibit seizures and cardiac arrhythmias. The seizures are characteristic of strychnine poisoning, which involves opisthotonos, extension of major extremities by dominant muscle groups, and respiratory arrest. If death does not occur, the sheep recover fully within 30 minutes.

Similar heightened responses have been reported in the pregnant rat.[22] In that study, pregnant and nonpregnant rats were infused with cocaine at 2 mg/kg per minute to observe the cardiotoxic and neurotoxic effects of higher-dose cocaine. Lower blood levels of cocaine were documented in pregnant rats during the onset of convulsions and cardiovascular depression, defined as hypotension or circulatory collapse, than in nonpregnant rats. Moreover, the time to cocaine neurotoxicity was shorter in pregnant than in nonpregnant rats. Yet, once neurotoxicity was noted, the time to circulatory collapse was equivalent between groups.

These data raise several questions. Are the cardiac manifestations of cocaine that have been seen in pregnant rats and sheep a result of cocaine's actions as a local anesthesic to block sodium channels or do they reflect an inability of the coronary circulation to meet the increased oxygen needs of the cocaine-stimulated heart? This latter phenomenon, described by Gradman[21] and observed clinically,[23] has not been addressed in any species during pregnancy. Species differences also may be significant. In sheep, cocaine-induced cardiac arrhythmias occasionally were seen at large doses (5 mg/kg iv) without seizures, whereas in the rat, neurotoxicity to infused cocaine preceded cardiac toxicity or circulatory collapse.[6,18]

Altered metabolism of cocaine during pregnancy may contribute to its enhanced cardiovascular effects in sheep. The cardiovascular toxicity noted in pregnant sheep was associated with a higher blood level of cocaine.[12] These findings suggested that despite similar milligrams per kilogram dosing as used in nonpregnant sheep, impaired metabolism allowed for a higher blood level of cocaine which in turn produced a greater cardiovascular effect. Cocaine metabolism differs among species and may only relate partially to effect. For example, plasma cholinesterase activity in sheep, important in hydrolysis of cocaine, is 13–25 times lower than that in humans and 10 times lower than levels in the rat.[18] Moreover, high cholinesterase levels may not offer protection during pregnancy. In the rat, cholinesterase levels were elevated in pregnant rats compared with nonpregnant ones. Neurotoxicity, however, was associated with lower blood cocaine levels in pregnant rats compared with nonpregnant ones.[22]

One could also argue that weight determinations in pregnant sheep, which include the adult sheep carcass plus amniotic fluid and fetal and placental weight, should increase the total dose of cocaine given, based on kilogram weight, compared with those in nonpregnant sheep. The expanded maternal blood volume and rapid placental transfer make this argument unlikely as an explanation for cocaine's enhanced actions during pregnancy.

Recently, cocaine metabolism in pregnant rats at each trimester was noted to change. In late gestation, cocaine conversion to benzolecgnonine was significantly greater than that observed early in pregnancy.[24] In that study, maternal cardiovascular responses at each trimester were not documented. It remains to be determined, therefore, if the enhanced cardiovascular effects of cocaine are consistent across all three trimesters and if altered metabolism of cocaine or changing responsiveness of the adrenergic system to cocaine's actions represents the underlying mechanism.

COCAINE'S EFFECTS ON PLACENTAL IMPLANTATION AND THE DEVELOPING EMBRYO

With the advent of ultrasound Doppler techniques, our knowledge of first trimester development of the placenta and developing embryo has undergone great change.[25,26] Proper implantation involves invasion of maternal tissue by two types of fetal trophoblast tissue, villous trophoblast and extravillous trophoblast.[27] Villous trophoblasts act as anchors to secure fetal villi to maternal tissue, whereas extravillous trophoblasts invade the maternal decidua, seeking to establish a vascular network with maternal vessels for the exchange of oxygen, nutrients, and cellular waste products.

But what controls the invasion process? It now appears that trophoblast tissue produces certain growth factors called integrins that promote invasion by extravillous trophoblast tissue. Initially, trophoblast tissue invades the smallest maternal blood vessels. These maternal vessels, in time, will carry oxygenated blood to the intervillous space of the placenta where oxygen and nutrient exchange with fetal capillaries within the intervillous space will occur. During this initial invasion, however, trophoblasts plug these invaded vessels, rendering them incapable of delivering oxygen to the developing placenta. But what does this mean regarding oxygen availability to the developing embryo?

Doppler flow analysis of the early first-trimester placenta demonstrates that intervillous blood flow, critical to delivery of oxygen to fetal villi, first appears at about 9–11 weeks' gestation, several weeks after structural development of the embryo is complete.[28] In fact, delayed formation of an intervillous flow pattern until late first trimester now appears to be important to stimulate proper invasion of trophoblasts, in anticipation of establishing adequate oxygen and nutrition exchange. Premature appearance of intervillous blood flow is associated with a significant increase in miscarriages early in pregnancy and impaired fetal growth or preeclampsia in later pregnancy.[29–32] These findings are significant for several reasons. First, they appear to link two late-gestation complications, preeclampsia and intrauterine growth restriction, to improper placental implantation. As significant, however, is the observation that the early embryo develops in an environment in which our traditional concept of oxygen delivery, that is, delivery via intervillous blood flow, is not applicable. When placental and endometrial pO_2 levels were measured *in vivo,* oxygen tension in these tissues was found to increase significantly only after 12–13 weeks' gestation.[8] These findings complement those of others that few red blood cells were noted in placental specimens obtained from first-trimester pregnancies[33] and that chorionic villous samples obtained prior to 12 weeks seldom contained red blood cells.[34]

Studies of the isolated trophoblast provide an even more intriguing picture of trophoblast differentiation. Until 7 or 8 weeks' gestation, experimental hypoxia has no negative effect on trophoblast differentiation and migration. Cultures of 10–12-week placentas, however, under hypoxic conditions, exhibit an impaired ability by trophoblasts to differentiation and to invade the extracellular matrix, whereas under normoxic conditions (consistent with the appearance of intervillous blood flow) differentiation and invasion occur normally.[27]

The consequences of cocaine's vasoconstrictive actions have undergone reanalysis as they apply to the developing embryo and its early placenta. Cocaine-induced tissue damage to the fetus traditionally has been attributed to ischemia secondary to vasospasm. In one series, in which cocaine was administered to pregnant rats on day 16, the rat pups that were delivered 48 hours later showed evidence of hemorrhage and edema. Delivery 5 days later produced pups with limb-reduction deformities.[35] These studies were performed to address mechanistically the clinical observations that cocaine abusers delivered newborns with cerebral infarction, urinary tract malformation, limb-reduction defects, and intestinal abscess or infarction.[36–38] Investigators now believe that tissue damage may occur as reperfusion follows cocaine-induced ischemia, introducing excessive oxygen and the release of reactive oxygen species into a fetal-placental system that is unprepared to control the tissue-damaging byproducts of oxygen toxicity.

Reactive oxygen species are molecules with one unpaired electron in their outer orbit, which are capable of existing independently for some time.[39] Examples of reactive oxygen species are superoxide, hydrogen peroxide, hydroxyl ions, nitric oxide, and hypochlorous acid. The two principal sources of reactive oxygen species are leakage from the mitochondrial electron transport system during cellular respiration and production by immune cells to destroy bacteria and viruses in the body. Some reactive oxygen species, such as superoxide, may survive up to 10 seconds but are considered reasonably harmless. Others, such as the hydroxyl radical, may exist for only 10^{-9} seconds, but are capable of initiating lipid peroxidation, disrupting cell membranes, altering protein, and damaging DNA and DNA repair enzymes. The body uses numerous antioxidant systems to neutralize reactive oxygen species, including endogenous enzymes such as superoxide dismutase, catalase, and glutathione peroxidase, as well as diet-acquired antioxidants such as α-tocopherol (vitamin E) and ascorbic acid (vitamin C). Unfortunately, after cocaine-induced ischemia and during reperfusion, the introduction of excessive oxygen may lead to the sudden appearance of oxygen-free radicals into tissues that are not properly equipped with antioxidants, leading to cell death and tissue destruction.

Several theories have arisen to explain mechanistically the consequences of free-radical injury after ischemia and reperfusion. Xanthine dehydrogenase is a critical enzyme in the mitochondrion for the transfer of free energy from glucose to the generation of adenosine triphosphate (ATP), the fuel for most cellular events. During hypoxia, ATP is converted to adenosine monophosphate (AMP) and then to hypoxanthine and xanthine. Moreover, under reduced oxygen conditions, xanthine dehydrogenase is converted to xanthine oxidase. As reperfusion occurs and oxygen is reintroduced, xanthine oxidase is reoxidized by molecular oxygen, generating the free radical superoxide.[7,40]

Hypoxia-reperfusion also has been shown *in vitro* to alter endothelial cell wall permeability. Cells in monolayer, when exposed to hypoxia, exhibited a 1.5-times increase in permeability to labeled albumen. Reoxygenation, in comparison, increased cell permeability 2.3 times.[41]

Finally, ischemia-reperfusion may lead to the release of several reactive oxygen species which, when combined, produce additional tissue-damaging molecules. Nitric oxide (NO), or endothelium-derived relaxing factor, is recognized as contributing to vascular smooth muscle relaxation during pregnancy.[42] Under optimal conditions, NO can be stimulated by superoxide.[43] In this setting, normal control of superoxide levels by antioxidants such as superoxide dismutase (SOD) allows superoxide and NO to participate in important physiologic processes.[44] If excessive superoxide is produced, however, as during reperfusion following an ischemic event, its relation to NO is altered. In this setting, NO and superoxide combine to form peroxynitrite or its acid, peroxynitrous acid, which is a reactive oxygen species capable of initiating lipid peroxidation and endothelial cell damage.[45]

Several investigations have shown that the early embryo is at risk for oxygen toxicity.[7] For example, significantly more mouse embryos, cultured in 5% oxygen with the antioxidant superoxide dismutase, survived to the blastocyst stage than those cultured in 5% oxygen without SOD or those cultured in 20% oxygen.[46] Fantel and coworkers[47] indicated that cocaine risk to the young embryo may be related directly to its lack of defenses against oxygen toxicity. Rat embryos cultured in cocaine *in vitro* under altered oxygen conditions exhibited damage to their mitochondrial respiratory electron transport when compared with embryos cultured in hypoxia alone. Thus, the investigators suggest that cocaine affects the developing embryo adversely by disrupting energy-producing mechanisms for cell metabolism. More recently, Fantel and coworkers[48] reported that fetal tissues differ in their capacity to tolerate oxygen stress. In a study of adult and rat embryos, the embryo's limb buds and central nervous system, while capable of generating reactive oxygen species, exhibited low antioxidant properties when compared with the fetal heart. By contrast, adult tissues exhibited a balance of oxidants and antioxidants in all tissues.

Lack of antioxidant properties in the first-trimester placenta may also influence fetal risk from cocaine-induced oxygen toxicity. Unlike the term placenta, which contains the important antioxidants copper/zinc superoxide dismutase (CuZn-SOD) and glutathione peroxidase, the first-trimester placenta develops antioxidant capabilities only by 10–12 weeks' gestation.[9,49] Copper/zinc superoxide dismutase was found in cytotrophoblasts at all stages of pregnancy. By contrast, CuZn-SOD was absent from the syncytiotrophoblast at 8 weeks, but was widespread by 12 weeks, a time when intervillous blood flow and increased oxygen availability have been noted. These findings provide further support that oxygen tension within the placenta is low throughout most of the first trimester and that antioxidant defenses are not needed before 12 weeks' gestation. During that initial period, oxygen reaching the young embryo does so largely by diffusion. After 12 weeks' gestation, as oxygenated maternal blood enters the intervillous space, however, antioxidants such as CuZn-SOD become necessary to prevent oxygen toxicity to the placenta and fetus.

AMNIOTIC FLUID EXPOSURE TO COCAINE

The third area involving prenatal cocaine abuse that deserves reevaluation is that of fetal exposure to cocaine. Due to limitations of blood sampling in smaller animals, such as the mouse and rat, most studies of cocaine transport by the placenta and its effects on the fetus have been carried out in catheterized pregnant ewes and fetuses in the third trimester and in the dually perfused human placental lobule.[50,51] The dynamics of amniotic-fluid generation during the first and second trimester make it imperative that we reexamine how the fetus is exposed to cocaine. This issue is important, because fetal neurotransmitter development within the nervous system is initiated in the first half of pregnancy, whereas most cocaine kinetic studies have been done in late gestation.

In fact, amniotic fluid may represent a significant repository for cocaine exposure to the fetus throughout pregnancy. Studies conducted in the guinea pig, sheep, and human, collectively, indicate that maternal cocaine use results in amniotic fluid cocaine concentrations that may prolong fetal exposure. In one series, pregnant guinea pigs were injected daily with 6 mg/kg cocaine intraperitoneally, and they were sacrificed 1 hour after the tenth-day injection. Cocaine concentrations in amniotic fluid were three to four times greater than those in fetal blood.[52]

Measurements of cocaine and metabolites in amniotic fluid from human pregnancies support data obtained from the animal model. In a study of 23 women with known cocaine use, benzoylecgonine levels ranged from 400 to over 5,000 ng/ml, while cocaine levels up to 250 ng/ml were documented.[53] In a follow-up case report by this group, benzoylecgonine was higher in amniotic fluid than in umbilical cord blood, whereas amniotic fluid cocaine levels were greater than newborn urine cocaine concentrations.[54]

That the fetus in the first half of pregnancy may be at equal or greater risk of cocaine exposure is extrapolated from studies of the premature human newborn. Water transport across the human fetal skin is unrestricted until after 24 weeks at which time cornification of the epithelium erects a barrier for water transport through the skin.[55] If cocaine enters the amniotic fluid in early pregnancy, its passage across the fetal skin could enhance fetal exposure markedly at a time when neurotransmitter development is being initiated.

Cocaine in amniotic fluid can access the near-term fetus.[56] In that series, an Alzet osmotic pump placed in the amniotic fluid delivered cocaine at 1 mg/kg per hour over a 7-day period, during which daily cocaine measurements from maternal and fetal blood and amniotic fluid were taken. Approximately 3% of amniotic fluid cocaine was detected in fetal blood, documenting entry of cocaine from amniotic fluid into the fetal circulation. In a subset of animals, esophageal ligature was performed before osmotic pump placement, to eliminate the role of fetal swallowing in fetal exposure. Both esophageal ligated and control animals, when exposed to amniotic fluid cocaine, exhibited similar blood levels, indicating that entry of cocaine occurred either across placental surface blood vessels or the umbilical cord or through the fetal skin. Both also exhibited comparable levels of metabolites in meconium, raising questions about how cocaine metabolites enter the gastrointestinal tract.

To determine if cocaine in amniotic fluid can enter the mid-gestation fetus, the protocol used by Mahone *et al.*[56] was modified. Alset osmotic pumps, delivering cocaine at 1 mg/hour, were placed in the amniotic fluid compartments of five pregnant sheep at 60–80 days' gestation. This dose was selected to deliver into the amniotic fluid a similar total dose of cocaine per 24 hours as calculated by Mahone *et al.* using milligrams per estimated kilograms fetal weight per hour in near-term fetal lambs weighing approximately 1 kg each. After 7 days, the animals were sacrificed, and samples of maternal and fetal blood and amniotic fluid were taken immediately for measurements of cocaine, benzoylecgonine, and ecgonine methyl ester. At sacrifice, all fetal umbilical vein

TABLE 1. Concentration (in ng/ml) of Cocaine and Metabolites from Near Term (n = 6) and Preterm (n = 5) Fetal Sheep to Seven Days of Intraamniotic Cocaine Administration[a]

	Cocaine	Benzoylecgonine	Ecgonine Methyl Ester
Amniotic Fluid			
Mid-gestation	1,118 ± 1,501	732 ± 781	1,628 ± 985
Late gestation	767 ± 417	175 ± 88	1,158 ± 607
	NS	p <0.001	NS
Fetal Plasma			
Mid-gestation	1 ± 4	55 ± 46	185 ± 132
Late gestation	33 ± 13	43 ± 48	Undetectable
	p <0.001	NS	p <0.05
Maternal Plasma			
Mid-gestation	8 ± 14	3 ± 7	145 ± 138
Late gestation	8 ± 2	14 ± 11	Undetectable
	NS	p <0.05	NS

[a]Values are mean ± SD. Statistical significance, p <0.05.

pH values were between 7.21 and 7.29. Fetal weights ranged from 125 to 360 g. The sensitivity and recovery yields for cocaine and its metabolites have been reported previously.[56] The results of this study are shown in TABLE 1. When these results were compared with those of near-term fetuses, several differences were noted. Cocaine was detected in amniotic fluid in concentrations similar to those in late gestation, but it was not detected in four mid-gestational fetuses and there was a trace (8 ng/ml) in the fifth fetus. Benzoylecgonine levels in amniotic fluid and fetal blood were comparable to those in late gestation. Most noteworthy, in late gestation, ecgonine methyl ester was the highest concentration of cocaine metabolites recorded in amniotic fluid but was undetectable in the fetus. In mid-gestation, all but one of the fetuses exhibited ecgonine methyl ester levels that were 10–50% of amniotic fluid levels. Lack of detectable cocaine but easily documented levels of benzoylecgonine and ecgonine methyl ester in the mid-gestation fetus indicate that cocaine metabolism in amniotic fluid or in the fetus in mid- and late gestation differs. Moreover, fetal skin or placenta and umbilical cord allow ready access of amniotic fluid cocaine or its metabolites into the fetal circulation in both mid- and late gestation.

SUMMARY

The biology of prenatal cocaine risk assessment deserves a critical review, which takes into consideration maternal cardiovascular adaptations during pregnancy, vulnerability of the first-trimester fetal-placental unit, and the role of amniotic fluid as a repository for enhanced fetal drug exposure. Appreciating these excess risks from prenatal cocaine use may contribute to our understanding of the true impact of cocaine abuse in pregnancy.

REFERENCES

1. RYAN R.M., WAGNER C.L., SCHULTZ J.M., VARLEY J., DIPRETA J., SHERER D.M., PHELPS D.L., KWONG T. 1994. Meconium analysis for improved identification of infants exposed to cocaine in utero. J. Pediatr. **125:** 435–440.

2. Cornelius M.D., Taylor P.M., Geva D., Day N.L. 1995. Prenatal tobacco and marijuana use among adolescents: Effects on offspring gestational age, growth, and morphology. Pediatrics **95:** 738–743.
3. McCalla, S., J. Feldman, H. Hebbeh, R. Admadi & H.L. Minkoff. 1995. Changes in perinatal cocaine use in an inner-city hospital 1988 to 1992. Am. J. Public Health **85:** 1695–1697.
4. NIDA News, April 1997, p. 12.
5. Woods, J.R. & M.A. Plessinger. 1990. Pregnancy increases cardiovascular toxicity to cocaine. Am. J. Obstet. Gynecol. **162:** 529–533.
6. Woods, J.R., M.A. Plessinger, K. Scott & R.K. Miller. 1989. Prenatal cocaine exposure to the fetus: A sheep model for cardiovascular evaluation. Ann. N.Y. Acad. Sci. **562:** 267–279.
7. Fantel, A.G. 1996. Reactive oxygen species in developmental toxicity. Review and hypothesis. Teratology **53:** 196–217.
8. Rodesch, F., P. Simon, C. Donner & E. Jauniaux. 1992. Oxygen measurements in the maternal-trophoblast border during early pregnancy. Obstet. Gynecol. **80:** 283–285.
9. Watson, A.L., M.E. Palmer, E. Jauniaux & G.J. Burton. 1997. Variations in expression of copper/zinc superoxide dismutase in villous trophoblast of the human placenta with gestational age. Placenta **18:** 295–299.
10. Rutter, N. 1987. Percutaneous drug absorption. Clin. Perinatol. **14:** 911–930.
11. Monga, M. & R.K. Creasy. 1994. Cardiovascular and renal adaptation to pregnancy. Chapter 46, *In:* Maternal-Fetal Medicine, 3rd Ed. R.K. Creasy & R. Resnik, Eds.: 758–767. W. B. Saunders Co. Philadelphia, PA.
12. Woods, J.R., K.J. Scott & M.A. Plessinger. 1994. Pregnancy enhances cocaine's action on the heart and within the peripheral circulation. Am. J. Obstet. Gynecol. **170:** 1027–1035.
13. Plessinger, M.A. & J.R. Woods. 1990. Progesterone increases cardiovascular toxicity to cocaine in nonpregnant ewes. Am. J. Obstet. Gynecol. **163:** 1659–1664.
14. Morishima H.O., H. Pedersen, M. Finster, H. Hiraoka, A. Tsuji, H.S. Feldman, G.R. Arthur & B.G. Covino. 1985. Bupivacaine toxicity in pregnant and non-pregnancy ewes. Anesthesiology **63:** 134–139.
15. Moller, R.A., S. Datta, J. Fox, M. Johnson & B.G. Covino. 1992. Effects of progesterone on the cardiac electrophysiologic action of Bupivacaine and Lidocaine. Anesthesiology **76:** 604–608.
16. Wood, R.W., J.F. Graefe, C.P. Fang, J. Shojaie, L.C. Chen & J. Willetts. 1996. Generation of stable test atmospheres of cocaine base and its pyrolyzate, methylecgonidine. Pharmacol. Biochem. Behav. **55:** 237–248.
17. Plessinger, M.A. & R.W. Wood. Effect of the "crack" cocaine pyrolysis product, methylecgonidine, in sheep (Abstr.). College of Problems of Drug Dependency, Nashville, Tennessee, June 1997.
18. Morishima, H.O., T.B. Cooper, T. Hara & E.D. Miller. 1992. Pregnancy alters the hemodynamic responses to cocaine in the rat. Dev. Pharmacol. Ther. **19:** 69–79.
19. Young, D. & J.J. Glanber. 1947. Electrocardiographic changes resulting from acute cocaine toxicity. Am. Heart J. **34:** 272–279.
20. Isner, J.M., N.A.M. Estes, P.D. Thompson, M.R. Costanzo-Nordin, R. Subramamanian, G. Miller, G. Katsas, K. Sweeney & W.Q. Sturner. 1986. Acute cardiac events temporally related to cocaine abuse. N. Engl. J. Med. **315:** 1438–1443.
21. Gradman, A.H. 1988. Cardiac effects of cocaine: A review. Yale J. Biol. Med. **61:** 137–147.
22. Morishima, H.O., T. Masaoka, T. Hara, A. Tsuji & T.B. Cooper. 1993. J. Lab. Clin. Med. **122:** 748–756.
23. Lange, R.A., R.G. Cigarroa, C.W. Yancy, J.E. Willard, J.J. Popma, M.N. Sills, W. McBride, A.S. Kim & L.D. Hillis. 1989. Cocaine-induced coronary-artery vasoconstriction. N. Engl. J. Med. **321:** 1557–1562.
24. Church, M.W. & M.G. Subramanian. 1997. Cocaine's lethality increases during late gestation in the rat: A study of "critical periods" of exposure. Am. J. Obstet. Gynecol. **176:** 901–906.
25. Aplin, J.D. 1996. The cell biology of human implantation. Placenta **17:** 269–275.

26. JAFFE, R., E. JAUNIAUX & J. HUSTIN. 1997. Maternal circulation in the first-trimester human placenta: Myth or reality? Am. J. Obstet. Gynecol. **176:** 695–705.
27. GENBACEV, O., R. JOSLIN, C.H. DAMSKY, B.M. POLLIOTTI & S.J. FISHER. 1996. Hypoxia alters early gestational human cytotrophoblast differentiation/invasion in vitro and models the placenta defects that occur in preeclampsia. J. Clin. Invest. **97:** 540–550.
28. JAFFE, R. & J.R. WOODS. 1993. Color Doppler imaging and *in vivo* assessment of the anatomy and physiology of the early uteroplacental circulation. Fertil. Steril. **60:** 293–297.
29. GERRETSEN, G., H.J. HUISJES & J.D. ELEMA. 1981. Morphological changes of the spiral arteries in the placental bed in relationship to pre-eclampsia and fetal growth retardation. Br. J. Obstet. Gynecol. **88:** 876–881.
30. KHONG, T.Y., F. DEWOLF, W.B. ROBERTSON & I. BROSEN. 1986. Inadequate maternal vascular response to placentation in pregnancies complicated by pre-eclampsia and by small-for-gestational age infants. Br. J. Obstet. Gynecol. **93:** 1049–1059.
31. KHONG, T.Y., H.S. LIDDEL & W.B. ROBERSON. 1986. Defective haemochorial placentation as a cause of miscarriage: A preliminary study. Br. J. Obstet. Gynecol. **94:** 649–655.
32. JAFFE, R. 1995. Color Doppler imaging of first trimester uteroplacental circulation and prediction of pregnancy outcome. Gynecol. Obstet. & Reprod. Med. **1:** 147–150.
33. BENIRSCHKE, K. & P. KAUFMANN. 1995. The Human Placenta. Springer-Verlag. Heidelberg.
34. HUSTIN, J. & J.P. SCHAAPS. 1987. Echogenic and anatomic studies of the maternotrophoblastic border during the first trimester of pregnancy. Am. J. Obstet. Gynecol. **157:** 162–168.
35. WEBSTER, W.S. & P.D.C. BROWN-WOODMAN. 1990. Cocaine as a cause of congenital malformation of vascular origin. Experimental evidence in the rat. Teratology **41:** 689–697.
36. CHASNOFF, I.J., M.E. BUSSEY, R. SAVICH & C.M. STACK. 1986. Perinatal cerebral infarct and maternal cocaine use. J. Pediatr. **106:** 456–459.
37. CHASNOFF, I.J., G.M. CHISUM & W.E. KAPLAN. 1988. Maternal cocaine use and genitourinary tract malformations. Teratology **37:** 201–204.
38. HOYME, H.E., K.L. JONES, S.D. DIXON, T. JEWETT, J.W. HANSON, L.K. ROBINSON, M.E. MSALL & J.E. ALLENSON. 1990. Prenatal cocaine exposure and fetal vascular disruption. Pediatrics **85:** 743–747.
39. HALLIWAY, B., J.M.C. GUTTERIDGE & C.E. CROSS. 1992. Free radicals, antioxidants, and human disease: Where are we now? J. Lab. Clin. Med. **114:** 598–620.
40. MCCORD, J.M. 1993. Human disease, free radicals and the oxidant/antioxidant balance. Clin. Biochem. **26:** 351–357.
41. INAUEN, W., D.K. PAYNE, P.R. KVIETYS & D.P. GRANGER. 1990. Hypoxia/reoxygenation increases the permeability of endothelial cell monolayers: Role of oxygen radicals. Free Rad. Biol. **9:** 219–223.
42. VEILLE, J.C., P. LI, J.C. EISENACH, A.G. MASSMANN, J.P. FIGUEROA. 1996. Effects of estrogen on nitric oxide and vasorelaxant activity in sheep uterine and renal arteries *in vitro.* Am. J. Obstet. Gynecol. **174:** 1043–1049.
43. STEMLER, J. 1996. A radical vascular connection. Nature **380:** 108–111.
44. PRYOR, W.A. & G.L. SQUADRITO. 1995. The chemistry of peroxynitrite: A product from the reaction of nitric oxide with superoxide. Am. J. Physiol. **268:** L699–L722.
45. BECKMAN, J.S., J.W. BECKMAN, J. CHEN, P.A. MARSHALL & B.A. FREEMAN. 1990. Apparent hydroxyl radical production by peroxynitrite: Implications for endothelial injury from nitric oxide and superoxide. Proc. Natl. Acad. Sci. **87:** 1620–1624.
46. UMAOKA, Y., Y. NODA, K. NARIMOTO & T. MORI. 1992. Effects of oxygen toxicity on early development of mouse embryos. Mol. Reprod. Dev. **31:** 28–33.
47. FANTEL, A.G., R.E. PERSON, C.J. BURROUGHS-GLEIM *et al.* 1990. Direct embryotoxicity of cocaine in rats: Effects on mitochondrial activity, cardiac function, and growth and development in vitro. Teratology **42:** 35–43.
48. FANTEL, A.G., R.E. PERSON, R.W. TUMBIC, T.D. NGUYEN & B. MACKLER. 1995. Studies of mitochondria in oxidative embryotoxicity. Teratology **52:** 190–195.
49. MANY, A., A. LARSON-WESTERHAUSEN, A. KAYBOUR-SHAKIR & J.M. ROBERTS. 1996. Xanthine oxidase: Dehydrogenase is present in human placenta. Placenta **17:** 361–365.

50. Woods, J.R., M.A. Plessinger & K.E. Clark. 1987. The effects of cocaine upon uterine blood flow and fetal oxygenation. JAMA **257:** 957–961.
51. Simone, C., L.O. Derewlany, M. Oskamp, B. Knie & G. Koren. 1994. Transfer of cocaine and benzoylecgonine across the perfused human placental cotyledon. Am. J. Obstet. Gynecol. **170:** 1404–1410.
52. Sanberg, J.A. & G.D. Olsen. 1992. Cocaine and metabolite concentrations in the fetal guinea pig after chorionic maternal cocaine administration. J. Pharmacol. Exp. Ther. **260:** 587–591.
53. Jain, L., W. Meyer, C. Moore, I. Tebbett, D. Gauthier & D. Vidyasagar. 1993. Detection of fetal cocaine exposure by analysis of amniotic fluid. Obstet. Gynecol. **81:** 787–790.
54. Moore, C.M., S. Brown, A. Negrusz, I. Tebbett, W. Meyer & L. Jain. 1993. Determination of cocaine and its major metabolite, benzoylecgonine, in amniotic fluid, umbilical cord blood, umbilical cord tissue and neonatal urine. J. Anal. Toxicol. **17:** 62.
55. Rutter, N. 1988. The immature skin. Br. Med. Bull. **44:** 957–969.
56. Mahone, P.R., K. Scott, G. Sleggs, T. D'Antoni & J.R. Woods. 1994. Cocaine and metabolites in amniotic fluid may prolong fetal drug exposure. Am. J. Obstet. Gynecol. **171:** 465–469.

Effects of Prenatal Cocaine on Hearing, Vision, Growth, and Behavior[a]

MICHAEL W. CHURCH,[b-d,f] WILLIAM J. CROSSLAND,[e] PAMELA A. HOLMES,[b] GEORGE W. OVERBECK,[b] AND JACQUELINE P. TILAK[b]

[b]*Department of Obstetrics & Gynecology;* [c]*Department of Otolaryngology, Head & Neck Surgery;* [d]*Department of Audiology, Speech and Language Pathology;* [e]*Department of Anatomy and Cell Biology, Wayne State University School of Medicine, Detroit, Michigan 48201, USA*

ABSTRACT: The illicit use of cocaine has increased dramatically over the last 10–12 years. There has been a corresponding increase in cocaine abuse among obstetric patients and in the number of "cocaine babies." According to some estimates, these children make up more than half of the drug-associated births. This problem is therefore a major public health concern. Consequently, our laboratory investigated the effects of prenatal cocaine exposure on hearing, vision, growth, and exploratory/stress behavior. This chapter summarizes the literature on animals and humans on these topics and presents new observations from our laboratory. In terms of maternal toxicity, prenatal cocaine exposure causes hypertension, placental abruption, spontaneous abortion, poor pregnancy weight gain, and undernutrition secondary to appetite suppression. Some offspring effects include *in utero* growth retardation, cephalic hemorrhage, fetal edema, altered body composition, congenital malformations, and even pre- and postnatal death. The offspring can also exhibit a variety of behavioral, visual, hearing, and language disorders. Differential effects of animal strain and late gestational cocaine exposure are discussed. Comparisons are made between prenatal cocaine, the fetal alcohol syndrome, and the effects of prenatal undernutrition. Recommendations for clinical assessment and intervention are made.

INTRODUCTION

Suspicion about the teratogenic potential of mind-altering drugs, particularly alcohol, stretches back many centuries.[1] However, not until recently has there been scientific evidence to substantiate this belief. It is now acknowledged by medical and scientific communities that many drugs of abuse are teratogenic in terms of both physical malformations and neurobehavioral effects. This is particularly true for alcohol, opiates, marijuana, phencyclidine, amphetamines, and nicotine.

Over the last 10–12 years, cocaine use has emerged as one of the nation's most important public health concerns, particularly in regards to its harmful effects on the mother and unborn child. For example, some inner-city hospitals report that 10–20% or more of their obstetric patients or newborn infants are positive for cocaine. (For a review, see ref. 1.) Cocaine can indirectly influence the unborn child through its hypertensive/vasoconstrictive/hypoxic effects on the uterus and placenta and its appetite-

[a] This work was supported by research grants from the National Institute on Drug Abuse (R01 DA05536), the National Institute on Alcohol Abuse and Alcoholism (P50 AA07606, R01 AA01941), and the National Eye Institute (EY04068).

[f] Address for correspondence: Dr. Michael W. Church, C.S. Mott Center, 275 E. Hancock Avenue, Detroit, MI 48201.

suppressing effects and increased energy demands on the mother.[1] Cocaine readily crosses the placenta and can thereby directly influence the unborn child through its vasoconstrictive effects on the conceptus vasculature, neurochemistry, and cellular growth and survival.[1]

Unlike the fetal alcohol syndrome (FAS), no one has fully described a specific pattern of defects in children born to cocaine-abusing women. Yet evidence is mounting that prenatal cocaine can cause a variety of morbidities. Some maternal complications include hypertension, placental abruption, spontaneous abortion, and premature delivery. Some pre- and neonatal effects include fetal edema, cephalic hemorrhage, sensory abnormalities, intrauterine growth retardation (IUGR), neurobehavioral and cognitive deficits, and occasionally craniofacial, skeletal, and internal organ anomalies.[1]

This chapter summarizes our research observations on growth, hearing, vision, and behavior in an animal (rat) model of prenatal cocaine exposure. We relate these observations to findings in the human and animal literature. This chapter also discusses the putative mechanisms of these cocaine-induced morbidities and the implications for clinical assessment and intervention and draws comparisons with the effects of prenatal alcohol and undernutrition.

MATERNAL OUTCOME

Animal Studies

We have observed that cocaine administration to pregnant rats results in a dose-dependent suppression of maternal weight gain and food consumption.[2–6] This is undoubtedly due to cocaine's appetite-suppressing effects and increased energy demands from cocaine stimulation. Curiously, maternal water consumption is increased over normal levels, starting about the fourth treatment day.[2–6] Cocaine, like some other drugs, may cause diuresis during pregnancy, possibly resulting in such complications as dehydration and electrolyte loss.[6]

Gestation length in the laboratory rat is not affected by cocaine administration,[2–6] but placental abruptions can occur if the dose is high enough.[2] Maternal mortality can also occur with high doses.[2,7] Both placental abruption and maternal mortality appear to be late gestational effects. These effects may be due to changes in the hormonal environment, such as increasing levels of progesterone and estrogen.[7] Indeed, there is good evidence that progesterone increases cocaine's cardiovascular toxicity.[8]

Strain-dependent differences in cocaine's maternal toxicity exist.[6] This may reflect genetic differences in cocaine metabolism and neurotoxicity. Individual, age- and ethnic-related differences in cocaine sensitivity in pregnant women have not been described, but these may be important variables in influencing cocaine-induced morbidities.

Human Studies

The human literature occasionally describes poor appetite, poor maternal weight gain, and placental abruption in cocaine-using women.[1] Although premature labor has been described occasionally, the evidence is mixed.[1] Mortality seems uncommon, but appears to occur mostly during late gestation in humans[1] just as it does in the laboratory rat. A more common effect in humans is a preeclamptic-like morbidity.[9] Whereas maternal cocaine intoxication can mimic the preeclamptic symptoms of hypertension, headaches, blurred vision, placental abruption, and the like, cocaine intoxication differs from preeclampsia in its effects on fibronectin levels/vascular damage[9] and mechanisms of uterine vasoconstriction.[10,11]

OFFSPRING OUTCOME

Animal Studies

We have observed that prenatal cocaine exposure in laboratory rats can cause dose-dependent decreases in birth weight (i.e., IUGR), prenatal and postnatal mortality, and postnatal growth.[2–6] Analyses of fetal body composition revealed proportionately lower levels of body fat,[6] protein, and calcium.[12] Magnesium, zinc, potassium, iron, and sodium content were not influenced.[12] The bone composition of adult offspring can also be altered in terms of mineral and organic matter content.[13] These effects are also seen to some degree in pair-fed control animals.[6,12,13] Such control animals mimic the undernutrition that accompanies cocaine intoxication. The topic of undernutrition is discussed in detail in Galler's chapter.

In terms of mechanisms, the reduction in fetal protein and body fat content in cocaine-exposed offspring suggests decreased protein and fat synthesis secondary to decreased placental transport of fatty acids and amino acids. This could result from reduced nutrient supplies in the maternal blood secondary to decreased maternal food consumption, increased maternal/fetal energy demands, and the uterine and placental vasoconstrictions that accompany cocaine intoxication. Decreased transport of amino acids, for example, has been observed in both animal[14] and human placentas[15] following cocaine exposure. Likewise, the reduction in fetal calcium levels in such fetuses may have been due to decreased placental transport secondary to reduced maternal food consumption, uterine vasoconstriction,[12] or even the chelation of calcium ions by cocaine.[16] Reduced blood flow is one of the main mechanisms of IUGR.[17,18]

It is also conceivable that the reduced protein, fat, and calcium levels may be secondary to fetal immaturity. That is, fetal weight, percent body fat, protein, and calcium concentrations increase with gestational age at the expense of body water.[17,18] Thus, the relatively decreased levels of these former substances in the cocaine and pair-fed fetuses resemble those in chemically and physically immature offspring.

Proteins and fatty acids are important sources of calories and structural components of organs, the nervous system, and hormones. Calcium is needed for bone growth and the excitability of nerves and muscles. Deficiencies in these nutrients can therefore result in IUGR, decreased internal organ size, decreased cell number, decreased skeletal growth, limb reduction, decreased intelligence, and increased pre- and postnatal mortality.[17,18]

The effects of prenatal cocaine on fetal body composition are important because such information can guide pre- and postnatal nutritional intervention. Such intervention would involve supplementation that provides the deprived nutrients.[19] Inasmuch as prenatal cocaine exposure is associated with decreased birth weight, body fat, protein, and calcium content, any pre- and postnatal supplementation should provide extra fats, proteins, and calcium.

In our experience, cocaine-induced birth defects in laboratory rats are occasionally seen, but only at relatively high dose levels (about 60 mg/kg/day or more). These include cephalic hemorrhage, anophthalmia, malformed or missing digits (FIGS. 1–3), and malformed jaws and ribs.[2–6,20,21] In terms of mechanisms, most of these effects were probably induced by cocaine's vasoconstrictive effects on either the uterus, placenta, or fetus which can lead to hypoxia, ischemia, and hemorrhage. Cocaine might also have some direct cytotoxic effects, causing reductions in cell numbers and disrupting cell migration.

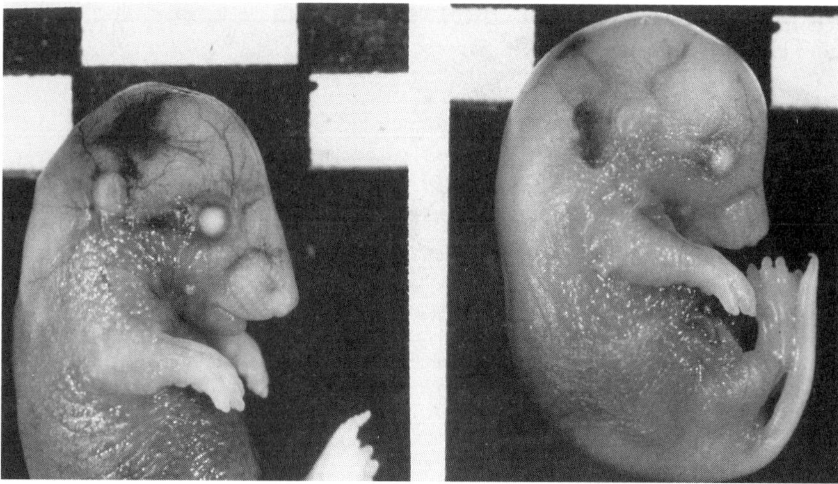

FIGURE 1. Rat fetuses with cephalic hemorrhages induced by prenatal cocaine exposure.

Human Studies

Low birth weight and pre- and postnatal mortality are occasionally reported in the human literature. Prenatal mortality is usually associated with placental abruption. Some of the postnatal deaths may have been due to sudden infant death syndrome (SIDS). The evidence for an increased incidence of SIDS among cocaine-exposed infants is mixed, however. Other factors could have played a role in these postnatal mortalities such as maternal neglect, overlaying (a sleeping parent accidentally rolling over

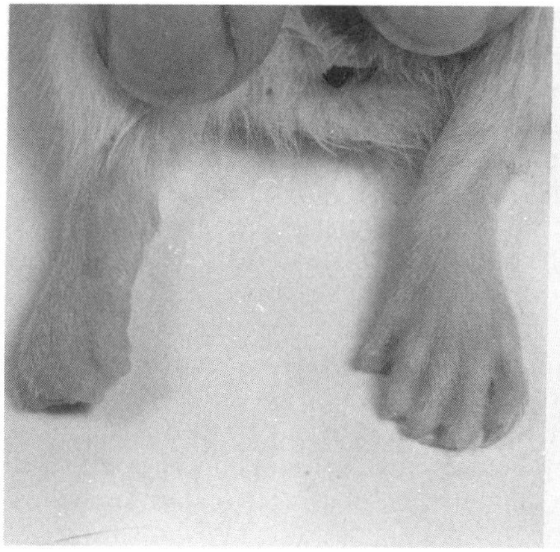

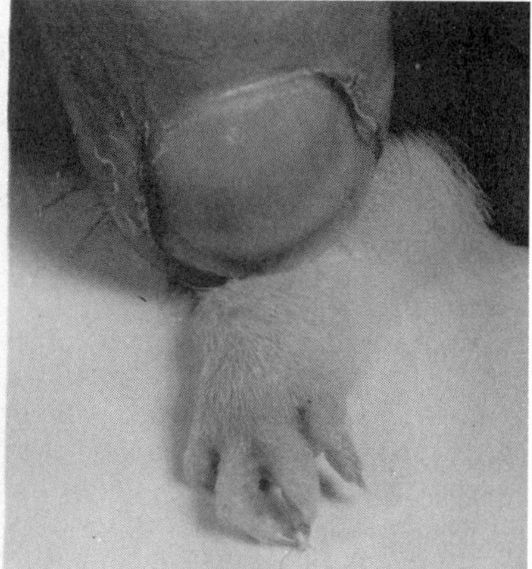

FIGURE 2. Ectrodactyly and camptodactyly induced by prenatal cocaine exposure.

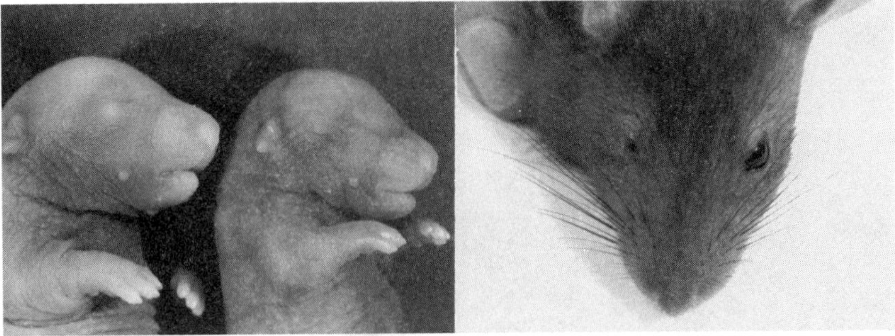

FIGURE 3. (Left) Unilateral anophthalmia (missing eye bud) in a rat fetus prenatally exposed to cocaine contrasted with an ostensibly normal littermate. **(Right)** Unilateral anophthalmia in an adult rat that was prenatally exposed to cocaine.

an infant), abuse, or postnatal cocaine exposure via the mother's milk or passive inhalation of crack cocaine fumes.[1]

Whereas various birth defects have been observed in cocaine-exposed neonates, these observations are confounded by exposure to other teratogens such as alcohol, cigarette smoking, opiates, and the adulterants used "to cut" the cocaine. Despite these considerations, there is a somewhat consistent pattern of gastroschisis, necrotizing enterocolitis, cephalic hemorrhage, and limb reduction in cocaine-exposed neonates. In terms of mechanisms, all of these morbidities could be the result of cocaine-induced vasoconstriction and subsequent vascular rupture and/or tissue necrosis.[1]

OFFSPRING BEHAVIOR

Animal Studies

Several different tests have been used to evaluate the effects of prenatal cocaine exposure on reflex development in laboratory rats. The tests include negative geotaxis (a measure of vestibular maturation), surface and free-fall righting reflexes, cliff avoidance, and acoustic startle. The reports on such testing are mixed in that some studies reported developmental delays or impairment while others did not.[1]

We and others have observed reduced activity levels in an open field test or similar conditions in periweanling and juvenile rats that were prenatally exposed to cocaine. Others have observed suppressed levels of juvenile play, attenuated behavioral responses to perioral stimulation and stimulant drug challenges, as well as decreased male sexual behavior, albeit some of these effects are rather mixed. (See ref. 22 for literature overview.)

The open-field test putatively provides a method for measuring individual differences in "emotionality." The emotional animal is one that has low activity, resulting from an increased duration of initial "freezing" behavior. This initial freezing is a species-specific defensive reaction of rats that is displayed in certain fearful situations. When it is displayed in response to a novel environment or stimulus, it is often described as a "neophobic response." The animal will show relatively decreased exploratory behavior for 15–30 minutes or so. Eventually, the animal habituates to the novel environment and moves about in a normal manner. While increased emotionality or neophobia is a common interpretation of decreased activity levels in a novel environment, it is also possible that the cocaine-exposed animals were behaviorally depressed, showing decreased play or other social behaviors, experiencing low arousal or a disrupted state control, lacking the motivation to explore their environment, or engaged in nonexploratory behaviors such as grooming, resting, or stereotypy.[22]

Recent research has provided a biological mechanism for prenatal cocaine's effects on locomotor activity. The brain's dopaminergic (DA) system is involved in the expression of active behavior such as motor and sexual behaviors. Thus, altered activity levels suggest a dysfunctional DA system. Indeed, there is considerable evidence for a dysfunctional DA system in the supraschiasmatic nucleus, striatum, substantia nigra, ventral tegmentum, and related structures resulting from prenatal cocaine exposure.[22]

In contrast to prenatal cocaine, prenatal alcohol usually results in rat offspring that are hyperactive in the open field or activity cage environment.[23] Prenatal undernutrition in laboratory rats has been associated with reduced activity levels. While our pair-fed (undernutrition) control animals did not show significantly reduced activity, the influence of prenatal undernutrition on offspring behavior merits consideration.

Another interest in our laboratory is the effects of cocaine and alcohol on the offspring's ability to cope with stress. Prenatal alcohol exposure can result in hyperresponsiveness, high anxiety, or poor stress adaptation in both humans and laboratory rats. Similarly, recent evidence indicates that prenatal cocaine exposure results in hyperresponsiveness to stress. Specifically, prenatal cocaine exposure in laboratory rats results in excessive fearfulness and frantic behavior.[24]

The forced swim test has become a widely used model for studying stress in animals. This test involves placing an animal in a cylinder of water and observing how long it remains immobile during the test period. The duration of immobility reflects the level of stress or fear in that the more the animal struggles to escape, the greater the stress or fear. Rats prenatally exposed to either cocaine or alcohol exhibit a heightened stress reaction in this test.[24] The topic of stress is further discussed in Spear's chapter in this volume.

Studies in our laboratory and others indicate that prenatal cocaine exposure in laboratory rats can cause learning and memory deficits. This topic is covered in detail in Harvey's chapter.

Human Studies

Like animal studies, human studies have shown that prenatal cocaine exposure can alter activity levels. For example, prenatal cocaine exposure can result in neonates who exhibit disrupted "state control," low arousal, and depressed interactive behavior. State control refers to the infants' ability to move appropriately through the various states of arousal in response to environmental demands. State control in cocaine-exposed infants can be poorly organized with infants spending most of their time in states that shut them off from external stimulation. Their state changes tend to be abrupt and inappropriate for the level of stimulation. For example, they may go into a deep self-protective sleep in response to initial stimulation. They may remain asleep but may startle, whimper, change color, breath irregularly, and thrash about with continued stimulation. They may also vacillate between sleeping and crying throughout examination without reaching an alert, responsive state. These abnormalities in state control, low arousal, and depressed interactive behavior may persist for the first month or so.[25]

Konkol *et al.*[26] described cocaine-exposed neonates as having two neurobehavioral patterns, excitable and depressed. The excitable phase was transient, probably reflecting acute intoxication and withdrawal. Coles *et al.*[27] described neonates prenatally exposed to cocaine as showing autonomic depression and an overall pattern of low arousal. Several studies observed depressed motor and interactive abilities in such infants[28] and toddlers.[29] Such children can also be hyperresponsive and difficult to calm down once excited.[29]

VISUAL DISORDERS

Animal Studies

Animal studies have implicated the embryonic/fetal visual system as a target for cocaine. We observed a developmental delay in eye maturation and several instances of unilateral anophthalmia in rats prenatally exposed to cocaine.[2–6] More recently, we observed abnormal electroretinograms and reduced retinal thickness[30] in rats prenatally or neonatally exposed to cocaine (FIGS. 4 and 5). These results indicate abnormal retinal function and structure, respectively. It should be noted that some ocular anomalies and abnormal electroretinograms can be caused by severe pre- and postnatal malnutrition (e.g., ref. 31).

Mahalik and colleagues[20,21] were perhaps the first group to systematically investigate the teratogenicity of cocaine. CF-1 mice were exposed on either gestational day 7, 8, 9, 10, 11, or 12. Anophthalmia was seen in 5–9% of the fetuses, malformed lens in 0–31%, and missing lens in 0–13%. These effects seemed equally pronounced across the different exposure days. A variety of other terata, including skeletal, digit, kidney, brain, and genital abnormalities, were observed.

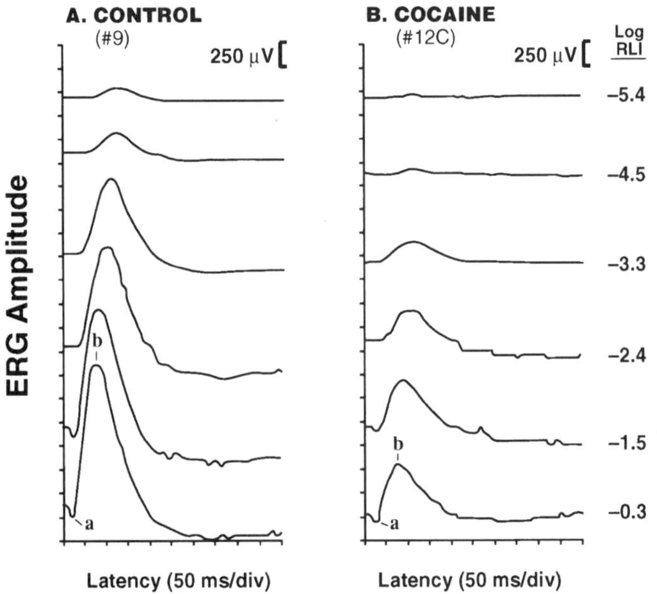

FIGURE 4. Serial electroretinograms (ERGs) in response to light flashes of graded intensities. A rat that was neonatally exposed to cocaine had a significantly altered ERG threshold and diminished ERG amplitudes as compared to controls, indicating impaired retinal functioning. The retinal histology for the cocaine-treated rat is shown in FIGURE 5. RLI = relative light intensity.

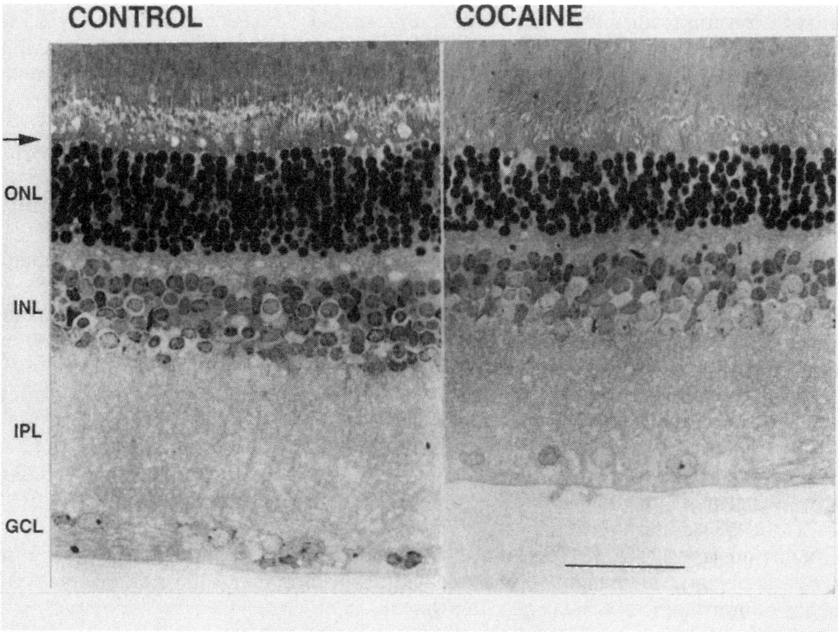

FIGURE 5. Histological sections through the central retina of a control rat (CONTROL) and a rat treated neonatally with cocaine (COCAINE). Retinas were embedded in epon-araldite, sectioned at 1 μm, and stained with toluidine blue. Retinas are aligned at the outer limiting membrane *(arrow)*. This figure illustrates the reduced thickness of the ONL, IPL, and overall retinal thickness of the cocaine-treated rat. The electroretinograms for this rat are illustrated in FIGURE 4. Scale bar equals 50 μm. ONL = outer nuclear layer; INL = inner nuclear layer; IPL = inner plexiform layer; GCL = ganglion cell layer.

Mendez-Armenta *et al.*[32] reported that rat fetuses, when prenatally exposed to cocaine, showed a variety of optic anomalies. These included decreased retinal cell numbers, areas of depleted retinal cells, interstitial edema, pyknotic (shrunken and dying) ganglion cells, necrotic areas in the photoreceptor and bipolar cell layers, areas of abnormal cell proliferation in the photoreceptor and ganglion layers, nuclear pyknosis, and cytoplasm destruction.

Silva-Araujo *et al.*[33] observed that prenatal cocaine exposure in Wistar rats caused increased numbers of ectopic photoreceptor-like cells in the retina's inner nuclear layer. This increase in ectopic photoreceptor-like cells was observed at postnatal day 14, but had dissipated by postnatal day 30. Although this abnormality was transitory and reflected a maturational delay, such an event can cause alterations in retinal circuitry organization. Retinal photoreceptor rosettes were present, reflecting areas of photoreceptor cell degradation. This effect was permanent. The cocaine group also showed reduced thickness of the retinal ganglion cell layer, smaller ganglion cell nuclear diameter, and higher ganglion cell linear density.[34] The latter-most effect dissipated somewhat from postnatal day 14 to 30. Cocaine's vascular disruptive effects were believed to be the cause of these anomalies.

Regarding nervous system development, the rat's neonatal period corresponds approximately to the third trimester of human pregnancy. Consequently, Silva-Araujo *et al.* also administered cocaine to neonatal rats. Such rats exhibited several changes in certain retinal cell layers and the optic nerve. The cocaine-treated group had a higher proportion of small axons, a lower proportion of large axons,[35] signs of optic nerve degeneration, a higher proportion of glial cells,[36] but no differences in the number of myelin lamellae per axon.[35] The retinas of such animals also showed decreases in ganglion cell, nerve fiber, and possibly the inner plexiform layers. In the ventral portion of the retina, such rats had reduced ganglion cell nuclear diameter, increased neuron packing density, increased prominence of smaller neurons,[35] and photoreceptor cell rosettes.[37]

Webster *et al.*[38] prenatally exposed Sprague-Dawley rats to cocaine, then examined the brains and eyes of a subgroup of fetuses that exhibited hemorrhages in the extremities. Several of these animals had severe retinal damage, retinal hemorrhages, and vacuolization of the lens. Mechanical constriction of the uterine vessel resulted in the same cluster of anomalies, suggesting the cocaine-induced effects were the result of vasoconstriction and subsequent ischemia/hypoxia damage. In an earlier study, Webster and Brown-Woodman[39] observed cocaine-induced hemorrhages in the eye as well as the cerebral hemispheres, upper lip, nose, mandible, digits, tail, and genital tubercle. These effects were ostensibly late gestational effects induced by cocaine's vasoconstrictive actions.[36,37]

Brittebo[40] reported that the pigmented epithelial layer of the fetal mouse's eye has a high binding for cocaine. This strongly implicates the pigmented epithelial layer as a target site for cocaine toxicity. The pigmented epithelial layer is important for the supply of nutrients to the retina (e.g., retinol), removal of waste products, maintenance of the blood-retinal barrier, absorption of scattered light, synthesis of proteins for the interphotoreceptor matrix, and retinal differentiation. Cocaine probably disrupts these pigmented epithelial layer functions.

Human Studies

Children with FAS are at increased risk for a variety of visual defects. These include severe myopia, severe astigmatism, strabismus, amblyopia, corneal opacities, retinal defects, hypoplastic optic disk, microphthalmia,[41–43] and impaired visuospatial abilities.[44] Prenatal exposure to cocaine appears to have effects on the human visual system as well.

In terms of visual abnormalities in infants born to cocaine-abusing women, Good *et al.*[45] described 13 such infants who had optic nerve hypoplasia ($n = 5$), delayed visual maturation ($n = 7$), and/or profound eyelid edema ($n = 4$). One child had severe bilateral optic atrophy. Another child had microphthalmia with colobomata (areas of missing retina). The eyelid edema persisted for at least 1 month. Facial characteristics included possible mild supraorbital ridge hypoplasia, flat nasal bridge, and zygomatic hypoplasia. Robin and Zackai[46] examined a dysmorphic infant born to a woman who abused both cocaine and alcohol. The infant had proptotic and widely spaced eyes with puffy eyelids as well as numerous craniofacial anomalies.

Dominguez *et al.*[47] observed optic nerve hypoplasia, nystagmus, and/or strabismus in 9 of 10 infants who were prenatally exposed to cocaine. Three of these infants also had abnormal optic disks, two being apparently blind. One infant had ptosis with third cranial nerve palsy in addition to nystagmus and strabismus. Isenberg *et al.*[48] found dilated and tortuous iris vessels in 6 of 13 such infants. Teske and Trese[49] examined one such infant who was born full-term. This infant had retinopathy of prematurity in one eye, whereas the other eye had corneal hypoplasia, microphthalmia, persistent hyperplastic primary vitreous (a fibrovascular stalk extending from the nerve head to the lens), and vitreous opacity. The authors suggested that the retinopathy of prematurity may have resulted from cocaine's vasoconstrictive effects, but that the hyperplastic primary vitreous was not. It is noteworthy, however, that the latter anomaly is indicative of disrupted cell differentiation and migration.

In a study of 70 children with prenatal cocaine exposure, one child was blind. Computerized tomography revealed bilateral infarctions cutting across each optic tract.[50] Several other children exhibited visual motor disturbances as evidenced by difficulties in copying straight lines, circles, and more complex forms. Many of the children also exhibited problems with language, motor skills, social skills, play behavior, and autism. Their mothers typically abused alcohol and other drugs, in addition to cocaine.

Vision was adversely affected in 16 full-term infants who had cocaine-positive urine tests shortly after birth. These infants had impaired visual attention/tracking as evidenced by the Brazelton Neonatal Assessment Scale (BNAS).[51] Eleven of 12 infants receiving further evaluation had abnormal visual evoked potentials. These disturbances persisted in six infants beyond the age of 4 months. Tenorio *et al.*[52] described an infant who had an *in utero* stroke and resulting porencephaly as a consequence of the mother's cocaine abuse. The infant had an abnormal visual evoked potential as well as an abnormal auditory brainstem response and electroencephalogram. Others have observed that such infants have poor visual fixation as assessed by the BNAS.[28,53]

Lessick *et al.*[54] observed an oculoauriculovertebral spectrum (a combination of eye, ear, vertebral, and facial anomalies) in one infant prenatally exposed to cocaine. The eye and periocular findings consisted of microphthalmia of the right eye, upward slanting palpebral fissures, and hypertelorism.

Block *et al.*[55] examined 55 infants who were prenatally exposed to cocaine and 100 control infants. Although there were no group differences for spherical refractive error, astigmatism, or anisometropia, the cocaine group had a significantly higher incidence of strabismus (27% versus 7%). Other ocular abnormalities in the cocaine group included optic nerve atrophy ($n = 1$), retinopathy of prematurity ($n = 2$), bilateral retinal coloboma with microcornea ($n = 1$), posterior staphyloma (a protrusion on the cornea or sclera) ($n = 1$), suspected glaucoma ($n = 1$), and left eye ptosis ($n = 1$).

Stafford *et al.*[56] evaluated 40 cocaine-exposed and 40 control infants and found no significant group differences in the incidence of eye defects such as congenital anomalies, subconjunctival hemorrhages, retinal hemorrhages, optic nerve abnormalities, or intraocular pressure. However, 11 of the control infants were positive for alcohol and/or other drug exposure, and optic nerve hypoplasia was suspect in three of the cocaine-exposed infants.

The studies observing ocular/visual problems in cocaine-exposed infants have attributed the effects to the vasoconstrictive, hypertensive, ischemic, hemorrhagic effects of cocaine in the fetus. Many of the infants in these studies were prenatally exposed to alcohol, heroin, and methadone in addition to cocaine. Strabismus, nystagmus, and retinal abnormalities are often observed in infants prenatally exposed to alcohol[44] and heroin/methadone.[57] Retinal, eyelid, vitreous, and optic nerve damage as well as strabismus sometimes occurs with the shaken baby syndrome and retinopathy of prematurity.[58] These confounding factors need to be considered when evaluating infants born to cocaine-abusing women.

HEARING DISORDERS

Animal Studies

Congenital craniofacial and ocular anomalies are traditionally associated with hearing disorders.[59] Although craniofacial and ocular anomalies in cocaine-exposed infants are admittedly uncommon, such anomalies do occur. Prenatal cocaine exposure is also associated with other risk factors for congenital hearing loss such as congenital cardiac anomalies, low birth weight, low Apgar scores, intracranial hemorrhages, and perinatal hypoxia.[60] Thus, it seems plausible that prenatal cocaine exposure may increase the neonate's risk for hearing disorders. Recent animal and human research by our group and others supports this conjecture.

In a series of animal studies, we sought to determine if prenatal exposure could adversely influence auditory/neurological function as assessed by the auditory brainstem response and if this effect was permanent or dissipated with maturation. The auditory brainstem response is a sensory-evoked potential elicited by a series of clicks or tone pips. In the rat, the auditory brainstem response is comprised of four vertex-positive waves labeled P1 through P4, occurring within 6 ms poststimulus. The chief neural generators in the rodent are the auditory nerve (P1), the cochlear nucleus (P2), the superior olivary complex (P3), and the inferior colliculus (P4). The human auditory brainstem response can have seven waveforms, and its neural generators are more complex. Clinically, auditory brainstem responses are used to evaluate peripheral and retrocochlear hearing loss, demyelinating diseases, and the effects of toxic agents. In terms of postnatal development, auditory brainstem response latencies decrease monotonically with increasing age in concert with the brain's maturation. Thus, auditory brainstem responses can provide a useful, noninvasive measure of peripheral and brainstem auditory pathway maturation and function.[61]

We observed that rats prenatally exposed to cocaine showed developmental delays in ear opening[2,4,61] and in auditory brainstem response maturation.[62] The latter observation was also made in an animal (rat) study conducted by Salamy *et al.*[63] Such a developmental delay in auditory brainstem response maturation can be caused by severe protein malnutrition.[64] A few of our animals had a persistence of abnormal auditory brainstem responses into adulthood. A follow-up study revealed that these particular animals had permanent sensorineural hearing loss as evidenced by the auditory brainstem response[65] (FIG. 6).

Burchfield[66] exposed fetal sheep to cocaine and examined brain metabolic rates as evidenced by glucose utilization. Reduced metabolic rates in the treated fetuses were observed in 33 of 34 structures as compared to controls. Affected areas included such auditory structures as the cochlear nucleus, superior olivary complex, lateral lemniscus, inferior colliculus, and auditory cortex. The author felt that such decreases in brain metabolic rates were the result of cocaine's vasoconstrictive/ischemic actions.

Dow-Edwards *et al.*[67] exposed neonatal rat pups to cocaine and examined the animals at 60 days of age for brain metabolic rates as evidenced by glucose utilization. Several brain areas showed altered metabolic rates including some auditory structures. Specifically, treated females had significantly increased metabolic rates in the medial geniculate nucleus, while treated males had significantly decreased metabolic rates in the auditory cortex. The inferior colliculus showed no cocaine treatment effect. Other auditory structures were not examined.

Human Studies

While a search of the literature produced only two reports of a "deaf" child born to a cocaine-abusing woman,[50,68] a number of scientific and clinical studies suggest that varying degrees of hearing impairment can be a consequence of prenatal cocaine exposure. For example, Cone-Wesson and her colleagues[69,70] observed abnormal auditory brainstem responses in neonates born to cocaine-abusing women. The auditory brainstem response abnormalities suggested otoneurological impairment or developmental compromise. The potential confounding influence of drugs other than cocaine was not systematically evaluated.

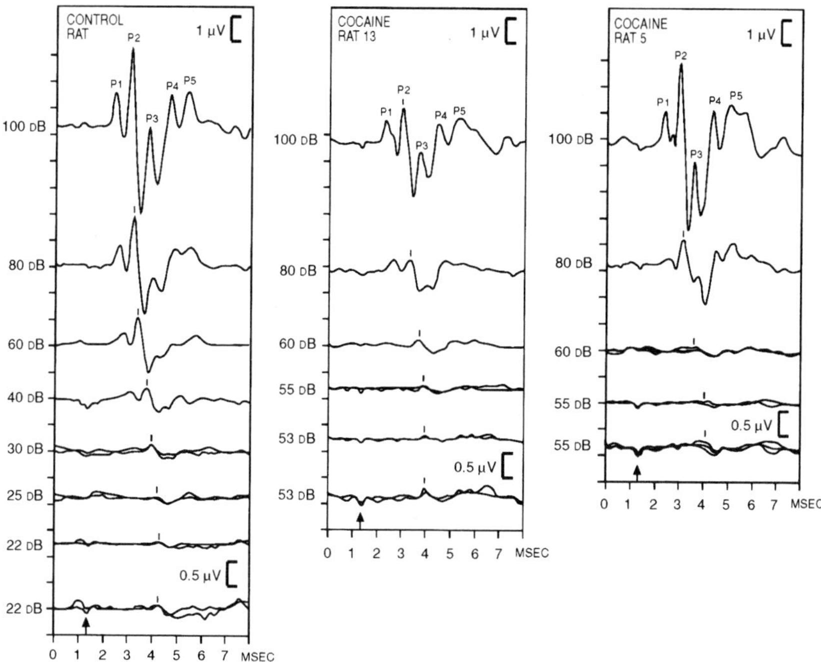

FIGURE 6. Serial auditory brainstem responses elicited by 8,000 Hz tone pips. **(Left)** The auditory brainstem responses from a typical control rat had a threshold at 22 dB. **(Middle and right)** The auditory brainstem responses from two rats prenatally exposed to cocaine had small amplitudes, prolonged latencies, and thresholds elevated to 53 and 55 dB, respectively. These threshold elevations suggest hearing losses of about 30 dB for the 8,000 Hz tone pips. (Modified from Church and Overbeck.[65])

In studies that more carefully controlled for other drug abuse, Salamy and Eldredge[71] found that cocaine-exposed neonates were four to five times more likely to have abnormal auditory brainstem responses than were controls and that such auditory brainstem response abnormalities indicated slowed brainstem transmission of the sensory information. This slowing seemed to dissipate with aging, suggesting a neurodevelopmental delay with subsequent normalization.[72] In a study of 14 cocaine-only and 18 cocaine-plus-alcohol infants, Fries *et al.*[73] reported a general finding of abnormal auditory brainstem responses in such infants, but provided no descriptive details. The cocaine-exposed infant described by Tenorio *et al.*[52] had an abnormal auditory brainstem response. We, too, have observed abnormal auditory brainstem responses in neonates prenatally exposed to cocaine and/or alcohol.[74]

Kankirawatana *et al.*[74] described Möbius syndrome in a cocaine-exposed infant. The infant had multiple craniofacial anomalies, multiple cranial nerve palsy, and abnormal auditory brainstem responses suggestive of peripheral hearing loss (probably sensorineural hearing loss). The authors pointed out that vascular injury is one of the favored theoretical mechanisms for both Möbius syndrome and cocaine-induced birth defects. Hearing loss is common in the Möbius syndrome.[59]

Carzoli *et al.*[76] evaluated the auditory brainstem responses of 50 full-term neonates born to cocaine-abusing women. This study did not find any abnormal auditory brainstem responses. Their neonates were relatively healthy in terms of standard neonatal assessments, however (e.g., normal Apgar scores, normal gestational age, normal birth weight, and no congenital anomalies).

A few studies have reported language disorders in cocaine-exposed children, which could reflect a hearing and/or cognitive impairment. Angelilli *et al.*[77] found more maternal cocaine use during pregnancy among language-delayed children than among controls. Bender *et al.*[78] observed that a group of 18 children prenatally exposed to cocaine had significantly worse receptive language ability than did controls. Similarly, several studies have reported language development deficits in children born to women who abused cocaine, methadone, and/or heroin during pregnancy.[25,50,79,80]

The developmental delays in auditory brainstem response maturation observed in both animal and human studies probably reflected impaired neural growth. The instances of sensorineural hearing loss in animals as well as peripheral hearing loss and deafness in humans probably resulted from damage to the auditory sensory receptor cells and/or the auditory nerve. The animal study findings of altered metabolic functioning in brainstem and cortical structures suggest the existence of central hearing disorders. The possibilities of conductive hearing loss, otitis proneness, and central hearing loss have yet to be investigated in children who were prenatally exposed to cocaine.

OTHER SENSORY DISORDERS

Brittebo[40] noted high concentrations of cocaine in the olfactory mucosa of the fetal mouse, suggesting that prenatal cocaine exposure might damage olfaction. Disappointingly little research has been done on olfactory damage in such animals. Spear *et al.*[81] observed altered behavior in an odor-association learning task in prenatally exposed rat pups. This effect, however, may have been due to impaired olfaction, impaired cognitive ability, or a combination. One recent animal study reported altered somatosensory (foot shock) reactions as a consequence of prenatal cocaine treatment,[82] while another did not.[81]

RECOMMENDATIONS AND CONCLUSIONS

Vascular disruption is probably the major mechanism underlying the visual, hearing, growth, and behavioral effects of prenatal cocaine exposure. Maternal/fetal undernutrition and dopaminergic dysfunction also contribute to the adverse effects on the offspring.

Adequate hearing is necessary for proper speech and language acquisition and comprehension. A child with a hearing loss, who is otherwise normal, will tend to exhibit behavioral problems such as hyperactivity, distractibility, withdrawal, and poor coping skills as well as language and learning disabilities if intervention is delayed beyond the critical period of speech and language development. Similarly, childhood visual impairments can cause permanent visuoperceptual, cognitive, and behavioral deficits. Problems with vision, hearing, language, behavior, and cognition can occur in the child prenatally exposed to cocaine. Although hearing and vision problems may not be the sole cause of such behavioral and cognitive problems, hearing and vision problems will worsen them. Thus, we recommend early identification and intervention for such disorders to help the child reach full potential.

Another recommendation is for hearing and visual assessments to occur before language, visuoperceptual, behavioral, and cognitive testing because hearing and visual deficits can invalidate such tests. Finally, we recommend that assessment and intervention for hearing, vision, behavioral, cognitive, and growth disorders occur as soon as possible after birth. The earlier the intervention, the better the patient outcome.

REFERENCES

1. Church, M.W. *et al.* 1991. Effects of prenatal cocaine exposure. *In* Biochemistry and Physiology of Substance Abuse, Vol. III. Chapter 8. R.R. Watson, Ed.: 179–204. CRC Press. Boca Raton, FL.
2. Church, M.W. *et al.* 1988. Dose-dependent consequences of cocaine on pregnancy outcome in the Long-Evans rat. Neurotoxicol. Teratol. **10:** 51–58.
3. Church, M.W. *et al.* 1988. The interactive effects of alcohol and cocaine on maternal and fetal toxicity in the Long-Evans rat. Neurotoxicol. Teratol. **10:** 355–361.
4. Church, M.W. *et al.* 1990. Prenatal cocaine exposure in the Long-Evans rat. I. Dose-dependent effects on gestation, mortality and postnatal maturation. Neurotoxicol. Teratol. **12:** 327–334.
5. Church, M.W. *et al.* 1991. Interactive effects of prenatal alcohol and cocaine exposures on offspring development and behavior in the Long-Evans rat. Neurotoxicol. Teratol. **13:** 377–386.
6. Church, M.W. *et al.* 1995. Comparative effects of prenatal cocaine, alcohol and undernutrition on maternal fetal toxicity and fetal body composition in the Sprague-Dawley rat with observations on strain dependent differences. Neurotoxicol. Teratol. **17:** 559–567.
7. Church, M.W. & M.G. Subramanian. 1997. Cocaine's lethality increases during late gestation in the rat: A study of "critical periods" of exposure. Am. J. Obstet. Gynecol. **176:** 901–906.
8. Plessinger, M.A. & J.R. Woods. 1991. The cardiovascular effects of cocaine use in pregnancy. Reprod. Toxicol. **5:** 99–113.
9. Church, M.W. & E.F. Mammen. 1997. The effect of cocaine treatment on plasma fibronectin levels in pregnant and nonpregnant rats does not mimick pre-eclampsia. Submitted.
10. Cook, J.L. & C.L. Randall. 1996. Cocaine does not affect prostacyclin, thromboxane or prostaglandin E production in human umbilical veins. Drug Alcohol Depend. **41:** 113–119.
11. Zhang, X. *et al.* 1997. Evidence for a serotonin-mediated effect of cocaine causing vasoconstriction and herniated umbilici in chicken embryos. Pharmacol. Biochem. Behav. In press.
12. Church, M.W. *et al.* 1998. Prenatal cocaine, alcohol and undernutrition differentially alter mineral and protein content in fetal rats. Pharmacol. Biochem. Behav. In press.
13. Seifert, M.F. & M.W. Church. 1991. Long term effects of prenatal cocaine exposure on femurs in rats. Life Sci. **49:** 569–574.
14. Novak, D.A. *et al.* 1995. Effect of chronic cocaine administration on amino acid uptake in rat placental membrane vesicles. Life Sci. **56:** 1779–1789.
15. Barnwell, S.L. & B.V.R. Sastry. 1983. Depression of amino acid uptake in human placental villus by cocaine, morphine and nicotine. Trophoblast Res. **1:** 101–120.
16. Misra, A.L. & S.J. Mulé. 1975. Calcium-binding property of cocaine and some of its active metabolites: Formation of molecular complexes. Res. Commun. Chem. Pathol. Pharmacol. **11:** 663–666.
17. Hohenauer, L. & W. Oh. 1969. Body composition in experimental intrauterine growth retardation in the rat. J. Nutr. **99:** 23–26.
18. Moghissi, K.S. 1977. Relationship of maternal amino acids and proteins to infant growth and mental development. *In* Nutritional Impacts on Women. K.S. Moghissi & T.N. Evans, Eds.: 86–106. Harper & Row Publishing. New York, NY.
19. Lechtig, A. & R.E. Klein. 1981. Pre-natal nutrition and birth weight: Is there a causal association? *In* Maternal Nutrition in Pregnancy: Eating for Two? J. Dobbing, Ed.: 131–155. Academic Press. New York, NY.
20. Mahalik, M.P. *et al.* 1980. Teratogenic potential of cocaine hydrochloride in CF-1 mice. J. Pharm. Sci. **69:** 703–706.

21. Mahalik, M.P. *et al.* 1984. Mechanisms of cocaine-induced teratogenesis. Res. Commun. Subst. Abuse **5:** 279–302.
22. Church, M.W. & J.P. Tilak. 1996. Differential effects of prenatal cocaine and retinoic acid on activity levels throughout the day and night. Pharmacol. Biochem. Behav. **55:** 595–605.
23. Bond, N.W. & E.L. Di Gusto. 1976. Effects of prenatal alcohol consumption on open-field behavior and alcohol preference in rats. Psychopharmacology. **46:** 163–168.
24. Bilitzke, P. & M.W. Church. 1992. Prenatal cocaine and alcohol exposures affect rat behavior in a stress test (the Porsolt swim test). Neurotoxicol. Teratol. **14:** 359–364.
25. Griffith, D.R. *et al.* 1994. Three-year outcome of children exposed prenatally to drugs. J. Am. Acad. Child. Adolesc. Psychiatry **33:** 20–27.
26. Konkol, R.J. *et al.* 1994. Cocaine metabolites in the neonate: Potential for toxicity. J. Child. Neurol. **9:** 242–248.
27. Coles, C.D. *et al.* 1992. Effects of cocaine and alcohol use in pregnancy on neonatal growth and neurobehavioral status. Neurotoxicol. Teratol. **14:** 23–34.
28. Chasnoff, I.J. *et al.* 1985. Cocaine use in pregnancy. New Engl. J. Med. **313:** 666–669.
29. Rodning, C. *et al.* 1989. Prenatal exposure to drugs and its influence on attachment. Ann. N.Y. Acad. Sci. **563:** 352–354.
30. Church, M.W. *et al.* 1996. Visual impairment from pre- and postnatal cocaine exposure: Critical periods of exposure. Teratology **53:** 108.
31. Bonavolonta, O. *et al.* 1989. Retinal and lens damages observed in young rats undergoing protein malnutrition in selected stages of their growth. Int. J. Nutr. Res. **59:** 117–121.
32. Mendez-Armenta, M. *et al.* 1997. Retinal lesions in rat fetuses prenatally exposed to cocaine. Neurotoxicol. Teratol. **3:** 199–203.
33. Silva-Araujo, A. *et al.* 1995. Effects of prenatal cocaine exposure in the photoreceptor cells of the rat retina. Molec. Neurobiol. **11:** 77–86.
34. Silva-Araujo, A. *et al.* 1995. Effects of prenatal cocaine exposure in the retinal ganglion cell layer of the rat. Molec. Neurobiol. **11:** 87–97.
35. Silva-Araujo, A. *et al.* 1993. Changes in the retinal ganglion cell layer and optic nerve of rats exposed neonatally to cocaine. Exp. Eye Res. **56:** 199–206.
36. Silva-Araujo, A. *et al.* 1991. Morphological changes in the optic nerve after chronic exposure of neonatal rats to cocaine and amphetamine. Ophthal. Res. **23:** 295–302.
37. Silva-Araujo, A. *et al.* 1994. Retinal changes induced by neonatal cocaine exposure in the rat. Graefe's Arch. Clin. Exp. Ophthalmol. **232:** 162–166.
38. Webster, W.S. *et al.* 1991. Fetal brain damage in the rat following prenatal exposure to cocaine. Neurotoxicol. Teratol. **13:** 621–626.
39. Webster, W.S. & P.D.C. Brown-Woodman. 1990. Cocaine as a cause of congenital malformations of vascular origin: Experimental evidence in the rat. Teratology **41:** 689–697.
40. Brittebo, E.B. 1988. Binding of cocaine in the liver, olfactory mucosa, eye, and fur of pigmented mice. Toxicol. Appl. Pharmacol. **96:** 315–323.
41. Church, M.W. *et al.* 1997. Hearing, speech, language, vestibular and dentofacial disorders in the Fetal Alcohol Syndrome. Alcohol Clin. Exp. Res. **21:** 227–237.
42. Church, M.W. & J.A. Kaltenbach. 1997. Hearing, speech, language and vestibular disorders in the Fetal Alcohol Syndrome: A literature review. Alcohol Clin. Exp. Res. **21:** 495–512.
43. Stromland, K. 1995. Ocular abnormalities in the fetal alcohol syndrome. Acta Ophthalmol. **63**(Suppl. 171): 1–50.
44. Aronson, M. *et al.* 1985. Children of alcoholic mothers. Acta Paediatr. Scand. **74:** 27–35.
45. Good, W.V. *et al.* 1992. Abnormalities of the visual system in infants exposed to cocaine. Ophthalmology **99:** 341–346.
46. Robin, N.H. & E.H. Zackai. 1994. Unusual craniofacial dysmorphia due to prenatal alcohol and cocaine exposure. Teratology **50:** 160–164.
47. Dominguez, R. *et al.* 1991. Brain and ocular abnormalities in infants with in utero exposure to cocaine and other street drugs. AJDC **145:** 688–695.
48. Isenberg, S.J. *et al.* 1987. Ocular signs of cocaine intoxication in neonates. Am. J. Ophthalmol. **103:** 211–214.
49. Teske, M.P. & M.T. Trese. 1987. Retinopathy of prematurity-like fundus and. persistent hy-

perplastic primary vitreous associated with maternal cocaine use. Am. J. Ophthalmol. **103:** 719–720.
50. DAVIS, E. *et al.* 1992. Autism and developmental abnormalities in children with perinatal cocaine exposure. J. Natl. Med. Assoc. **84:** 315–319.
51. DIXON, S.D. *et al.* 1987. Visual dysfunction in cocaine-exposed infants. Pediatr. Res. **21:** 359A (abstr.).
52. TENORIO, G.M. *et al.* 1988. Intrauterine stroke and maternal polydrug abuse. Clin. Pediatr. **27:** 565–567.
53. MOROCHNICK, M. *et al.* 1991. Circulating catecholamine concentrations in cocaine-exposed neonates: A pilot study. Pediatrics **88:** 481–485.
54. LESSICK, M. *et al.* 1991. Severe manifestations of oculoauriculovertebral spectrum in a cocaine exposed infant. J. Med. Genet. **28:** 803–804.
55. BLOCK, S.S. *et al.* 1997. Visual anomalies in young children exposed to cocaine. Optom. Vision Sci. **74:** 28–36.
56. STAFFORD, J.R., JR. *et al.* 1994. Prenatal cocaine exposure and the development of the human eye. Ophthalmology **101:** 301–308.
57. NELSON, L.B. *et al.* 1987. Occurrence of strabismus in infants born to drug-dependent women. Am. J. Dis. Child. **141:** 175–178.
58. GIESE, M.J. 1994. Ocular findings in abused children and infants born to drug abusing mothers. Optom. Vision Sci. **71:** 184–191.
59. NORTHERN, J.L. & M. DOWNS. 1984. Hearing In Children, 3rd Ed. Williams & Wilkins. Baltimore, MD.
60. JOINT COMMITTEE ON INFANT HEARING 1990 POSITION STATEMENT. 1991. Am. Speech Hear. Assoc. **33**(Suppl. 5): 3–6.
61. MOLLER, A.R. 1993. Neural generators of auditory evoked potentials. *In* Principles & Applications in Auditory Evoked Potentials. J.T. Jacobson, Ed.: 23–46. Allyn and Bacon. Boston, MA.
62. CHURCH, M.W. & G.W. OVERBECK. 1990. Prenatal cocaine exposure in the Long-Evans rat. III. Developmental effects on the brainstem auditory evoked potential. Neurotoxicol. Teratol. **12:** 345–351.
63. SALAMY, A. *et al.* 1992. Perinatal cocaine exposure and functional brainstem development in the rat. Brain Res. **598:** 307–310.
64. PLANTZ, R.G. *et al.* 1981. Effects of undernutrition on development of far-field auditory brain stem responses in rat pups. Brain Res. **213:** 319–326.
65. CHURCH, M.W. & G.W. OVERBECK. 1991. Sensorineural hearing loss as evidenced by the auditory brainstem response (ABR) following prenatal cocaine exposure in the Long-Evans rat. Teratology **43:** 561–570.
66. BURCHFIELD, D.J. 1995. Effects of cocaine on fetal brain metabolism and behavioral state in the sheep model. NIDA Monograph **158:** 58–66.
67. DOW-EDWARDS, D.L. *et al.* 1988. Stimulation of brain metabolism by perinatal cocaine exposure. Dev. Brain Res. **42:** 137–141.
68. TOUFEXIS, A. 1991. Innocent victims: Damaged by the drug their mothers took, crack kids will face social and educational hurdles and must count on society's compassion. Time Magazine, May 13: 56–60.
69. SHIH, L. *et al.* 1988. Effects of maternal cocaine abuse on the neonatal auditory system. Inter. J. Pediatr. Otorhinolaryngol. **15:** 245–251.
70. CONE-WESSON, B. & A. SPINGARN. 1993. Effects of maternal cocaine abuse on neonatal auditory brainstem responses. Am. J. Audiol., Nov.: 48–54.
71. SALAMY, A. & L. ELDREDGE. 1994. Risk for ABR abnormalities in the nursery. Electroencephalogr. Clin. Neurophysiol. **92:** 392–395.
72. SALAMY, A. *et al.* 1990. Clinical and laboratory observations: Brain-stem transmission time in infants exposed to cocaine in utero. J. Pediatr. **4:** 627–629.
73. FRIES, M.H. *et al.* 1993. Facial features of infants exposed prenatally to cocaine. Teratology **48:** 413–420.
74. RINTELMANN, W.F. *et al.* 1994. Effects of maternal alcohol and/or cocaine on neonatal ABRs. Am. Speech Hear. Assoc., October: 85.

75. Kankirawatana, P. *et al.* 1993. Möbius syndrome in infant exposed to cocaine in utero. Pediatr. Neurol. **9:** 71–72.
76. Carzoli, R.P. *et al.* 1991. Evaluation of auditory brain-stem response in full-term infants of cocaine-abusing mothers. Am. J. Dis. Child. **145:** 1013–1016.
77. Angelilli, M.L. *et al.* 1994. History of in utero cocaine exposure in language-delayed children. Clin. Pediatr. **33:** 514–516.
78. Bender, S.L. *et al.* 1995. The developmental implications of prenatal and/or postnatal crack cocaine exposure in preschool children: A preliminary report. Dev. & Behav. Pediatr. **16:** 418–424.
79. Nulman, I. *et al.* 1994. Neurodevelopment of adopted children exposed in utero to cocaine. Can. Med. Assoc. **151:** 1591–1597.
80. Van Baar, A. 1990. Development of infants of drug dependent mothers. Child Psychol. Psychiatry **31:** 911–920.
81. Spear, L.P. *et al.* 1989. Effects of prenatal cocaine exposure on behavior during the early postnatal period. Neurotoxicol. Teratol. **11:** 57–63.
82. Smith, R.F. *et al.* 1989. Alterations in offspring behavior induced by chronic prenatal cocaine dosing. Neurotoxicol. Teratol. **11:** 35–38.

The Effects of Prenatal Protein Malnutrition and Cocaine on the Development of the Rat[a]

J. R. GALLER[b] AND J. TONKISS

Center for Behavioral Development and Mental Retardation, M923, Boston University School of Medicine, 80 E. Concord St., Boston, Massachusetts 02118, USA

INTRODUCTION

There has been considerable interest in documenting the effects of cocaine exposure during pregnancy on the physical, neurologic, and behavioral development of the offspring.[1-4] Results of human studies have often been contradictory and confusing. The wide range of outcomes reported in different clinical settings may be the result of factors other than cocaine, including concomitant abuse of alcohol and other drugs, poor nutrition of the mother and fetus, and compromised conditions in the home and rearing environment of the baby. Moreover, the ability to document retrospective patterns of drug abuse by the pregnant mother is imprecise at best. Animal models have contributed to our understanding of the effects of cocaine because they have made it possible to isolate the effects of cocaine abuse independent of other confounding variables.[5] However, there are several features of reported models that differ from the human condition, and these differences may obscure our understanding of the impact of the drug as it pertains to human populations. The first pertains to the duration of cocaine exposure. In human populations, drug habits are generally well established prior to pregnancy. However, cocaine exposure in animal studies is typically begun during pregnancy at a time following neural tube closure in the developing offspring.[6-10] The prolonged drug abuse that is characteristic of drug-addicted humans may have different effects on the development of the offspring than the more limited exposure given in the animal models.

A second important distinction between the human condition and animal studies of prenatal cocaine exposure is the underlying nutritional status of the drug-exposed individual. A recent study in Tenerife, Spain[11] has provided evidence that the nutritional status of drug-addicted individuals is significantly compromised. Although not specifically cocaine addicts, more than 70% of a population of drug-addicted patients admitted to the hospital for detoxification treatment weighed less than 90% of the mean weight for the general population when matched for sex and height. About one third weighed below 80% of the mean weight and, by subjective assessment, approximately one fifth were "deeply malnourished." Importantly, the nutritional status of female drug addicts was poorer than that of males and their drug abuse was more severe. By contrast, animal studies of prenatal cocaine abuse other than our own have provided subjects with good quality diets only. Thus, although animal models are deliberately constructed to identify the independent effects of cocaine, they may not be directly comparable to human populations, in which cocaine exposure and poor nutritional status generally go hand in hand. The coexistence of malnutrition and drug abuse in females raises two possibilities: (1) that some of the effects observed in the offspring that

[a] This research was supported by Research Grants HD22539 (JRG) and DA07934 (JRG) from the National Institutes of Health.

[b] Phone, 617/638–4840; fax, 617/638-4843; e-mail, jgaller@bu.edu

are generally attributed to prenatal drug exposure may instead be related to the compromised nutritional status of the mother during pregnancy, or (2) that malnutrition may potentiate the detrimental impact of prenatal cocaine on the development of the offspring.

Finally, the concomitant presence of malnutrition in drug abusers may reflect the low socioeconomic status of the chronic drug abuser. It may also partially be explained by the anorexia associated with cocaine abuse. In rats, compensatory increases in the consumption of carbohydrate and fat, but not of protein, have been observed following suppression of food intake by cocaine.[12] Pair feeding in which control subjects are provided with the same amount of food as that consumed by cocaine-exposed animals may therefore not be an adequate model. Given our own extensive data demonstrating significant changes in brain development and behavior caused by maternal protein malnutrition,[13–16] there can be little doubt that (among numerous nutritional and nonnutritional factors) an inadequate protein intake in pregnancy represents a significant risk factor for the offspring of drug-abusing mothers.

In a series of four published reports,[17–20] we compared the separate and combined effects of protein malnutrition and cocaine exposure on the growth and behavioral development of rats, using a model in which both insults were present before and during pregnancy. The chronic exposure to these insults better approximates the human situation than do animal models restricting these conditions to pregnancy only. We have also selected a dose of cocaine (30 mg/kg) that produces blood levels typically found in human drug abuse. We have previously reported that this dose (in contrast to 40 mg/kg) did not increase fetal mortality and was not toxic to the developing fetus.[17] We have relied heavily on methods and procedures used in extensive published studies on the effects of prenatal protein malnutrition on the developing rat.

RESEARCH DESIGN

A 2 × 2 research design was used in which female Sprague-Dawley (viral and antibody-free, VAF plus) rats were assigned to one of two nutritional groups (malnourished or well nourished) and one of two drug groups (cocaine versus saline). Both conditions were imposed beginning 5 weeks prior to mating and throughout the duration of pregnancy. During the experimental period, the *nutritional treatment* was as follows: rats were provided with either a diet of low protein (6% casein) or high protein (25% casein) content. The specific composition of the diets is given in a previous paper.[21] Although varying in protein content, the two diets were isocaloric, and they also had the same vitamin, mineral, and fat content.

The *drug treatment* was as follows: within each diet group, rats were subdivided into those receiving cocaine injections and those receiving saline injections (controls). Rats received either cocaine or saline injections at a frequency of two times per week prior to pregnancy and daily from day 3 to day 18 of pregnancy. A mixed route of administration of cocaine, namely, intraperitoneal (ip) before pregnancy and subcutaneous (sc) during pregnancy, was applied. This approach minimized cocaine-associated skin lesions and anorexia and spared the fetus from any potential damage during pregnancy. We used a dose of 30 mg/kg cocaine in a volume of 1 ml/kg of 0.9% saline for ip injections and the same dose in a volume of 3 ml/kg for sc injections. At this dose, the number of fetal deaths was minimal in contrast to 40 mg/kg, which we have shown to be fetotoxic.[17]

At birth, rats in all groups were fostered to well-nourished drug-free mothers from the 25% casein group and provided with a standard lab chow after weaning. Thus, exposure of the offspring to a nutritionally inadequate diet and cocaine was limited to the gestational period. All litters were culled to eight pups (six males and two females) and fostered as whole litters within 24 hours of birth. Pups were selected for fostering based on their proximity to the litter mean body weight for each sex. Sample sizes used in the studies to be described was adequate. In most cases, 10 litters or more per treatment group were used. To control for possible litter effects, developmental studies used the mean value for each litter as the basis for data analyses. For all behavioral studies, only one male rat per litter was tested. In all studies, the tester was blind to the treatment group of the rat to exclude the possibility of tester bias.

RESULTS

Prenatal Measures

Maternal Weight Gain and Food Intake. The aim of this first set of studies was to compare the effects of prenatal malnutrition or cocaine exposure on maternal weight gain during pregnancy, food intake, and duration of pregnancy. Weight gain for the 5-week period prior to pregnancy was sensitive to the effects of diet but not cocaine administration. Thus, rats from the low protein (6% casein) group gained approximately 20 g less than did rats provided with the 25% casein diet. By contrast, nutrition group and cocaine exposure both affected weight gain during pregnancy. Rats provided with the low protein diet gained considerably less weight than did rats provided with the high protein diet (110 versus 78 g). Cocaine treatment reduced weight gain in the well-nourished (25% casein) group by 20 g and in the malnourished (6% casein) group by 10 g. Thus, a low protein diet was strongly associated with reduced weight gain both before and during pregnancy, whereas cocaine exposure had no impact prior to pregnancy but had some effects during pregnancy, especially in well-nourished pregnant females.

In a companion study, we showed that weight gain during pregnancy was not explained by changes in food intake. We previously reported that the protein content of the diet does not affect food intake during pregnancy in our model.[22] However, in this study, and possibly due to the use of saline even in control animals, we did report a difference in the two nutrition groups, notably an increase in the food consumption of low protein rats on days 8–11. Cocaine administration reduced food intake in both nutrition groups. When we corrected for the higher consumption in the 6% versus the 25% casein (non-cocaine) group on days 8–11, a reduction in food intake following cocaine exposure was present only on days 4–5, regardless of nutrition group. Thus, reduced food intake may partly account for the reduction in weight gain observed in the cocaine-treated animals. However, it did not fully explain the pattern of weight gain following cocaine exposure. Of note, the anorexic effects of cocaine in this study were far less than those reported in other studies restricted to cocaine exposure during pregnancy, probably because the rats were acclimated to cocaine prior to pregnancy.

Finally, length of gestation was only minimally affected by the conditions of this study. Thus, gestation was reduced by a half day out of 21 days following cocaine exposure in comparison with the other treatment groups. This difference did not impact birth weight or other developmental outcomes.

Postnatal Development from Birth to Weaning

Pup Weights. Prenatal malnutrition significantly reduced both litter size (from 15 to 13 pups per litter) at birth. Despite smaller litters, average pup weights at birth were also lower in the 6% casein group versus the 25% group (5.2 and 5.8 g, respectively). Prenatal cocaine did not impact litter size, but did reduce average birth weights in the malnourished group (from 5.4 to 4.9 g) and in the well-nourished group (from 6.0 to 5.8 g). Thus, there appears to be an addictive effect of the two prenatal conditions with respect to birth weight. However, prenatal cocaine did not have sustaining effects on weight after birth. By contrast, during the postnatal period, pup weights continued to be reduced in the low protein (6% casein) group relative to the well-nourished pups. This difference persisted until weaning, but was no longer present in adulthood.

Physical Development and Developmental Milestones. We first measured the extent of developmental delays in rat pups attributable to the maternal exposure to cocaine or malnutrition or their combination. At birth, the extent of *skeletal maturation* was measured. Although no malformations were observed, both prenatal cocaine and malnutrition resulted in striking delays on all three measures of skeletal maturation, including number of stained phalanges per hind limb, heel bones, and caudal vertebrae. For example, cocaine reduced the proportion of well-nourished pups showing alizarin red staining of the heel-bone from 100% to 42%. In the malnourished group, all rat pups showed only 20% staining, regardless of whether they were exposed to cocaine or not. The difference of 22% in the well-nourished cocaine group versus the malnourished cocaine group is evidence of additive effects of the two insults.

TABLE 1 shows the mean day of appearance of *physical and reflexive milestones,* which were selected because they covered the span of postnatal development. With re-

TABLE 1. Age of Appearance of Milestones (Days ± SE)

	6% Casein		25% Casein	
	Saline (6)	Cocaine (8)	Saline (9)	Cocaine (8)
Milestones: Physical				
Pinna unfolding	2.28 (± 0.21)	2.82 (± 0.29)	2.60 (± 0.22)	3.08 (± 0.38)
Tooth eruption	9.25 (± 0.36)	9.33 (± 0.35)	8.97 (± 0.27)	9.57 (± 0.39)
Eye opening (first signs)	13.13 (± 0.18)	13.45 (± 0.30)	13.21 (± 0.23)	13.64 (± 0.26)
Eye opening (fully open)	13.73 (± 0.18)	13.93 (± 0.33)	13.66 (± 0.20)	14.06 (± 0.30)
Milestones: Reflexive				
Righting reflex	1.17 (± 0.17)	1.41 (± 0.21)	1.11 (± 0.06)	1.25 (± 0.09)
Cliff avoidance	3.63 (± 0.40)	3.93 (± 0.50)	3.81 (± 0.34)	3.22 (± 0.24)
Negative geotaxis	4.71 (± 0.35)	4.88 (± 0.60)	4.36 (± 0.32)	4.59 (± 0.47)
Vibrissae placing	8.46 (± 0.57)	9.15 (± 0.37)	8.01 (± 0.26)	8.31 (± 0.48)
Auditory startle	12.63 (± 0.28)	13.80 (± 0.40)	12.89 (± 0.34)	13.03 (± 0.39)
Visual placing	15.08 (± 0.20)	15.43 (± 0.25)	15.31 (± 0.31)	15.57 (± 0.32)
Free-fall righting	15.17 (± 0.15)	15.68 (± 0.35)	15.61 (± 0.22)	15.64 (± 0.29)

spect to the physical milestones, pinna unfolding and eye opening (first appearance and full) were all significantly delayed by prenatal cocaine exposure. However, prenatal malnutrition either alone or in conjunction with cocaine did not alter the date of appearance of these landmarks. As may also be seen in the table, the development of several early reflexes was sensitive to the delaying effects of cocaine, especially the righting reflex and also the auditory startle reflex. Prenatal malnutrition significantly delayed vibrissae placement. TABLE 1 also shows that for most of the early reflexes (except one), the greatest delays were present in the group exposed to the combination of malnutrition and cocaine (column two). To summarize, during the postnatal period, the effect of prenatal cocaine on the development of reflexes and physical milestones was especially prominent. However, the effects of prenatal malnutrition were greater than those of cocaine exposure on weight gain during pregnancy and in the postnatal period of the developing rat pup. However, at birth and during the postnatal period, the exposure to both insults combined appeared to have more effects than did either insult alone on a range of developmental measures.

Homing Behavior. We also evaluated the behavioral development of rat pups during the suckling period, using a test of home orientation. This test, which measures the progressive ability of the young pups to locate the nest when displaced from it, has been found to be a sensitive indicator of postnatal development in both felines and rodents.[23,24] In normal rats, there is an increased attraction to the nest over postnatal days 7–11, which is disrupted by both prenatal and postnatal malnutrition[25,26] and malnutrition present over many generations.[27,28] Prenatal cocaine also disrupts olfactory orientation to the home cage in rat pups,[29] especially in rats exposed to the drug treatment early in pregnancy during prenatal days 7–13. The aim of our study was to examine home orientation in rats exposed to prenatal cocaine and malnutrition.[19] Methods included transferring bedding from the nest region of the home cage into one corner of a clean test cage.[30] Fresh bedding was placed into the opposite corner of the test cage. On postnatal days 7, 9, and 11, a single pup from each litter was placed into the center of the cage and its path traced over a 3-minute test period. The latency to reach home bedding, the number of quadrants traversed during the 3-minute test, and the time spent in different parts of the test cage were measured. Because of the number of behaviors tested and the possibility that some of these were related to one another, the data were analyzed using factor analysis. This procedure groups related behavioral observations and thereby eliminates the possibility of random findings. Two main factors were derived, one describing the pup's attraction to the nest and the other referring to activity level.

Independent effects of prenatal malnutrition and cocaine exposure were present for each of the two factors. Prenatal malnutrition alone resulted in a reduced attraction to the nest bedding. Thus, prenatally malnourished pups showed increased latency to approach their nest bedding, reduced time spent on this bedding, and a decreased number of entries into the sector containing the home bedding on all days of testing. We also found that prenatal cocaine had a significant effect on factor scores derived from the activity factor, whereas malnutrition did not. Reduced activity levels associated with prenatal cocaine exposure were most pronounced on postnatal day 7, less striking on day 9, and completely absent by day 11. Thus, the effect of cocaine was transient. On the activity factor only, we found evidence of additive effects of the two insults. In the well-nourished group, the number of entries into the half of the cage containing fresh bedding (one of two behaviors contained in this factor grouping) was reduced from 4.8 ± 1.1 to 2.3 ± 0.6 in response to cocaine exposure. In the malnourished group, these values were reduced from 4.6 ± 1.1 to 1.3 ± 0.4 by cocaine. Thus, on day 7 only, the least active group of all four appeared to be the group exposed to both insults. In summary, the test showed an independent effect of prenatal malnutrition on the development of nest orientation and a transient effect of cocaine on activity, which was also sensitive to the combined insults.

Mother-Pup Interaction. Delays in the physical and behavioral development of pups exposed to malnutrition or cocaine may have contributed to changes observed in mother-pup interaction. Thus, pup characteristics play an important role in determining the social milieu of the suckling period. It has long been recognized that disruption of early litter environment of the developing rat pup may influence its long-term development independent of any direct effects of the insult on brain and behavior.[31,32] Recent animal studies have sought to document the effects of cocaine treatment during pregnancy or the suckling period on mother-pup interaction.[33,34] However, the majority of these studies have included mothers who themselves were exposed to cocaine with cocaine-exposed offspring. Only one investigation has been conducted using healthy foster mothers,[33] and this study concluded that there were no significant differences in home cage behavior on postnatal day 4, in pup retrieval on day 5, or maternal aggression towards an intruder female on postnatal day 10 between foster mothers rearing prenatally cocaine-exposed pups or control pups. However, as only selected time points were used in that study a difference in maternal behavior on other days may have been overlooked. The aim of our study was to record the profile of mother-pup interaction over the entire course of the suckling period from postnatal day 2 to day 21.[18] Daily observations were made of litters containing well-nourished, drug-free foster mothers and pups derived from each of the four treatment groups. Measures of active nursing, passive nursing, contact between mother and young, time spent in nest, and nest ratings were made.

Mother-infant interaction was affected by cocaine exposure and also the combination of cocaine and malnutrition. However, there were no significant effects of malnutrition alone. Dams showed a 50% increase in the percentage of time spent in contact with cocaine-exposed pups as compared with non-drug–exposed pups during the second postnatal week. In the case of passive nursing, we found a significant interaction between cocaine and malnutrition for the duration of the suckling period. Passive nursing refers to pup-initiated suckling in which the mother remained in a passive position, either lying on her side or engaged in other activities in the home cage. Finally, there was also a tendency for pups with both prenatal insults to be groomed less often by foster mothers than were pups from the three other groups, especially pups exposed only to prenatal malnutrition. Thus, foster mothers responded differently to pups with different prenatal insults and also appeared to be sensitive to animals with the double insult of both cocaine and malnutrition.

The increased contact between cocaine-exposed infants and their foster mothers is consistent with the larger number of developmental delays in the cocaine-exposed pups during the second week of life. These delays are likely to increase maternal responsiveness to her pups, as the suckling dam continues responding to them as she would to younger pups. Moreover, we found a greater delay in the appearance of reflexes throughout the postnatal period in the group exposed to both malnutrition and cocaine insults. These delays may explain the finding of a drug x diet interaction in the case of passive nursing, which was most increased in the combined insult group. Developmentally delayed pups may attach more vigorously as a compensatory response to improve the chances for additional milk, warmth, and other stimulation. In contrast to our previous report,[21] there was no increase in passive nursing among foster mothers rearing prenatally malnourished pups. However, pregnant dams in our earlier study did not experience daily saline injections, and the results of the two studies may have differed because of this procedure.

Development after Weaning and in Adulthood

Morris Maze Performance. The effects of prenatal cocaine exposure and protein malnutrition on the development of spatial navigation were assessed in rats at two stages of development: immediately following weaning (days 21–30) and again in adulthood (day 70). The Morris water maze[35,36] is a commonly used test of cognitive functioning in rodents, which has proven sensitive in revealing impaired performance following septo-hippocampal damage and following the administration of centrally acting drugs.[38] Animals are required to swim in a large tank of water to find a "hidden" escape platform located just below the surface at a fixed position relative to remote visual cues in the vicinity of the tank. The rats are placed into the tank at different start positions which requires them to learn to navigate to the platform by the flexible use of multiple cues. Prenatal cocaine was reported to produce a limited impact upon acquisition of this task in mature rats.[9] Differences were confined to the initial period of testing,[38,39] with gender playing an important role.[39,40] However, another study using this procedure failed to detect any significant effects of prenatal cocaine exposure on spatial learning performance.[9] The effect of prenatal cocaine during the earliest development of this behavior, at around postnatal day 25–27,[41,42] has not been examined. Thus, the aim of the present study was to examine the separate and combined effects of prenatal cocaine and protein malnutrition on the development of spatial navigation abilities.

On postnatal days 21, 25, and 30, rats were first tested for their ability to locate the submerged platform in the Morris water maze. Rats showed improved performance (i.e., shorter swim distances) over days of testing. By day 30, all rats had learned this task, but the best performance was found in the well-nourished control rats. A significant interaction between cocaine and malnutrition was found on this phase of the test. Prenatal cocaine (1,005 ± 23 cm) increased the total mean distance swum of well-nourished rats relative to saline controls (907 ± 37 cm). Prenatal malnutrition (1,011 ± 38 cm) was also associated with longer swim paths, similar to levels seen in the cocaine-exposed rats. However, rats exposed to both prenatal cocaine and malnutrition (944 ±34 cm) had values that were intermediate between 25% casein controls and the rats exposed to either insult alone. Neither prenatal insult affected the accuracy of spatial navigation at these ages, as determined by their search pattern when the platform was removed.

The Morris maze test was also administered to rats at day 70. Using the submerged platform, rats (males and females) with prenatal cocaine had impaired spatial performance on the first of 2 days of testing. This finding suggests a temporary delay in the acquisition of the spatial navigation task following prenatal cocaine administration. The absence of any effects of prenatal malnutrition at this age is similar to our findings in an earlier report.[42] As in the case of the younger animals, there were no differences in search pattern when the platform was removed at these later ages. These results suggest a long-term deficit from postweaning to adulthood on the spatial navigation test specifically associated with prenatal cocaine exposure. By adulthood, the deficit is less enduring. Malnutrition effects were limited to the earlier stage of development, and this finding is at variance with our earlier published report of no effects in the water maze.[42] However, as just noted, animals in the current series of studies received saline injections, which may have introduced stress not observed in our earlier studies.

Radial Arm Maze. We supplemented the Morris water maze test with an additional test of spatial orientation, the radial arm maze.[43] In contrast to the Morris water maze, an advantage of the radial arm maze is that individual components of memory (i.e., working and reference memory) can easily be examined.[44] This is accomplished by baiting only half of the arms in the maze. The test was originally used to study the effects of malnutrition. However, the results are not clear. Malnutrition imposed prenatally and continuing through suckling impaired the acquisition of spatial learning in adulthood in 8- and 16-arm maze configurations.[45] However, other studies with more stringent controls showed no effects in either 8- or 12-arm configurations.[46,47] The radial arm maze has been used to study the effects of cocaine. A significant impairment in task acquisition among prenatally cocaine-exposed females was found, whereas males were not significantly impaired.[41] In our study, a rigorous criterion was applied in an effort to reveal subtle differences in acquisition due to these prenatal insults. Male rats were tested at 130 days of age, using the 8-arm radial maze with four baited arms. They were required to collect all four food pellets within 5 minutes to complete a trial. Subjects were tested for one trial/day until they met the criterion for successful acquisition of the task. Criterion was attained when the rat collected three out of the four food pellets within its first four arm entries within a trial (while still completing the trial) with this level of performance being maintained for three consecutive trials.

The results showed a clear dissociation between the effects of prenatal malnutrition and those of prenatal cocaine. Prenatally malnourished rats required a greater number of trials to criterion, made more reference memory errors (but not working memory errors), and exhibited increased latency to complete a trial when compared to controls. The effects of prenatal malnutrition were present only when the rats were required to perform to this strict criterion, whereas there were no differences attaining the first two out of four entries. These deficits arose from errors in reference (long-term) memory, not working memory. Although these effects did not appear to be appetitively motivated, further studies are needed. It is known that previously malnourished rats are more motivated by a food reward, but comparable studies have not been performed in rats exposed to prenatal cocaine. In contrast to the striking effects of prenatal malnutrition, we found no deficits due to prenatal cocaine on any measure, and there were no additive effects with prenatal malnutrition. Of note, we used male rats only. Given the previous report of significant findings of cocaine in females, it will be necessary to repeat this study in females.

CONCLUSIONS

Our series of studies confirm the presence of significant effects of both prenatal malnutrition and cocaine during pregnancy and the early postnatal period. In the offspring, this presented as significant delays in skeletal maturation and the age of appearance of physical and reflexive milestones. Independent effects of cocaine and malnutrition were present, as shown specifically in the case of homing behavior. However, there were also many instances of additive effects when the rat pup was exposed to both insults in combination. For example, reflexive development showed a number of such effects of the two insults together.

Similarly, performance on tests of spatial orientation in adulthood were also impacted by prenatal cocaine and malnutrition. We found an interaction between cocaine and malnutrition on the acquisition of the Morris water maze task in the postweaning period when the rat normally develops the ability to learn this task. In adulthood, a transient deficit was attributable to cocaine exposure alone. Performance on the radial arm maze was altered by malnutrition alone, whereas cocaine had no effect on this test. However, additive effects were generally not observed at the later ages on the tasks. It is, however, possible that these may be present in other domains not tested in the present series of studies. Future studies will focus on social development and attention which have been selectively identified as long-term sequelae of malnutrition[48–50] and cocaine in human populations.

ACKNOWLEDGMENT

All procedures described in this paper were approved by the Institutional Animal Care and Use Committee (Boston University School of Medicine, Laboratory Animal Science Center; *Approval #92-003, #95-027*).

REFERENCES

1. AZUMA, S.D. & I.J. CHASNOFF. 1993. Outcome of children prenatally exposed to cocaine and other drugs: A path analysis of three-year data. Pediatrics **92:** 396–402.
2. CHURCH, M. W. *et al.* 1991. Effects of prenatal cocaine exposure. *In* Biochemistry and Physiology of Substance Abuse. R. R. Watson, Ed.: 179–204. CRC Press. Boca Raton, FL.
3. GRIFFITH, D.R., S.D. AZUMA & I.J. CHASNOFF. 1994. Three-year outcome of children exposed prenatally to drugs. J. Am. Acad. Child Adolesc. Psychiatry **33:** 20–27.
4. NEUSPIEL, D.R. & S.C. HAMEL. 1991. Cocaine and infant behavior. J. Dev. Behav. Pediatrics **12:** 55–64.
5. SPEAR, L.P. 1993. Missing pieces of the puzzle complicate conclusions about cocaine's neurobehavioral toxicity in clinical populations: Importance of animal models. Neurotoxicol. Teratol. **15:** 307–309.
6. CHURCH, M.W. & H.C. RAUCH. 1992. Prenatal cocaine exposure in the laboratory mouse: Effects on maternal water consumption and offspring outcome. Neurotoxicol. Teratol. **14:** 313–319.
7. DOW-EDWARDS, D. 1990. Fetal and maternal cocaine levels peak rapidly following intragastric administration in the rat. J. Subst. Abuse **2:** 427–437.
8. HUTCHINGS, D.E., T.A. FICO & D.L. DOW-EDWARDS. 1989. Prenatal cocaine: Maternal toxicity, fetal effects and locomotor activity in rat offspring. Neurotoxicol. Teratol. **11:** 65–69.
9. RILEY, E.P. & J.A. FOSS. 1991. Exploratory behavior and locomotor activity: A failure to find effects in animals prenatally exposed to cocaine. Neurotoxicol. Teratol. **13:** 553–558.
10. SPEAR, L.P., C.L. KIRSTEIN & N.A. FRAMBES. 1989. Cocaine effects on the developing central nervous system: Behavioral, psychopharmacological and neurochemical studies. Ann. N.Y. Acad. Sci. **562:** 290–307.
11. SANTOLARIA-FERNÁNDEZ, F.J., J.L. GÓMEZ-SIRVENT, C.E. GONZÁLEZ-REIMERS, J.N. BATISTA-LÓPEZ, J.A. JORGE-HERNÁNDEZ, F. RODRÍGUEZ-MORENO, A. MARTÍNEZ-RIERA & M.T. HERNÁNDEZ-GARCÍA. Nutritional assessment of drug addicts. Drug Alcohol Depend. **38:** 11–18.
12. BANE, A.J., J.G. MCCOY, B.S. STUMP & D.D. AVERY. 1993. The effects of cocaine on dietary self-selection in female rats. Physiol. Behav. **54:** 509–513.
13. GALLER, J.R., J.S. SHUMSKY & P.J. MORGANE. 1996. Malnutrition and brain development. *In* Chapter 14:196–212. Nutrition in Pediatrics: Basic Science and Clinical Application. 2nd Ed. J.B. Decker Europe, Inc. W.A. Walker & J.B. Watkins, Eds. Neuilly-sur-Seine; France.
14. MORGANE, P.J., J.D. BRONZINO, R.J. AUSTIN-LAFRANCE, J. TONKISS & J.R. GALLER. 1992. Malnutrition and the developing central nervous system. *In* The Vulnerable Brain and Environmental Risks, Vol. 1. Malnutrition and Hazard Assessment. R. Isaacson & K. Jensen, Eds. Chapter 1, 3–44. Plenum Press. New York.
15. MORGANE, P.J., R.J. AUSTIN-LAFRANCE, J.D. BRONZINO, J. TONKISS, S. DIAZ-CINTRA, L. CINTRA & J.R. GALLER. 1993. Prenatal malnutrition and development of the brain. Neurosci. Biobehav. Rev. **17:** 91–128.
16. TONKISS, J., J.R. GALLER, P.J. MORGANE, J.D. BRONZINO & R.J. AUSTIN-LAFRANCE. 1993. Prenatal protein malnutrition and postnatal brain function. Ann. N. Y. Acad. Sci. **678:** 215–227.
17. TONKISS, J., P.L. SHULTZ, J.S. SHUMSKY, S. BLEASE, T. KEMPER & J.R. GALLER. 1995. The

effects of cocaine exposure prior to and during pregnancy in rats fed low or adequate protein diets. Neurotoxicol. Teratol. **17:** 593–600.

18. TONKISS, J., J.S. SHUMSKY, P.L. SHULTZ, S.S. ALMEIDA & J.R. GALLER. 1995. Prenatal cocaine but not prenatal malnutrition affects foster mother-pup interactions in rats. Neurotoxicil. Teratol. **17:** 601–608.
19. TONKISS, J., R.H. HARRISON & J.R. GALLER. 1996. Differential effects of prenatal protein malnutrition and prenatal cocaine on a test of homing behavior in rat pups. Physiol. Behav. **60:** 1013–1018.
20. TONKISS, J., P.L. SHULTZ, J.S. SHUMSKY & J.R. GALLER. 1997. Development of spatial navigation following prenatal cocaine and malnutrition in rats: Lack of additive effects. Neurotoxicol. Teratol. **19:** 363–372.
21. GALLER, J. R. & J. TONKISS. 1991. Prenatal protein malnutrition and maternal behavior in Sprague-Dawley rats. J. Nutr. **121:** 762–769.
22. KANAREK, R.B., P.M. SCHOENFELD & P.J. MORGANE. 1986. Maternal malnutrition in the rat: Effects on food intake and body weight. Physiol. Behav. **38:** 509–515.
23. ROSENBLATT, J.S., G. TURKEWITZ & T.C. SCHNEIRLA. 1969. Development of home orientation in newly born kittens. Ann. N.Y. Acad. Sci. **31:** 231–250.
24. TURKEWITZ, G. 1966. The development of spatial orientation in relation to the effective perceptual environment in rats. Unpublished doctoral dissertation, New York University.
25. ALTMAN, J., K. SUDARSHAN, G.P. DAS, N. MCCORMICK & D. BARNES. 1971. The influence of nutrition on neural and behavioral development. III. Development of some motor, particularly locomotor patterns during infancy. Dev. Psychobiol. **4:** 97–114.
26. FLEISCHER, S.F. & G. TURKEWITZ. 1979. Effect of neonatal stunting on development of rats: Large litter rearing. Dev. Psychobiol. **12:** 137–149.
27. GALLER, J.R. 1979. Home orientation in nursling rats: The effects of rehabilitation following intergenerational malnutrition. Dev. Psychobiol. **12:** 499–508.
28. GALLER, J.R. 1980. Home-orienting behavior in rat pups surviving postnatal or intergenerational malnutrition. Dev. Psychobiol. **13:** 563–572.
29. VORHEES, C.V., T.M. REED, K.D. ACUFF-SMITH, M.A. SCHILLING, G.D. CAPPON, J.E. FISHER & C. PU. 1995. Long-term learning deficits and changes in unlearned behaviors following *in utero* exposure to multiple daily doses of cocaine during different periods and maternal plasma cocaine concentrations. Neurotoxicol. Teratol. **17:** 253–264.
30. GALLER, J.R., J. TONKISS & C.S. MALDONADO-IRIZARRY. 1994. Prenatal protein malnutrition and home orientation in the rat. Physiol. Behav. **55:** 993–996.
31. GALLER, J.R., H.N. RICCIUTI, M.A. CRAWFORD & L.T. KUCHARSKI. 1984. The role of the mother-infant interaction in nutritional disorders. *In* Nutrition and Behavior. J.R. Galler, ed.: 269–304. Plenum Press. New York. 1984.
32. LEVINE, S. & S. WIENER. 1976. A critical analysis of data on malnutrition and behavioral deficits. Adv. Pediatr. **22:** 113–136.
33. HEYSER, C.J., V.A. MOLINA & L.P. SPEAR. 1992. A fostering study of the effects of prenatal cocaine exposure: I. Maternal behaviors. Neurotoxicol. Teratol. **14:** 415–421.
34. JOHNS, J.M., L.R. NOONAN, I. ZIMMERMAN, L. LI & C.A. PEDERSEN. 1994. Effects of chronic and acute cocaine treatment on the onset of maternal behavior and aggression in Sprague-Dawley rats. Behav. Neurosci. **108:** 107–112.
35. MORRIS, R. G. M. 1981. Spatial localization does not require the presence of local cues. Learn. Motiv. **12:** 239–260.
36. MORRIS, R. G. M. 1984. Developments of a water-maze procedure for studying spatial learning in the rat. J. Neurosci. Methods **11:** 47–60.
37. BRANDEIS, R., Y. BRANDYS & S. YEHUDA. 1989. The use of the Morris water maze in the study of memory and learning. Int. J. Neurosci. **48:** 29–69.
38. SMITH, R. F., K. M. MATTRAN, M. F. KURKJIAN & S. L. KURTZ. 1989. Alterations in offspring behavior induced by chronic prenatal cocaine dosing. Neurotoxicol. Teratol. **11:** 35–38.
39. HEYSER, C. J., N. E. SPEAR & L. P. SPEAR. 1995. Effects of prenatal exposure to cocaine on Morris water maze performance in adult rats. Behav. Neurosci. **109:** 734–743.
40. LEVIN, E. D. & F. J. SEIDLER. 1993. Sex-related spatial learning differences after prenatal cocaine exposure in the young adult rat. Neurotoxicol. Teratol. **14:** 23–28.

41. TONKISS, J., P. SHULTZ & J. R. GALLER. 1992. Long-Evans and Sprague-Dawley rats differ in their spatial navigation performance during ontogeny and at maturity. Dev. Psychobiol. **25:** 567–579.
42. TONKISS, J., P. SHULTZ & J. R. GALLER. 1994. An analysis of spatial navigation in prenatally protein malnourished rats. Physiol. Behav. **55:** 217–224.
43. OLTON, D. S. & R. J. SAMUELSON. 1976. Remembrance of places passed: Spatial memory in rats. J. Exp. Psychol. **2:** 97–116.
44. OLTON, D. S. & B. C. PAPAS. 1979. Spatial memory and hippocampal function. Neuropsychologia **17:** 669–682.
45. JORDAN, T. C., S. E. CANE & K. F. HOWELLS. 1981. Deficits in spatial memory performance induced by early undernutrition. Dev. Psychobiol. **14:** 317–325.
46. HALL, R. D. 1983. Is hippocampal function in the adult rat impaired by early protein or protein-calorie deficiency? Dev. Psychobiol. **16:** 395–411.
47. WOLF, C., C. R. ALMLI, S. FINGER, S. RYAN & P. J. MORGANE. 1986. Behavioral effects of severe and moderate early malnutrition. Physiol. Behav. **38:** 725–730.
48. GALLER, J.R., F. RAMSEY, G. SOLIMANO & W.E. LOWELL. 1983. The influence of early malnutrition on subsequent behavioral development: II. Classroom behavior. J. Am. Acad. Child Psychiatry **22:** 16–22.
49. GALLER, J.R., F. RAMSEY, D.S. MORLEY & E. ARCHER. 1990. The long-term effects of early kwashiorkor compared with marasmus. IV. Performance on the national high school entrance examination. Pediatr. Res. **28:** 235–239.
50. RICHARDSON, G. A., M. L. CONROY & N. L. DAY. 1996. Prenatal cocaine exposure: Effects on the development of school-age children. Neurotoxicol. Teratol. **18:** 627–634.

Neonatal Neurobehavioral and Neuroanatomic Correlates of Prenatal Cocaine Exposure

Problems of Dose and Confounding

DEBORAH A. FRANK,[a] MARILYN AUGUSTYN, AND BARRY S. ZUCKERMAN

Child Development, Boston Medical Center; Department of Pediatrics, Boston University School of Medicine; Department of Public Health, Boston University of Public Health; Boston, Massachusetts 02118, USA

ABSTRACT: Complex methodologic challenges face researchers studying the effects of prenatal cocaine exposure on infant outcome. These include unavoidable imprecision in ascertaining the gestational timing and dose of cocaine to which the fetus was exposed and difficulties in identifying and quantifying the confounding, mediating, and moderating variables. Review of research on neonatal behavioral and cranial ultrasound findings following *in utero* cocaine exposure is used to illustrate these issues. We conclude that there are measurable but not dramatic dose-related effects of prenatal cocaine exposure on infant central nervous system structure and function. The effects of dose of prenatal cocaine exposure on later child development remain to be determined. Such research would be facilitated by a scientific consensus delineating relative doses of prenatal cocaine exposure.

INTRODUCTION

Many complex methodologic issues contribute to scientific uncertainty regarding the effects of prenatal cocaine exposure in free living human populations.[1,2] Unlike those using animal models, researchers with human samples still struggle to refine methods to ascertain accurately whether cocaine exposure occurred at all as well as to determine gestational timing of exposure and the acute and cumulative doses to which the fetus was exposed. In addition, identification and quantification of pharmacologic, biologic, and social variables that may confound, mediate, or moderate drug effects pose a formidable methodologic challenge. To illustrate how these two methodologic issues influence interpretation of human neonatal neurobehavioral outcome studies, we focus on findings of the Neonatal Behavioral Assessment Scales[3–13] and on neonatal cranial ultrasounds.[14–20] These outcomes have been measured in multiple studies for nearly a decade.

IDENTIFICATION OF COCAINE DOSE

Many different methods, all with intrinsic limitations, have been used in research projects to identify human prenatal cocaine exposure. The first is to ascertain substance exposure based on interviews conducted by clinicians and noted in medical records. Clinical ascertainment of the use of illicit substances in pregnancy has repeatedly been demonstrated as inadequate, consistently identifying less than half the users identified

[a] Address for correspondence: Deborah A. Frank, MD, FGH-3, 818 Harrison Avenue, Boston, MA 02118. Phone, 617/534–5251; fax, 617/534–7047; e-mail, dafrank@bu.edu

by other methods.[21,22] Under research conditions using trained interviewers with stringent assurances of confidentiality, more respondents will acknowledge cocaine use.[5,23] However, research has shown that without biologic markers, even the most skilled research interviewer will underidentify cocaine-exposed mother/infant dyads.[24]

The lack of standardization of potency and purity of illegal drugs further detracts from the usefulness of self-report. Even if a respondent is willing, within the limits of memory, to make every effort to provide an accurate account of her illicit substance use during pregnancy, the substance that she has used may vary from day to day, from place to place, and from year to year. By contrast, self-report of the use of legal psychoactive substances such as ounces of wine or beer or number of cigarettes permits more accurate calculations of the average volume of alcohol or nicotine to which child and mother were exposed, regardless of where or when the substance was used. No such standardization exists for purity or potency in lines of cocaine. Moreover, respondents may be completely unaware of potential contaminants that have been introduced into illegal drugs, contaminants that may have active toxic effects of their own.

Self-report, however, should never be omitted from research on prenatal cocaine exposure because it also offers some unique advantages. First, clinical interviewing by a skilled interviewer is more equitable than selective urine screening in clinical settings which may be based on provider expectation of drug use rather than actual drug use.[22,25] Secondly, maternal report is the only way to ascertain lifetime use before conception or use within the first trimester of pregnancy.[26] Self-report also identifies route of drug administration and whether the drug is used in a "binge" pattern.[26] Self-report can delineate patterns of simultaneous or sequential psychoactive substance use (e.g., cocaine and alcohol use), which also may have important physiologic implications.[29] Furthermore, self-report scales are low in cost, readily available, generally well standardized, and easily administered.

Supplementing interview data with biologic markers enhances ascertainment of newborns exposed to cocaine *in utero*.[21,22,24,25] Unfortunately, no biologic marker yet developed permits precise quantification of the dose of cocaine exposure throughout all trimesters of pregnancy. Until recently the most widely used biologic marker for cocaine exposure in clinical or research settings was assays of maternal or infant urine, either during pregnancy or at delivery.[28] The addition of urine assay does enhance ascertainment of infant effects in pregnancies exposed to cocaine. In fact, in a study conducted by our research group, if maternal urine assay had not been used, the cocaine effect on infant size at birth would not have been identified, because so many users would have been misclassified as nonusers.[24]

Despite its widespread application and demonstrated usefulness, urine assay for drug metabolites poses difficulties. Cocaine metabolites appear in maternal and infant urine for only 24–72 hours after the last dose; therefore, if a mother does not present to a research or clinical setting to provide urine samples relatively close to the time of drug use, such use may not be identified.[28] In addition, urine assays are not useful for identification of dose of drug exposure. The concentration of cocaine metabolites in urine varies with the hydration status of the subject.

The short window of identification and inability to use urine assay as an indicator of dose has led to many studies exploring other biologic tissues, including maternal and infant hair and infant meconium. A few studies have used assays of umbilical cord blood and amniotic fluid, but their collection requires sufficiently controlled conditions in the delivery room as to eliminate their usefulness in large epidemiologic studies.[29,30] The use of maternal or neonatal hair[31] to identify drug exposure, whether prenatal or otherwise, has been a matter of controversy. Whereas some researchers suggest that segmenting the maternal hair is a reliable way to identify exposure over time,[22] other investigators working with nonpregnant samples found that rates of appearance of radioactive labeled cocaine show wide individual variability.[32,33] In addition, hair assays may inadvertently create ethnic and age biases in research data, such that dose of exposure in underestimated in fair haired samples. Hair with high concentrations of melanin binds cocaine metabolites more readily than does blond or white hair.[34] Environmental contamination may be reflected in assays of adult hair, contamination that cannot be completely removed by washing techniques.[32] Cosmetic treatments of hair also alter drug concentration in that hair.[32,34] Therefore, the use of maternal hair for identifying the timing and amount of illicit cocaine exposure during pregnancy must be considered approximate at best.

Fetal hair is considered by some to be a more promising medium than maternal hair, because the issues of cosmetic interference and environmental contamination do not apply.[31] However, in many clinical settings mothers may be reluctant to consent to hair being cut from the head of their newborn.[22] Assaying newborn hair does not identify exposure before the second trimester when fetal hair begins to grow and does not have 100% congruence with other measures.[31,35] However, one study of dose effects of prenatal cocaine use correlated concentration of cocaine metabolites in fetal hair with fetal head growth.[35]

Meconium is currently a relatively widely used biologic marker for ascertaining prenatal cocaine exposure for research purposes.[21] Although some investigators have reported that drug metabolites can be excreted into meconium as early as 15 prenatal weeks,[36] others have been unable to show any accumulation in infants of known users until 3 weeks prior to delivery.[30] Meconium is still a controversial medium for measuring dose of cocaine exposure, because in clinical settings the cocaine concentration may be altered by admixture of infant urine which contains cocaine metabolites from recent maternal use.[37] Nevertheless, meconium has in several studies proved useful for a heuristic rank ordering of exposure.[12,13,38] Neither meconium assay nor other biologic markers currently available permit a precise determination of threshold and dose response or of gestational timing of exposure.

CONFOUNDING AND MODERATING VARIABLES

A second major area of difficulty in research on teratology of illegal drug use in the human population is the problem of confounding and moderating variables.[1] In animal studies, these issues are controlled by pair feeding and by standardizing rearing conditions between exposed and unexposed animals. However, in human samples, pregnant women who use cocaine tend to use multiple illicit substances as well as toxic but not illegal substances such as nicotine and alcohol.[1,24,39,40] As interest in dose has emerged, it has become clear that those who are heavy users of one substance are also likely to be heavy users of another.[13] Although cumulative adverse effects on birth weight have been described,[41] little is known about the antagonism or synergy of commonly used psychoactive substances during pregnancy in determining fetal outcome. For example, the teratologic effects of cocaethylene are not yet delineated in humans. Cocaethylene, which is synthesized by the liver with the simultaneous use of cocaine and alcohol, has been found in adults to have enhanced cardiotoxicity and longer duration of action than does cocaine used alone.[27,42]

In addition to pharmacologic confounding, researchers on human infants must deal with a large array of other potential biologic and social confounders. These include factors preceding conception such as maternal age, education, nutritional status, gravidity, and parity.[40] Other confounders during gestation include infectious disease (particularly sexually transmitted infections such as HIV and syphilis),[40] lead exposure,[41] malnutrition, and trauma.[40]

Besides biologic confounding and mediating variables, many psychosocial variables must be assessed repeatedly in evaluating the long-term outcome of cocaine-exposed children. These include parental comorbid psychiatric pathology, homelessness, and exposure to violence.[1] Moreover, the researcher in human populations must account for the possible effects of planned (but not usually randomly assigned) interventions both before delivery (prenatal care, drug treatment)[6] and after, such as home visiting developmental or educational intervention targeted to at-risk infants and children,[43] maternal drug treatment,[6] or placement of the child away from the mother.

NEONATAL BEHAVIOR AND CRANIAL ULTRASOUNDS

To illustrate how variability in measurement of dose and of confounding or mediating variables contributes to inconsistencies in studies evaluating whether prenatal cocaine exposure exerts independent negative neurobehavioral and neuroanatomic effects on human neonates, we focus on findings on neonatal behavioral assessment scales and neonatal cranial ultrasounds, which have been measured in multiple studies for nearly a decade.

As TABLE 1 shows, Brazelton's Neonatal Behavioral Assessment Scale[3] (NBAS) was performed in seven independent samples without regard to dose.[4,6–11] No consistent behavioral profile emerged in the immediate neonatal period. Two of these studies which assessed both newborn behavior and behavior at 2–4 weeks of life found no effects in the first 3 days of life, but detected effects later in the first month.[8,10] TABLE 2 summarizes three[5,12,13] studies using the NBAS to assess outcome after some estimation of dose of prenatal cocaine exposure. Each study uses a different method. For example, Delaney-Black *et al.*[12] perform continuous correlation with concentration of cocaine metabolites in meconium; Tronick *et al.*[13] ordinally rank exposure by a combination of meconium metabolites and the number of self-reported days of cocaine use; and Richardson *et al.*[5] by the use of one or more lines of cocaine a day during the first two trimesters of pregnancy. Again, although all of these studies attempt to address dose, no cocaine effect is found in all three studies, although state regulation is less optimal following *in utero* cocaine exposure in two samples out of three.[12,13] In addition, the Delaney-Black *et al.*[12] and Richardson *et al.*[5] studies do not follow up children beyond the first week of life, although the Richardson study showed washout of the negative effects found on Day 2 by Day 3.

The data on cranial ultrasound outcome after prenatal exposure to cocaine is even more difficult to interpret, because in many studies covariates are not controlled. In published studies correlating cocaine exposure with neonatal ultrasound lesions, only one controlled for *in utero* cigarette or marijuana exposure[16]; two controlled for *in utero* opiate exposure[16,18] and one for alcohol.[19] Thus, misattribution to cocaine of the effects of other psychoactive substances on ultrasound findings cannot be ruled out from published data.

Despite case reports of catastrophic central nervous system infarction and malformations following *in utero* cocaine exposure,[44,45] the findings in large controlled samples with comparison groups are much less striking, with three studies finding an increase in low grade intraventricular hemorrhage among cocaine-exposed children of various gestational ages,[14,18,19] whereas four did not[15–17,20] (TABLE 3). None of these studies controlled for maternal cigarette use; the other variables controlled varied from study to study. We recently reanalyzed a dataset in which no differences were found among 241 term infants in ultrasound lesions if they were categorized only as cocaine exposed or unexposed.[46] The increased risk for grade I intraventricular hemorrhage was found

TABLE 1. Cocaine Effects on Brazelton Neonatal Behavioral Assessment Score in Term Infants Not Exposed to Opiates

Study	Habituation	Orientation	Motor	State Range	State Regulation	Autonomic Regulation	Abnormal Reflexes
Chasnoff (1989) (*n* = 79)	0	+	+	0	+	0	+
Eisen (1991) (*n* = 52)	+	0	0	0	0	0	0
Neuspiel (1991) (*n* = 111)	0	0	+*	0	0	0	0
Coles (1992) (*n* = 107)	0	0	0	0	+*	+*	+*
Mayes (1993) (*n* = 86)	+	0	0	0	0	0	0
Scafidi (1996) (*n* = 60)	0	0	0	+	+	0	0
Phillips (1996) (*n* = 50)	0	0	0	+	+	0	0

[+] 1 to 3 days.
[+*] 2–4 weeks.

TABLE 2. Cocaine Dose Effects on Brazelton Neonatal Behavioral Assessment Scores

Study	Habituation	Orientation	Motor	State Range	State Regulation	Autonomic Regulation	Abnormal Reflexes
Tronick* (*n* = 251)	0	0	0	0	+	0	0
Richardson[+] (*n* = 165)	0	0	+	0	0	+	+
Delaney-Black (*n* = 52)	0	0	+	0	+	0	0

*At 3 weeks only.
[+]Present on day 2, not day 3.

TABLE 3. Findings on Neonatal Echosonography after *in Utero* Cocaine Exposure without Regard to Dose

	Dixon & Bejar (1989)	Heier *et al.* (1994)	Dusick *et al.* (1993)	Dogra *et al.* (1994)	Singer *et al.* (1994)	King *et al.* (1996)
Cocaine exposed (*n*)	50	43	41	40	86	39
% African American	50%	84%	100%	NR	93%	63%
Controls (*n*)	87 19 well	62	41	84	146	39
% African American	94% 0	76%	100%	NR	86%	77%
% Preterm	0	Median GA both groups, 31 weeks	100% <1,500 g	27%	100% <1,500 g	Median GA 39 weeks
Urine toxic screen	100% cases	58%	85%	100% cases	100% cases	100% cases and controls
Meconium cases	NR	No	No	No	30%	No
Controls	No	24%	No	100%	100%	No
Cigarettes %	NR	NR NR controls	78% cocaine	NR	NR	NR
Controlled analysis?	No	No	No	No	No	No
Alcohol %	NR	NR 6% controls	46% cocaine NR controls	47% cocaine	NR	NR
Controlled analysis?	No	No	No	Yes	No	No
Marijuana	NR	NR 0% controls	36% cocaine	No	NR	NR
Opiates	45%	NR	None	No	NR	NR
Grade I, II, IVHs	10% cases 3.4% sick Controls 5.4% Well cases	35% cases 31% controls	42% cases 20% controls	7.5% cases 0 controls	36% cases 35% controls	11% cases 11% controls
Other CNS findings increased in cocaine exposed	White matter cavities; white matter densities; acute infarction; subarachinoid hemorrhage; ventricular enlargement	Cortical infarction (17%); congenital CNS abnormality (12%)	None	Echolucencies in basal ganglia (25% vs 0)	Seizures (17% vs 5%)	Increase in cerebral blood flow day 1 to day 2
Notes	All cocaine exposed in normal nursery	All in NICU	All in NICU	All had prenatal care and AGA term with more lesions than preterm	17% cases used alcohol, opiates, marijuana	All in normal nursery

only among the most heavily cocaine exposed (top quartile by days of self-reported use or concentration of cocaine metabolites in meconium), in whom the odds of such a hemorrhage were 3.88 (95% CI 1.45, 10.35, two-tailed $p = 0.007$) compared to those of unexposed after covariate control (including cigarettes, alcohol, and marijuana).[47] The more lightly exposed did not differ from the unexposed. This lesion is clinically silent at birth and has unknown long-term implications for developmental outcomes.

When all these studies are reviewed together, the perinatal effects of prenatal cocaine exposure on human central nervous system structure and function, once confounding variables are considered, appear to be small but detectable. Unlike the narcotic abstinence syndrome, prenatal cocaine exposure is not associated with a clinically obvious, consistent neurobehavioral profile; however, subtle adverse effects on state regulation have been described in more than half the published studies, both those measuring dose effect[12,13] and those analyzing cocaine exposure as an all or none variable.[4,6,9,10] Structural alterations in the neonatal central nervous system are also inconsistent from sample to sample.[14–20]

CONCLUSIONS

The popular perception is that *any* prenatal exposure to cocaine is almost certainly associated with devastating effects on the neonate. However, these data suggest that most potentially detrimental effects (including neonatal size,[38] neonatal behavior,[12,13] and central nervous system lesions[47]) of prenatal cocaine exposure occur disproportionately among the heaviest users, a phenomenon also noted for alcohol and cigarette exposure.[23] This dose effect requires further replication, because it has only been explored in a few samples.

To enhance the field of investigation into *in utero* exposure to illicit drugs in general and cocaine in particular, a consensus must evolve in defining what is heavy use. Currently, it is not clear whether the heavy users in one population are comparable to the heavy users in another, given the geographic variability in potency and routes of administration and the different modes of ascertainment of dose of prenatal cocaine exposure. Moreover, some of the current interview criteria for quantifying heavy dose (using more than 2 days a week[23] or more than one line a day[5]) conflate frequency and quantity. In alcohol research, because of the standardization of alcohol content under government supervision, the problem of comparative dose has been addressed more systematically, although imprecision for the purpose of teratologic studies remains. There is consensus that more than five drinks on a single occasion constitute a "binge." The most familiar type of index of substance use has been used to quantify drinking behavior. One measure is the Quantity-Frequency index of Strauss and Bacon[48] which was modified by Mulford and Miller.[49] This tool used the average amount per drinking occasion as the measure of quantity, thus making no distinction between the person who achieves a certain average quantity by drinking extremely large amounts on some occasions and very small amounts on others and the one who achieves the same average quantity through drinking the same amount on each occasion. A second index, developed by Cahalan and Cisin,[50] is the Volume-Variability Index which attempts to compare massed versus spaced drinking which holds volume constant. The basic technique of this index entails a two step operation: (1) to classify each respondent according to his average daily volume and (2) to divide each of several daily-volume groups into subgroups according to how variable the person is in his/her intake from day to day. The latter scale can differentiate people who drink only medium amounts of alcoholic beverages in terms of total consumption, depending on whether they drink in a massed or spaced-out pattern.[50] There is as yet no comparable consensus in cocaine research.

In addition, the precision of dose quantification in humans for cocaine is not yet adequate for statements to be made regarding whether the pattern of the effect is continuous or whether there is an actual threshold beyond which effects occur. Great caution must be exercised in drawing health education and public policy conclusions from available information regarding dose. For instance, several studies define heavy users as those who use more than twice a week,[13,23] but this is a not a true threshold. One cannot be sure that less frequent use would not have detrimental effects. In addition, dose may vary throughout pregnancy; most investigators find that women's use decreases as the pregnancy progresses.[5] It is not yet known whether the primary determinant of adverse outcome is cumulative dose, which is only approximately reflected in meconium[21] or neonatal hair,[31] or maximum dose used on a single occasion, which usually occurs earlier in pregnancy and may not be reflected in available biologic markers.

Even if a standardized mode of quantifying prenatal cocaine exposure develops, the phenomenon of dose response is not always straightforward. Simple linear models (the more exposure, the worse the outcomes) may not be adequate to describe the actual relationships, which may be nonlinear or even paradoxical (some is worse than none or a lot).[53] Moreover, the possible explanations for such paradoxical effects vary and include biologic and social mechanisms. For example, a larger cocaine dose may produce greater placental vasoconstriction with less metabolite transferred to the fetus.[51] One could speculate that repeated use might upregulate enzymatic pathways of detoxification, decreasing effects with higher cumulative use.[52] There is also the question of a "healthy user" effect, with women with better overall health tolerating higher doses than women with other adverse health conditions which may place the fetus at risk.[53]

There are also potential social mediators of possible paradoxical dose effects, if women with better education or more economic resources obtain more doses of an illicit drug. This phenomenon has been described in Jamaica where compared to infants of nonusers, infants of heavy marijuana users had more optimal behavioral findings at 1 month of age.[54] In the United States, because heavier users and their infants may be more readily detected by clinicians, they may be given preferential access to compensatory services such maternal drug treatment or infant developmental intervention, leading to a more optimal long-term outcome than that of infants exposed to a lower dose who receive no compensatory care.[6,43,55]

Currently available human research suggests that after confound control, there is a cocaine dose effect on neonatal size at birth, with the more heavily exposed infants in any sample being smaller in all parameters than those less heavily exposed. Dose effects have also been detected on neonatal behavior and on cranial ultrasound findings, but these results must be considered tentative until replicated because they have only been reported in one or two samples. The effects of dose after the neonatal period have been explored in only two samples,[23,56] one of which found negative effects of higher dose exposure on infant information processing,[23] whereas the other found no effect on cognitive test scores at 4 years.[56] More information is needed on potential dose effects on long-term outcome such as cognitive test scores, attention, behavior, affect regulation, and physical growth after the first year of life. As these areas evolve, defining dose and documenting mediating and confounding biologic and social variables will continue to pose major challenges.

REFERENCES

1. Frank, D.A., K. Bresnahan & B. Zuckerman. 1993. Maternal cocaine use: Impact on child health and development. Advances in Pediatrics. **40:** 65–99. Mosby-Year Book, Inc. St. Louis, MO.

2. LESTER B.M., L. LAGASSE & S. BRUNNER. 1997. Data base of studies on prenatal cocaine exposure and child outcome. J. Drug Issues **27:** 487–499.
3. BRAZELTON, T.B. (Ed.) 1984. Neonatal Behavioral Assessment Scale. 2nd ed. Spastics International. London, England.
4. SCAFIDI, F.A., T.M. FIELD, A. WHEEDEN *et al.* 1996. Cocaine-exposed preterm neonates show behavioral hormonal differences. Pediatrics **97:** 851–855.
5. RICHARDSON, G.A., S.C. HAMEL, L. GOLDSCHMIDT & N.L. DAY. 1993. The effects of prenatal cocaine use on neonatal neurobehavioral status. Neurotoxicol. Teratol. **18:** 519–528.
6. CHASNOFF, L.J., D.R. GRIFFITH, S. MACGREGOR, K. DRIKES & K.A. BURNS. 1989. Temporal patterns of cocaine use in pregnancy. JAMA **261:** 1741–1744.
7. MAYES, L.C., R.H. GRANGER, M. FRANK, R. SCHOTTENFELD & M.H. BORNSTEIN. 1993. Neurohaviorial profiles of neonates exposed to cocaine prenatally. Pediatrics **9:** 778–783.
8. NEUSPIEL, D.R., S.C. HAMEL, E. HOCHBERG, J. GREEN & D. CAMPBELL. 1991. Maternal cocaine use and infant behavior. Neurotoxicol. Teratol. **13:** 229–233.
9. PHILLIPS, R.B., R. SHARMA, B.R. PREMACHANDRA, A.J. VAUGHN & M. REYES-LEE. 1996. Intrauterine exposure to cocaine effect on neurohehavior of neonates. Infant Behav. Dev. **19:** 71–81.
10. COLES, C.D., K.A. PLATZMAN, L. SMITH, M.A. JAMES & A. FALEK. 1992. Effects of cocaine and alcohol use in pregnancy on neonatal growth and neurobehavioral status. Neurotoxicol. Teratol. **14:** 23–33.
11. EISEN, L.N. T.M. FIELD, E.S. BANDSTRA, J. ROBERTS, C. MORROW, S.K. LARSON & B. STEELE. 1991. Perinatal cocaine effects on neonatal stress behavior and performance on the Brazelton scale. Pediatrics **88:** 477–480.
12. DELANEY-BLACK, V., C. COVINGTON, E. OSTREA, JR. *et al.* 1996. Prenatal cocaine and neonatal outcome: Evaluation of dose-response relationship. Pediatrics **98:** 735–740.
13. TRONICK, E.Z., D.A. FRANK, H. CABRAL, M. MIROCHNICK & B. ZUCKERMAN. 1996. Late dose-response effects of prenatal cocaine exposure on newborn neurobehavioral performance. Pediatrics **98:** 76–83.
14. SINGER, L.T., T.S. YAMASHITA, S. HAWKINS, D. CAIRNS, J. BALEY & R. KLIENMAN. 1994. Increased incidence of intraventricular hemorrhage and developmental delay in cocaine-exposed, very low birth weight infants. J. Pediatr. **124:** 765–771.
15. HEIER, L.A., C.R. CARPANZANO, J. MAST, P.W. BRILL, P. WINCHESTER & M.D.F. DECK. 1991. Maternal cocaine abuse: The spectrum of radiologic abnormalities in the neonatal CNS. AJR **157:** 1105–1110.
16. DUSICK, A.M., R.F. COVERT, M.D. SCHREIBER *et al.* 1993. Risk of intracranial hemorrhage and other adverse outcomes after cocaine exposure in a cohort of 323 very low birth weight infants. J. Pediatr. **122:** 438–445.
17. MCLENAN, D.A., O.A. AJAUI, R.J. RYDMAN & R.S. PILDES. 1994. Evaluation of the relationship between cocaine and intraventricular hemorhage. J. Natl. Med. Assoc. **86:** 281–287.
18. DIXON, S.D. & R. BEJAR. 1989. Echoencephalographic findings in neonates associated with maternal cocaine and methamphetamine use: Incidence and clinical correlates. J. Pediatr. **115:** 770–778.
19. DOGRA, V.S., J.M. SHYKEN, P.A. MENON, J. POBLETE, D. LEWIS & J.S. SMELTZER. 1994. Neurosonographic abnormalities associated with maternal history of cocaine use in neonates of appropriate size for their gestational age. Am. J. Neuroradiol. **15:** 697–702.
20. KING, T.A., J.M. PERLMAN, A.R. LAPTOOK, N. ROLLINS, G. JACKSON & B. LITTLE. 1995. Neurologic manifestations of in utero cocaine exposure in near-term and term infants. Pediatrics **96:** 259–264.
21. OSTREA, E.M., M.J. BRADY, S. GAUSE, A.L. RAYMUNDO & M. STEVENS. 1992. Drug screening of newborns by meconium analysis: A large-scale, prospective, epidemiologic study. J. Pediatr. **89:** 107–113.
22. KLINE J., S.K.C. NG, M. SCHITTINI, B. LEVIN & M. SUSSER. 1997. Cocaine use during pregnancy: Sensitive detection by hair assay. Am. J. Public Health **87:** 352–358.
23. JACOBSON, S.W., J.L. JACOBSON, R.J. SOKOL, S.S. MARITER & L.M. CHIODO. 1996. New evidence for neurobehavioral effects of in utero cocaine exposure. J. Pediatr. **129:** 581–590.

24. Zuckerman, B., D.A. Frank, R. Hingson *et al.* 1989. Effects of maternal marijuana and cocaine use on fetal growth. N. Engl. J. Med. **320:** 763–768.
25. Chasnoff, I.J., H. Landress & M. Barett. 1990. The prevalence of illicit drug or alcohol use during pregnancy and discrepancies in mandatory reporting in Pinellas County, Florida. N. Engl. J. Med. **322:** 120–126.
26. McLellan, A.T., H. Kushner, D. Metzger *et al.* 1992. The fifth edition of the addiction severity index. J. Subst. Abuse Treat. **9:** 199–213.
27. Perez-Reyes, M. 1994. The order of drug administration: Its effects on the interaction between cocaine and ethananol. Life Sci. **55:** 541–550.
28. Osterloh, J.D. & B.L. Lee. 1989. Drug screening in mothers and newborns. Am. J. Dis. Child. **143:** 791–793.
29. Winecker, R.E., B.A. Goldberger, I. Tebbett, M. Behnke, F. D. Eyler, M. Conlon, K. Wobie, J. Karlix & R.L. Bertholf. 1997. Detection of cocaine and its metabolites in amniotic fluid and umbilical cord tissue. J. Analyt. Toxicol. **21:** 97–104.
30. Casanova, O.Q., N. Lombardero, M. Behnke, F.D. Eyler, M. Conlon & R.L. Bertholf. 1994. Detection of cocaine exposure in the neonate. Analyses of urine, meconium, and amniotic fluid from mothers and infants exposed to cocaine. Arch. Pathol. Lab. Med. **118:** 988–993.
31. Koren, G. 1995. Measurement of drugs in neonatal hair; a window to fetal exposure. Forensic Sci. Int. **70:** 77–82.
32. Welch, M. J., L.T. Sniegoski, C.C. Allgood & M. Habram. 1993. Hair analysis for drugs of abuse: Evaluation of analytical methods, environmental issues, and development of reference materials. J. Analyt. Toxicol. **17:** 389–398.
33. Henderson, G.L., M.R. Harkey, C. Zhou, R.T. Jones & P. Jacob. 1996. Incorporation of isotopically labeled cocaine and metabolites in human hair. 1. Dose-response relationships. J. Analyt. Toxicol. **20:** 1–12.
34. Reid, R.W., F.L. O'Connor & J.W. Crayton. 1994. The in vitro differential binding of benzoylecgonine to pigmented human hair samples. J. Toxicol. Clin. Toxicol. **32:** 405–410.
35. Sallee, F.R., L.P. Katikaneni, P.D. McArthur, H.M. Ibrahim, L. Nesbitt & G. Sethuraman. 1995. Head growth in cocaine-exposed infants: Relationship to neonate hair level. J. Dev. Behav. Pediatr. **16:** 77–81.
36. Ostrea, E.M., A. Romero, K. Knapp, A.R. Ostrea, J.E. Lucena & R.B. Utarnachitt. 1994. Postmortem drug analysis of meconium in early gestation human fetuses exposed to cocaine: Clinical implications. J. Pediatr. **124:** 477–479.
37. Rosengren, S.S., D. B. Longobucco, B. A. Bernstein, S. Fishman, E. Cooke, F. Boctor & S.C. Lewis. 1993. Meconium testing for cocaine metabolite: Prevalence, perceptions, and pitfalls. Am. J. Obstet. Gynecol. **168:** 1449–1456.
38. Mirochnick, M., D.A. Frank, H. Cabral, A. Turner & B. Zuckerman. 1995. Relation between meconium concentration of the cocaine metabolite benzolecgonine and fetal growth. J. Pediatr. **126:** 636–638.
39. Hurt, H., N. Brodsky, L. Braitman & J. Giannetta. 1995. Natal status of infants of cocaine users and control subjects: A prospective comparison. J. Perinatol. **15:** 297–304.
40. Frank, D.A., B. Zuckerman, H. Amaro *et al.* 1988. Cocaine use during pregnancy: Prevalence and correlates. Pediatrics **82:** 888–895.
41. Neuspiel, D.R., M. Markowitz & E. Drucker. 1994. Intrauterine cocaine, lead, and nicotine exposure and fetal growth. Am. J. Public Health **84:** 1492–1495.
42. McCance, E.F., L.H. Price, T.R. Kosten & P.I. Jatlow. 1995. Cocaethylene: Pharmacology, physiology, and behavioral effects in humans. J. Pharmacol. Exp. Ther. **274:** 215–223.
43. Hofkosh, D., J.L. Pringle, H.L. Wald, J. Swital, S.A. Hinderliter & S.C. Hamel. 1995. Early interactions between drug involved mothers and infants. Arch. Pediatr. Adolesc. Med. **149:** 665–672.
44. Chansnoff, I.F., M.E. Bussey, R. Savich *et al.* 1987. Perinatal cerebral infarction and maternal cocaine use. J. Pediatr. **111:** 571–578.
45. Dominquez, R., A.A. Vila-Coro, J.M. Slopis *et al.* 1991. Brain and ocular abnormalities in infants with in utero exposure to cocaine and other street drugs. Am. J. Dis. Child. **145:** 688–695.
46. Frank, D.A., K. McCarten, H. Cabral, S. M. Levenson & B. Zuckerman. 1992. Cra-

nial ultrasound in term newborns: Failure to replicate excess abnormalities in cocaine exposed (abstr.). Pediatr. Res. **31:** 247A.

47. FRANK, D.A., K. MCCARTEN, H. CABRAL, S.M. LEVENSON & B. ZUCKERMAN. 1994. Association of heavy in utero cocaine exposure with caudate hemorrhage in term newborns (abstr.). Pediatr. Res. **35:** 269A.
48. STRAUSS, R. & S. BACON. 1953. Drinking in College. Yale University Press. New Haven, CT.
49. MULFORD, H. & D. MILLER. 1960. Drinking in Iowa. II. The extent of drinking and selected sociocultural categories. Q. J. Stud. Alcohol **21:** 26–39.
50. CAHALAN, D. & H. CISIN. 1967. American drinking practices: Summary of findings from a national probability sample. Q. J. Stud. Alcohol **28:** 642–656.
51. POTTER, S., J. KLEIN, G. VALIANTE, D.M. STACK, A. PAPAGEORGIOU, W. STOTT, D. LEWIS, G. KOREN & P.R. ZELAZO. 1994. Maternal cocaine use without evidence of fetal exposure. J. Pediatr. **125:** 652–654.
52. SIMONE, C., L. O. DEREWLANY, M. OSKAMP, B. KNIE & G. KOREN. 1994. Transfer of cocaine and benzoylecgonine across the perfused human placental cotyledon. Am. J. Obstet. Gynec. **170:** 1404–1410.
53. DECOUFLE, P. & C. BOYLE. 1997. Dose response analyses of women's alcohol use during pregnancy and children's cognitive functioning. Am. J. Public Health **87:** 299.
54. DREHER, M.C., K. NUGENT & R. HUDGINS. 1994. Prenatal marijuana exposure and neonatal outcomes in Jamaica: An ethnographic study. Pediatrics **93:** 254–260.
55. OLDS, D.L., C.R. HENDERSON & R. TATELBAUM. 1994. Prevention of intellectual impairment in children of women who smoked during pregnancy. Pediatrics **93:** 228–233.
56. HURT, H., E. MALMUD, L. BETANCOURT, L.E. BRAITMAN, N. BRODSKY & J. GIANNETTA. 1997. Children with in utero cocaine exposure do no differ from control subjects on intelligence testing. Arch. Pediatr. Adolesc. Med. **151:** 1237–1241.

Selective Direct Toxicity of Cocaine on Fetal Mouse Neurons

Teratogenic Implications of Neurite and Apoptotic Neuronal Loss

MARIE-CÉCILE NASSOGNE,[a,b,c] PHILIPPE EVRARD,[b] AND PIERRE J. COURTOY[a]

[a]*Cell Biology Unit, Christian de Duve Institute of Cellular Pathology, 75, avenue Hippocrate, B-1200 Brussels, Belgium*

[b]*Service de Neurologie Pédiatrique, Saint Luc Hospital, University of Louvain Medical School, B-1200 Brussels, Belgium*

ABSTRACT: This chapter reviews epidemiologic clinical surveys and experimental animal studies, indicating that cocaine may induce severe teratogenic effects on the developing brain. Evidence for direct toxic effects is next presented. Using cocultures of embryonic brain cells, we demonstrate that cocaine selectively affects neuronal cells, first causing a dramatic reduction in the number and length of neurites, then extensive neuronal death by apoptosis. By contrast, cocaine affected neither the abundance of astroglial cells nor their glial fibrillary acidic protein content. These effects are not due to cocaine metabolites. The contributions of indirect and direct effects that could account for cocaine neuroteratogenicity are finally discussed.

CLINICAL EVIDENCE OF TERATOGENIC EFFECTS OF COCAINE ON THE DEVELOPING BRAIN

Estimation of the Prevalence of Cocaine Exposure in Utero

In various US studies, the prevalence of maternal cocaine use, based on urine tests and/or history reports, ranges from 0.3–19.7% in the general population,[1–7] but approaches 62% in women with no prenatal care. Few data are available on cocaine prevalence in Europe.[5] The high variability in reports of prevalence underlines the difficulties of obtaining reliable information about drug use during pregnancy. Altogether, the prevalence of cocaine abuse of 1% in the total US population appears to be a conservative estimate.

Newborn Outcome upon Cocaine Exposure in Utero

Low Birth Weight and Intrauterine Growth Retardation

About 25 reports have shown that cocaine use during pregnancy is associated with lower infant weight for gestational age. In all but one study with a sample size of over

[c] Address for correspondence: M. C. Nassogne, Cell Biology Unit, University of Louvain Medical School & Christian de Duve Institute of Cellular Pathology, Avenue Hippocrate 75, 1200 Brussels, Belgium. Phone, 32 2 764 75 41; fax, 32 2 764 75 43; e-mail, Nassogne@cell.ucl.ac.be

100 cases, there was a positive correlation between maternal cocaine use during pregnancy and a lower infant birth weight (for a review, see ref. 8). Whereas unadjusted analyses found significant deficits in mean birth weight ranging from 265–610 g, multivariate analyses that take into account gestational age and other variables, such as maternal age, parity, alcohol and tobacco use, multiple drug use, hypertension, and prenatal care, estimate the deficit attributable to cocaine at between 80 and 380 g.[9]

A poor pregnancy nutritional status, as assessed by a lower prepregnancy weight or a lower body mass index and/or decreased maternal nutrient intake due to the anorexigenic effects of cocaine, may play a role in the fetal growth retardation found in the babies of cocaine users.[9,10] Fetal growth retardation due to prenatal cocaine exposure may also be due to chronic fetal hypoxia and impaired maternal delivery of nutrients secondary to vasoconstriction of uterine vessels. Moreover, activation of the sympathetic nervous system in the fetus by cocaine should increase basal metabolism and deplete nutrient stores, accounting for fetal malnutrition in excess over that predicted from maternal malnutrition. Indeed, cocaine-exposed infants often show lower fat stores. A study reported that the pattern of growth retardation is symmetric, implying that the cocaine effect operates for a prolonged time during gestation and/or starts early in gestation or suggesting a direct effect on brain development.[11] The symmetric pattern of intrauterine growth retardation was associated with a worse prognosis for postnatal growth and neurobehavioral function than either asymmetric intrauterine growth retardation or normal intrauterine growth.

Brain Disturbances

The first clinical evidence of cocaine effects on the developing brain is the presence of microcephaly in children exposed *in utero* to cocaine. Impairment of intrauterine brain growth, manifested as microcephaly, is the most common brain abnormality in infants born to cocaine-abusing mothers.[12] When confounding variables such as maternal undernutrition, intrauterine infection, the use of other illicit drugs, or smoking during pregnancy are controlled, the incidence of microcephaly after prenatal cocaine exposure persists. The effects of cocaine on the fetal brain may be related to either destructive lesions or perturbations of the development of the fetal brain (teratogenic effects).

Destructive Brain Defects

Exposure of the fetus to cocaine may lead to serious destructive effects in the brain, principally due to ischemic or hemorrhagic mechanisms. Cerebral infarction in the distribution of major brain vessels, usually the middle cerebral artery, has been identified in numerous infants exposed prenatally to cocaine.[13–16] According to clinical and radiographic measures, the time of the infarction varied from hours to months before delivery. Some infants had a well-established porencephaly,[17] compatible with an event occurring weeks or months earlier, whereas others had cerebral edema indicative of a recent event.[13] A similar prenatal origin was apparent in an infant with hydrocephalus related to the destruction of the cerebral hemispheres in the distribution of the middle and anterior cerebral arteries, during a pregnancy under marked cocaine exposure.[18] Data obtained from cranial ultrasonography in the first days of life reveal that 22–35% of cocaine-exposed neonates had abnormalities (echolucent "cavities" or acute infarction) compatible with acute or old infarctions.[19] Regarding the genesis of the ischemic lesions, vasospasm may be crucial, as in the genesis of ischemic cerebrovascular phenomena in cocaine-exposed adults.

Hemorrhagic lesions have also been described in the subarachnoid, subependymal, or intraventricular space.[14,20–23] Fetal hypoxemia caused by disturbances of placental blood flow likely results in impaired fetal cerebral autoregulation, making the fetus particularly vulnerable to changes in arterial blood pressure. The abrupt increase in blood pressure in hypoxic brains, caused by catecholamines transferred across the placenta or produced in the fetus after transplacental transfer of cocaine, may lead to rupture of immature arteries. Intracranial hemorrhage can also occur in the immediate neonatal period, as elevation in blood pressure and increase in blood flow have been documented in the first days of life in infants who had been exposed to cocaine *in utero.*

Teratogenic Brain Effects

The potential teratogenic effects of cocaine should be considered in the context of the major events in brain development and their timing as well as of the clinical abnormalities reported after intrauterine exposure to cocaine. Disturbances in midline prosencephalic development including agenesis of the corpus callosum, absence of the septum pellicidum, and septo-optic dysplasia have been described.[17] Neuronal migration is also impaired by prenatal cocaine exposure in humans, resulting in schizencephaly, neuronal heterotopias, and pachygyria.[15,17,24] Disturbances of neuronal differentiation were demonstrated by immunochemical and histologic findings in the cerebral cortex of three infants exposed to cocaine *in utero.*[25]

Postnatal Signs of Intrauterine Cocaine Exposure

Neonatal Neurological and Neurophysiological Features

Infants exposed to cocaine *in utero* frequently exhibit abnormal neurobehavioral signs in the neonatal period, usually including the motor and regulation of NBAS state clusters.[27] During sleep-wake behavior observations, they show difficulties in maintaining alert states and in self-regulating their behavior. They also have decreased periods of quiet sleep and increased levels of agitated behavior, including tremulousness, mouthing, multiple limb movements, and clenched fists.[23] Several studies also documented dose-response effects of *in utero* cocaine exposure on the neurobehavioral score of human infants.[26,27]

Long-Term Neurological and Cognitive Outcomes

There are few published controlled longitudinal studies on the long-term development of children exposed prenatally to cocaine. Chasnoff and colleagues studied three groups of infants from birth to 2 years of age[28] and then to 3 years of age.[29] The first group was exposed to cocaine as well as alcohol, marijuana, phencyclidine, or amphetamines; the second to marijuana and alcohol but not to cocaine; and the third group consisted of children not exposed to cocaine, alcohol, or marijuana during pregnancy. Both cocaine-exposed and alcohol/marijuana-exposed groups demonstrated catch-up in weight from growth deficits during the early months of life to normal overall growth at 18 months. However, at all ages studied, the first two groups had significantly lower mean head circumferences than did unexposed infants and did not differ from one another.

This lack of catch-up in head size growth provides a strong indicator of potential problems, as it is well known that subnormal head size or microcephaly is predictive of poor subsequent performance. Whereas no significant differences were noted in global measures of intellectual development among the two drug groups and the control group, the cocaine/polydrug group received significantly lower scores on verbal reasoning tasks while the noncocaine/polydrug group scored lower on abstract/visual reasoning. Other investigators found lower scores in cocaine-exposed infants, using the Bayley Mental Scale at 6 and 12 months of age[30] and the Fagan Test of Infant Intelligence at 18 and 24 months of age,[31] as well as poor motor performance.[32] Long-term educational defects observable in school-age children that are attributable to prenatal cocaine exposure include attention deficits, language delays, difficulties with affect regulation, and poor social skills. These children also display high susceptibility to the environment including irritability, agitation, and aggression.[33]

Clearly, evaluation of the long-term consequences of prenatal cocaine is difficult. Multiple confounding prenatal variables (use of other illicit drugs, smoking, alcohol, prematurity, etc.) may be additive to, if not potentiate, the specific effects of cocaine. Postnatal outcome is likewise, worsened by combined environmental problems such as low socioeconomic status, continued maternal cocaine use, maternal psychological characteristics, or poor mother-infant interactions.[34,35] For instance, "cocaine babies" are at a substantially higher risk for both maltreatment and changes in the primary caretaker during the first 24 months of life.[36]

EXPERIMENTAL EVIDENCE OF NEUROTERATOGENIC EFFECTS OF COCAINE IN ANIMAL MODELS

Contribution of Animal Models

While providing useful information about the potentially adverse effects of prenatal cocaine exposure, human studies have several shortcomings. For instance, data were generally collected from small and probably biased populations and were often obscured by such confounding variables as maternal age and undernutrition, varying concentrations and availability of cocaine, multiple drug use, poor pre- and postnatal care, and the presence of toxic adulterants mixed with or used to process cocaine (e.g., amphetamines, procaine, talc, solvents, heroin, and phenylcyclidine). Animal studies make it possible to control for many of these confounding variables. Moreover, fine alterations in brain observed in infants who had been exposed to cocaine *in utero* have been reproduced in primates and mice.

Vascular Changes

Several early studies demonstrated that acute maternal cocaine exposure in conscious pregnant sheep produces several maternal and fetal vascular effects, including decreased uterine blood flow, maternal and fetal hypertension, fetal hypoxemia, and vasoconstriction of fetal cerebral arteries inducing decreased cerebral blood flow.[37–40] Autoradiographic patterns confirmed decreased local cerebral glucose utilization typical of ischemia in conscious fetal sheep after ewes were injected with cocaine.[41] However, these conclusions were recently challenged by two recent reports concluding that acute cocaine administration in early-gestation fetal sheep does not produce fetal hypoxemia or impede blood flow and oxygen delivery to the brain and heart.[42]

Neuroanatomic Lesions and Altered Gene Expression

Studies in primates[43] and rodents[12,44–47] clearly demonstrate the potential for cocaine to disturb the structural integrity of the developing cerebral cortex. In rhesus monkeys, chronic intermittent prenatal exposure to cocaine produces highly abnormal tissular characteristics in cerebral cortices, particularly distortion of laminar architecture with a significant increase in the number of cells in the underlying white matter. (^{3}H)Thymidine labeling further demonstrates that many cortical cells do not reach their proper destination and glial fibrillary acid protein (GFAP) labeling reveals a decreased density of cortical glial elements.[43]

Mice embryos exposed *ex vivo* to cocaine at the 7-somite stage display a prosencephalon deprived of almost all glial cytological features during the entire culture period, although the other developmental parameters evolve normally.[44] Prenatal cocaine exposure of mice *in vivo* induces a decrease in glial fascicle density, a delay in gliogenesis, and a disorganization of the axonal-dendritic bundles as well as the horizontal lamination of the neuropil.[12,44,45]

In rats, prenatal cocaine exposure also inhibits DNA synthesis throughout the developing brain during the period of rapid cell replication,[48] and delays normal astroglial maturation and the development as well as the outgrowth of neurons.[46,47] During rat brain development, cocaine produced brain region-specific and developmental age-specific induction of *c-fos, c-jun,* and zif/268 mRNAs. At each age, acute cocaine administration resulted in a cell-specific pattern of *c-fos* mRNA induction and *c-fos* expression in the striatum, with activation of related proteins to DNA binding sites, called AP-1. At each age examined, substance P-positive striatal neurons were the predominant class of cells in which cocaine induced *c-fos* gene expression.[49,50] Activation by cocaine of immediate early genes in the developing brain by cocaine could alter programs of neural gene expression and, thereby, neuronal phenotype and function.

Effects on Neurotransmitters

Cocaine is known to inhibit the uptake of monoamine neurotransmitters by presynaptic nerve terminals and thus to increase synaptic concentrations of norepinephrine, serotonin, and dopamine. Because cocaine easily gains access to the fetal brain, alterations of monoaminergic neurotransmitters therein may, in turn, perturb several neurodevelopmental aspects, including cell division,[51] astrocyte formation,[52] and migration of cortical neurons. Many reports highlighted the effects of prenatal cocaine on the different neurotransmitters. Prenatal cocaine exposure decreased spontaneous activity in dopaminergic cells in the substantia nigra pars compacta and the ventral tegmental area of adult rat offsprings[53] and was associated with a 50% diminution of basal dopamine release. Cocaine exposure during early gestation in rabbits reduced striatal dopamine and its metabolite DOPAC (3,4-dihydroxyphenylacetic acid) in the newborn.[54] Intermittent cocaine treatment in pregnant monkeys reduced tyrosine hydroxylase mRNA in 60-day-old fetal macaques.[55] Taken together, these data are consistent with a deleterious effect of prenatal cocaine exposure on the development and maturation of the dopamine system.

With the use of a rabbit model of prenatal cocaine exposure (2–4 mg/kg, iv, twice daily, E_8-E_{21}), defined disturbances on neurotransmitters could be demonstrated.[56,57] In the mature central nervous system of rabbits exposed prenatally to cocaine, dendrites of pyramidal neurons in layers III and V were 30–50% longer in the anterior cingulate cortex, a target region of dense input of dopaminergic neurons (DA). In the same region, an increased number of GABA-immunoreactive neurons was visible and was accompanied by a dramatic downregulation of $GABA_A$ receptors, as evidenced by a reduction in mRNA coding the α_1 and β_2 subunits of these receptors. The predicted functional consequences of these anatomical changes would include impaired attentional mechanisms.

Biochemical Abnormalities

Chronic exposure of rats to cocaine during pregnancy results in elevated levels of both neutral glycosphingolipids and gangliosides in brain at postnatal day 1. However, by postnatal day 11, these two compounds return to control levels.[58] Neuronal migration and differentiation in the developing central nervous system involve delicately timed sequences of molecular signals. Membrane glycoconjugates are known to act as recognition signals in many cellular systems. Abnormal increases in neutral glycosphingolipid and ganglioside content at an improper developmental stage may shift the timed appearance of a necessary signal, with subsequent deleterious effects on the formation of neuronal connections.

Cocaine exposure of the fetal guinea pig results in significant alterations in brain Na+, K+-ATPase activity, consistent with a change in cell membrane function, without affecting brain cell membrane structure.[59] This observation suggests that the mechanism by which cocaine affects the fetal brain is independent of its action as a vasoconstrictor or of hypoxic injury.

DIRECT COCAINE EFFECTS ON EMBRYONIC NEURONAL CELLS

Rationale and Experimental Strategy

All the alterations reported so far could be due to either vascular or hypoxic effects, indirect local effects due to the accumulation of neurotransmitters, or direct toxic effects of cocaine itself or of its metabolites generated elsewhere in the body. Inhibition of macromolecular syntheses, especially of thymidine and uridine incorporation, has been reported in cultured glioblastoma cells and neocortical glial cells exposed to cocaine.[60] In serum-free medium, differentiation of neuroblastoma cells by NGF and proliferation stimulated by IGF-I are both impaired by cocaine.[61] In cultured embryonic GABAergic-neurons, cocaine induced a drastic decrease in the number of neurons and the degeneration of their processes.[62]

To test whether cocaine may itself cause direct toxic effects on brain cells independently of excitotoxicity, we used the embryonic mouse coculture system of neuronal and glial cells[63] that maintains communication between these two major populations of cerebral cells and we tested for toxicity of cocaine concentrations that can be reached in the fetal brain upon severe maternal abuse. The system of cultured cells not only bypasses possible vascular and hypoxic effects, but also eliminates the most important presynaptic sites of cocaine action, namely, the reuptake of neurotransmitters as well as the metabolic and degradative pathways of cocaine present in systemic and brain parenchymal compartments.

Neurons and glial cells were obtained from brain hemispheres of 15-day-old mouse embryos and were cocultured for up to 6 days with Minimum Essential Medium supplemented by heat-inactivated fetal calf serum. After 2 days and daily thereafter, freshly dissolved cocaine was added to the culture at various concentrations, and medium was renewed daily. Once such cultures were established (after 2 days), neurons laid and extended neurites on a flat layer of glial cells.

Direct and Selective Toxicity of Cocaine on Embryonic Neurons

The effects of cocaine were first examined by immunofluorescence. After 6 days of coculture, control preparations showed neurons with extensive neurites and prominent MAP2 labeling, well spread over a flat layer of glial cell, labeled for GFAP (FIG. 1A). After 4 days of exposure to 100 μM cocaine, neurites became scanty and less branches (FIG. 1B). At 250 μM, the number of neurites per cell had largely decreased, producing an aspect of bi- and unipolar cells (FIG. 1C). At 500 μM, neurites had almost completely vanished and very few scattered MAP2-labeled round cell bodies persisted (FIGS. 1D and 2). By contrast, the number of glial cells remained unchanged in control and treated cultures; however, the drug caused some cell flattening and a discrete alteration in their fibrillar structure (FIG. 1F-G). When cells were exposed to cocaine for only 2 days and further cultured in cocaine-free medium for 2 additional days, the remaining cells could reextend neurites, although a definitive loss of cells was evident (FIG. 1E). Quantitative immunoassays confirmed the morphological findings (FIG. 3).

Thus, in embryonic cerebral cocultures, cocaine induces major neurite perturbations followed by neuronal death without affecting the survival of glial cells.[64] We therefore undertook to investigate the mechanism whereby cocaine causes neuronal disappearance, using neuron-enriched preparations.[65]

Cocaine Induces Neuronal Apoptosis

In sectioned pellets of such preparations, control cultures almost exclusively displayed cells with large nuclei containing well-developed nucleoli and dispersed euchromatin. By contrast, upon exposure to cocaine, a large fraction of nuclei appeared on the light microscope as denser and smaller or fragmented. By transmission electron microscopy, cocaine-treated cells exhibited nuclei with remarkably condensed and marginated chromatin and no visible nucleoli, whereas mitochondrial morphology remained essentially normal. Such alterations, indicative of apoptosis, were observed after 2 days in the presence of cocaine and became most prominent after 4 days of exposure.

The effect of cocaine on the integrity of genomic DNA was next examined by agarose electrophoresis (FIG. 4). The characteristic formation of oligonucleosome-sized fragments of multiples of 180–200 bp, producing typical DNA "ladders" that are the biochemical hallmark of apoptosis, were detected after 60 hours of culture in the presence of cocaine and persisted thereafter for 48 hours, indicating that cocaine-exposed neurons undergo asynchronous apoptosis. By contrast, the bulk of chromosomal DNA from control cultures remained of high molecular throughout culture. As an independent confirmation of apoptosis, multiple fragmentation of nuclear DNA was detected cytochemically in neurons by specific *in situ* labeling of DNA breaks (FIG. 5, TUNEL method).

To investigate whether the death of cocaine-treated neurons is an active process requiring protein synthesis, cultures were incubated concomitantly with 500 μM cocaine and 1 μM cycloheximide. Cycloheximide, which by itself did not affect neuronal viability, fully preserved neurons against cocaine toxicity for up to 3 days, as demonstrated by similar MAP2 content and by indistinguishable morphologic characteristic compared with those of control cells not exposed to cocaine. Thus, cocaine-induced neuronal apoptosis depends on protein synthesis.

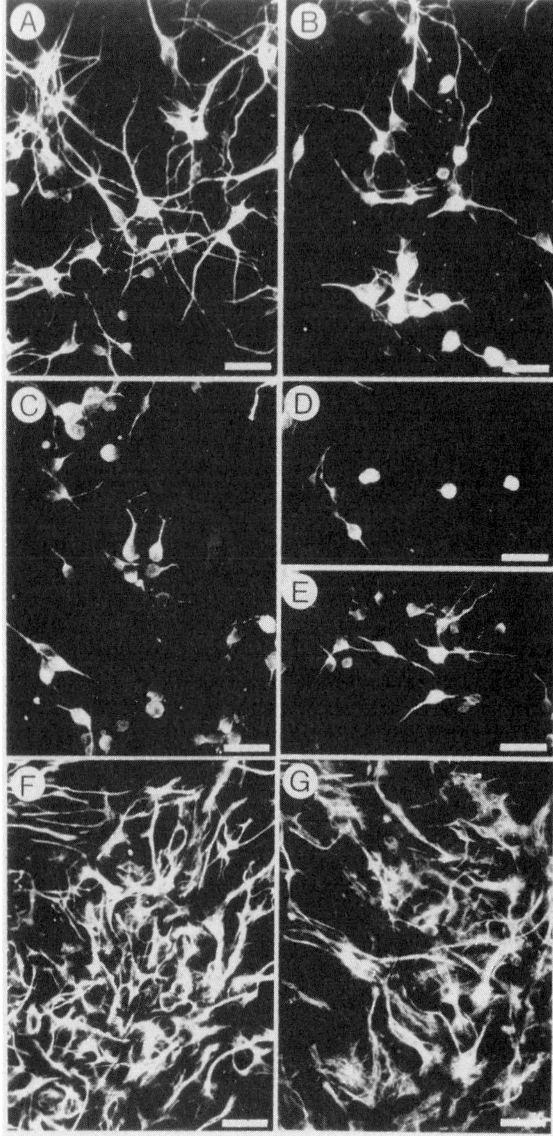

FIGURE 1. Effect of cocaine on MAP2 and GFAP immunolabeling. Cocultures of embryonic cerebral cells were established for 2 days, cultured for an additional 4 days in control medium **(A** and **F)** or in medium supplemented with 100 μM **(B)**, 250 μM **(C)**, and 500 μM **(D** and **G)** cocaine, fixed, and immunolabeled. Parallel cultures were exposed to 500 μM cocaine only during days 3 and 4 and were further incubated in a cocaine-free medium for 2 additional days prior to fixation **(E)**. **(A–E)** MAP2 labeling. **(F** and **G)** GFAP labeling. All fields were photographed at the same magnification and exposure. (Bars = 25 μm). Reproduced from ref. 64 with permission.

FIGURE 2. Scanning electron microscopy. Cocultures were established for 2 days, cultured for 4 additional days in control medium **(A)** or in medium with 500 μM cocaine **(B** and **C)**, fixed, and processed for scanning electron microscopy. (Bars = 5 μM). Reproduced from ref. 64 with permission.

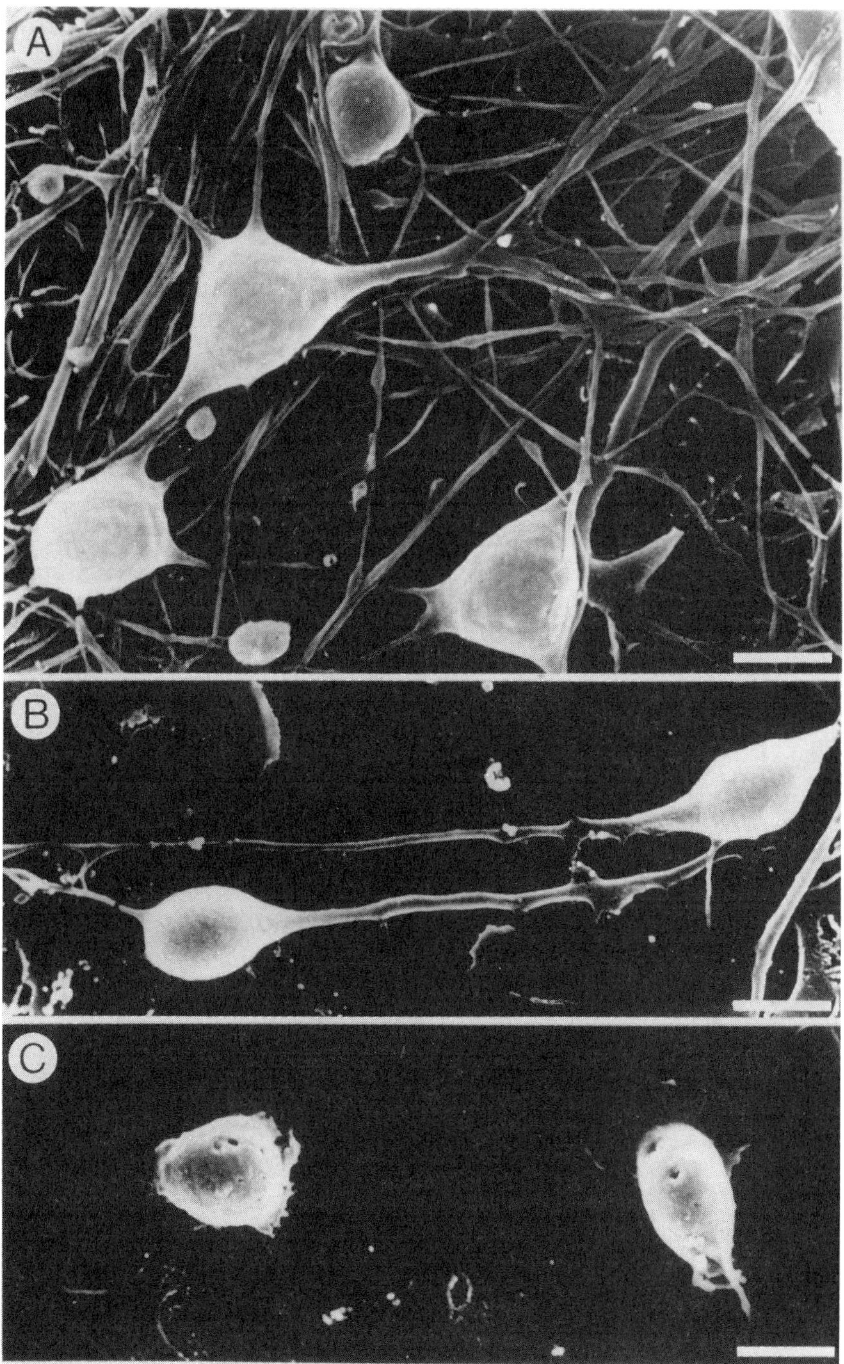

FIGURE 2. *See legend on facing page.*

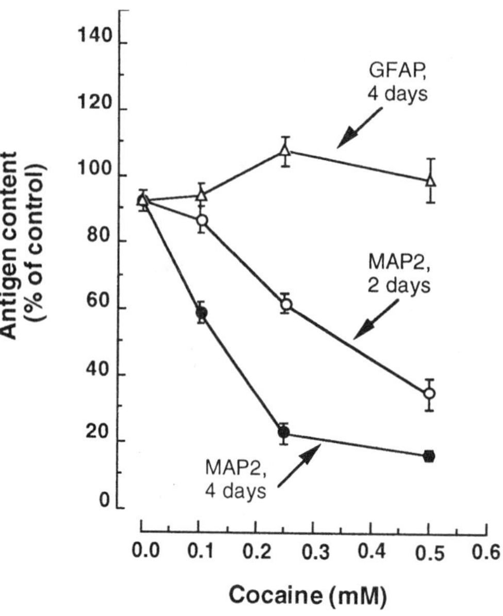

FIGURE 3. Quantitation of MAP2 and GFAP immunolabeling upon cocaine exposure. GFAP *(open triangles)* and MAP2 *(circles)* content was measured by immunoassay after 2 *(open circles)* or 4 *(filled circles)* days of incubation with the indicated cocaine concentrations. Results are expressed as percentages of control cultures and are means ± SEM (n = 6–8 dishes pooled from two separate isolates). Reproduced from ref. 64 with permission.

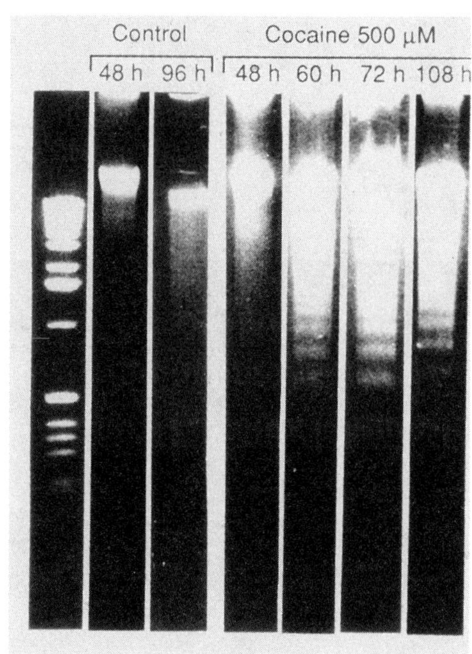

FIGURE 4. Biochemical evidence of DNA fragmentation after cocaine exposure. Cocultures were first established for 2 days in MEM supplemented by 10% fetal calf serum, and cultured for the indicated times in daily renewed Neurobasal® medium supplemented by B27 with or without 500 μM cocaine. Total genomic DNA of cultures was extracted and run on agarose gel. Molecular weight markers were loaded in the *left lane.* Note typical "ladders" after 60–108 hours of cocaine treatment. Reproduced from ref. 65 with permission.

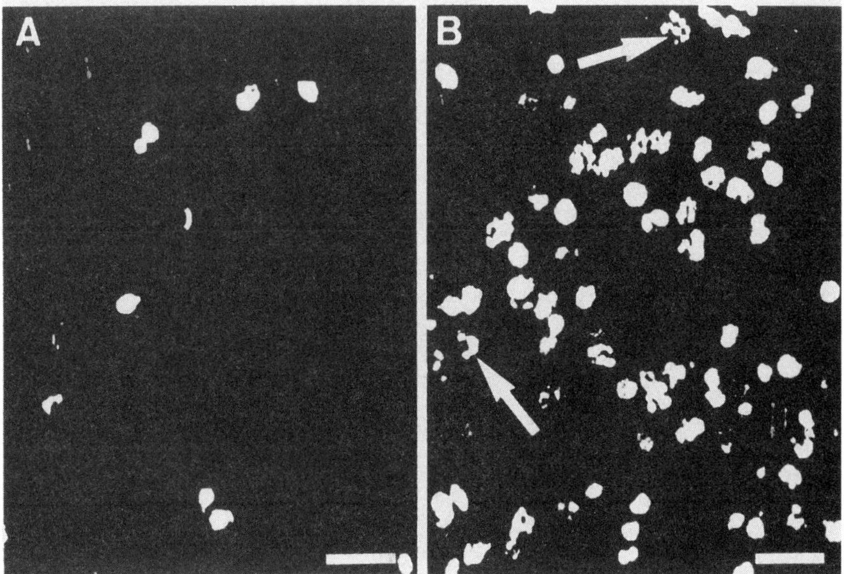

FIGURE 5. *In situ* histochemical evidence of DNA fragmentation after cocaine exposure. Cocultures were first established for 2 days in MEM supplemented by 10% fetal calf serum and cultured for 4 additional days in daily renewed Neurobasal® medium supplemented by B27 without **(A)** or with **(B)** 500 μM cocaine. After cells were fixed, DNA nick-end labeling of fragmented nuclear DNA (TUNEL method) was performed and detected by confocal microscopy. Cocultures were photographed at the level of the neuronal layer. Note the prominent labeling in the vast majority of treated cells, including those showing nuclear fragmentation *(arrows),* in contrast with the homogeneous labeling of but a few control cells (bars = 20 μm). Reproduced from ref. 65 with permission.

Neuronal Apoptosis Is Due to Cocaine Itself

The unusually long delay between induction of apoptosis after cocaine exposure, as compared with that of other agents inducing apoptosis, suggests an indirect effect. The possibility of the delayed conversion of cocaine into metabolites (ecgonine, methylecgonine, and ecgonine methylester) was tested by adding these compounds directly to the culture. For comparison, norcocaine was also investigated; however, it could not be produced from cocaine in our culture conditions. Only cocaine and norcocaine, but none of the major cocaine metabolites that are no longer cationic amphiphiles, significantly decreased MAP2 content (FIG. 6). This suggests that the apoptotic cascade might require intracellular penetration of cocaine and its trapping in an acidic compartment.

MECHANISMS OF NEUROTERATOGENIC EFFECTS OF COCAINE

Cocaine Accessibility to the Placenta and the Fetal Brain

Data from human and experimental animal studies have demonstrated that cocaine easily crosses the placenta.[66–68] The rapid transport of cocaine across the placenta can

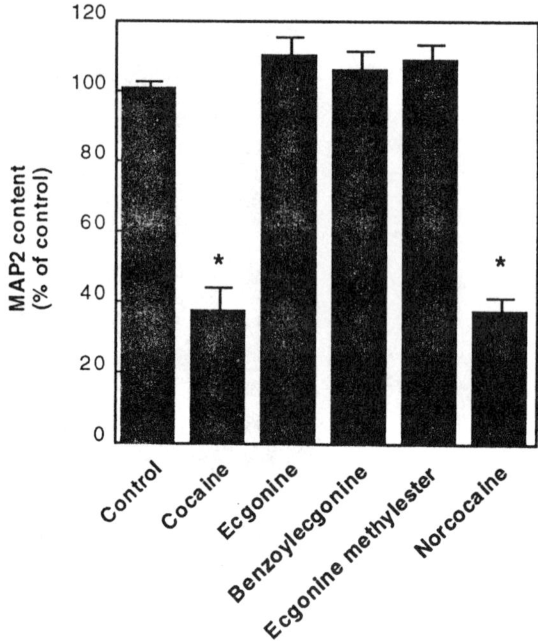

FIGURE 6. Toxicological comparison of cocaine and its metabolites. Cocultures were established for 2 days in MEM supplemented by 10% fetal calf serum and cultured for 3 additional days in daily renewed Neurobasal® medium supplemented by B27 without any drug or with 500 μM of the indicated compounds. Whereas norcocaine was equally active as cocaine, no significant difference was noted between control cultures and cultures exposed to the three major metabolites (*p <0.05, Student's t test). Results are means ± SEM (n = 6 dishes pooled from two different experiments). Reproduced from ref. 65 with permission.

be explained by limited binding of cocaine to human plasma (8–10% is protein bound) as well as by the low molecular weight and amphiphilic nature of the drug. Moreover, concentration of serum esterases involved in cocaine metabolism is diminished during pregnancy and is low in fetal serum.[69] As a result, a given dose of cocaine in a pregnant female may produce higher and more sustained blood levels in the fetus as compared with a nonpregnant adult level.

Transplacental transfer of norcocaine and cocaethylene is also very rapid.[70] By contrast, the rate of benzoylecgonine transfer across the human cotyledon is significantly lower, a finding that can be explained in part by its greater hydrophilicity. Significant amounts of maternal cocaine and benzoylecgonine are retained by the placenta and later leach out into both fetal and maternal circulations. This phenomenon may be significant for the fetal toxicity of cocaine and benzoylecgonine, whose effects are thus prolonged.[68,70] In addition, cocaine could perturb placental function, as indicated by a reduction in permeability to inulin and a diminution in HCG release into the maternal circulation.[71]

Altogether, it is clear that cocaine and at least some of its metabolites may accumulate in the amniotic fluid. This places the fetus at increased risk because (1) during the first half of pregnancy, drugs may diffuse the fetal skin and thus enhance fetal exposure to cocaine; and (2) the human fetus swallows amniotic fluid and is exposed to cocaine and its metabolites through absorption in the gut.

Human and animal studies have also demonstrated that cocaine gains further access to fetal brain tissue shortly after maternal uptake.[68,70] Although actual concentrations in the maternal and especially the fetal brain are difficult to assess, we could extrapolate some information. Serum levels of cocaine in human volunteers receiving a dose of 0.5 mg/kg ranged between 10^{-7} and 10^{-6} *M*,[72] but are often considerably higher in active abusers, reaching the 10^{-4} *M* level.[73] Moreover, cocaine readily crosses the blood-brain-barrier and accumulates in the central nervous system, generally resulting in brain concentrations that remain for an extended period at five times the peak plasma concentration. After acute intoxication, levels within the central nervous system may be up to 20-fold higher than those in the plasma. Thus, effects observed *in vitro* at the 10^{-4} level are likely to be clinically relevant.

Indirect and Direct Effects of Cocaine on the Developing Brain

Cocaine could perturb the developing brain by both indirect mechanisms and direct effects.

Indirect Effects at the Maternal and Placental Levels

Cocaine increases maternal circulating catecholamine levels, resulting in the physiological sequelae of prolonged vasoconstriction episodes, accelerated heart rate, and hypertension. The placental vasculature is also affected by these effects. Following administration of cocaine to pregnant ewes, cocaine induced a dose-dependent decrease in uterine blood flow accompanied by fetal hypoxemia, tachycardia, and hypertension.[37,38] Impaired placental blood flow could also disturb the transfer of nutrients to the fetus.

Indirect Effects at the Fetal Level

As already discussed, cocaine easily crosses the placental barrier and is concentrated within the fetal milieu. There too, cocaine could directly block catecholamine reuptake, resulting in increased heart rate and higher blood pressure also in the fetus. These effects were reproduced by the direct injection of cocaine into ewe fetuses.[38] In humans, disturbances in catecholamines were recorded in neonates who had been exposed prenatally to cocaine.[74]

Indirect Effects in the Fetal Brain

Cocaine further crosses the fetal blood-brain-barrier without restriction. In the brain, cocaine could prevent the reuptake of neurotransmitters or exert direct effects on neuronal and glial cells. Because neurotransmitters act as trophic factors early in development, the fetus might be particularly at risk for abnormal neuronal growth and differentiation, altered migrational events, or abnormal glial function.[51,52] Neuronal excitotoxicity is a possible additional mechanism of neuronal injury in fetuses exposed to cocaine. In neuronal cell cultures, catecholamines can lead to neuronal death, principally by acting as a glutamate agonist, especially in dopaminergic neurons and their projection targets. Moreover, glutamate-receptor antagonists markedly reduced the occurrence of cocaine-induced seizures and death in mice.[75]

Direct Effects in the Fetal Brain

At last, but not at least, cocaine could directly perturb glial and neuronal cells. Indeed, both neuroblastoma and glial cells were sensitive to cocaine *in vitro.*[60,61] By using embryonic mouse primary cocultures of embryonic mouse neuronal and glial cells, we demonstrated that (1) cocaine selectively affects embryonic neuronal cells, causing first a dramatic reduction in both number and length of neurites and then extensive neuronal death; and (2) disappearance of neurons upon cocaine exposure is caused by apoptosis, based on morphology of apoptotic neuronal nuclei and typical laddering fragmentation of DNA. Neuronal cell death on cocaine exposure is prevented by cycloheximide, suggesting involvement of a cascade of proteins, including newly synthesized one(s).

Consequences of Neuronal Toxicity on Brain Development

Consequences of the Loss of Neurites

These results emphasize that in addition to the known vascular effects that produce gross structural defects in the developing brain, cocaine may independently cause direct toxic effect at the level of individual neurons and thereby impair cortical development. An alteration in neurite outgrowth would obviously alter subsequent synaptogenesis during the critical period of cell differentiation and rapid axonal as well as dendritic expansion. Furthermore, a disturbed neuronal differentiation could alter neuronal-glial interactions that are critical for the correct radial migration of neurons during corticogenesis, resulting in malformation if not absence of specific neuronal pathways. Disturbances in neuronal migration that are well known in animal models of cocaine toxicity,[44,45] are evidenced in the brain of infants born to cocaine-addicted mothers by schizencephaly and neuronal heterotopias.[15,17,24]

Consequences of the Loss of Neurons

In addition to perturbations of neurite outgrowth, our results further demonstrate that cocaine can induce apoptosis of neuronal cells. Apoptosis, or programmed cell death, is a fundamental process during different stages of brain development, particularly immediately after the arrival of axons in the postsynaptic target fields, leading to disappearance of neurons in excess. Thus, apoptosis appears essential in the normal framing of local brain networks and in the general organization of the central nervous system. Conversely, enhancement of apoptosis or its inappropriate timing could severely perturb the neurodevelopmental program and contribute to the quantitative and qualitative neuronal defects that are too frequently reported after *in utero* exposure to cocaine.

Perspectives for Future Work

Further work should define the molecular pathway(s) involved in cocaine-induced apoptosis. Many regulatory mechanisms are implicated in the triggering of apoptosis in neuronal cells,[76–78] several of which could be implicated in the initiation of apoptosis by cocaine. (1) As a local anesthetic, cocaine interferes with transmembrane movements of sodium, calcium, and potassium, by binding to the transmembrane channel. In several experiments, changes in cytosolic calcium ion concentration appear to play a key role in the early signaling event of apoptosis.[77,78] (2) During the immediate postnatal period of rat brain development, cocaine activates immediate early genes such as c-*fos,* c-*jun,* and *zif268,* which have been implicated in certain forms of spontaneous neuronal apoptosis in neurons.[12] (3) It is also conceivable that cocaine, which partitions into membranes, could activate the neutral sphingomyelinase and lead to the accumulation of ceramide, a membrane lipid that triggers apoptosis.[79]

Although a direct effect of cocaine on developing cerebral cells in culture has been demonstrated in this work, it remains essential to determine if neuronal apoptosis is similarly induced *in vivo.* This will require quantitation of apoptosis in defined regions of the brain in the offspring of mice and possibly at autopsy of human children born to cocaine-exposed mothers.

REFERENCES

1. Chasnoff, I.J., H.J. Landress *et al.* 1990. The prevalence of illicit-drug or alcohol use during pregnancy and discrepancies in mandatory reporting in Pinellas County, Florida. N. Engl. J. Med. **322:** 1202–1206.
2. George, S.K., J. Price *et al.* 1991. Drug abuse screening of childbearing-age women in Alabama public health clinics. Am. J. Obstet. Gynecol. **165:** 924–927.
3. Miller, J.M., Jr., M.C. Boudreaux *et al.* 1995. A case-control study of cocaine use in pregnancy. Am. J. Obstet. Gynecol. **172:** 180–185.
4. Ostrea, E.M., M. Brady *et al.* 1992. Drug screening of newborns by meconium analysis: A large-scale, prospective, epidemiologic study. Pediatrics **89:** 107–113.
5. Martinez Crespo, J.M., E. Antolin *et al.* 1994. The prevalence of cocaine abuse during pregnancy in Barcelona. Eur. J. Obstet. Gynecol. Reprod. Biol. **56:** 165–167.
6. Chasnoff, I.J., K.A. Burns *et al.* 1987. Cocaine use in pregnancy: Perinatal morbidity and mortality. Neurotoxicol. Teratol. **9:** 291–293.
7. Mc Gregor, S.N., L.G. Keith *et al.* 1989. Cocaine abuse during pregnancy: Correlation between prenatal care and perinatal outcome. Obstet. Gynecol. **74:** 882–885.
8. Holzman, C. & N. Paneth. 1994. Maternal cocaine use during pregnancy and perinatal outcomes. Epidemiol. Rev. **16:** 315–334.
9. Zuckerman, B., D.A. Frank *et al.* 1989. Effects of maternal marijuana and cocaine use on fetal growth. N. Engl. J. Med. **320:** 762–768.
10. Kosofsky, B.E., A.S. Wilkins *et al.* 1994. Transplacental cocaine exposure: A mouse model demonstrating neuroanatomic and behavioral abnormalities. J. Child Neurol. **9:** 234–241.
11. Richardson, G.A. & N.L. Day. 1991. Maternal and neonatal effects of moderate cocaine use during pregnancy. Neurotoxicol. Teratol. **13:** 455–460.
12. Frank, D.A., H. Bauchner *et al.* 1990. Neonatal body proportionality and body composition after *in utero* exposure to cocaine and marijuana. J. Pediatr. **117:** 622–626.
13. Chasnoff, I.J., M.E. Bussey *et al.* 1986. Perinatal cerebral infarction and maternal cocaine use. J. Pediatr. **108:** 456–459.
14. Dixon, S.D. & R. Bejar. 1989. Echoencephalographic findings in neonates associated with maternal cocaine and methamphetamine use: Incidence and clinical correlates. J. Pediatr. **115:** 770–778.
15. Heier, L.A., C.R. Carpanzano *et al.* 1991. Maternal cocaine abuse: The spectrum of radiologic abnormalities in the neonatal CNS. Am. J. Neuroradiol. **12:** 951–956.
16. Dusick, A.M., R.F. Covert *et al.* 1993. Risk of intracranial hemorrhage and other adverse outcomes after cocaine exposure in a cohort of 323 very low birth weight infants. J. Pediatr. **122:** 438–445.
17. Dominguez, R., A. Aguirre Vila-Coro *et al.* 1991. Brain and ocular abnormalities in in-

fants with *in utero* exposure to cocaine and other street drugs. Am. J. Dis. Child. **145:** 688–695.
18. VOLPE, J.J. 1995. Teratogenic effects of drugs and passive addiction. *In* Neurology of the Newborn: 811–850. W.B. Saunders Co. Philadelphia.
19. DOGRA, V.S., J.M. SHYKEN *et al.* 1994. Neurosonographic abnormalities associated with maternal history of cocaine use in neonates of appropriate size for their gestational age. Am. J. Neuroradiol. **15:** 697–702.
20. KAPUR, R.P., C.M. SHAW *et al.* 1991. Brain hemorrhages in cocaine-exposed human fetuses. Teratology **44:** 11–18.
21. COHEN, H.L., J.H. SLOVES *et al.* 1994. Neurosonographic findings in full-term infants born to maternal cocaine abusers: Visualization of subependymal and periventricular cysts. J. Clin. Ultrasound. **22:** 327–333.
22. TSAY, C.H., J.C. PARTRIDGE *et al.* 1996. Neurologic and ophthalmologic findings in children exposed to cocaine *in utero.* J. Child Neurol. **11:** 25–30.
23. SCAFIDI, F.A., T.M. FIELD *et al.* 1996. Cocaine-exposed preterm neonates show behavioral and hormonal differences. Pediatrics **97:** 851–855.
24. GOMEZ-ANSON, B. & R.G. RAMSEY. 1994. Pachygyria in a neonate with prenatal cocaine exposure: Magnetic resonance features. J. Comput. Assisted Tomogr. **18:** 637–639.
25. KAUFMANN, W.E. 1990. Developmental cortical abnormalities after prenatal exposure to cocaine. Soc. Neurosci. Abstr. **16:** 305.
26. JACOBSON, S.W., J.L. JACOBSON *et al.* 1996. New evidence for neurobehavioral effects of *in utero* cocaine exposure. J. Pediatr. **129:** 581–590.
27. NAPIORKOWSKI, B., B.M. LESTER *et al.* 1996. Effects of *in utero* substance exposure on infant neurobehavior. Pediatrics **98:** 71–75.
28. CHASNOFF, I.J., D.R. GRIFFITH *et al.* 1992. Cocaine/polydrug use in pregnancy: Two-year follow-up. Pediatrics **89:** 284–289.
29. AZUMA, S.D. & I.J. CHASNOFF. 1993. Outcome of children prenatally exposed to cocaine and other drugs: A path analysis of three-year data. Pediatrics **92:** 396–402.
30. SINGER, L.T., R. ARENDT *et al.* 1992. Development of infants exposed *in utero* to cocaine. Pediatr. Res. **31:** 260A.
31. STRUTHERS, J.M. & R.L. HANSEN. 1992. Visual recognition memory in drug-exposed infants. Dev. Behav. Pediatr. **13:** 108–111.
32. FETTERS, L. & E.Z. TRONICK. 1996. Neuromotor development of cocaine-exposed and control infants from birth through 15 months: Poor and poorer performance. Pediatrics **98:** 938–943.
33. SCHERLING, D. 1994. Prenatal cocaine exposure and childhood psychopathology: A developmental analysis. Am. J. Orthopsychiatry **64:** 9–19.
34. FRANK, D.A., K. BRESNAHAN *et al.* 1993. Maternal cocaine use: Impact on child health and development. Adv. Pediatr. **40:** 65–99.
35. SINGER, L. & R. ARENDT. 1993. Neurodevelopmental effects of cocaine. Clin. Perinatol. **20:** 245–262.
36. WASSERMAN, D.R. & J.M. LEVENTHAL. 1993. Maltreatment of children born to cocaine-dependent mothers. Am. J. Dis. Child. **147:** 1324–1328.
37. MOORE, T.R., J. SORG *et al.* 1986. Hemodynamic effects of intravenous cocaine on the pregnant ewe and fetus. Am. J. Obstet. Gynecol. **155:** 883–888.
38. WOODS, J.R., JR., M.A. PLESSINGER *et al.* 1989. Prenatal cocaine exposure to the fetus: A sheep model for cardiovascular evaluation. Ann. N. Y. Acad. Sci. **562:** 267–279.
39. DOLKART, L.A., M.A. PLESSINGER *et al.* 1990. Effect of alpha-1 receptor blockade upon maternal and fetal cardiovascular responses to cocaine. Obstet. Gynecol. **75:** 745–751.
40. COVERT, R.F., M.D. SCHREIBER *et al.* 1994. Hemodynamic and cerebral blood flow effects of cocaine, cocaethylene and benzoylecgonine in conscious and anesthetized fetal lambs. J. Pharmacol. Exp. Ther. **270:** 118–126.
41. BURCHFIELD, D.J. & R.M. ABRAMS. 1993. Cocaine depresses cerebral glucose utilization in fetal sheep. Dev. Brain Res. **73:** 283–288.
42. BURCHFIELD, D.J., A. PENA *et al.* 1996. Cocaine does not compromise cerebral or myocardial oxygen delivery in fetal sheep. Reprod. Fertil. Dev. **8:** 383–389.

43. LIDOW, M.S. 1995. Prenatal cocaine exposure adversely affects development of the primate cerebral cortex. Synapse **21:** 332–341.
44. GRESSENS, P., F. GOFFLOT *et al.* 1992. Early neurogenesis and teratogenesis in whole mouse embryo cultures. Histochemical, immunocytological and ultrastructural study of the premigratory neuronal-glial units in normal mouse embryo and in mouse embryos influenced by cocaine and retinoic acid. J. Neuropathol. Exp. Neurol. **51:** 206–219.
45. GRESSENS, P., B.E. KOSOFSKY *et al.* 1992. Cocaine-induced disturbances of corticogenesis in the developing murine brain. Neurosci. Lett. **140:** 113–116.
46. AKBARI, H.M., P.M. WHITAKER-AZMITIA *et al.* 1994. Prenatal cocaine decreases the trophic factor S-100beta and induced microcephaly: Reversal by postnatal 5-HT_{1A} receptor agonist. Neurosci. Lett. **170:** 141–144.
47. CLARKE, C., K. CLARKE *et al.* 1996. Prenatal cocaine delays astroglial maturation: Immunodensitometry shows increased markers of immaturity (vimentin and GAP-43) and decreased proliferation and production of the growth factor S-100. Brain Res. Dev. Brain Res. **91:** 268–273.
48. ANDERSON-BROWN, T., T.A. SLOTKIN *et al.* 1990. Cocaine acutely inhibits DNA synthesis in developing rat brain regions: Evidence for direct actions. Brain Res. **537:** 197–202.
49. KOSOFSKY, B.E., L.M. GENOVA *et al.* 1995. Postnatal age defines specificity of immediate early gene induction by cocaine in developing rat brain. J. Comp. Neurol. **351:** 27–40.
50. KOSOFSKY, B.E., L.M. GENOVA *et al.* 1995. Substance P phenotype defines specificity of c-fos induction by cocaine in developing rat striatum. J. Comp. Neurol. **351:** 41–50.
51. LIDOW, M.S. & P. RAKIC. 1995. Neurotransmitter receptors in the proliferative zones of the developing primate occipital lobe. J. Comp. Neurol. **360:** 393–402.
52. WHITAKER-AZMITIA, P.M., A.V. SHEMER *et al.* 1990. Role of high affinity serotonin receptors in neuronal growth. Ann. N. Y. Acad. Sci. **600:** 315–330.
53. MINABE, Y., C.R. ASHBY, JR. *et al.* 1992. The effects of prenatal cocaine exposure on spontaneously active midbrain dopamine neurons in adult male offspring: An electrophysiological study. Brain Res. **586:** 152–156.
54. WEESE-MAYER, D.E., J.M. SILVESTRI *et al.* 1993. Effect of cocaine in early gestation on striatal dopamine and neurotrophic activity. Pediatr. Res. **34:** 389–392.
55. RONNEKLEIV, O.K. & B.R. NAYLOR. 1995. Chronic cocaine exposure in fetal rhesus monkey: Consequences for early development of dopamine neurons. J. Neurosci. **15:** 7330–7343.
56. WANG, X.-H., P. LEVITT *et al.* 1995. Intrauterine cocaine exposure of rabbits: Persistent elevation of GABA-immunoreactive neurons in anterior cingulate cortex but not visual cortex. Brain Res. **689:** 32–46.
57. LEVITT, P., J.A. HARVEY *et al.* 1997. New evidence for neurotransmitter influences on brain development. Trends Neurosci. **20:** 269–274.
58. LESKAWA, K.C., G.H. JACKSON *et al.* 1994. Cocaine exposure during pregnancy affects rat neonate and maternal brain glycosphingolipids. Brain Res Bull. **33:** 195–198.
59. LIEN, R., O.P. MISHRA *et al.* 1994. Alteration of brain cell membrane function following cocaine exposure in the fetal guinea pig. Brain Res. **637:** 249–254.
60. GARG, U.C., H. TURNDORF *et al.* 1993. Effect of cocaine on macromolecular syntheses and cell proliferation in cultured glial cells. Neuroscience **57:** 467–472.
61. ZACHOR, D., J.K. CHERKES *et al.* 1994. Cocaine differentially inhibits neuronal differentiation and proliferation in vitro. J. Clin. Invest. **93:** 1179–1185.
62. ALTER-YABLONSKY, E., I.I. GLEZER *et al.* 1995. Cocaine adversely affects development of embryonic neurons *in vitro:* Immunocytochemical study of calcium-binding proteins. Soc. Neurosci. Abstr. **21:** 705.
63. CULICAN, S.M., N.L. BAUMRIND *et al.* 1990. Cortical radial glia: Identification in tissue culture and evidence for their transformation to astrocytes. J. Neurosci. **10:** 684–692.
64. NASSOGNE, M.C., P. EVRARD *et al.* 1995. Selective neuronal toxicity of cocaine in embryonic mouse brain cocultures. Proc. Natl. Acad. Sci. USA **92:** 11029–11033.
65. NASSOGNE, M.C., J. LOUAHED *et al.* 1997. Cocaine induces apoptosis in cortical neurons of fetal mice. J. Neurochem. **68:** 2442–2450.
66. SPEAR, L.P., N.A. FRAMBES *et al.* 1989. Fetal and maternal brain and plasma levels of cocaine and benzoylecgonine following chronic subcutaneous administration of cocaine during gestation in rats. Psychopharmacology **97:** 427–431.

67. Wiggins, R.C., C. Rolsten *et al.* 1989. Pharmacokinetics of cocaine: Basic studies of route, dosage, pregnancy and lactation. Neurotoxicology **10:** 367–381.
68. Simone, C., L.O. Derewlany *et al.* 1994. Transfer of cocaine and benzoylecgonine across the perfused human placental cotyledon. Am. J. Obstet. Gynecol. **170:** 1404–1410.
69. Fleming, J.A., R. Byck *et al.* 1990. Pharmacology and therapeutic applications of cocaine. Anesthesiology **73:** 518–531.
70. Schenker, S., Y. Yang *et al.* 1993. The transfer of cocaine and its metabolites across the term human placenta. Clin. Pharmacol. Ther. **53:** 329–339.
71. Malek, A., Ivy D., E. Blann *et al.* 1995. Impact of cocaine on human placental function using an *in vitro* perfusion system. J. Pharmacol. Toxicol. Methods **33:** 213–219.
72. Cone, E.J. 1995. Pharmacokinetics and pharmacodynamics of cocaine. J. Anal. Toxicol. **19:** 459–478.
73. Albuquerque, M.L.C. & C.D. Kurth. 1993. Cocaine constricts immature cerebral arterioles by a local anesthetic mechanism. Eur. J. Pharmacol. **249:** 215–220.
74. Mirochnick, M., J. Meyer *et al.* 1997. Elevated plasma norepinephrine after *in utero* exposure to cocaine and marijuana. Pediatrics **99:** 555–559.
75. Shimosato, K., R.J. Marley *et al.* 1995. Differential effects of NMDA receptor and dopamine receptor antagonists on cocaine toxicities. Pharmacol. Biochem. Behav. **51:** 781–788.
76. Sanders, E.M. & M.A. Wride. 1995. Programmed cell death in development. Int. Rev. Cytol. **163:** 105–173.
77. Hale A.J., C.A. Smith *et al.* 1996. Apoptosis: Molecular regulation of cell death. Eur. J. Biochem. **236:** 1–26.
78. Vaux, D.L. & A. Strasser. 1996. The molecular biology of apoptosis. Proc. Natl. Acad. Sci. USA **93:** 2239–2244.
79. Hannun, Y.A. & L.M. Obeid. 1995. Ceramide: An intracellular signal for apoptosis. Trends Cell. Biol. **5:** 73–77.

Round Table 1. Drug Interactions in Cocaine Abuse: Methodologic Concerns in Human and Animal Studies

Moderators: STEVEN E. HYMAN, BARRY ZUCKERMAN

Panelists: JAMES R. WOODS, JR., MICHAEL W. CHURCH, JANINA R. GALLER, DEBBIE FRANK

Discussants: JOHN HARVEY, BARRY KOSOFSKY, BARRY LESTER (BROWN), JEROME MEYER (UMASS), PAT LEVITT (PITTSBURGH), ABIGAIL SNYDER-KELLER (ALBANY)

STEVEN E. HYMAN: Dr. Frank, one of the issues you raised very directly was that of sensitivity of the behavioral tests and also their relevance. At the time you examine these babies, and often with the animal tests, the behavioral repertoires may be relatively limited. It's clear that there are many neurobehavioral disorders in which the seeds, we believe, are planted early, but serious behavioral symptoms might arise later. The most speculative such disorder is schizophrenia, but there are cases as dramatic as autism in which an abnormality would not be detected in the first postnatal days or even months of life. Would you comment on strategies for dealing with that kind of problem.

DEBBIE FRANK: I do longitudinal studies and so I will put in a plug for those. Many of us now have kids who are in the 4–6 year age range. There is a huge need for longitudinal studies, but the problem of confounders becomes massive, and the further out you go, the more confounding it gets, such as how many foster home changes and who saw who kill whom. A few years ago I had a wonderful conversation with Dr. Chasnoff at a meeting, saying these kids are driving us nuts with their ear infections. I asked him if he thought cocaine did something to their immune system? He said that since all their mothers smoke, it is the most likely cause of the increased incidence of ear infection.

But in fact there are cumulative insults, both biologic and social, that are difficult to document. You've got to try, as that may be what clouds the signal or exacerbates the signal. We have data to suggest that kids who get intervention early, within the first 6 months, seem to have a much more positive outcome. We can say without contradiction that the *Rolling Stone* magazine idea that these kids are born hopeless is really "off the table."

BARRY ZUCKERMAN: I want to turn that question back to you, Steve. Given what you spoke about regarding expression of genes and dopamine receptors, what would one expect to see, at what age might you see it, and are there any measurements to identify it?

STEVEN E. HYMAN: Well, let me give you an abstract answer, as the same issues confound the examination of animal models. Brain development does not terminate at birth. Indeed in humans, brain development continues, I hope, at least into the mid-40s. And the expression of subtle abnormal behavioral signs and symptoms especially may appear only with brain maturation. However, insults very early in life may be setups for this. One issue, therefore, is the need for appropriate longitudinal studies, and I do respect the issue of confounds.

The other issue not addressed by this theoretical idea, however, is what are the appropriate behavioral tests. Will what you do in the clinic, which is cheap and efficient, really tell us something about how a child is behaving in an "open field" or in the home? There are famous, overdramatized stories of highly impaired adults with frontal lobe syndromes who were not "picked up" in the neurologist's office, but if you go home with the patient, the problem is immediately obvious. So there really is a second tier of issues about not only when to do the tests, but also how to pick up life-altering abnormalities that may not be apparent in the clinic.

BARRY ZUCKERMAN: The only other thing I would add to the longitudinal aspect is the interactions that one would see with hormonal changes in puberty. For example, what about subsequent drug use when the person becomes an adolescent. Are there different thresholds of susceptibility? I've always wondered about gender effects, because the dopamine system is involved and females seem to suffer depression more than do males. Might there be an interactive effect by gender mediated by some other genetic or hormonal mechanisms?

JOHN HARVEY: I wanted to reintroduce a question that was raised somewhat tangentially a little earlier. No one indicated the dose of cocaine and the route of administration, even those using animal models where they should be able to specify. What I'm raising is the issue of pharmacokinetics. You can easily have a U-shaped dose-effect curve. In fact, when you give a large dose of cocaine, you get a lot of vasoconstriction, slowing down drug entry into the fetus. If you give a smaller dose and it's easily transported, a much higher percentage may enter the infant.

The other factor is the route of administration. Following sniffing, smoking, or IV injection, pharmacokinetics are totally different than those after subcutaneous, intramuscular, or intraperitoneal injection. Depending on the species, no cocaine may be found in the bloodstream as early as 15 minutes after iv injection.

From what was said here, very high doses were being used, which is very important if we want to find out the upper level. Even if the effects are totally nonspecific, at least you are getting effects. And then the other question is, what's the very lowest dose? If we don't know that and try to compare things, we're going to be in serious trouble.

The other thing is that if a person setting up a behavioral animal model does not pay attention to the clinician, they're going to be in serious trouble. But if the clinician doesn't pay attention to the animal model, they can be in serious trouble because it is characteristically the only way we can define neurotoxicity. If you want to know if something produces cancer, you go to an animal model to find out what the thresholds are, is it cumulative, and so on. Therefore, if we can't get some comparability between what you measure in the human situation and in the animal, we're going to be faced constantly with the problem of trying to understand why one person got one thing and another something else.

DEBBIE FRANK: The complication beyond that is that things you want to know about in humans, such as language and executive function, are not measurable in animals.

JOHN HARVEY: You can certainly measure language in animals. You simply give them a language to use. It's called a conditioned stimulus.

JAMES R. WOODS, JR.: I guess I need to get my pregnant population into this discussion. Going back to your question of how these humans use the drug, it is fascinating that in focus groups where we brought together addicts to find out what's really going on in their lives, there are extenuating circumstances that make the analysis even more complicated. There are those who only use drugs when they can get their hands on them and they use as much as they can get. There are others who titrate it. But there's a factor that I never appreciated, that within the social groups in which they exist, cocaine is doled out in many ways like cigarettes. For all of us who are ex-smokers, you'd sit down with a group of friends and you'd throw your cigarette pack out in the middle and everybody would have a cigarette. This sharing of cocaine seems to be a pattern of behavior that I never appreciated in the past.

When doing these sheep studies, we were giving very consistent doses, some very high. In the first couple of days there was an enormous reaction and then there was a rapid attenuation. Unfortunately our animal data led us to believe that you could get the same vascular responses from these chronic cocaine users as you could get out of these animals who had never seen cocaine and were suddenly given this blast of it; from this, we extrapolated those observations. For these women who use cocaine, some high, some low doses depending on what they can access, they're still probably not the same as a naive animal that receives a drug as a bolus. We make these wonderful graphs to publish, but in fact, they may not have any relevance. That's what led us to look at this ischemia issue; it isn't really always there and maybe it's not there a lot. There may be steady passage of cocaine into the fetus, working its actions on the fetal side as opposed to the uterine vasculature.

JERRY MEYER: Some important, possible mechanisms of cocaine action have been discussed including effects on the vasculature and certainly possible direct effects on the fetal brain. I want to add one to the list that we haven't talked about, that is, the possible effects of cocaine on the placental trophoblastic cells. Work in the last few years has shown that in human syncytial trophoblast cells there are transporters for norepinephrine and serotonin. Ours and several other laboratories have found these transporters in animal models. These transporters are situated to take up catecholamines and serotonin from the maternal circulation and also possibly, and likely, from the fetal circulation. We don't know at this point exactly what this uptake is accomplishing, but there are some speculations. But just to raise one possibility, we know that placental cells possess adrenergic receptors, and we know that those receptors are involved in regulating the secretion of some placental hormones such as HCG and steroid hormones. In our laboratory we found that just 3 days of continuous cocaine exposure led to a very large upregulation of the norepinephrine transporter in rat placenta. So I think that another emerging target of cocaine in the maternal-fetal unit is the placenta itself, not just in terms of vascular effects, which had been discussed and are obviously important, but also in terms of effects on the placental trophoblastic cells.

SPEAKER: I am going to steal a page out of Dr. Koren's laboratory to mention one of the most interesting single case reports they published. They gave chronic cocaine to a human placenta that was being perfused and looked at the accumulation of cocaine in the placenta as opposed to passage onto the fetal side, comparing that against placentas that had never been exposed to cocaine before. They found that the placenta chronically exposed to cocaine acted as a sink to reduce the amount of cocaine that passed to the fetus, while increasing the accumulation of cocaine within the placenta itself. That raises a question: Does a chronic cocaine user actually have a different placenta from that of some of these animal models that we are using to identify transport across a placenta naive to drug.

PAT LEVITT: The relevance of animal models from my perspective is not whether the models are modeling what's happening in the human condition, but whether it's modeling or trying to model the underlying biologic mechanisms for what could effect very specific developmental events. If you approach animal models from that perspective, as you would approach understanding the regulation of the cell cycle and how that relates to understanding cancer, there wouldn't be debates about whether we are looking at appropriate animal models to explain a specific clinical effect. We all agree that if we look at the distribution of reuptake molecules for the monoamines and their receptors and innervation patterns, almost every cell in the organism could be identified as a potential target. The relevant aspect is to actually do some cell biology and to understand what mechanisms are operative. To state that there's a vascular effect, that's a phenomenon; that there's a brain effect, that's a phenomenon. But what are the underlying mechanisms, the molecular and cellular changes in each of these areas that we are all focusing on. We'll never model what happens clinically. If we get beyond that, perhaps in the 3 days of this conference, we could talk about the potential range of effects at the cellular level and what that means developmentally. What was striking about this first session, except for one illustration, was that there was no reference to a specific developmental timeline about what's happening. I think that's really critical to emphasize over these 3 days.

JANINA GALLER: The earlier comment that the human clinician and the basic scientist and rat investigator all need to be talking to one another is very salient. I don't think that someone dealing with molecular biology and looking at upregulation issues, etc, should be unaware of what a reasonable model for a human population is. In fact, we've struggled very hard to do that. It has taken us a number of years to come up with a model of cocaine administration to rats that in fact does not just represent a spurious response or potential adaptation which is indeed possible. I don't think you have to limit yourself that way; I think it's possible to do both. It's possible to take a slice and to perfuse and expose it to cocaine and look at what the intrinsic membrane properties are. You can at the same time also look in the integrated, intact, whole animal model as a way of answering different parts of the question. One is of no merit without the other. You need to do both.

PAT LEVITT: I would disagree, but maybe members of the panel can comment. It's not clear to me if any animal model presented would go unscathed in terms of criticism and in terms of an inability to model the clinical problem. Therefore, it diverts the attention of those of us who are doing animal model work who are trying to get at cellular mechanisms. I'll give you an example with cancer. You can modify a cell cycle under conditions of malnutrition and hormonal state, etc. That doesn't preclude the benefits of understanding the basic mechanisms of how the cell cycle is regulated to understand what happens when that goes wrong in the state of cancer. So we can continually argue about what is appropriate: whether it is 60 mg or 10 mg; IV, IP, IG, or SC injections; 2 or 3 days of administration.

BARRY ZUCKERMAN: Let me just add to the confusion by pointing out that we are talking about different mechanisms. I think that you were referring to direct mechanisms when you spoke about the molecular level and that in addition we have indirect mechanisms such as ischemia and malnutrition that are indirectly related to the effects of cocaine.

Just two other comments. One related to mechanism, although you could also call it a confounder, is the genetics of the mother and father. If you buy some aspect of the self-medication theory of drug use, cocaine may to some extent "treat" depression and ADHD. Maybe the parents who get addicted to cocaine have that sort of genetic loading and therefore too has the baby. Then you get a synergistic effect or perhaps you are just seeing the genetic aspects. That genetic load may have consequences at the molecular level.

Finally, we talked about reward mechanisms and Steve mentioned the importance of context. We also know that dopamine has to do with affect. Any behavioral measure that we'll see in a human is just a meta-phenomenon for maybe some underlying function of that. And one question is, how do we measure those very important functions early on, let alone how are they going to be confounded later on? We have to be aware that there's not a direct link. Maybe we are looking in the wrong place—where the "light is" because we have measurement tools—but that may not be where the answer is.

BARRY KOSOFSKY: Pat Levitt and I, who have worked for many years in the field of monoamines, have been up against this for 20 years. The neurochemical systems that release norepinephrine, serotonin, and dopamine are divergent, but not diffuse. They comprise very discrete presynaptic neurochemical systems and postsynaptic signal transduction pathways. And at the next level that Steve talked about, given the coupling proteins and the convergence of postsynaptic responses, a whole other level of specificity exists. Identifying what dopamine does or what norepinephrine does is very hard on the mechanistic level, and when one tries to add to this an understanding at the developmental, behavioral, and clinical levels, it's next to impossible.

I wanted to ask Dr. Galler a question. You so elegantly showed in an animal model how malnutrition's effects are dissociable and distinct from cocaine's effects, and almost mutually exclusive in terms of the sets of deficits that were represented. But then you alluded to going to clinical meetings where people talk about the same sets of behaviors that are altered in children who are alcohol exposed or cocaine exposed or malnourished. So I want to frame the question at the level that Steve was talking about.

We know in the adult that there is plasticity of "brain reward" systems, and there are convergent mechanisms through which such systems can be altered by nicotine, alcohol, marijuana, etc. Are there similar convergent mechanisms during development? Are there final common pathways mediating altered brain function and behavior that are altered? Or are we just not yet clever enough as clinicians to take behavior and to reduce it to the fundamental elements, such as Dr. Robbins has done in preclinical models. Can we make meaningful clinical distinctions, and do we have instruments, scans, or approaches which at each level of analysis allow us to better understand drug-induced changes in brain structure and function? Will we become more sophisticated, and how can we promote that process? We know that alterations in monoaminergic systems may have hard to detect but profoundly important consequences. Affect, attention, and arousal are very subtle human behaviors, hard to define in the adult. If those are the areas of concern for drug-exposed children that are identified in preclinical models, how can we capitalize in designing clinical studies that characterize and discriminate such subtleties?

JANINA GALLER: I think you've just basically answered the question for yourself. Those of us who work with both human and rat models get frustrated on both ends. On the one hand, you have a very narrow focus when you are dealing with a laboratory rat. You can administer 10, 20, 30, 40, 60, or 80 mg and obtain a very nice dose response curve for all of the above and a wide range of behaviors. Even in that setting it is not particularly clear as to what you are dealing with. But I think really there are two answers to what you are questioning.

Number one, I think interdisciplinary research is the order of the day. The only way that the proper questions and therefore the proper answers will be obtained is by having basic scientists merge with people involved in clinical outcomes studies to be able to apply more specificity to the underlying outcomes. That's very much the case; otherwise, you are dealing in the dark. It's a major advantage at this point in time that to obtain as much specificity as you can to suggest some of those responses. But there is no simple answer in terms of the human condition because of everything everyone else has been saying. Even in dealing with our longitudinal nutritional studies we have had to resort to extraordinary statistical methods to come up with conclusions that would allow you to isolate independent effects of particular variables.

What it takes is to sit around a very long time with a population, to have a very large population, and to have excellent control of that population. For instance, in the Barbados situation, we were very lucky that after 30 years we still have 85% of the population, because where do you go other than into the sea or to somewhere in the United States. It's unusual to lose people for migration purposes. But that will be very unlikely with the cocaine longitudinal studies. In fact, Debbie Frank, Barry Zuckerman, and I have frequently talked about why we have not become involved in more of this research in Boston, and the reason is that after 6 weeks you can't find a lot of your population. That's very true in terms of some of the questions you are asking.

DEBORAH FRANK: You can find them, but it's expensive.

JANINA GALLER: Like Debbie Frank, I think more funds have to be channeled into interdisciplinary research which takes into account the basic mechanisms and appropriate questions in human models. More money has to be channeled into supporting interdisciplinary, longitudinal studies of a proper nature which means not just 10 kids per group but large samples where, in fact, ultimate statistical treatment will help, at least, to address some of these questions somewhat better. The other very important issue is the length of the study. That takes money and support, but I think the issue has been raised by a number of the investigators, including yourself, that sometimes some of these effects are simply not present until later in life. We, in fact, in looking at the early impact of nutrition at this point, are very intrigued with the possibility now, with the population hitting their 30s, that we may be able to pick up an escalated incidence of schizophrenia in the population, something we could never have looked at previously. With some of these early toxic exposures, those are indeed in and of themselves very interesting questions.

So that's where the animal model becomes so important, because you can't do this easily and reasonably economically in the current era. But you can do it in rat studies. You can at least begin to get some answers from looking in the very long haul and looking broadly in that setting.

STEVEN HYMAN: One thing that has to go into this mix is understanding interactions in complex systems. We've been talking longitudinally, but something I'm very mindful of, in terms of studies that NIMH funds, for example, the search for genes that involve behavior, let alone about rather dramatic and obvious forms of mental illness, is that we've recognized very clearly that no one mechanism, no one gene, for example, has the lion's share in the behavioral outcome. It's really critical that what has just been presented reminds us that there is a panoply of potentially relevant mechanisms, vascular mechanisms, mechanisms with respect to the placental cells, and mechanisms with respect to the developing brain, each of which is going to change over time, and what we've been calling confounds are actually the fellow travelers very much like the genes that might be needed to develop depression plus the environmental insults, maybe five or ten genes each contributing only a twofold recurrence risk. And we really have to resolve these problems, unless this whole group is missing something about a single, major effector—the elephant sitting in the room that we are not noticing—and actually think about the complex interaction of many, many factors that will sum not even in a simple linear way, but that will have temporal dynamics and synergies and additions and subtractions, and there'll be modifier genes that are protective, not only deleterious. So that's not to make people pessimistic, but we really have to be very mindful of the complexity of putting these things together.

ABIGAIL SYNDER-KELLER: My question relates to the issue of funding. A question that I repeatedly get asked as somebody who uses the animal model, is why are we not studying binge exposure and why are we not studying a combination of cocaine and alcohol or other drugs. I would like to answer my own question by suggesting that it's partly because studies like that are not funded, and I would like to ask why?

STEVEN HYMAN: Your question gets to the issue of complex systems. In the general scientific opportunity, the ability to solve a problem and take the next step depends on an effect size that you can isolate, and all of us are very, very nervous about systems that are more and more complex. Indeed, the whole reason for intermediate models, taking a putatively simple problem like human memory. . . . people argue about whether we should be studying molecules such as Creb or cultured cells, or slice preparations, or knockout animals, or animals with lesions, or animals . . . what does this have to do with the human with amnesia? The virtue of finding simple, intermediate models where we can control all the variables is that we can get very certain effects.

We increasingly get calls for interdisciplinary research and research that recognizes the difficulties of crossing levels, of attributing causality across levels, and research that brings together many, many factors. Certainly with respect to mental illness, we cannot solve these problems with the hoped for simple answer; some main effector is simply not there for many of the problems we are most interested in. We can't fault the review process regarding who reviews (it's you who review). What we can fault is the process for being timid. We also have to be very careful about the ability to get a real signal rising above the noise. We are going to get there. Different institutes have different strategies for bringing together interdisciplinary research, to analyze complex systems in genetics. I don't have a simple, off-the-shelf answer because we are balancing the ability to answer the questions that we are really interested in against the possibility of making real progress that is going to stick and not wash away with the next study.

ABIGAIL SNYDER-KELLER: I would like to press the clinicians to tell us what they would like to see being done in an animal model. Would it be more appropriate to study a binge pattern? That sort of input would be valuable.

STEVEN HYMAN: It is obviously the peer community that decides in study sections and foundation committees, in some sense, what they pay for in this area, so if nothing else, this is a very healthy discussion.

BARRY KOSOFSKY: I want to thank Steve Hyman and our panel of presenters. Debbie Frank asked the question why was she up first and why was she a "human in the midst of animals"? The goal was to get the issues out on the table and we've done that. We've seen the problem in all its ugliness and we've seen the problem of comparing what's good and what's bad about clinical and preclinical studies, and the importance of this communication. We thank this first group for doing such a marvelous job of laying out the entire spectrum of topics that we're going to be discussing. We hope to take this up at the next level of analysis in terms of animal models, discussing functional deficits and developmental mechanisms and then longitudinal studies and interventions. We want to thank everybody for actively participating in this conference.

* * * * *

Animal Behavior Models

Increased Sensitivity to Stressors and Other Environmental Experiences after Prenatal Cocaine Exposure[a]

LINDA P. SPEAR,[b] JAMES CAMPBELL, KRISTYN SNYDER, MARISA SILVERI, AND NINA KATOVIC

Department of Psychology and Center for Developmental Psychobiology, Binghamton University, Binghamton, New York 13902–6000, USA

ABSTRACT: Neural compensations occurring after prenatal cocaine exposure may often permit some functional recovery, although the cost of this reorganization may be a decrease in adaptability. As we have seen in our rodent model of prenatal cocaine exposure, latent deficits may become unmasked when offspring are exposed to cognitive and environmental demands and stressors. In adolescence and adulthood, offspring exposed gestationally to cocaine exhibit characteristic decreases in stress-induced immobility along with increases in aggression under the demands of social competition. Recently, we observed that cocaine-exposed offspring are also unusually sensitive to the long-term effects of early manipulation (noninvasive heart rate testing at 16 days of age). When tested in adulthood, cocaine-exposed offspring not receiving this early experience exhibited less immobility when tested in the presence of intermittent footshock or when subsequently examined in an open field as well as more locomotion in the open field than control offspring, findings reminiscent of previous work. By contrast, these effects were normalized (shock-induced immobility) or reversed (open field immobility and locomotion) in cocaine-exposed animals given the early experience. This marked susceptibility to the effects of early manipulation was less evident in control offspring and even in a group of stunted nutritional controls. Thus, cocaine-exposed offspring may exhibit increased sensitivity not only to environmental demands and stressors, but also to the potential moderating or beneficial effects of early experiences.

INTRODUCTION

Over the last decade, conclusions regarding the consequences of prenatal cocaine exposure have undergone predictable transformation reminiscent of early phases of research with other developmental toxicants such as lead and alcohol.[1] In initial work examining a suspected developmental toxicant, there is often a flurry of clinical case studies and preliminary reports suggesting marked adverse effects; some of these findings may be sensationalized in the popular press. This initial "rush to (negative) judgment"[2] is typically followed by a second phase of reevaluation and criticism in which some researchers question the validity of early work which, by its preliminary nature, may well have been inadequately designed and controlled. This skepticism may also receive notable attention in the popular press. A characteristic third phase of well-

[a] This work was supported in part by Grants R01 DA04478 and K02 DA00140 from the National Institute on Drug Abuse.

[b] Address for correspondence: Linda P. Spear, Ph.D., Department of Psychology and Center for Developmental Psychobiology, Binghamton University, Box 6000, State University of New York, Binghamton, NY 13902-6000. Phone, 607/777-2825; fax, 607/777-6418; e-mail, lspear@binghamton.edu

controlled studies then gradually emerges that serves to redefine the field, confirming some initial reports, failing to replicate others, and increasing the breadth and age range of the research being conducted. The results of the New York Academy of Sciences' conference summarized in this volume[3] convincingly document that research examining the developmental toxicology of cocaine is now firmly established in this third phase. Although in some respects the consequences of developmental cocaine exposure have been somewhat more subtle than expected, as amply substantiated in this volume,[3] consistent patterns of neurobehavioral findings are beginning to emerge in both clinical studies and experiments with various animal models.

In our work using a rodent model of prenatal cocaine exposure, we have been struck by the remarkable plasticity of the developing nervous system in seemingly compensating for some cocaine-induced perturbations early in life. Yet, there appears to be a cost to this compensation, an increased vulnerability to environmental and cognitive demands and stressors. Interestingly, these themes of increased susceptibility to stressors and vulnerability to the environment have also emerged in studies with clinical populations.[4] This chapter reviews findings from our animal studies showing alterations in cocaine-exposed offspring in their responsiveness to environmental stressors and challenges. In this discussion, we also highlight the intriguing results of a recent preliminary study suggesting that these animals may be differentially sensitive to the effects of an early experience. As a background for this discussion, we first briefly consider the issue of compensatory systems as modulators of the functional expression of early insults.

The cocaine exposure regimen used in the work reported in this chapter consists of chronic exposure of Sprague-Dawley rat dams from gestational days 8–20 via daily subcutaneous injections of 40 mg/kg cocaine, a dose that produces plasma cocaine levels in the high human use range.[5] This exposure paradigm is below threshold for producing maternal toxicity and reducing offspring body weight,[6] but, as outlined below, it is clearly above threshold for inducing neurobehavioral alterations in exposed offspring. In our work litters are typically fostered to untreated surrogate mothers at birth to control for possible residual effects of cocaine exposure on subsequent maternal behavior. Cocaine-exposed offspring are compared with various groups of control offspring; experimenters conducting all tests are unaware of the prenatal treatment group to which the animals are assigned.

COMPENSATORY PROCESSES AND THEIR IMPACT ON EXPRESSION OF COCAINE-RELATED NEUROBEHAVIORAL EFFECTS

Compensatory processes are pervasive in the nervous system, particularly during ontogeny. Without such ongoing microadjustments and compensations occurring normally during the process of development, it is difficult to envision how the multitudes of neurons and their billions of interconnections could be ontogenetically elaborated in a manner that, for the most part, rarely results in conspicuous functional impairments. Following early drug or toxin insults, these pervasive compensatory mechanisms may promote substantial recovery within the compromised systems or realignments within other neural systems to allow for substantial retention or return of some functions.[7] There may be a long-term cost, however, to such neural reorganization: a decrease in adaptability of the organism. That is, although certain behavioral and physiological functions may appear "normal" under basal testing conditions, deficits may become "unmasked" when these rectified neural systems would ordinarily be taxed by stressors and other challenges. (See refs. 7 and 8 for further discussion.)

In terms of prenatal cocaine exposure, we observed in numerous studies that exposed offspring exhibit conditioning deficits along with alterations in dopaminergic (DA) and other neuronal systems when tested during the early postnatal period; some of these alterations appear relatively transient and are less evident when offspring are examined later in life. (See refs. 1 and 9 for review.) In testing conducted in adulthood, exposed offspring do exhibit a decrease in the number of spontaneously active neurons per electrode tract in both the A9 and A10 dopamine (DA) cell body regions.[10] Although these electrophysiological data suggest a rather notable and long-lasting decrease in DA neuronal activity following gestational cocaine exposure, this fundamental alteration in DA activity has proved difficult to detect neurochemically under baseline conditions in adulthood. Our working hypothesis is that neural compensatory processes may mask this fundamental electrophysiologic deficit in the functioning of the DA system under resting conditions. However, when this fundamentally compromised DA system would ordinarily be activated by stressors or other challenges, it may not be able to respond appropriately, resulting in the emergence of behavioral deficits indicative of DA dysfunction. Indeed, when cocaine-exposed offspring are subjected to pharmacologic, cognitive, or stressful challenges in adulthood, they exhibit behavioral alterations reminiscent of those observed after damage to forebrain DA systems. (See refs. 1 and 11 for review.) These alterations include deficits in reversal performance[12] and attenuation in the rewarding efficacy of cocaine[13] as well as alterations in responsivity to stressor.

STRESS RESPONSIVITY

Cocaine-exposed offspring differ behaviorally from control animals in their response to many stressful and environmentally challenging situations. They also appear to be differentially responsive to the effects of early environmental manipulation.

Passive Behavioral Responses to Stress: Immobility

When exposed to a stressful situation such as a forced swim or intermittent footshock, normal adult rats first try to escape. If that is impossible, they typically will exhibit an increase in immobility which may be adaptive in serving to conserve energy. This increase in immobility is seen not only during the stressful circumstance, but also frequently after the stressor when animals are subsequently confronted with a novel but otherwise unstressful situation such as an open field. We[14] and others[15] have shown that adult offspring exposed gestationally to cocaine exhibit markedly less of this immobility response. For instance, FIGURE 1 shows immobility measured during a 5-minute forced swim (FIG. 1a) and in response to intermittent footshocks (FIG. 1b) by offspring of dams exposed to 40 mg/kg cocaine during pregnancy (C40) as well as control dams that were injected with saline solution and pair fed (PF) or were untreated and given free access to lab chow (LC). In both of these situations, C40 offspring exhibited significantly less stress-induced immobility than did control offspring. Twenty-four hours later, when the animals were placed in a novel open field (OF) for 5 minutes, LC and PF animals exposed previously to footshock exhibited a significant increase in OF immobility relative to their nonstressed counterparts. By contrast, prior stressor exposure did not significantly alter OF immobility in C40 offspring (FIG. 1c).

Thus, in several situations (exposure to a forced swim, intermittent footshock, or post-stressor OF testing), cocaine-exposed offspring fail to exhibit elevations in immobility evident in control offspring. Interestingly, this effect appears to be age-dependent. Preweanling offspring exposed prenatally to cocaine conversely exhibit more immobility than do control offspring[16]; by adolescence, the adult-typical pattern of attenuated immobility is evident.[17] Similar ontogenetic reversals in stress-related response measures have been reported after other insults. For instance, Weinberg[18] showed that offspring exposed prenatally to alcohol exhibit suppressed adrenocortical stress responses during the preweanling period, these stress responses being normalized around the time of weaning and enhanced thereafter.

Other Stress-Related Behaviors

It is not the case, however, that all behavioral responses to stressors are affected by prenatal cocaine exposure. For instance, we found no evidence that cocaine-exposed offspring differ from controls in terms of tail-pinch–induced oral behaviors or probe burying (Campbell *et al.*, in preparation). It is not simply passive behavioral responses to stress such as immobility, however, that are altered. As a striking example, consider the following work showing an unusual response of cocaine-exposed offspring to the stress of social competition.

Altered Responsivity to Environmental Demands

As part of our research examining social behavior in offspring exposed gestationally to cocaine,[17,19] we included assessment of social competition in thirsty animals competing for a single water source. Offspring were tested in adolescence in age-matched triads, each triad consisting of one same-sexed offspring from each prenatal treatment group (C40, PF, and LC).[20] Other animals from each prenatal treatment group were tested in adulthood when they competed for water in dyads with an untreated, same sex competitor. During the 5-minute tests conducted daily for 5 days, both adolescent and adult C40 offspring were just as successful as other animals in competing for the sole water source. Surprisingly, however, substantially more adolescent C40 animals developed aggression over the 5 days of this test than did their age-matched control counterparts (FIG. 2a); increased aggression was also evident in male cocaine-exposed animals tested in adulthood (FIG. 2b). Heightened aggression was not evident, however, when cocaine-exposed offspring were tested in less stressful social interaction tests that did not involve the multiple stressors of water deprivation, single housing, and competition for a limited water source.[19] Therefore, it is not simply that cocaine-exposed animals are generally more aggressive, but rather that they appear to be particularly sensitive to environmental demands in the production of this aberrant aggression.

These findings of increased susceptibility to environmental demands are akin to those observed in clinical populations by Mayes.[4] She reported that infants and preschool-aged children exposed gestationally to cocaine exhibit a lower threshold for activation of "stress circuits" when exposed to novel challenges and hence may be particularly vulnerable to the detrimental effects of stressful environmental conditions. She has hypothesized that monoaminergic dysfunction disrupts arousal regulation in these offspring, resulting in overarousal in the face of novel/stressful circumstances and consequent increased vulnerability to stressful conditions. Thus, in addition to the converging clinical and animal data suggesting alterations in stress responsivity in offspring exposed gestationally to cocaine, hypotheses regarding these effects from both our laboratory and the Mayes group[4] have focused on neural dysfunctions in the dopaminergic (and potentially other monoaminergic) systems.

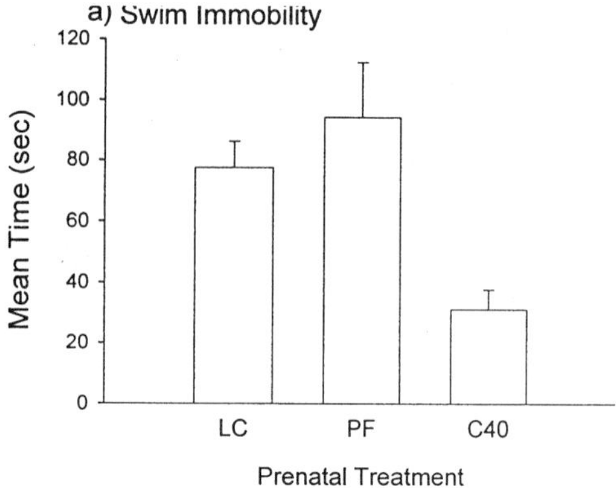

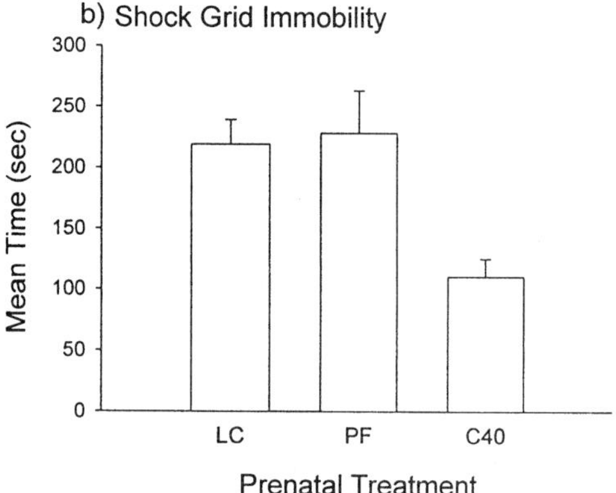

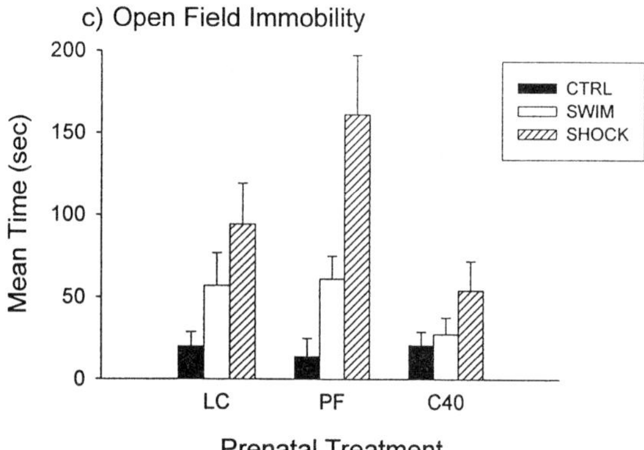

FIGURE 1. *See legend on facing page.*

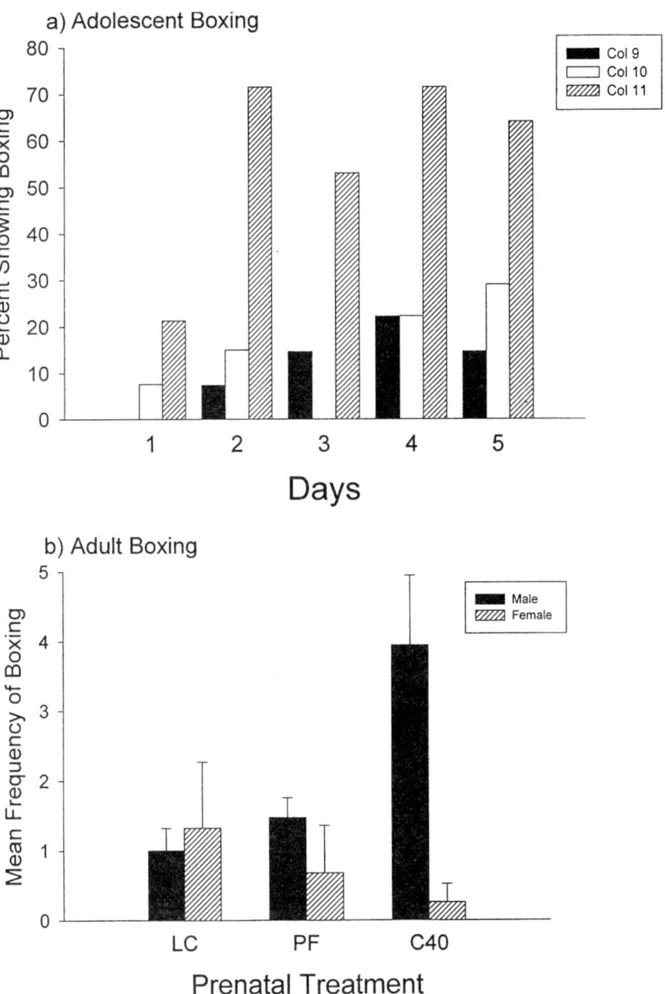

FIGURE 2. **(a)** Percentage of adolescent animals from each of the prenatal treatment groups (LC = nontreated control; PF = pair-fed control; C40 = prenatal cocaine) exhibiting boxing on each of the 5 test days. Data were collapsed across sex, as there were no significant sex differences in this measure. **(b)** Mean frequency of boxing in adult male and female offspring from each of the prenatal treatment groups. Data were collapsed across test day as prenatal treatment did not interact with test day in the analysis of this measure. Error bars indicate SEMs. Data are derived from ref. 20.

←

FIGURE 1. Mean time (in seconds) spent in immobility by animals from each prenatal treatment group examined during **(a)** a 5-minute forced swim test; **(b)** a 10-minute intermittent footshock session (during which animals received 20 1-mA 1-second shocks); and **(c)** a subsequent open field test conducted 24 hours later. Prior to open field testing, animals either were not stressed (CTRL) or were exposed to the forced swim (SWIM) or footshock (SHOCK) sessions. Error bars indicate SEMs. LC = nontreated control; PF = pair-fed control; C40 = prenatal cocaine. Data are derived from ref. 14.

Sensitivity to the Effects of Early Experience

Reminiscent of findings that cocaine-exposed offspring exhibit increased sensitivity to environmental demands, we recently obtained intriguing, although preliminary, data to support the suggestion that cocaine-exposed offspring may also be differentially sensitive to the effects of an early experience. In this study, we examined immobility during intermittent footshock exposure as well as immobility and other behaviors in an open field subsequent to shock exposure in adult cocaine-exposed and control offspring. There were two unusual aspects to this study. First, we attempted to control for nutritional effects using a procedure other than pair-feeding by diluting the diet of a group of nutritional control (NC) dams with cellulose in an attempt to match their food intake to that of C40 dams while avoiding explicit food restriction. Although we were reasonably successful in using this procedure in the past,[21] we were less fortunate in this project. For reasons that are not completely clear, NC neonates weighed notably less (5.37 ± 0.54 g) than C40 (6.86 ± 0.11) and LC (7.15 ± 0.17) pups. Consequently, the NC group in this experiment represents a deprived, stunted group of offspring rather than a nutritional control per se.

The second unusual aspect of this study was that whereas we typically only test animals at one age and do not expose them to longitudinal testing, approximately one half the litters from each prenatal treatment group in this experiment were exposed to early testing. This early test consisted of a noninvasive and presumably minimally stressful study of heart rate (HR) conditioning to a tone at postnatal day (P) 16. In this ongoing project, preweanlings at P16 were given two 20-minute assessments of HR, with the two sessions separated by a 4-hour interval. For each test session, subcutaneous electrodes were attached to the pups, and HR responses to 10 presentations of a 10-second 2,000-Hz pulsating 80-dB tone were measured. Between the two sessions, pups were either returned to the dam and littermates or maintained at 32 ± 1°C in isolation. Due to limitations in sample sizes in this ongoing HR experiment, for the discussion of these findings in adulthood, data were collapsed across test and intersession variables to derive a single subset of animals in each prenatal treatment group exposed to early heart rate testing.

As adults (beginning at P76–81), offspring from each litter were singly housed and placed in one of three treatment groups: chronic footshock exposure (9 consecutive daily 15-minute sessions during each of which animals were given 1-second 1-mA footshocks on a VI 30-second schedule), acute footshock exposure (one 15-minute session of footshock using the same parameters as with the chronic group), and a group not exposed to footshock. On each day of the chronic period, immobility during the footshock sessions was assessed. In addition, 24 hours after the last shock session, animals were tested in a well-illuminated open field for 5 minutes, and several open field measures were assessed.

The results were interesting in several respects. First, in open field testing, there was no evidence of adaptation to the chronic shock. Although animals not exposed to shock differed from shocked animals, no difference was noted between acutely and chronically shocked animals in their open field behavior, with shocked animals exhibiting less locomotion, rearing, and grooming and more immobility than nonshocked animals. These findings differ from our previous work showing adaptation after chronic footshock in LC (but not C40 or PF animals) and may be related to the use of a dimly lit OF in our prior study.[22]

More germane to the present discussion were the interactions observed between prenatal treatment and early experience. Much to our surprise, the pattern of behavioral alterations observed in C40 offspring varied, depending on whether or not the animals were exposed to the early testing experience. For instance, when examining animals not manipulated early in life (see left side of FIG. 3), C40 offspring in adulthood exhibited less shock-induced immobility during the first footshock session than did either LC or the stunted NC offspring, replicating previous findings.[14] Rather surprisingly perhaps, the stunted NC animals behaved like LC control animals in this regard. However, in animals given the early experience of HR testing on P16, no differences were seen among the treatment groups; as can be seen on the right side of FIGURE 3, the behavior of LC and NC animals was not influenced by whether or not they had the early experience, whereas the early experience reversed the reduction in immobility typically seen in C40 offspring.

This effect, although significant, was not large and might have gone relatively unnoticed, except that similar findings were obtained in open field testing. Among animals not exposed to the early experience, the C40 and the NC groups both exhibited significantly less OF immobility than did LC control offspring (left side of FIG. 4). No such reductions are seen in animals given the early experience (right side of FIG. 4); the early experience normalized the amount of immobility seen in the stunted NC animals and significantly *increased* the amount of immobility exhibited by the cocaine offspring. Thus, the nature of the alterations observed in these adult cocaine-exposed offspring varied depending on whether or not they had received the early experience.

A similar response pattern was seen when other response measures were examined. For example, in terms of OF locomotion (FIG. 5), among animals not exposed to the early experience, both C40 and NC animals exhibited significantly more forward locomotion than did LC animals. This hyperactivity was no longer evident in the NC animals that had received the early experience and was actually *reversed* in C40 animals, with cocaine-exposed animals that received the early manipulation being significantly less active than LC and NC control animals and than C40 animals not receiving the early experience.

Thus, in two different testing situations and with several behavioral measures, the long-term outcome of prenatal cocaine exposure was found to be notably altered by an

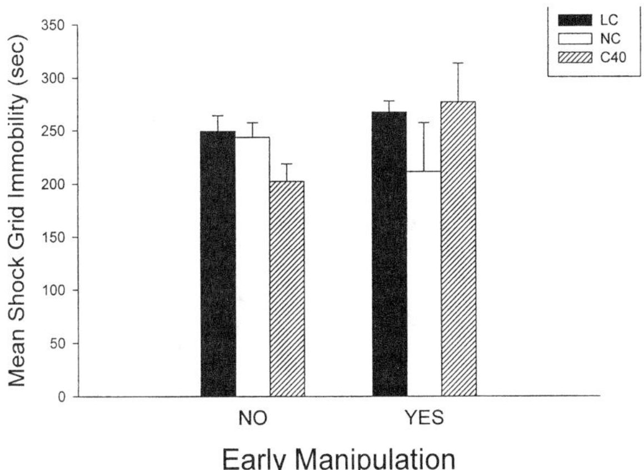

FIGURE 3. Mean duration (in seconds) of immobility displayed during the first footshock session by adult animals from each of the prenatal treatment groups (LC = nontreated control; NC = stunted nutritional control; C40 = prenatal cocaine) as a function of whether they experienced the preweanling manipulation (heart rate testing on P16). Error bars indicate SEMs.

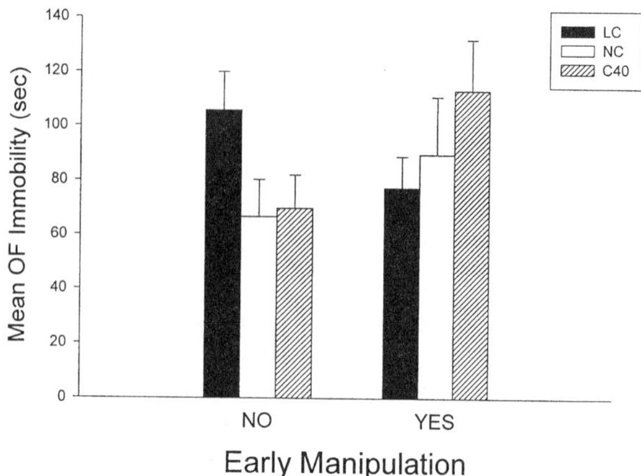

FIGURE 4. Mean duration (in seconds) of immobility displayed in the open field 24 hours after footshock exposure by adult animals from each of the prenatal treatment groups (LC = non-treated control; NC = stunted nutritional control; C40 = prenatal cocaine) as a function of whether they experienced the preweanling manipulation (heart rate testing on P16). Error bars indicate SEMs.

acute manipulation early in life that seemed to have less pronounced effects on LC control and perhaps even stunted NC animals. Early experience during the preweanling period was previously shown to have long-lasting consequences on neurobehavioral function (see, for example, refs. 23 and 24) and to modify adverse behavioral outcomes associated with prenatal stress[25] or prenatal exposure to ethanol.[26] We are currently pur-

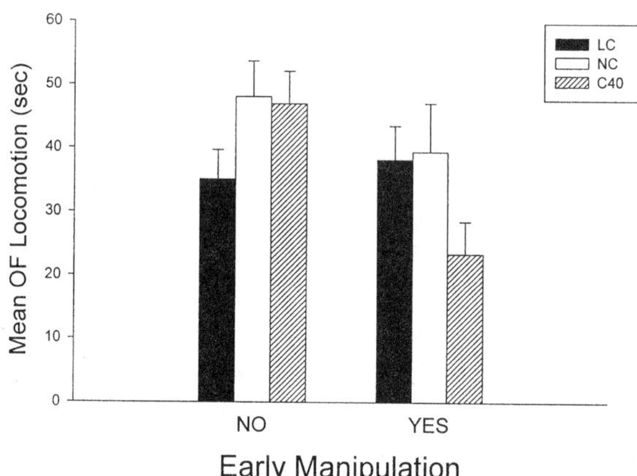

FIGURE 5. Mean duration (in seconds) of locomotion displayed in the open field 24 hours after footshock exposure by adult animals from each of the prenatal treatment groups (LC = non-treated control; NC = stunted nutritional control; C40 = prenatal cocaine) as a function of whether they experienced the preweanling manipulation (heart rate testing on P16). Error bars indicate SEMs.

suing these intriguing findings by using a more traditional early experience (handling) that has been well characterized in terms of its long-term behavioral, physiologic, and hormonal consequences (see, for example, refs. 27 and 28). Eventually, work of this nature may provide an important complement to preliminary clinical studies suggesting that developmentally supportive environments may promote age-appropriate developmental skills in substance-exposed infants.[29]

COMMENTS ON PAIR-FEEDING AND OTHER NUTRITIONAL CONTROL PROCEDURES

In our examinations of stress responsivity, we have become increasingly perplexed about appropriate controls for nutritional effects. Food restriction such as that associated with pair-feeding and other forms of nutritional restriction is a known stressor,[30] and there is ample evidence that prenatal stress induces neurobehavioral teratogenic effects (see, for example, refs. 31–33). Given that stress selectively stimulates many of the same neural regions as does cocaine (e.g., mesocortical and mesolimbic DA terminal regions[34]), pair-feeding during the prenatal period might be expected to elicit similar consequences in some respects to those of prenatal cocaine exposure. However, prenatal malnutrition has been reported to produce effects that are different from, and not interacting with, those associated with prenatal cocaine exposure per se.[35] Indeed, in several dozen of our early investigations of prenatal cocaine, we found pair-feeding and other nutritional controls to have little impact on neurobehavioral functioning. Only when we began to include assessments of stress responsivity did PF and NC effects sometimes begin to emerge; however, these effects were not always in the same direction or of the same magnitude as were effects observed in C40 offspring (e.g., see previous section on Early Experience). This sensitivity of measures of stress responsivity to pair-feeding effects perhaps should not be surprising, in that alterations in later responsivity to stressors are a particular hallmark of the consequences of prenatal stressors (see, for example, refs. 32, 33, and 36).

We have not yet resolved this nutritional control issue to our satisfaction. On the one hand, when conducting follow-up experiments using dependent measures in which there is a substantial prior database showing that prenatal cocaine effects are unrelated to nutritional consequences of the drug exposure, we have begun to question whether the automatic inclusion of PF or other nutritional controls is justified in terms of cost and animal use. On the other hand, when prenatal stressors are known to influence the dependent measures under examination, positive results in nutritional control offspring are difficult to interpret and could reflect either the nutritional consequences of the diet per se or the stressful nature of the associated dietary restriction. This makes it difficult to interpret findings in the situation when similar results are seen in cocaine-exposed and nutritional control offspring, which rather defeats the purpose associated with inclusion of pair-fed or other nutritional controls. Thus, whereas inclusion of pair-fed controls is often considered *de rigueur* when designing studies of developmental toxicants, we are beginning to reassess the implications associated with the routine and unvarying use of this control procedure.

SUMMARY AND CONCLUSIONS

In many respects we found that cocaine-exposed offspring differ from controls in their response to environmental demands and stressors. They exhibit characteristic alterations in stress-induced immobility that are seen in a number of test situations and that undergo ontogenetic reversal. Increases in aggression are also seen under the demands of social competition, and these offspring may also be differentially sensitive to the effects of early experience. Taken together, these findings reinforce our working hypothesis that prenatal cocaine exposure may be associated with increased vulnerability of exposed offspring to environmental stressors and demands in the production of abnormal behavior; similar conclusions have also been reached in longitudinal studies in clinical populations.[4] Whether or not these offspring are also particularly sensitive to early experience effects is an intriguing question that, although supported by initial work, needs to be examined further. In ongoing work with cocaine-exposed offspring examining other stressor responses, the impact of early experiences on such behavioral expression, and the physiologic substrates underlying this altered responsivity, we will continue to weigh various strategies for addressing nutritional control issues.

This theme of increased vulnerability to stressors and other challenges as a long-term consequence of early insults is not specific to cocaine, but it is one that has emerged following a variety of early insults such as prenatal exposure to alcohol[37] or diazepam[38] and early postnatal stress.[39] The presence of these common vulnerabilities does not imply that the neural systems affected by these different insults would necessarily be the same. Numerous neural systems modulate the organism's response to stressors and other challenges, and insult-induced compensations in any of them could decrease the capacity of those systems to mount an adequate response to later challenges. Thus, although the specific neural systems involved may vary with the insult, any of a variety of early insults may elicit compensatory processes, with the net result of increased vulnerability of the organism to later stressors and other challenges.

Prenatal cocaine exposure appears to be but one of many such risk factors to which children reared in adverse circumstances may be exposed. Although adverse sociocultural difficulties may exacerbate the effects (i.e., increase the magnitude of the "signal") resulting from prenatal cocaine exposure, these adversities also may increase the strength of the "noise," reducing the likelihood of detection of a significant effect attributable specifically to this or any other particular risk factor. (See ref. 40, for an enlightening discussion of this issue with regard to early lead exposure, and also ref. 41.) The interaction of various risk and protective factors in the production of increased vulnerability to later challenges and stressors remains an important issue for future research with both clinical populations and laboratory animal studies to explore toxicant/environment interactions.

ACKNOWLEDGMENT

Our thanks to Patricia Heebner for her assistance in the preparation of this manuscript.

REFERENCES

1. Spear, L. P. 1995. Alterations in cognitive function following prenatal cocaine exposure: Studies in an animal model. *In* Mothers, Babies and Cocaine: The Role of Toxins in Development. M. Lewis & M. Bendersky, Eds.: 207–227. Lawrence Erlbaum Associates. Hillsdale, NJ.
2. Mayes, L. C., R. H. Granger, M. H. Bornstein & B. Zuckerman. 1992. The problem of prenatal cocaine exposure: A rush to judgment. J. Am. Med. Assoc. **267:** 406–408.
3. Harvey, J. A. & B. E. Kosofsky. 1998. Cocaine: Effects on the Developing Brain. Ann. N.Y. Acad. Sci. This volume.

4. MAYES, L. C., C. GRILLON, R. GRANGER & R. SCHOTTENFELD. 1998. Regulation of arousal and attention in preschool children exposed to cocaine prenatally. *In* Cocaine: Effects on the Developing Brain. J. A. Harvey & B. E. Kosofsky, Eds. Ann. N.Y. Acad. Sci. This volume.
5. SPEAR, L. P., N. A. FRAMBES & C. L. KIRSTEIN. 1989. Fetal and maternal brain and plasma levels of cocaine and benzoylecgonine following chronic subcutaneous administration of cocaine during gestation in rats. Psychopharmacology **97:** 427–431.
6. SPEAR, L. P. & C. J. HEYSER. 1992. Cocaine and the developing nervous system: Laboratory findings. *In* Maternal Substance Abuse and the Developing Nervous System. T. A. Slotkin & I. S. Zagon, Eds.: 155–175. Academic Press. Orlando, FL.
7. HUGHES, J. A. & S. B. SPARBER. 1978. D-Amphetamine unmasks postnatal consequences of exposure to methylmercury in utero: Methods for studying behavioral teratogenesis. Pharmacol. Biochem. Behav. **8:** 365–375.
8. SPEAR, L. P. 1997. Neurobehavioral abnormalities following exposure to drugs of abuse during development. *In* Drug Addiction and its Treatment: Nexus of Neuroscience and Behavior. B. A. Johnson & J. D. Roache, Eds.: 233–255. Lippincott-Raven Publishers. Philadelphia, PA.
9. SPEAR, L. P. 1996. Neurobehavioral consequences of gestational cocaine exposure: Studies using a rodent model. *In* Prenatal Cocaine Exposure. R. J. Konkol & G. D. Olsen, Eds.: 169–181. CRC Press, Inc. Boca Raton, FL.
10. MINABE, Y., C. R. ASHBY, JR., C. HEYSER, L. P. SPEAR & R. Y. WANG. 1989. The effects of prenatal cocaine exposure on spontaneously active midbrain dopamine neurons in adult male offspring: An electrophysiological study. Brain Res. **586:** 152–156.
11. SPEAR, L. P. 1996. Assessment of the effects of developmental toxicants: Pharmacological and stress vulnerability of offspring. *In* Behavioral Studies of Drug-Exposed Offspring: Methodological Issues in Human and Animal Research. C. L. Wetherington, V. L. Smeriglio & L. P. Finnegan, Eds.: 125–145. NIDA Research Monograph 164.
12. HEYSER, C. J., N. E. SPEAR & L. P. SPEAR. 1992. Effects of prenatal exposure to cocaine on conditional discrimination learning in adult rats. Behav. Neurosci. **106:** 837–845.
13. HECHT, G. S., N. E. SPEAR & L. P. SPEAR. 1998. Alterations in the reinforcing efficacy of cocaine in adult rats following prenatal exposure to cocaine. Behav. Neurosci. In press.
14. MOLINA, V. A., J. M. WAGNER & L. P. SPEAR. 1994. The behavioral response to stress is altered in adult rats exposed prenatally to cocaine. Physiol. Behav. **55:** 941–945.
15. BILITZKE, P. J. & M. W. CHURCH. 1992. Prenatal cocaine and alcohol exposures affect rat behavior in a stress test (the Porsolt Swim Test). Neurotoxicol. Teratol. **14:** 359–364.
16. GOODWIN, G. A., T. BLIVEN, C. KUHN, R. FRANCIS & L. P. SPEAR. 1997. Immediate early gene expression to examine neuronal activity following acute and chronic stressors in rat pups: Examination of neurophysiological alterations underlying behavioral consequences of prenatal cocaine exposure. Physiol. Behav. **61:** 895–902.
17. WOOD, R. D., V. A. MOLINA, J. M. WAGNER & L. P. SPEAR. 1995. Play behavior and stress responsivity in periadolescent offspring exposed prenatally to cocaine. Pharmacol. Biochem. Behav. **52:** 367–374.
18. WEINBERG, J. 1993. Neuroendocrine effects of prenatal alcohol exposure. Ann. N.Y. Acad. Sci. **697:** 86–96.
19. WOOD, R. D. 1996. Prenatal Cocaine and Social Behaviors Over Ontogeny. Ph.D. thesis, Binghamton University, New York.
20. WOOD, R. D. & L. P. SPEAR. 1998. Prenatal cocaine alters social competition of infant, adolescent and adult rats. Behav. Neurosci. In press.
21. SPEAR, L. P. & C. J. HEYSER. 1993. Is use of cellulose-diluted diet a viable alternative to pair-feeding? Neurotoxicol. Teratol. **15:** 85–89.
22. CAMPBELL, J., T. BLIVEN, M. SILVERI, K. SNYDER & L. P. SPEAR. 1996. Effects of prenatal cocaine on later behavioral adaptations to chronic stressors (abstr.). International Behavioral Neuroscience Society. Cancun, Mexico.
23. MEANEY, M. J., D. H. AITKEN, C. VAN BERKEL, S. BHATNAGAR & R. M. SAPOLSKY. 1988. Effect of neonatal handling on age-related impairments associated with the hippocampus. Science **239:** 766–768.
24. CHEVINS, P. F. D. 1990. Early environmental influences on fear and defence in rodents. *In*

Fear and Defence (Ettore Majorana International Life Sciences Series, Vol. 8). P. F. Brain, S. Parmigiani, R. J. Blanchard & D. Mainardi, Eds.: 269–288. Harwood Academic Publications. London.

25. Wakshlak, A. & M. Weinstock. 1990. Neonatal handling reverses behavioral abnormalities induced in rats by prenatal stress. Physiol. Behav. **48:** 289–292.
26. Weinberg, J., C. K. Kim & W. Yu. 1995. Early handling can attenuate adverse effects of fetal ethanol exposure. Alcohol **12:** 317–327.
27. Meaney, M. J., D. H. Aitken, V. Viau, S. Sharma & A. Sarrieau. 1989. Neonatal handling alters adrenocortical negative feedback sensitivity and hippocampal type II glucocorticoid receptor binding in the rat. Neuroendocrinology **50:** 597–604.
28. Costela, C., P. Tejedor-Real, J. A. Mico & J. Gibert-Rahola. 1995. Effect of neonatal handling on learned helplessness model of depression. Physiol. Behav. **57:** 407–410.
29. Hofkosh, D., J. L. Pringle, H. P. Wald, J. Switala, S. A. Hinderliter & S. C. Hamel. 1995. Early interactions between drug-involved mothers and infants: Within-group differences. Arch. Pediatr. Adolesc. Med. **149:** 665–672.
30. Weinberg, J., T. B. Sonderegger & I. J. Chasnoff. 1992. Methodological issues: Laboratory animal studies of perinatal exposure to alcohol or drugs and human studies of drug use during pregnancy. *In* Perinatal Substance Abuse. T. B. Sonderegger, Ed.: 13–20. The Johns Hopkins University Press. Baltimore, MD.
31. Ward, I. L. 1984. The prenatal stress syndrome: Current status. Psychoneuroendocrinology **9:** 3–11.
32. Deminière, J. M., P. V. Piazza, G. Guegan, N. Abrous, S. Maccari, M. Le Moal & H. Simon. 1992. Increased locomotor response to novelty and propensity to intravenous amphetamine self-administration in adult offspring of stressed mothers. Brain Res. **586:** 135–139.
33. Takahashi, L. K., J. G. Turner & N. H. Kalin. 1992. Prenatal stress alters brain catecholaminergic activity and potentiates stress-induced behavior in adult rats. Brain Res. **574:** 131–137.
34. Dunn, A. J. & N. R. Kramarcy. 1984. Neurochemical responses in stress: Relationships between the hypothalamic-pituitary-adrenal and catecholamine systems. *In* Handbook of Psychopharmacology, Vol. 18. L. L. Iversen, S. D. Iversen & S. H. Snyder, Eds.: 455–515. Plenum Publishing Corporation. New York, NY.
35. Galler, J. R. 1998. Prenatal exposure to cocaine and malnutrition in a rat model: Developmental consequences. *In* Cocaine: Effects on the Developing Brain. J. A. Harvey & B. E. Kosofsky, Eds. Ann. N.Y. Acad. Sci. This volume.
36. Henry, C., M. Kabbaj, H. Simon, M. Le Moal & S. Maccari. 1994. Prenatal stress increases the hypothalamo-pituitary-adrenal axis response in young and adult rats. J. Neuroendocrinol. **6:** 341–345.
37. Riley, E. P. 1990. The long-term behavioral effects of prenatal alcohol exposure in rats. Alcohol Clin. Exp. Res. **14:** 670–673.
38. Kellogg, C. K. 1991. Postnatal effects of prenatal exposure to psychoactive drugs. Pre-Post-Natal Psychol. **5:** 233–251.
39. Cabib, S., S. Puglisi-Allegra & F. R. D'Amato. 1993. Effects of postnatal stress on dopamine mesolimbic system responses to aversive experiences in adult life. Brain Res. **604:** 232–239.
40. Bellinger, D. C. 1995. Interpreting the literature on lead and child development: The neglected role of the "Experimental System." Neurotoxicol. Teratol. **17:** 201–212.
41. Koren, G. 1998. The Toronto adoption study after *in utero* cocaine exposure: Biological markers of intrauterine cocaine exposure. *In* Cocaine: Effects on the Developing Brain. J. A. Harvey & B. E. Kosofsky, Eds. Ann. N.Y. Acad. Sci. This volume.

Prenatal Cocaine Exposure: Long-Term Deficits in Learning and Motor Performance[a]

ANTHONY G. ROMANO[b] AND JOHN A. HARVEY

Department of Pharmacology, Allegheny University of the Health Sciences, Philadelphia, Pennsylvania 19129, USA

ABSTRACT: We have developed a rabbit model of *in utero* exposure to intravenous injections of cocaine given twice daily to dams from gestational days 8–29. At the doses employed (4 mg/kg, injected twice daily), no differences were found in the body weight gain of dams, time to delivery, litter size, and body weight or other physical characteristics of the offspring. However, cocaine-exposed pups displayed an abnormal structural and neurochemical development of the anterior cingulate cortex which persisted into adulthood. In agreement with the known functions of the anterior cingulate cortex, we found that adult, sexually mature rabbits, exposed to cocaine prenatally, demonstrate impairments in motor function, alterations in associative learning and severe impairments in discrimination learning. Moreover, the alterations in discrimination learning were interpreted to be due to deficits in attentional processes. Specifically, cocaine progeny preferentially attend to more salient stimuli even when these are not relevant to the task. Consequently they have difficulty in attending to less salient but relevant stimuli when more salient but irrelevant stimuli occur in the same context. We concluded that the learning deficits are a reflection of the morphologic and neurochemical abnormalities of the anterior cingulate cortex. Alterations in dopamine function of the caudate nucleus may also contribute to the deficits in motor performance.

INTRODUCTION

For the last several years, a group of us at Allegheny University of the Health Sciences have documented the long-term neuroanatomical, neurochemical, and behavioral consequences of prenatal cocaine exposure in rabbits.[1,2] This chapter focuses on some of the long-term behavioral consequences of prenatal cocaine exposure in the rabbit model. Additional behavioral and CNS effects in the rabbit model are described by our colleagues elsewhere in this volume.[3–6]

RABBIT MODEL FOR PRENATAL EXPOSURE TO COCAINE

Selection of the Rabbit

The rabbit was chosen for these studies for a variety of reasons: (1) the sensitivity of the rabbit to the behavioral effects of various drugs which is similar to that of humans[7,8]; (2) the ease of performing multiple drug injections via the marginal ear vein and thus mimicking the pharmacokinetics of smoking "crack" cocaine, the primary

[a] This research was supported by a National Institutes of Health grant from the National Institute on Drug Abuse (DA11164-01).

[b] Address for correspondence: Anthony G. Romano, Department of Pharmacology, Allegheny University of the Health Sciences, 3200 Henry Avenue, Philadelphia, PA 19129.

route of administration by pregnant women[9]; (3) the history of the rabbit as a model of behavioral teratology following drug treatment[7,10–12]; (4) the metabolism by the rabbit of dopamine, the neurotransmitter through which cocaine is believed to act, in a similar manner to that in humans and other primates[13]; (5) the exhibition by rabbits of patterns of brain development and growth that parallel those of humans[11,14]; and (6) classical conditioning of the rabbit's nictitating membrane (NM) response exhibiting all of the cognitive processes that have been observed in humans.[8,15]

Treatment Protocol

TABLE 1 summarizes the treatment protocol for breeding and the drug injection procedure. Saline or cocaine injections began 8 days after breeding, at the time of implantation. This delay was used because cocaine is known to inhibit mating-induced ovulation in the rabbit[16] while having no effect on implantation.[17] Two injections of cocaine (4 mg/kg each) were administered daily for a total daily dose of 8 mg/kg. Injections were ended on gestational day 29 and normal delivery took place on days 30–31. With these procedures, no significant or consistent differences were noted between cocaine- and saline-injected dams in body weight gain or in the duration of pregnancy.[1] There were also no detectable effects of prenatal exposure to cocaine on: (1) litter size; (2) ratio of male to female births; (3) brain or body weights of the kits at birth or during subsequent postnatal development; (4) frequency of birth abnormalities; or (5) any other grossly observable physical characteristics.

Developmental Abnormalities of the Anterior Cingulate Cortex in Cocaine Progeny

Although prenatal cocaine exposure produced no gross teratologic effects in the rabbit, our group noted permanent developmental abnormalities in the anterior cingulate cortex that could be observed from birth up to the greatest age tested, 144 days after birth. These long-term morphologic and neurochemical effects of cocaine on the development of the anterior cingulate cortex are summarized in TABLE 2. Further details can be found elsewhere.[2,3,5]

Behavioral Functions of the Anterior Cingulate Cortex

There is an extensive literature on the behavioral functions of the anterior cingulate cortex and associated structures. Lesion studies in rodents[18], rabbits,[19–22] cats,[23]

TABLE 1. Protocol for Breeding of Dutch Belted Rabbits[a]

Gestational/ Postnatal Days		Protocol
Gestational day	0	Proven breeders are mated using natural breeding methods
Gestational day	8	Intravenous cocaine or saline injections (twice a day) begin
Gestational day	29	Last injection day
Gestational day	30–31	Kits are born. Birthday is considered to be postnatal day 0
Postnatal day	56	Kits are weaned and housed one per cage
Postnatal day	90–144	Behavioral testing begins

[a]For further details see Murphy *et al.*[1]

TABLE 2. Permanent Abnormalities of the Anterior Cingulate Cortex in Rabbits Prenatally Exposed to Cocaine[a]

- Anomalous neuronal development: dendrites of pyramidal neurons in layers III and V are 30–50% longer than those in controls[2,72]
- Increased number of GABA-immunoreactive cells in the cytoplasm of cortical interneurons[73]
- Lamina specific downregulation of mRNAs that encode the α_1 and β_2 subunits of the heteromeric $GABA_A$ receptor, suggesting that there has been a lamina-specific downregulation of $GABA_A$ receptors[74]
- Increased parvalbumin immunostaining in secondary and tertiary dendrites of a subset of GABA interneurons[75]
- Reduced D_1 DA receptor-Gi protein coupling[3,69,70]

[a]For further details see Levitt *et al.*[2]

nonhuman primates,[18] and humans[18,19,24] have clearly demonstrated that prefrontal cortex lesions or more restricted damage to the anterior cingulate cortex results in impairments in associative learning, attentional processes, and motor function. Supporting these findings are studies in normal rabbits demonstrating that neurons in the anterior cingulate cortex begin to respond differentially to a CS+ and CS– just prior to the acquisition of a discrimination, a task requiring attentional focus.[19,25,26] Similarly, in humans, imaging studies have demonstrated robust activation of the anterior cingulate cortex during the performance of tasks that provide measures of attentional processes such as the Stroop attentional conflict task,[27] a noun-verb conflict task,[28] or a stimulus change detection task.[29] These observations led us to examine the possibility that the morphologic and neurochemical abnormalities in the anterior cingulate cortex of rabbits exposed prenatally to cocaine might have a functional relevance for tasks involving measures of associative learning, attentional processes, and motor function.

LONG-TERM EFFECTS OF PRENATAL COCAINE ON LEARNING IN THE RABBIT

Alterations in Associative Learning

The first set of experiments was concerned with the effects of prenatal cocaine on associative learning as measured by the rate of acquisition of the rabbit's classically conditioned nictitating NM response.[30] Rabbits were trained using both a 75-dB tone conditioned stimulus (CS) and a flashing houselight CS. Each CS was paired with a corneal air puff unconditioned stimulus (US) for a total of 30 pairings in each of 10 daily sessions. The rate of acquisition to each of the two conditioned stimuli is shown in FIGURE 1. Note that both saline and cocaine progeny showed a faster rate of conditioned response (CR) acquisition to the tone CS compared to the light CS. By convention, this difference in the rate of learning given different conditioned stimuli has been attributed to differences in stimulus salience. The CS associated with the faster rate of conditioning (in this case, the tone) is said to be the more salient of the two. Analysis of the data depicted in FIGURE 1 showed that cocaine offspring learned significantly faster than did saline offspring when rate of learning was assessed in the presence of the more salient, tone CS, whereas no difference was noted in the rate of CR acquisition to the less salient light CS.

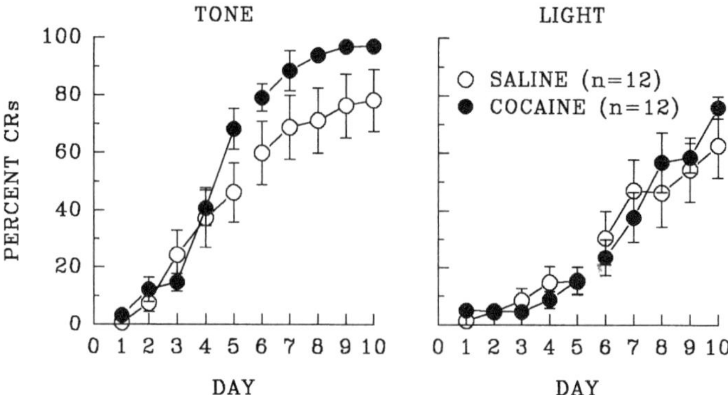

FIGURE 1. Conditioned response (CR) acquisition to tone and light conditioned stimuli (CSs). Data are presented as mean percentage of CRs to each of the two conditioned stimuli. Cocaine progeny acquired CRs to the salient tone CS significantly faster than did saline progeny. (Reprinted with permission from Romano *et al.*[30])

Absence of Effects on Nonassociative Learning

A number of nonassociative factors could have contributed to the accelerated rate of learning we observed in the previous experiment. For example, sensitized or pseudoconditioned responding in the presence of the tone may have contributed to the increased frequency of responding. The traditional control procedure for assessing these nonassociative influences in classical conditioning experiments is to assess the effects of unpaired CS and unconditioned stimulus (US) presentations on responding.[15] We examined the effects of unpaired CS and US presentations in two more groups of saline and cocaine offspring. Cocaine and saline animals were not significantly different from each other with respect to baseline response frequency, as shown in the top panel of FIGURE 2, neither did the two groups differ with respect to nonassociative responding in the presence of the light CS, as shown in the middle panel. More importantly, nonassociative responding in the presence of the tone, shown in the bottom panel, was unaffected by prenatal cocaine exposure.

Absence of Effects on Auditory Conditioned Stimulus Processing

The results of the unpaired procedure led us to conclude that the accelerated rate of acquisition to the tone CS could not be attributed to an increase in nonassociative responding. It was possible, however, that prenatal cocaine exposure had affected sensory processing of the tone CS, effectively increasing the animal's sensitivity to auditory stimuli. If so, then the intensive properties of the CS would be increased, leading to a faster rate of acquisition, and the function relating the frequency of CRs to tone CS intensity should also be altered. That is, cocaine offspring would be expected to exhibit more frequent CRs at lower CS intensities than would saline offspring.

To test the possibility that the intensive properties of the tone CS had been altered in cocaine animals, we assessed the CR frequency/CS intensity function in cocaine and saline animals previously trained using a 90-dB CS. Because asymptotic performance levels would be influenced by the different rates of learning in cocaine and saline animals, we trained the two groups of offspring to a common acquisition criterion of 80% CRs in a single session. As shown in FIGURE 3, cocaine offspring again showed an accelerated rate of acquisition. Cocaine animals required significantly fewer trials to achieve learning criteria of 5 and 10 consecutive CRs as compared to saline offspring. On average, cocaine animals required between 35 and 40 fewer trials to achieve these criteria than did saline offspring. However, because we restricted the amount of training each animal received, there was no difference in asymptotic performance; both groups responded at an average of 89% CRs the day before CS intensity testing was conducted.

FIGURE 4 shows the percentage of CRs as a function of CS intensity for both groups of animals. CS intensity was varied between 50 and 90 dB, and each intensity was presented a total of 10 times. As expected, CR frequency was a direct function of CS intensity. However, prenatal cocaine exposure failed to shift or otherwise alter that function. At 50 dB, responding for both groups was indistinguishable from the baseline rate obtained at 0 dB, and conditioned responding increased to nearly 100% at the 90-dB tone.

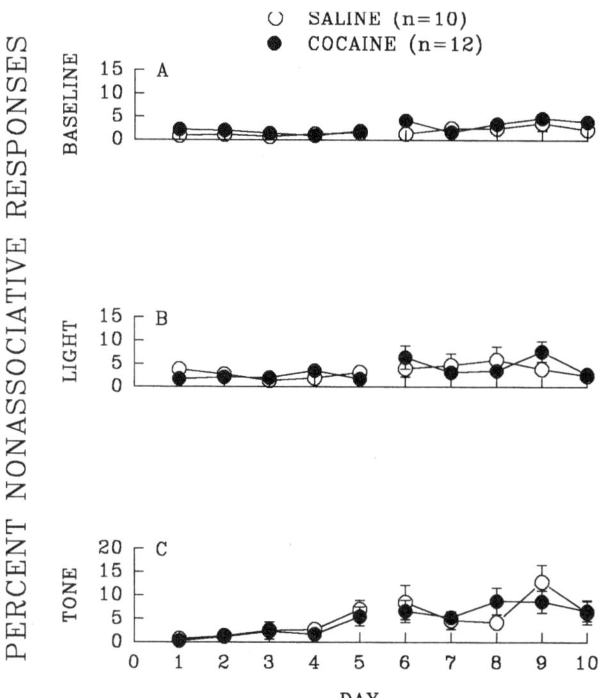

FIGURE 2. Responding during unpaired presentations of tone and light CSs and air puff unconditioned stimulus (US). Data are presented for baseline responding during the 800 ms preceding US onset **(A)**, and responding during the 800 ms presentations of the light **(B)** and tone **(C)** stimuli. There were no significant differences between cocaine and saline progeny on any measure of nonassociative responding. (Reprinted with permission from Romano *et al.*[30])

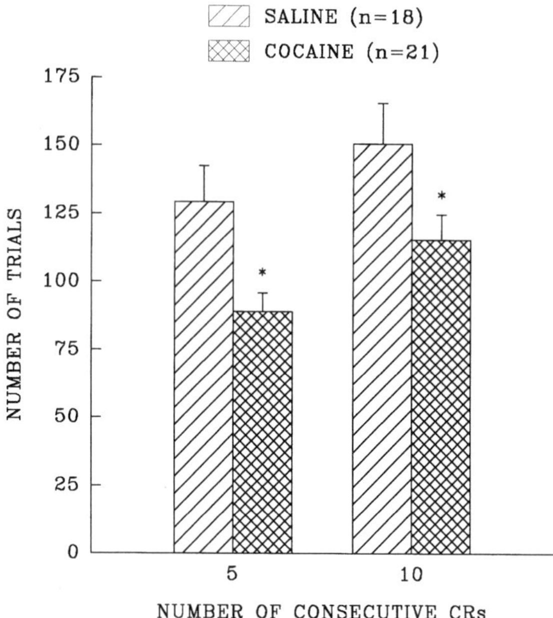

FIGURE 3. Rate of criterion CR acquisition to a tone CS expressed as the mean number of trials required to reach criteria of 5 or 10 consecutive CRs. *Asterisk* denotes a significant difference between the two groups with cocaine progeny showing the faster rate of learning. (Reprinted with permission from Romano *et al.*[30])

Alterations in Associative Learning Are Related to Attentional Processing

The results of these studies confirmed our hypothesis that prenatal exposure to cocaine would have functional consequences on the acquisition of CRs. Adult rabbits that had been exposed to cocaine prenatally acquired CRs to a tone CS at an accelerated rate and achieved higher asymptotic levels of responding than did saline-exposed animals. The effect of prenatal exposure to cocaine was not due to some general effect on learning, because acquisition of CRs to a light CS was not affected. The accelerated rate of CR acquisition to the tone CS exhibited by cocaine-exposed rabbits represented an increase in associative learning, because a control experiment involving unpaired presentations of the CSs and US indicated that no increase occurred in nonassociative responding to the tone. Furthermore, the accelerated rate of CR acquisition to the tone CS by cocaine-exposed rabbits did not appear to be due to alterations in the sensory properties of the tone CS, because both cocaine- and saline-exposed rabbits demonstrated similar psychophysical functions relating CR frequency to tone CS intensity. The fact that prenatal exposure to cocaine had no effect on the intensive properties of the tone CS, and the absence of any general effect on learning, suggests that the accelerated rate of CR acquisition in cocaine-exposed offspring was due to an alteration in attentional processing which is most evident when particularly salient stimuli are employed as CSs. Thus, an alteration in attentional processing of the salient tone CS could account for the more rapid entry of the tone CS into associative learning.

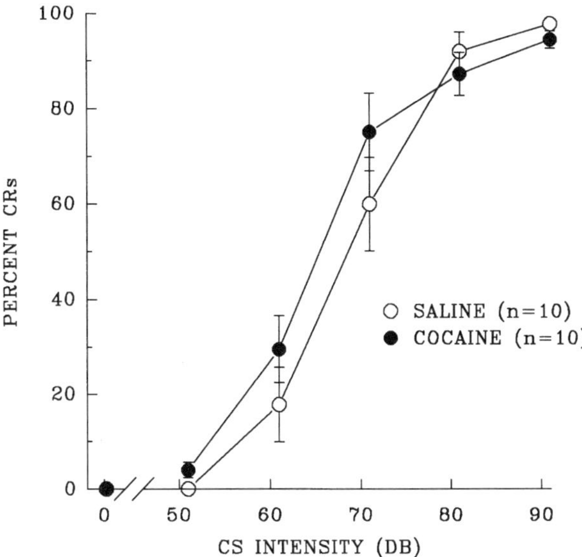

FIGURE 4. Function relating the frequency of conditioned responding to the intensity of the tone CS following asymptotic learning. Cocaine and saline progeny were not significantly different from each other in this assessment of auditory processing. (Reprinted with permission from Romano *et al.*[30])

In summary, our results at this point indicated that prenatal exposure to cocaine produced a modality-specific acceleration of classical conditioning which could not be attributed to an increase in nonassociative responding or to an alteration in the intensive properties of the auditory stimulus. Given these results, we hypothesized that prenatal cocaine exposure was affecting attentional processing, and it was the alteration in attentional processing which led to an accelerated rate of associative learning.

Discrimination Learning

To test our hypothesis that prenatal exposure to cocaine had affected attentional processing, we turned to discrimination learning tasks. These are tasks in which attentional processing plays a more critical role than that in simple acquisition of the CR. In the simplest discrimination learning task, two CSs are employed. One CS, designated the CS+, is consistently paired with the US, whereas the other CS, designated the CS–, is never paired with the US. A commonly held view of discrimination learning is that successful discrimination involves learning to attend and respond to the CS+ and learning to ignore and not respond to the CS–.[31] If attentional processing is altered as a consequence of prenatal cocaine exposure, then we would expect to see some alteration in discrimination learning as well.

Cross-modal discrimination: Salient CS+. The first discrimination task we examined involved the same tone and flashing light we used for simple acquisition.[32] For the present experiment, animals were trained with the relatively salient tone as the CS+ and

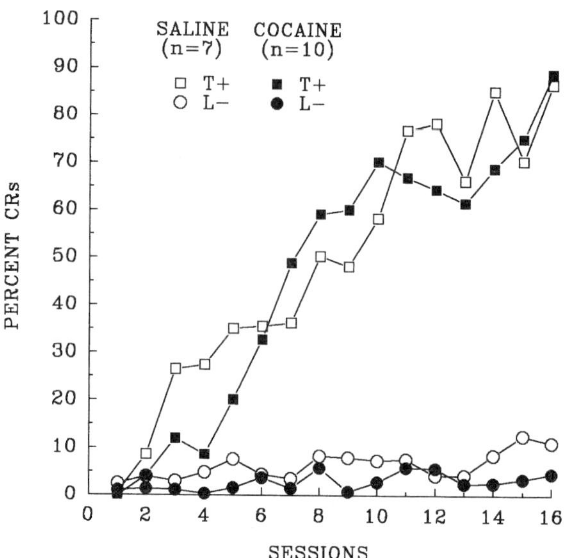

FIGURE 5. Percentages of discriminative responses to tone as a CS+ (T+) and light as a CS− (L−). The performance of cocaine progeny was normalized in the presence of the salient tone CS+ compared to FIGURE 1. (Reprinted with permission from Romano & Harvey.[32])

the less salient light as the CS–. Recall that relative salience of the tone and light was established in the first experiment we described above; in that experiment, CR acquisition was faster using the tone CS compared to the light CS regardless of prenatal condition. FIGURE 5 shows the results of the tone CS+/light CS– discrimination training procedure. Note that the rate of CR acquisition to the tone CS+ in this task was somewhat slower than it was when both tones and lights were paired with the US (FIG. 1). In that experiment, saline animals were responding at about 80% to the tone CS+ after 10 days of training, whereas saline animals in the present study are responding on about 60% of the tone CS+ trials after 10 days. Although the additional attentional demands in this task slowed the rate of learning for both groups, that effect was more pronounced in the cocaine offspring. Thus, it appears that the performance of cocaine animals was normalized when the task involved a salient CS+ and less salient CS–. Now instead of showing more rapid acquisition than normal, cocaine animals have slowed their rate of learning so that they now are no different from saline animals.

Cross-modal discrimination: Salient CS–. In the next experiment, conducted in separate groups of animals, the roles of the tone and light were switched.[32] The light now served as the CS+ and the more salient tone served as the CS–. As shown in FIGURE 6, this discrimination task was more difficult than the previous one; both groups required more sessions to achieve asymptotic performance when the CS– was the more salient stimulus. More importantly, cocaine-exposed animals were significantly retarded in their ability to acquire CRs to the less salient, light CS+. For example, on Day 10 of training, cocaine animals were responding at 21% to the light CS+ as compared to 43% of saline progeny.

Intramodal auditory discriminations. We conducted two more discrimination experiments, this time involving discrimination between two tones differing in both fre-

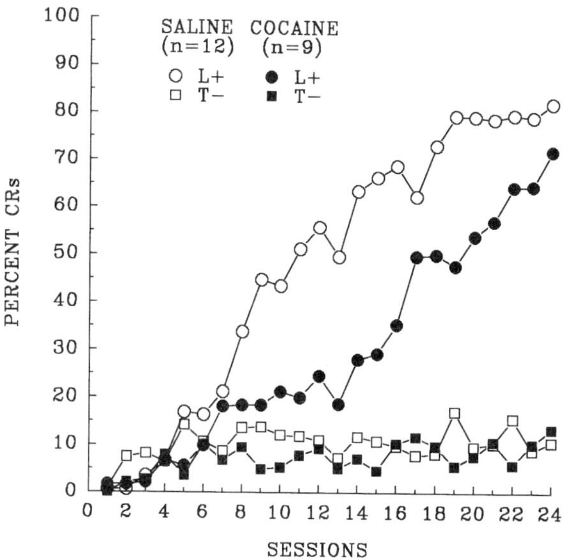

FIGURE 6. Percentages of discriminative responses to light as a CS+ (L+) and tone as a CS– (T–). Adult rabbits exposed to cocaine *in utero* were significantly retarded in acquiring CRs to the less salient light CS+. (Reprinted with permission from Romano & Harvey.[32])

quency and intensity.[33] The intensity dimension was manipulated to produce differences in stimulus salience between the two tones, because it seemed that differences in stimulus salience rather than modality were contributing to the attentional alterations seen in cocaine-exposed animals. In the first experiment, a 1-kHz tone of moderate intensity served as the CS+ and an 8-kHz tone of weaker intensity served as the CS–. For comparison purposes, we combined the results of the intramodal discrimination experiment with those of the cross-modal discrimination where the 1-kHz tone served as the CS+. The data in both experiments were collapsed over quarterly stages of training to adjust for unequal rates of learning across the two experiments. FIGURE 7 plots the data for CS+ responding only. Clearly, prenatal exposure to cocaine had no effect on cross-modal or intramodal discrimination learning when the CS+ was more salient or intense than the CS–. In the second intramodal discrimination experiment, the weaker intensity 8-kHz tone served as the CS+ and the louder 1-kHz tone served as the CS–. FIGURE 8 contrasts the results with the analogous cross-modal discrimination experiment involving a salient CS–. Regardless of the nature of the discrimination, either cross-modal or intramodal, prenatal cocaine exposure significantly retarded the rate of CR acquisition to the CS+ when a more salient stimulus served as the CS–.

Summary of Effects of Prenatal Cocaine Exposure on Learning

In summary, the three learning alterations noted above, (1) accelerated acquisition to a tone but not a light CS, (2) impaired discrimination between a light CS– and a tone CS+, and (3) impaired discrimination between a soft tone CS+ and a loud tone CS–,

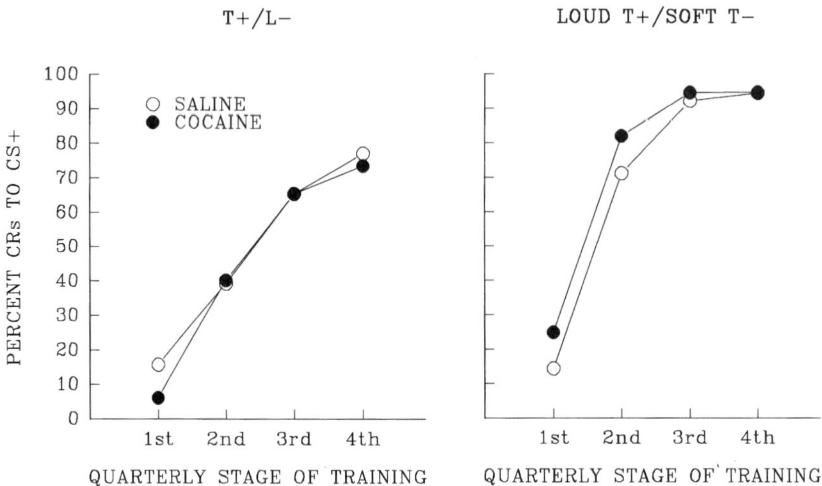

FIGURE 7. **(Left panel)** Percentages of CRs to a tone CS+ during tone CS+/light CS– (T+/L–) discrimination training. **(Right panel)** Percentages of CRs to a loud, 1-kHz tone CS+ (loud T+) during discrimination training between the loud tone and a soft, 8-kHz tone CS– (soft T–). No significant differences were noted between cocaine and saline progeny when the CS+ was the more salient cue. (Reprinted with permission from Wilkins *et al.*[33])

can all be attributed to an attentional deficit in processing stimuli differing in salience. Simple acquisition of a defensive CR was accelerated in a modality-specific and salience-dependent fashion. As the attentional demands of the learning task were increased, cocaine progeny showed some degree of normalization, learning a simple discrimination between a salient CS+ and a less salient CS– at the same rate as controls. However, when a more difficult discrimination was required, that is, between a less salient CS+ and a more salient CS–, cocaine progeny showed a retarded rate of learning. The retardation in learning suggests impaired ability to attend to a relevant stimulus when a more salient, but irrelevant, stimulus occurs in the same context.

Deficits in discrimination learning and other learning phenomena dependent upon attentional factors occur in a variety of species following prenatal exposure to cocaine. In most instances, an increase in the demands of the task have led to an increase in the severity of deficits seen in cocaine progeny, similar to what we observed in our rabbit NM preparation. Thus, it was reported[34] that first-order odor conditioning was intact in infant rats prenatally exposed to cocaine, whereas sensory preconditioning was impaired. Similarly, adult rats exposed prenatally to cocaine were able to form a conditional discrimination based on odor cues but showed a significantly slower reversal of that discrimination than did control animals.[35] The mouse model described elsewhere in this volume[36] shows a similar pattern of apparently normal learning during a simple acquisition task but impaired learning when greater attentional demands are placed on the organism. Adult mice exposed to cocaine prenatally demonstrate normal aversion to an odor paired with a footshock but fail to show blocking of associative learning when a redundant CS is added to the original odor-footshock pair.[33,37] Blocking of

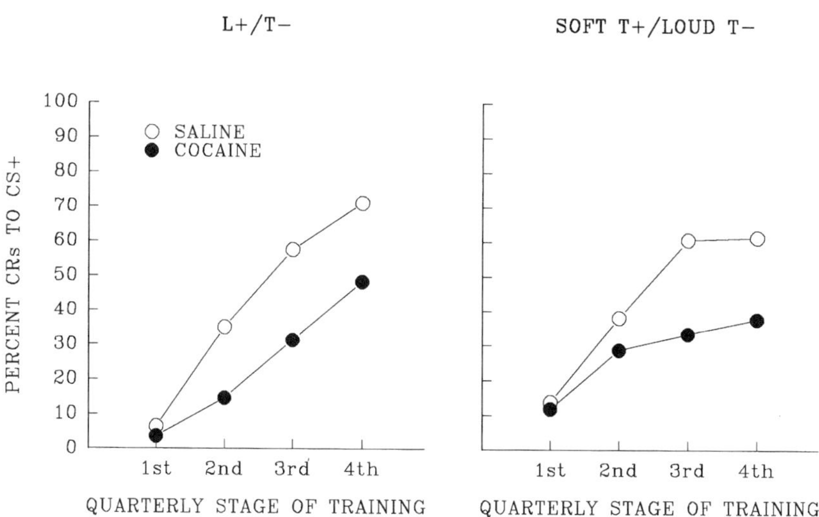

FIGURE 8. (Left panel) Percentages of CRs to a light CS+ during light CS+/tone CS− (L+/T−) discrimination training. **(Right panel)** Percentages of CRs to a soft, 8-kHz tone CS+ (soft T+) during discrimination training between the soft tone and a loud, 1-kHz tone CS− (loud T−). Cocaine progeny acquired CRs to the CS+ at a significantly slower rate than did saline progeny when the CS+ was the less salient cue. (Reprinted with permission from Wilkins *et al.*[33])

associative learning when a redundant CS is added to an already established CS-US association is often regarded as an attentional phenomenon whereby animals learn to ignore the redundant CS.[31]

Most of the cognitive behavioral deficits just described suggest that prenatal exposure to cocaine disrupts learned, attentional processing. Other learned behaviors, less dependent upon attentional processing, should therefore be spared. Spatial learning appears to fall into such a category. Mixed results have been reported in spatial learning tasks such as the Morris water maze and eight-arm radial maze. Cocaine progeny sometimes fail to show deficits in the Morris water maze[38] of if they do show deficits, these deficits appear to be short lived[39–41] and/or gender-dependent.[41] Similarly, spatial learning in the eight-arm radial maze is either unaffected by prenatal cocaine exposure[39] or impaired in only one gender.[42]

Relationship of Deficits in Attentional Processing to Abnormalities in Anterior Cingulate Cortex

The behavioral findings just described clearly indicate a deficit in learned attentional processes and both morphologic and neurochemical abnormalities in the anterior cingulate cortex. As noted earlier in this chapter (see section on Behavioral Functions of the Anterior Cingulate Cortex) considerable evidence exists from animal and human studies that the anterior cingulate cortex plays an important role in tasks requiring attentional focus. Therefore, a colleague, Michael Gabriel, carried out a set of experiments to determine whether the attentional deficits that we observed in discrimination tasks were in fact associated with alterations in stimulus processing within the anterior cingulate cortex. Previous research from Gabriel's laboratory had demonstrated that in normal rabbits, neurons in the anterior cingulate cortex begin to respond differentially to a CS+ and CS– just prior to behavioral acquisition of an instrumental discrimination.[4,25] In a series of experiments, neuronal responses of the anterior cingulate cortex during discrimination training were carried out in saline and cocaine progeny provided by our laboratory. It was found that cocaine progeny demonstrated a deficit in the development of differential neuronal responding in anterior cingulate cortex to the CS+ and CS– as compared with controls.[4] These findings allow us to conclude that prenatal exposure to cocaine produces an identifiable behavioral deficit in attentional processing that is the result of structural, neurochemical, and electrophysiologic abnormalities within a specific brain region.

LONG-TERM SENSORIMOTOR EFFECTS OF PRENATAL EXPOSURE TO COCAINE

Motor Performance

Not all of the behavioral anomalies we observed in the preceding experiments could be attributed to a deficit in learned attentional processing. In this regard, we noted that cocaine progeny given unpaired presentations of the tone and light CSs and the air puff US showed a consistent but nonsignificant reduction in the amplitude of the NM reflex across 10 days of testing.[30] Several experiments were designed to follow up on the preceding observation to determine if elicitation or modification of the defensive NM reflex was altered by prenatal exposure to cocaine.[43]

The motor performance of cocaine and saline progeny was assessed by comparing the functions relating NM reflex frequency and NM reflex amplitude to the intensity of the US. FIGURE 9 shows the results of this experiment. The intensity of the air puff US was manipulated by altering its duration in the range of 20–100 ms. As shown in FIGURE 9, both the percentages and amplitudes of NM responses increased significantly with increases in US intensity. More importantly, both measures were significantly reduced by prenatal cocaine exposure. Thus, the mean percentage of NM responses collapsed across US intensities was 80% for saline animals compared to 59% for cocaine animals, and response amplitudes averaged 3.22 mm for saline animals and 1.99 mm for cocaine animals. The shapes of the two functions, however, did not differ between the two groups. Thus, no significant interaction was noted between prenatal treatment condition and US intensity for either the percentage of NM responses or NM response amplitude. The motor performance of cocaine progeny suggests that prenatal cocaine exposure produced long-term consequences for neurobehavioral function which were detectable as an alteration in an aversive, tactile reflex. Other reflex systems have been examined in other species following prenatal exposure to cocaine and varying results have been reported. The variability in results is not surprising given that different species, drug dosages, routes of administration, and postnatal ages at testing have been employed. For example, the amplitude of the reflexive eyeblink elicited by glabellar tap is increased in human infants exposed to cocaine *in utero,*[44] whereas neither tail-flick latencies of weanling rats nor footshock sensitivity of 12-day-old rat pups are affected by prenatal exposure to cocaine.[45,46] Mixed results have also been reported for adult animals. Prenatal exposure to cocaine altered tail-flick latencies and footshock sensitivity in adult rats,[47] but the acoustic startle reflex was either unaffected following

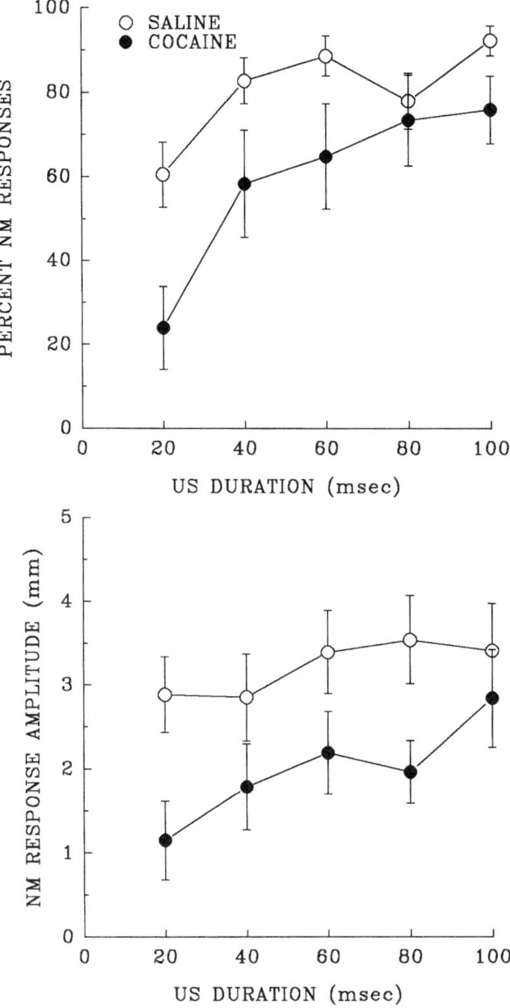

FIGURE 9. (Top panel) Mean percentages of reflex NM responses as a function of US duration. **(Bottom panel)** Mean amplitudes of the NM reflex as a function of US duration. The 20-, 40-, 60-, 80-, and 100-ms USs corresponded to air puff pressures of 63, 104, 139, 166, and 200 g/cm^2. Both the percentages of NM reflex responses and their amplitudes were significantly reduced in cocaine versus saline progeny. (Reprinted with permission from Romano & Harvey.[43])

prenatal cocaine exposure[48] or yielded inconsistent results[49] or results that were gender dependent.[50] Thus, it appears that human infants and adult rats and rabbits exhibit altered responses to tactile and/or nociceptive stimuli following prenatal exposure to cocaine, but their sensitivity to other, nontactile stimuli may be unaltered. The findings reported by Mayes in this volume[51] are consistent with altered tactile responsiveness in human infants exposed to cocaine *in utero.*

Sensorimotor Gating

A second experiment in this series assessed sensorimotor gating using the reflex modification paradigm.[43] Reflex modification is an unlearned behavioral phenomenon and has been demonstrated in a wide variety of mammalian species.[52] The paradigm is formally similar to the classical conditioning paradigm in that it involves presentations of a reflex-eliciting stimulus preceded by another, usually innocuous stimulus. Such paired stimulus presentations produce reliable alterations in the topography of the reflex compared to the topographies observed when the reflex-eliciting stimulus is presented by itself. Reflex modification is regarded as a form of sensorimotor gating[53–55] or pre-attentive stimulus filtering.[56] In rats, reflex modification is typically measured as inhibition of startle amplitude although, under appropriate conditions, a reduction of reflex latency or a facilitation of startle amplitude can also be obtained.[52,57,58] In rabbits and humans, reflex modification is typically measured using the eye-blink component of the startle reflex. The eye-blink reflex in humans and the eye-blink/NM reflex in rabbits can be elicited by tactile stimuli in the eye region such as puffs of air directed towards the cornea, a mild electric shock, or a mechanical tap.[56,59–63] Like the startle reflex in rats, the blink reflex in rabbits and humans shows both inhibition and facilitation of magnitude as well as a reduction in latency.[56,59–64] One of the most potent variables affecting the magnitude and direction of reflex modification is the interstimulus interval, the interval of time separating the reflex-eliciting stimulus from the antecedent stimulus. Rabbits typically show augmentation of NM reflex amplitude and reduction of NM reflex latency when that reflex is preceded by a moderate intensity tone at intervals in the range of 200–800 ms.[61,63–66] There have been mixed reports of reflex modification effects in rats and human infants following prenatal exposure to cocaine.[44,49–51]

FIGURE 10 shows the results of manipulating the interstimulus interval between a moderate intensity tone and reflex-eliciting air puff on modification of NM reflex amplitudes. As shown in the top panel of FIGURE 10, the amplitude of the NM reflex was augmented at all intervals relative to baseline US-alone trials. Although the percentage of reflex facilitation appeared to be greater in cocaine progeny (top panel, FIG. 10), raw response amplitudes were lower in cocaine progeny than in saline progeny (bottom panel, FIG. 10). However, unlike the results of the previous experiment, the difference in response amplitudes between the two groups did not achieve statistical significance. Moreover, there was no evidence of a significant interaction between the interstimulus interval and prenatal treatment condition, suggesting that modification of NM reflex amplitude was unaffected by prenatal cocaine exposure.

A similar lack of effect of prenatal cocaine exposure on reflex modification can be seen in FIGURE 11. Although the latency of the reflex was significantly reduced as a function of increases in the interstimulus interval, the shape of that function did not differ significantly between the two groups. However, cocaine progeny showed a consistent delay in their reaction time to the reflex-eliciting stimulus, responding, on average, 31 ms later than did saline progeny. Our reflex modification results are comparable to those reported for human infants. Cocaine-exposed infants showed an increase in the amplitude of the eyeblink elicited by glabellar tap, but the effect of antecedent stimulation did not interact with cocaine exposure.[44] That is, the amount of change in reflex amplitude as a consequence of antecedent stimulation was the same for normal and cocaine-exposed infants. Similar results were found in the present study: no significant effect on reflex amplitude, a significant increase in reflex latency as a consequence of prenatal exposure to cocaine, but no interaction between prenatal treat-

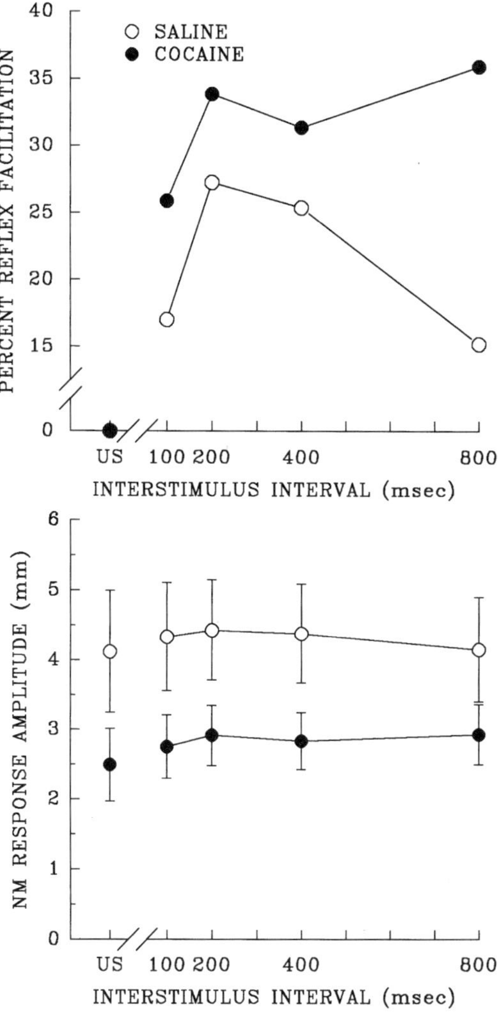

FIGURE 10. (Top panel) Modification of NM reflex amplitude expressed as the percentage of reflex facilitation during tone-air puff presentations relative to air puff alone (US) presentations. SEMs have been eliminated for illustrative purposes. **(Bottom panel)** Mean NM reflex amplitudes (corresponding to *top panel*) as a function of the tone-air puff interstimulus interval. NM reflex amplitudes were significantly altered as a function of the interstimulus interval but prenatal cocaine exposure had no effect on the reflex modification function. (Reprinted with permission from Romano & Harvey.[43])

ment condition and antecedent stimulus conditions. Thus, prenatal cocaine exposure altered the intensity threshold for eliciting a tactile, defensive reflex, retarded the reaction time of that reflex, but did not appear to affect sensorimotor gating of that reflex.

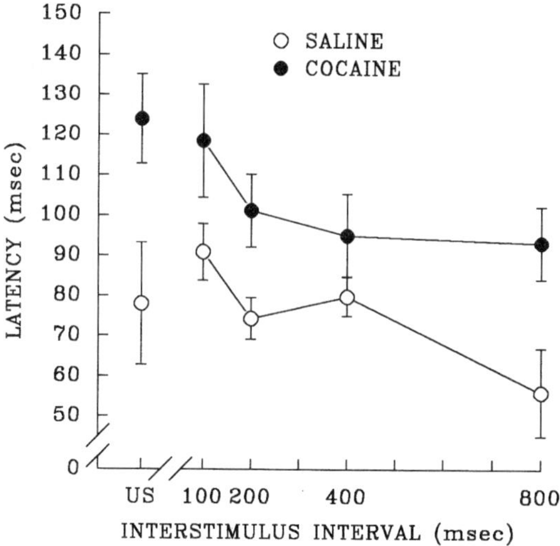

FIGURE 11. Mean NM reflex latencies as a function of the interstimulus interval or in response to air puff alone (US) presentations. Reflex latencies were significantly reduced when the air puff was preceded by a tone, and the amount of decrease was an increasing function of an increase in the interstimulus interval. Although cocaine progeny showed significantly longer reaction times than did saline progeny at all interstimulus intervals, the amount of latency reduction across the interstimulus intervals did not vary between the two groups. (Reprinted with permission from Romano & Harvey.[43])

Relationship of Deficits in Motor Function to Neural Abnormalities

We had earlier presented evidence that the deficits in attentional processes demonstrated by cocaine progeny were due to impaired functioning of the anterior cingulate cortex (see section on Relationship of Deficits in Attentional Processing to Abnormalities in Anterior Congulate Cortex). A number of investigators have demonstrated that lesions to the prefrontal cortex including the anterior cingulate cortex can also produce impairments in motor function,[18] and so it is possible that the abnormalities noted in the anterior cingulate cortex of cocaine progeny might also be involved in the motor deficits that we just mentioned. It should be noted that the anterior cingulate cortex has strong reciprocal connections with a number of other structures that are importantly involved in motor function, the caudate nucleus and the red nucleus, and so the alterations in anterior cingulate cortex seen in cocaine progeny might affect the functioning of those two regions. For example, it is known that optimal performance of the NM reflex of the rabbit involves activity of the caudate nucleus and red nucleus.[67,68] Motor function is also known to be critically dependent on the normal functioning of the dopamine system which projects powerfully to the caudate nucleus as well as to the anterior cingulate cortex. The decreased functioning of the dopamine D_1 receptor due to an uncoupling from its Gi protein occurs not only in the anterior cingulate cortex of cocaine progeny but also in the caudate nucleus.[3,69,70] This uncoupling in the caudate nucleus has been shown to have a functional consequence in that D-amphetamine fails to elicit a motor response that is dependent on activation of the D_1 receptor in the caudate nucleus.[6,71] It would appear therefore that the uncoupling of the D_1 receptor in the anterior cingulate cortex and caudate nucleus along with possible changes in functioning of the red nucleus might form the anatomic basis for the motor deficits observed in cocaine progeny.

SUMMARY

- Prenatal exposure to cocaine alters attentional processing in rabbits so that conditioned stimuli become associated with unconditioned stimuli at abnormal rates.
- Cocaine progeny have difficulty in preferentially attending to less salient but relevant stimuli when more salient, irrelevant stimuli occur in the same context.
- Prenatal exposure to cocaine impairs the elicitation and reaction time of a motor reflex but does not affect sensorimotor gating of that reflex.
- The attentional deficits and alterations in motor function demonstrated by cocaine progeny are linked to the developmental abnormalities of the anterior cingulate cortex and caudate nucleus.

REFERENCES

1. Murphy, E.H., J.G. Hammer, M.D. Schumann, M.Y. Groce, X.-H. Wang, L. Jones, A.G. Romano & J.A. Harvey. 1995. The rabbit as a model for studies of cocaine exposure *in utero.* Lab. Anim. Sci. **45:** 94–101.
2. Levitt, P., J.A. Harvey, E. Friedman & E.H. Murphy. 1997. New evidence for neurotransmitter influences on brain development. TINS **20:** 269–274.
3. Friedman, E. & H.-Y. Wang. 1998. Prenatal cocaine exposure alters signal transduction in the brain D_1 dopamine receptor system. *In* cocaine: Effects on the Development Brain. Ann. N.Y. Acad. Sci. In press.
4. Gabriel, M. & C. Taylor. 1998. Prenatal exposure to cocaine impairs neuronal coding of attention and discrimination learning. *In* Cocaine: Effects on the Developing Brain. Anna. N.Y. Acad. Sci. This volume.
5. Levitt, P., E.H. Murphy & D.R. Grayson. 1997. *In utero* cocaine causes targeted changes in cortical development. *In* Cocaine: Effects on the Developing Brain. Conference, N.Y. Acad. Sci.
6. Simansky, K.J., G. Baker, W.J. Kachelries, H. Hood, A.G. Romano & J.A. Harvey. 1996. Prenatal exposure to cocaine reduces dopaminergic D_1-mediated motor function but spares the enhancement of learning by D-amphetamine in rabbits. In: Cocaine: Effects on the Developing Brain. Ann. N.Y. Acad. Sci. In press.
7. Denenberg, V.H., L.P. Zeidner, E.B. Thoman, P. Kramer, J.C. Rowe, A.F. Philipps & J.R. Raye. 1982. Effects of theophylline on behavioral state development in newborn rabbit. J. Pharmacol. Exp. Ther. **221:** 604–608.
8. Harvey, J.A. 1987. Effect of drugs on associative learning. *In* Psychopharmacology, The Third Generation of Progress. H. Meltzer, Ed.: 1485–1491. Raven Press. New York.
9. Jones, R.T. 1990. The pharmacology of cocaine smoking in humans. *In* Research Findings on Smoking of Abused Substances, National Institute on Drug Abuse Research Monograph 99. Chiang, C.N. & Hawks, R.L. (Eds). U.S. Government Printing Office. Washington, DC.
10. Kasirsky, G. & M.F. Tansy. 1971. Teratogenic effects of methamphetamine in mice and rabbits. J. Am. Osteopath. Assoc. **70:** 1119–1120.
11. Hartman, H.A. 1974. The fetus in experimental teratology. *In* The Biology of the Laboratory Rabbit. R.E. Flatt & A.L. Kraus, Eds.: 92–144. Academic Press, Inc. New York, NY.
12. Hudson, R. & H. Distel. 1986. The potential of the newborn rabbit for behavioral teratological research. Neurobehav. Toxicol. Teratol. **8:** 209–212.
13. Reader, T.A. & K.M. Dewar. 1989. Endogenous homovanillic acid levels differ between rat and rabbit caudate, hippocampus, and cortical regions. Neurochem. Res. **14:** 1137–1141.

14. Harel, S., K. Watanabe, I. Linke & R.J. Schain. 1972. Growth and development of the rabbit brain. Biol. Neonate **21:** 381–399.
15. Romano, A.G. & J.A. Harvey. 1992. Drug effects on sensorimotor integration in a model system. *In* Drugs of Abuse and Neurobiology. R.R. Watson, Ed.: 23–37. CRC Press. Boca Raton, FL.
16. Kaufmann, R.A., R.T. Savoy-Moore, A.G. Sacco & M.G. Subramanian. 1990. The effect of cocaine on oocyte development and the follicular microenvironment in the rabbit. Fertil. Steril. **54:** 921–926.
17. Atlas, S.J. & E.E. Wallach. 1991. Effects of intravenous cocaine on reproductive function in the mated rabbit. Am. J. Obstet. Gynecol. **165:** 1785–1790.
18. Kolb, B. 1990. Animal models for human PFC-related disorders. *In* Progress in Brain Research. Vol. **85:** 501–519. Elsevier Science Publishers B.V. New York.
19. Vogt, B.A., D.M. Finch & C.R. Olson. 1992. Functional heterogeneity in cingulate cortex: The anterior executive and posterior evaluative regions. Cerebral Cortex **2:** 435–443.
20. Buchanan, S.L. & D.A. Powell. 1982. Cingulate cortex: Its role in Pavlovian conditioning. J. Comp. Physiol. Psychol. **96:** 755–774.
21. Gabriel, M. 1990. Functions of anterior and posterior cingulate cortex during avoidance learning in rabbits. *In* Progress in Brain Research. Vol. **85:** 467–483. Elsevier Science Publishers B.V. New York.
22. Gabriel, M., Y. Kubota, S. Sparenborg, K. Straube & B.A. Vogt. 1991. Effects of cingulate cortical lesions on avoidance learning and training-induced unit activity in rabbits. Exp. Brain. Res. **86:** 585–600.
23. Irle, E. & H.J. Markowitsch. 1982. Single and combined lesions of the cat's thalamic mediodorsal nucleus and the mammillary bodies lead to severe deficits in the acquisition of an alternation task. Behav. Brain Res. **6:** 147–165.
24. Mesulam, M.M. & N. Geschwind. 1978. On the possible role of neocortex and its limbic connections in the process of attention and schizophrenia: Clinical cases of inattention in man and experimental anatomy in monkey. J. Psychiat. Res. **14:** 249–259.
25. Gabriel, M., K. Foster, E. Orona, S.E. Saltwick & M. Stanton. 1980. Neuronal activity of cingulate cortex, anteroventral thalamus, and hippocampal formation in discriminative conditioning: encoding and extraction of the significance of conditional stimuli. *In* Progress in Psychobiology and Physiological Psychology. Vol. **9:** 125–231. Academic Press. New York.
26. Gibbs, C.M. & D.A. Powell. 1991. Single-unit activity in the dorsomedial prefrontal cortex during the expression of discriminative bradycardia in rabbits. Behav. Brain Res. **43:** 79–92.
27. Pardo, J.V., P.J. Pardo, K.W. Janer & M.E. Raichle. 1990. The anterior cingulate cortex mediates processing selection in the Stroop attentional conflict paradigm. Proc. Natl. Acad. Sci. USA **87:** 256–259.
28. Petersen, S.E., P.T. Fox, M.I. Posner, M. Mintum & M.E. Raichle. 1988. Positron emission tomographic studies of the cortical anatomy of single-word processing. Nature **331:** 585–589.
29. Corbetta, M., F.M. Miezin, S. Dobmeyer, G.L. Shulman & S.E. Petersen. 1991. Selective and divided attention during visual discriminations of shape, color, and speed: functional anatomy by positron emission tomography. J. Neurosci. **11:** 2383–2402.
30. Romano, A.G., W.J. Kachelries, K.J. Simansky & J.A. Harvey. 1995. Intrauterine exposure to cocaine produces a modality specific acceleration of classical conditioning in adult rabbits. Pharmacol. Biochem. Behav. **52:** 415–420.
31. Mackintosh, N.J. 1975. A theory of attention: Variations in the associability of stimuli with reinforcement. Psychol. Rev. **82:** 276–298.
32. Romano, A.G. & J.A. Harvey. 1996. Prenatal exposure to cocaine disrupts discrimination learning in adult rabbits. Pharmacol. Biochem. Behav. **53:** 617–621.
33. Wilkins, A.S., B.E. Kosofsky, A.G. Romano & J.A. Harvey. 1996. Transplacental cocaine exposure: Behavioral consequences. *In* Prenatal Cocaine Exposure. R.J. Konkol & G. Olsen, Eds.: 149–165. CRC Press Inc. Boca Raton, FL.
34. Heyser, C.J., W.-J. Chen, J. Miller, N.E. Spear & L.P. Spear. 1990. Prenatal cocaine ex-

posure induces deficits in Pavlovian conditioning and sensory preconditioning among infant rat pups. Behav. Neurosci. **104:** 955–963.
35. Heyser, C.J., N.E. Spear & L.P. Spear. 1992. Effects of prenatal exposure to cocaine on conditional discrimination learning in adult rats. Behav. Neurosci. **106:** 837–845.
36. Kosofsky, B.E. 1998. Structural and functional correlates of cocaine induced brain maldevelopment. Ann. N.Y. Acad. Sci. In press.
37. Wilkins, A.S., L.M. Genova, W. Posten & B.E. Kosofsky. 1998. Transplacental cocaine exposure. 1. A rodent model. Neurotoxicol. Teratol. **20:** 1–11.
38. Johns, J.M., M.J. Means, D.R. Anderson, L.W. Means & B.A. McMillen. 1992. Prenatal exposure to cocaine. II. Effects on open-field activity and cognitive behavior in Sprague-Dawley rats. Neurotoxicol. Teratol. **14:** 343–349.
39. Cutler, A.R., A.E. Wilkerson, J.L. Gingras & E.D. Levin. 1996. Prenatal cocaine and/or nicotine exposure in rats: Preliminary findings on long-term cognitive outcome and genital development at birth. Neurotoxicol. Teratol. **18:** 635–643.
40. Heyser, C.J., N.E. Spear & L.P. Spear. 1995. Effects of prenatal exposure to cocaine in Morris water maze performance in adult rats. Behav. Neurosci. **109:** 734–743.
41. Voorhees, C.V., T.M. Reed, K.D. Acuff-Smith, M.A. Schilling, G.D. Cappon, J.E. Fisher & C. Pu. 1995. Long-term learning deficits and changes in unlearned behaviors following *in utero* exposure to multiple daily doses of cocaine during different exposure periods and maternal plasma cocaine concentrations. Neurotoxicol. Teratol. **17:** 253–264.
42. Levin, E.D. & F.J. Seidler. 1993. Sex-related spatial learning differences after prenatal cocaine exposure in the young adult rat. Neurotoxicol. Teratol. **14:** 23–28.
43. Romano, A.G. & J.A. Harvey. 1996. Elicitation and modification of the rabbit's nicitating membrane reflex following prenatal exposure to cocaine. Pharmacol. Biochem. Behav. **53:** 857–862.
44. Anday, E.K., M.E. Cohen, N.E. Kelley & D.S. Leitner. 1989. Effect of *in utero* cocaine exposure on startle and its modification. Dev. Pharmacol. Ther. **12:** 137–145.
45. Kunko, P.M., D. Moyer & S.E. Robinson. 1993. Intravenous gestational cocaine in rats: Effects on offspring development and weanling behavior. Neurotoxicol. Teratol. **15:** 335–344.
46. Spear, L., C.L. Kirstein, J. Bell, V. Yoottanasumpun, R. Greenbaum, J. O'Shea, H. Hoffman & N.E. Spear. 1989. Effects of prenatal cocaine exposure on behavior during the early postnatal period. Neurotoxicol. Teratol. **11:** 57–63.
47. Smith, R.F., K.M. Mattran, M.F. Kurkjian & S.L. Kurtz. 1989. Alterations in offspring behavior induced by chronic prenatal cocaine dosing. Neurotoxicol. Teratol. **11:** 35–38.
48. Foss, J.A. & E.P. Riley. 1991. Failure of acute cocaine administration to differentially affect acoustic startle and activity in rats prenatally exposed to cocaine. Neurotoxicol. Teratol. **13:** 547–551.
49. Foss, J.A. & E.P. Riley. 1991. Elicitation and modification of the acoustic startle reflex in animals prenatally exposed to cocaine. Neurotoxicol. Teratol. **13:** 541–546.
50. Hughes, H.E., L.M. Donohue & D.L. Dow-Edwards. 1996. Prenatal cocaine exposure affects the acoustic startle response in adult rats. Behav. Brain Res. **75:** 83–90.
51. Mayes, L.C., C. Grillon, R. Granger & R. Schottenfeld. 1998. Regulation of arousal and attention in preschool children exposed to cocaine prenatally. *In* Cocaine: Effects on the Developing Brain. J.A. Harvey & B.E. Kosofsky, Eds. Ann. N.Y. Acad. Sci. In press.
52. Hoffman, H.S. & J.R. Ison. 1980. Reflex modification in the domain of startle. I. Some empirical findings and their implications for how the nervous system processes sensory input. Psychol. Rev. **87:** 175–189.
53. Braff, D.L. & M.A. Geyer. 1990. Sensorimotor gating and schizophrenia: Human and animal model studies. Arch. General Psychiatry **47:** 181–188.
54. Geyer, M.A., N.R. Swerdlow, R.S. Mansbach & D.L. Braff. 1990. Startle response models of sensorimotor gating and habituation deficits in schizophrenia. Brain Res. Bull. **25:** 485–498.
55. Swerdlow, N.R., D.L. Braff, N. Taaid & M.A. Geyer. 1994. Assessing the validity of an animal model of deficient sensorimotor gating in schizophrenic patients. Arch. Gen. Psychiatry **51:** 139–154.
56. Graham, F.K. 1975. The more or less startling effects of weak prestimulation. Psychophysiology **12:** 238–248.

57. ISON, J.R. & G.R. HAMMOND. 1971. Modification of the startle reflex in the rat by changes in the auditory and visual environments. J. Comp. Physiol. Psychol. **75:** 435–452.
58. ISON, J.R., D.W. MCADAM & G.R. HAMMOND. 1973. Latency and amplitude changes in the acoustic startle reflex of the rat produced by variation in auditory prestimulation. Physiol. Behav. **10:** 1035–1039.
59. ANTHONY, B.J. 1985. In the blink of an eye: Implications of reflex modification for information processing. *In* Advances in Psychophysiology. P. K. Ackles, J. R. Jennings & M. G. H. Coles, Eds. Vol. 1: 167–218. JAI Press, Inc. Greenwich, CT.
60. BOLINO, F., V. DI MICHELE, V. MANNA, L. DI CICCO, M.V. ISIDORI & M. CASACCHIA. 1993. Acoustic and electrically elicited startle reaction: Similar patterns of habituation and reflex modifications in humans. Int. J. Neurosci. **73:** 13–21.
61. ISON, J.R. & D.W. LEONARD. 1971. Effects of auditory stimuli on the amplitude of the nictitating membrane reflex of the rabbit *(Oryctolagus cuniculus)*. J. Comp. Physiol. Psychol. **75:** 157–164.
62. KRAUTER, E.E., D.W. LEONARD & J.R. ISON. 1973. Inhibition of the human eye blink by a brief acoustic stimulus. J. Comp. Physiol. Psychol. **84:** 246–251.
63. YOUNG, R.A., C.F. CEGAVSKE & R.F. THOMPSON. 1976. Tone-induced changes in excitability of abducens motoneurons and of the reflex path of the nictitating membrane response in the rabbit *(Oryctolagus cuniculus)*. J. Comp. Physiol. Psychol. **90:** 424–434.
64. WEISZ, D.J. & C. WALTS. 1990. Reflex facilitation of the rabbit nictitating membrane response by an auditory stimulus as a function of interstimulus interval. Behav. Neurosci. **104:** 11–20.
65. HARVEY, J.A., I. GORMEZANO & V.A. COOL-HAUSER. 1985. Relationship between heterosynaptic reflex facilitation and acquisition of the nictitating membrane response in control and scopolamine-injected rabbits. J. Neurosci. **5:** 596–602.
66. HARVEY, J.A., I. GORMEZANO, V.A. COOL-HAUSER & C.W. SCHINDLER. 1988. Effects of LSD on classical conditioning as a function of CS-UCS interval: Relationship to reflex facilitation. Pharmacol. Biochem. Behav. **30:** 433–441.
67. STEINMETZ, J.E. 1996. The brain substrates of classical eyeblink conditioning in rabbits. *In* The Acquisition of Motor Behavior in Vertebrates. J.R. Bloedel, T.J. Ebner & S.P. Wise, Eds.: 89–114. MIT Press. Cambridge, MA.
68. BRACHA, V. & J.R. BLOEDEL. 1996. The multiple-pathway model of circuits subserving the classical conditioning of withdrawal reflexes. *In* The Acquisition of Motor Behavior in Vertebrates. J.R. Bloedel, T.J. Ebner & S.P. Wise, Eds.: 175–204. MIT Press. Cambridge, MA.
69. WANG, H-Y., S. RUNYAN, E. YADIN & E. FRIEDMAN. 1995. Prenatal exposure to cocaine selectively reduces D_1 dopamine receptor-mediated activation of striatal Gs proteins. J. Pharmacol. Exp. Ther. **273:** 492–498.
70. FRIEDMAN, E., E. YADIN & H.-Y. WANG. 1996. Effect of prenatal cocaine on dopamine receptor-G protein coupling in mesocortical regions of the rabbit brain. Neuroscience **70:** 739–747.
71. SIMANSKY, K.J. & W.J. KACHELRIES. 1996. Prenatal exposure to cocaine selectively disrupts motor responding to D-amphetamine in young and mature rabbits. Neuropharmacology **35:** 71–78.
72. JONES, L., I. FISCHER & P. LEVITT. 1996. Nonuniform alteration of dendritic development in the cerebral cortex following prenatal cocaine exposure. Cereb. Cortex **6:** 431–445.
73. WANG, X.-H., P. LEVITT, D.R. GRAYSON & E.H. MURPHY. 1995. Intrauterine cocaine exposure of rabbits: Persistent elevation of GABA immunoreactive neurons in anterior cingulate cortex but not visual cortex. Brain Res. **689:** 32–46.
74. GRAYSON, D.R., Y. WU, A.A. BOOK & E.H. MURPHY. 1996. Alterations in $GABA_A$ receptor β2 mRNA levels in the anterior cingulate cortex of rabbits exposed prenatally to cocaine. Soc. Neurosci. Abstr. Vol. **22** (No. 762.9): 1941.
75. WANG, X.-H., A.O. JENKINS, L. CHOI & E.H. MURPHY. 1997. Altered neuronal distribution of parvalbumin in anterior cingulate cortex of rabbits exposed *in utero* to cocaine. Exp. Brain Res. **112:** 359–371.

Neurological Correlates of Fetal Cocaine Exposure[a]

CLAUDIA A. CHIRIBOGA[b]

Division of Pediatric Neurology, Department of Neurology, College of Physicians and Surgeons, Columbia University, and Harlem Hospital Center, New York, New York 10032, USA

ABSTRACT: Cocaine is a highly psychoactive substance with numerous effects that readily crosses the placenta, achieving variables levels in the fetus. Determining whether prenatal exposure to cocaine and its metabolites damages the developing human nervous system is hindered by the multiple intervening factors (confounders) that plague clinical settings, which warrant consideration in controlled studies. Prenatal cocaine exposure has been linked to numerous adverse neonatal outcomes, affecting fetal growth (i.e., low birth weight, intrauterine growth retardation, and small head size) and neurobehavior. These neurobehavior effects span the gamut from no abnormalities to impairments in arousal, neurological function, neurophysiological function, and state regulation. Strokes and possibly seizures are also noted. Dose-response effects of fetal cocaine exposure on fetal growth and neonatal neurobehavior are reported using quantitative methods of ascertainment. In early infancy, irritability and hypertonia are also described. Most cocaine associations are transient and resolve in infancy and early childhood. Whether such transient abnormalities place infants at increased risk for later neurodevelopmental impairments is not known. Controlled studies have found no cognitive differences related to prenatal cocaine exposure among toddlers or school age children, except as mediated through effects on head growth. Anecdotally, cocaine-exposed children seem to suffer from neurobehavioral abnormalities, but to date controlled studies have not established an association between cocaine and behavioral disorders, except for inattentiveness. Despite encouraging reports, the question of whether cocaine exerts long-term adverse effects on the developing human nervous system has not yet been resolved, largely because of the limitations of existing studies that rely on inadequate, mostly qualitative ascertainment of cocaine exposure as well as the dearth of studies in older children. Such methodological limitations may have compromised our ability to identify cocaine-exposed children at most risk.

INTRODUCTION

The 1980s were marred by an unprecedented level of cocaine abuse as "crack" cocaine found its way into urban America. At the height of the epidemic, about 30% of young adults reported using cocaine at least once.[1] Although cocaine use began to decline after 1987, it is still a major public health problem, especially in urban centers. Early in the epidemic the medical and lay press prognosticated, with little substantiation, that infants born to women using crack/cocaine (the so-called "crack/cocaine babies") were likely to suffer life-long developmental, learning, and behavioral handicaps. A decade later such dire predictions have been challenged by the results of carefully designed cocaine neurodevelopment studies that provide a more realistic, albeit still incomplete, understanding of the spectrum of the neurobehavioral teratology of cocaine exposure *in utero*.

[a] This work was supported by NINDS Grant K08-NS01528.

[b] Address for correspondence: Neurological Institute, 710 West 168th Street, New York, NY 10032. Phone, 212/305-8549; fax, 212/305-7036; e-mail, cac3@columbia.edu

Determining whether prenatal exposure to cocaine damages the developing human nervous system is hindered by the myriad of intervening factors (confounders) that plague clinical settings, where in addition to the effects of the drug of interest, behavioral correlates of drug use, such as poor prenatal care or sexually transmitted diseases (HIV or congenital syphilis), may be more harmful to the offspring than the drug under study. Collectively the plethora of concomitant risk factors including poor nutrition, social chaos, poor parenting, and multiple drug exposures help explain why the offspring of alcohol- and drug-abusing women tend to fair less well neurodevelopmentally than do other children of similar socioeconomic background. However, the net effect of any single drug is substantially diminished once these confounding factors are taken into account. Hence applying epidemiological methods in clinical cocaine studies is important, as they provide the means for separating cocaine effects from those elicited by other factors. These efforts notwithstanding, the erratic high risk behaviors associated with drug use may introduce additional elements that make inferences in clinical studies regarding drug-related associations more vulnerable to bias, for example, selection bias resulting from a high level of attrition. This chapter discusses the salient neurological, developmental, and behavioral findings in humans exposed prenatally to cocaine.

PHARMACOLOGY

Cocaine is a highly psychoactive substance with numerous effects.[2] It inhibits postsynaptic reuptake of catecholamines, dopamine, and tryptophan and blocks sodium ion permeability, thus acting as a local anesthetic agent. In addition to the multiple effects exerted by the parent compound, cocaine has active metabolites (e.g., benzoylecgonine, benzoylnorecgonine) of similar or even more powerful pharmacological activity. Many of these substances are independently neurotoxic and may be responsible for perceived cocaine effects.[3,4] Cocaine and its metabolites readily pass the placenta, achieving variables levels in the fetus.[5] The mechanism by which cocaine affects the fetus is not fully known but is postulated to result from either a direct effect to the fetus or an indirect effect mediated through the maternal autonomic and cardiovascular system, especially at the level of the uterus.[6]

The two most common forms of cocaine used by addicts are cocaine hydrochloride, a water-soluble salt, and crack/cocaine, a free-base alkaloid.[7] Cocaine hydrochloride can be used intranasally by snorting the powder, by applying it to various mucosal membranes (oral or genital), or by injecting it intravenously. Crack/cocaine, volatile when heated, is administered by smoking.

COCAINE ADDICTION

In adults, cocaine use produces a state of euphoria characterized by increased energy and enhanced alertness. According to classic and operational conditioning theory the degree of euphoria, which depends on the speed of delivery and cerebral concentrations attained by cocaine, is a prominent positive reinforcer. Because crack/cocaine is smoked, this preparation delivers the highest levels of cocaine to the brain in the most expedient fashion,[8] thus producing a more intense euphoria than that of other methods of delivery, such as snorting or injecting. This intense sensation, described by addicts as a "rush" of pleasure, gradually gives way to dysphoria, an equally intense but opposite sensation that is described as a "crash" from cocaine. Dysphoria is characterized by a strong craving for the drug, a depressed state, and hypersomnia; it acts as a powerful negative reinforcer. Fluctuations in postsynaptic levels of dopamine are postulated to account for the reinforcing properties of cocaine.[9] Converging lines of evidence support a dopaminergic hypothesis of cocaine addiction related to a mesocortical limbic reward system.[10,11]

Abrupt cessation of cocaine use does not elicit severe physical withdrawal symptoms; however, it does generate an unwavering craving for the drug. The overpowering grip of cocaine addiction is evident in experimental models in which animals allowed to self-administer cocaine will do so compulsively and at the expense of food intake and to the point of toxicity or death.[12] The powerful addiction produced by crack/cocaine tends to render crack-addicted women unable to curtail its use during pregnancy despite the hazards posed to their fetuses and the risk of losing custody of their offspring. The human correlates of such addiction-related behaviors during pregnancy have obvious detrimental consequences to the fetus.

METHODOLOGICAL CONSIDERATIONS

In interpreting the results of clinical studies, in addition to study design issues, the reader must bear in mind the method of determining cocaine use (e.g., urine toxicology vs meconium analyses), the population under study (e.g., heavy users vs casual users), and the instrument and outcome measure used. Methodological considerations of these factors warrant discussion, as they are key to explaining many of the apparent discrepancies between studies and underscore the inadequacy of extrapolating findings from one study to another, even if they are drawn from the same institution.

Ascertainment. Self-report during interview and urine toxicological testing are the traditional methods of ascertaining drug and alcohol use. The information gleaned from structured interviews allows researchers to quantify and assess patterns of drug use over time, especially during the first trimester. Because of the stigma and legal ramifications attached to drug abuse during pregnancy (e.g., loss of child custody), maternal self-report of drug use is often inaccurate. Urine toxicology assays can confirm drug use, but inform solely about recent use. As cocaine is rapidly metabolized, it is detected in urine for 6–8 hours, whereas its metabolites are detected for up to 6 days.[13] However, in exceptional cases of prolonged heavy cocaine use, metabolites have been detected in urine up to 22 days after use.[14]

New methods of drug ascertainment, hair radioimmunoassay and meconium analysis, allow determination of more remote use of drugs, yet to date few studies have been published using these more accurate methods of ascertainment. Hair radioimmunoassay determines the past use of a number of drugs, including marijuana, cocaine, opiates, and phenylcyclidine.[15] Analysis of each 3.9 cm of maternal hair informs on drugs used during the previous 3 months. External contamination of the hair sample is readily avoided by washings. Hair that is chemically treated may bind cocaine metabolites less avidly and thus underestimate the true level of exposure. Meconium, which develops at about 18 weeks of gestational age, acts as a reservoir of drugs used by the mother. Analysis of meconium specimens collected during the first 2 days of life identifies chronic drug exposure during the latter half of fetal life.[16] These methods of ascertainment diminish the degree of misclassification of cocaine use otherwise expected, as exemplified in a study using hair radioimmunoassay (RIAH), in which 60% of women who denied using cocaine during pregnancy tested positive for it in the last trimester.[17] By the same token, ascertainment of cocaine exposure based entirely on self-report without external validation is inevitably prone to misclassification.

Prevalence. The prevalence of cocaine use during pregnancy varies across the United

States and is predicated on a number of demographic factors, including race, urban dwelling, and socioeconomic status. Although drug use is distributed equally across racial lines, urban blacks are more likely to use cocaine than other drugs.[18] Prevalence estimates of cocaine use are also influenced by the method of ascertainment. For example, rates of cocaine use among women giving birth in two urban hospitals were 9 and 13% using only urine toxicology.[19,20] Rates increased to 18% with both self-report and urine testing.[21] With meconium analysis 31% of infants born to women from a high risk urban population tested positive for cocaine.[22]

Risk factors associated with the highest rates of cocaine use during pregnancy are poor prenatal care and syphilis. About 30–50% of urban women who lack prenatal care will have a positive urine toxicology for cocaine at the time of delivery.[23] Rates reach 70–80% with the use of meconium or hair analysis.[24] The profile that emerges of women most likely to use cocaine during pregnancy are those living in inner cities who are single, black, older, of low socioeconomic status, and have syphilis, HIV, or poor prenatal care.

Other Risk Factors. In addition to specific drug effects, exposed infants are at increased risk because of behaviors related to drug abuse. Women who use drugs intravenously are at risk for systemic and cutaneous infection, including hepatitis B, bacterial endocarditis, brain abscess, HIV infection, and AIDS. They also tend to exchange sex for drugs, thereby increasing their risk for sexually transmitted diseases, especially HIV[25] and syphilis.[26]

Maternal Nutrition. The nutritional status of drug users is poor, because meager resources are spent procuring cocaine instead of food and cocaine suppresses appetite. Low serum folate and ferritin levels are often found among cocaine-positive pregnant women.[27] Poor weight gain during pregnancy, reflecting poor maternal nutrition, exerts a significant and independent effect on neonatal motor performance, visual habituation, orientation, and reflexes on the Brazelton Neonatal Behavioral Assessment Scale (BNBAS).[28,29]

Low Birth Weight. Low birth weight, frequently observed among drug-exposed infants, can result from prematurity or intrauterine growth retardation. Infants born prematurely are at risk for cerebral palsy, developmental delay, behavioral impairments, and learning difficulties,[4,30] and infants who are small for gestational age are also at risk for cognitive and neurological impairments in later life compared to infants who are appropriate for gestational age, especially if fetal brain growth is proportionately impaired (symmetrically or proportionally small for gestational age).[31]

Polysubstance Abuse. Women who use one drug are more likely to abuse multiple drugs, smoke cigarettes, and drink alcohol. Polydrug use is a major confounder of fetal drug effects, as many of the adverse outcomes described, such as low birth weight, intrauterine growth retardation, malformations, and neurobehavioral abnormalities, are common with prenatal exposure to other substances of abuse. The reader is referred to a review article for a more detailed discussion on the topic.[32]

COCAINE

Pregnancy Effects

Cocaine use during pregnancy has been linked to spontaneous abortion, abruptio placenta, stillbirths, fetal distress, meconium staining, and premature delivery.[33–36] These adverse effects, which are attributed to vasoconstrictive cocaine effects on uterine vessels,[6] are important because of their potential impact on subsequent infant neurobehavior and developmental outcome.

Neonatal Effects

Intrauterine Growth. Higher rates of low birth weight and intrauterine growth retardation are reported among cocaine-exposed infants.[19,21,22,37] Growth effects require either high levels or more prolonged cocaine exposure, as they are not seen in offspring exposed exclusively in the first trimester.[37] Cocaine impairs fetal brain growth independently of somatic growth and gestational age.[17,21] Two studies, one using meconium[38] and the other RIAH,[17] reported dose-response effects of cocaine exposure on fetal growth, including brain. In the latter study, the odds ratio of small head size associated with low levels of cocaine exposure was 3.3 and the odds ratio associated with high levels of cocaine exposure was 6.1 (χ^2 for trend $p = 0.000002$) (TABLE 2).[17] As discussed below, cocaine-related impairment of head growth is relevant because of its adverse impact on cognitive function (see neurodevelopmental effects).

Neurobehavior. Altered neonatal behavioral patterns and neurological findings have been linked to fetal cocaine exposure (TABLE 1).[37,39–42] Difficulties in regulation of neonatal behavioral state are well described among cocaine-exposed children; however, findings are inconsistent. Some reports describe that irritability and excitability,[41] poor feeding, and sleep disturbances[43] occur more frequently among cocaine- and cocaine/methamphetamine-infants[40] than among control infants. These infants also show motor and movement abnormalities including excessive tremor, hypertonia, and hyperreflexia.[42,44] Because of the similarity between these neurological signs and opiate withdrawal signs, cocaine-related findings were interpreted by some as indicative of a withdrawal syndrome. Another study found that newborns exposed to cocaine and alcohol alternated between an excitable and a lethargic state.[44] Other studies, however, found no evidence of withdrawal or excitability. Instead, infants were depressed and exhibited a poor organizational response state and impaired orientation on the Brazelton Scale (BNBAS).[37,39] In these early studies, most infants were examined shortly after birth, cocaine exposure was assessed by urine toxicology, and small sample size prevented controlling for confounding variables.

Later controlled studies obtained conflicting results. One noted depressed habituation and a greater amount of stress-related behaviors among cocaine-exposed infants on the Brazelton Scale (BNBAS) than among a control group.[45] Two other studies, one based on a nonselected cohort that was more representative of the community, found

TABLE 1. Neurological Fetal Cocaine Effects and Associations

Neonatal Period	**Abnormal neurobehavior**
Microcephaly	Impaired organizational state
Vascular abnormalities	Depressed sensorium
Stroke	Hypertonia
Porencephaly	Coarse tremor
Intraventricular hemorrhage	Irritability/excitable state
Seizures	**Other effects**
Brain malformations	Brainstem conduction delays
Agenesis of corpus callosum	Sudden infant death syndrome
Septo-optic dysplasia	Excessive startle
Skull defects	***Infancy and Childhood***
Encephalocele	Hypertonia in infancy
	Inattentiveness
	?Aggressive behavior
	?Dysphoria

TABLE 2. Newborn Anthromorphic Measures and Neurological Function Associated with Increasing Levels of Cocaine Exposure Based on Combined Upper and Lower Quartiles of RIAH Cocaine Values

Infant Characteristics	Unexposed (*n* = 136)		Exposed Low (2–66 NG) (*n* = 52)		Exposed High (81–4457 NG) (*n* = 53)		*P* Value
Growth Parameters							
Birth length (cm) ± sd	51.5 ± 2.6		50.4 ± 3.3		49.0 ± 2.7		0.000*
Birth weight (g) ± sd	3,369 ± 471		3,259 ± 546		2,934 ± 416		0.000*
Birth head size (cm) ± sd	34.7 ± 1.4		34.2 ± 1.5		33.4 ± 1.4		0.000*
Ponderal Index ± sd	2.5 ± 0.3		2.5 ± 0.4		2.5 ± 0.3		0.315
	n	(%)	*n*	(%)	*n*	(%)	
SGA head size	8	(6.9)	9	(17.3)	15	(28.8)	0.00012*
SGA birth weight	9	(6.6)	7	(13.5)	18	(34.0)	0.00001*
Neurological Findings							
Fixates on examiner	14	(10.7)	19	(37.3)	16	(32.7)	0.00004*
Does not follow face	23	(17.3)	10	(19.2)	20	(40.8)	0.00280*
Hypertonia	15	(11.0)	15	(28.8)	18	(34.6)	0.00029*
Coarse tremors	20	(15.0)	21	(40.4)	21	(40.4)	0.00006*
Extensor posture	6	(4.4)	7	(13.7)	13	(25.5)	0.00018*

Ponderal index = (birth weight/birth length)^3 × 100. SGA = small for gestational age as determined by measure <10th percentile according to norms by Miller *et al.*[105] Plus/minus represent standard deviations. Adapted from Chiriboga *et al.*[17]

no neurobehavioral effects with the Brazelton Scale at age 2–3 days in cocaine-exposed infants after controlling for confounders.[38,46]

The timing of the neonatal assessment may explain these disparate findings. Neuspiel *et al.*[46] found significant differences in motor clusters between cocaine-exposed and unexposed infants when the Brazelton Scale (BNBAS) was administered at 11–30 days after birth. No differences were noted, however, in any of the clusters when the BNBAS was administered within 72 hours of birth, suggesting that neurobehavioral abnormalities may be late in emerging. Along these lines, a controlled study by Tronick *et al.*[38] documented significant differences in state regulation and excitability on the BNBAS among heavily cocaine-exposed infants at 3 weeks of age but not at 3 days of age.

Based on the timing of onset of symptoms these divergent results have been attributed to two distinct types of neurobehavior: (1) a *rare* early depressed state occurring immediately after birth and resolving within 1–2 days, and (2) a late emerging excitable phase with variable onset ranging from 3–30 days.[47] The early depressed state usually coincides with recent cocaine exposure[39] and may be either the neonatal equivalent of the "crash"-like withdrawal observed in adult cocaine addicts or a direct toxic effect of cocaine or its metabolites.[48] The late excitable phase with its variable onset and prolonged duration is not a withdrawal syndrome, but it probably reflects a direct cocaine effect on the developing brain, whereby increases in postsynaptic concentration of monoamines during critical periods of neural development may alter the circuitry of these systems in fetal brain. In addition, a transitional intermediate phase in which state alternates between excitability and lethargy may lie interspersed between these two phases.

Dose-response effects of cocaine on neurobehavior are also reported. Using quantification of "lines" of cocaine used during pregnancy, Jacobson noted a modest dose-response effect with cocaine exposure. Tronick *et al.*[38] detected neurobehavioral abnormalities at age 3 weeks, but only among heavily exposed infants. Using RIAH to determine exposure, Chiriboga *et al.* reported muscle tone and movement abnormalities among cocaine-exposed newborns assessed at age 3 days which increased in dose-response fashion; the odds ratio associated with each of three levels of cocaine exposure (absent, low, and high) for global hypertonia was 1.0, 3.3, and 4.3 (χ^2 for trend p <0.001); for extensor leg posturing, 1.0, 3.4, and 7.4 (χ^2 for trend p <0.001); and for coarse tremor, 1.0, 3.8, and 3.8 (χ^2 for trend p <0.001) (TABLE 2).[17] In this controlled study cocaine exposure remained significantly associated with neurological abnormalities in logistic regression equations that controlled for 10 or more variables.

Strokes. Clinical reports describe neonatal strokes associated with prenatal cocaine exposure.[49,50] In animal models, cocaine and its metabolites exert a vasoconstrictive effect on fetal cerebral vasculature, resulting in decreased cerebral blood flow.[3] However, both direct and indirect mechanisms are invoked in the genesis of neonatal stroke related to fetal cocaine exposure. An indirect mechanism of stroke was likely involved in the initial clinical report which described a stroke in a severely asphyxiated newborn.[49] Thus, to some extent cocaine-related strokes appear mediated by other stroke risk factors, such as abruptio placentae or birth asphyxia, which are also linked to cocaine effects on uterine vasculature. A direct mechanism of neonatal stroke mediated by cocaine vasoconstriction on cerebral vessels is supported by a report by Dominguez *et al.*[51] describing porencephaly and bland infarcts among cocaine-exposed neonates, who had uncomplicated deliveries. Reports of high rates of intracranial hemorrhage and cystic lucencies among cocaine-exposed neonates[52,53] are unsubstantiated by other studies involving both term and premature infants.[54,55]

Seizures. Electroencephalographic tracings in cocaine-exposed newborns show conflicting results. One study showed marked central nervous system irritability, with bursts of sharp waves and spikes that were mostly multifocal and did not correlate with clinical seizures or neurological abnormalities. EEG findings resolved completely within 3–12 months.[56] Another study reported no frank EEG abnormalities but did find evidence of electroclinical sleep discordance, with cocaine-exposed infants displaying more mature, continuous slow wave sleep than a comparison group.[57]

Focal seizures are common in cocaine-exposed newborns with strokes. A higher incidence of neonatal seizures related to fetal cocaine exposure in the absence of strokes has not been established. One uncontrolled retrospective study determined subtle seizures among cocaine-exposed infants based on a correlation between stereotypic movements and "ictal" discharges.[58] Most "seizures" were treated with anticonvulsants without improvement. It is highly likely that such behaviors were not epileptic, but rather cocaine-related neurobehaviors. A study that assessed intracranial hemorrhage in premature infants found a three-fold higher rate of seizure among cocaine-exposed infants than among control infants.[55] Because seizures were not a study end-point and were not systematically evaluated, this finding should be taken with caution. In clinical practice seizures resulting from prenatal cocaine exposure, in the absence of stroke, are rare.

Malformations. Cocaine has been linked to numerous congenital malformations, including genitourinary anomalies,[41,59,60] limb reduction deformities, intestinal atresia,[61] and single cardiac ventricle.[62] These anomalies are ascribed to vascular disruption resulting from cocaine-induced vasoconstriction occurring during different periods of organogenesis.[61] Cocaine has also been implicated in the genesis of brain and eye malformations. Brain malformations include skull defects, exencephaly, encephaloceles, and delayed ossification[41,63] as well as septo-optic dysplasia and agenesis of the corpus callosum.[51] Reported ocular anomalies include strabismus, nystagmus, hypoplastic disks, persistent eyelid edema, delayed visual maturation, tortuous abnormally dilated iris vessels, and a persistent hyperplastic primary vitreous with retinopathy of prematurity-like findings.[51,64–66]

In rodents high doses of cocaine can induce urogenital, cardiac, cerebral, and limb reduction anomalies. Mahalik *et al.*[67] reported a high incidence of malformations induced by cocaine in CF-1 mice which mirrored those reported in human infants, namely, skeletal defects, exencephaly, ocular malformations, hydronephrosis, and delayed ossification. Nevertheless, the teratogenic potential for cocaine effects in animal studies is inconsistent and occurs with doses much larger than those encountered in clinical settings.

The teratogenicity of cocaine in humans, with the exception of urogenital malformations, has yet to be established by large scale epidemiological studies. Most reports on cocaine-related malformations are case reports or series, in which ascertainment bias is surely operant as cases are collected in a nonblinded, nonsystematic fashion based on exposure status; the few available population-based studies have not controlled for the effects of fetal alcohol exposure, a well-known teratogen. The influence of confounders on cocaine-related teratogenic effects is exemplified in a study by Zuckerman *et al.*[21] in which cocaine-exposed infants had significantly higher rates (14%) of three minor or one major congenital anomalies compared to cocaine-unexposed infants (8%); the difference disappeared, however, after controlling for confounders, including alcohol.[21]

One of the problems in making causal associations between cocaine and malformations in nonpopulation-based studies is that both cocaine use and malformations of any type are common in clinical practice. The high frequency of both cases and exposure makes associations between the two likely the result of chance and nullifies the rare disease assumption, which states that if a disease is rare (less than 5% prevalence) the odds ratio (the measure of association in case-control studies) will approximate the risk ratio (the measure of association in prospective cohort studies). Without such an approximation, the odds ratio may therefore not be a valid measure of the true association between cocaine exposure and malformations in case-controlled studies.[68]

SIDS and Other Effects. Studies on sudden infant death syndrome (SIDS) and fetal cocaine exposure have yielded somewhat discrepant results. Whereas several studies have reported an association between prenatal cocaine exposure and SIDS,[69–71] others have not found such linkage.[72] The rarity of SIDS may have made findings unstable, especially in smaller studies. A large population-based study found a 1.6-fold elevation in the risk of SIDS linked to cocaine, which reached statistical significance but was much lower than that noted with fetal opiate exposure.[69]

In pneumographic studies involving term infants, those with cocaine exposure exhibited increased episodes of longest apnea, bradycardia, and less periodic breathing than did control infants.[73] A cocaine effect on the norepinephrine system at the level of the locus coeruleus, which is believed responsible for arousal from sleep-related apnea, has been invoked in the genesis of SIDS.[74]

Adverse cocaine effects on the auditory system have also been described, with separate reports showing among cocaine-exposed infants prolonged interpeak latencies I through V on brainstem auditory evoked responses that persisted up to age 3 months.[75,76] An increased startle response was also reported among cocaine-exposed neonates.[77] Collectively, these studies suggest that cocaine affects the central pathways of the developing brain at the level of the brainstem.

Long-Term Neurodevelopment

The mechanism(s) by which fetal cocaine exposure affects the developing brain is not known. Neither is it known whether effects are related to cocaine or to one of its metabolites. Postulated mechanisms of action, discussed in detail elsewhere in this volume, include hypoxia,[6] direct toxicity, cortical dysgenesis,[78] and alterations of monoaminergic (norepinephrine, dopamine, and serotonin)[79–83] or other neural pathways.

Anecdotally, cocaine-exposed children seem to suffer from neurobehavioral abnormalities. Sleep disturbances, especially night terrors or inverted sleep patterns, unexplained unconsolable daytime crying, and an excessive startle response are commonly observed in a subset of cocaine-exposed infants and young children. In an uncontrolled study, high rates of autism and developmental abnormalities were reported among cocaine-exposed infants referred to a developmental clinic.[84]

Cognitive Effects. Several prospective studies have dealt with prenatal cocaine exposure and long-term neurodevelopment.[36,85–90] Most have involved infants or toddlers,[36,85–88] and two reports refer to the same cohort of children.[85,86] Although none of these studies reported cognitive differences related to cocaine, in the Chicago cohort fetal cocaine exposure was the best predictor of small head size, which in turn correlated with poor developmental outcome.[85,86]

Only two studies have addressed cognition and prenatal cocaine exposure among school-aged children. One report by Richardson, Conroy, and Day,[89] which comprised mostly white women with light to moderate cocaine hydrochloride use, found no differences in intellectual ability or academic achievement in exposed offspring at age 6 years. This study, however, suffered from limited statistical power, for although the study enrolled a large number of children, only 28 were cocaine exposed. It also involved a low risk population that is unlikely to show substantial cocaine-related problems. The other study by Wasserman *et al.*[90] found that school-age IQ was significantly associated with home environment, caretaker intelligence, and head size, but not with prenatal cocaine exposure. It involved inner-city children, many of whom were exposed to crack/cocaine. Of note, the cocaine-exposed children had over twice the rate of microcephaly as did the unexposed group.[91]

The practice followed by most, if not all, cocaine studies of controlling for head size in order to assess the effect of cocaine on cognition raises questions regarding the introduction of bias. It is well recognized that controlling for factors that lie in the causal pathway of disease (intervening factors) may lead to bias, often towards the null. Because little is known of the pathophysiology of cocaine's effects, it is possible that impairment of head growth lies within the causal pathway of cocaine's effects on neurodevelopment or that a common factor is responsible for both impaired brain growth and impaired neurodevelopment (FIG. 1). For instance, it is biologically plausible that cocaine impairs these two factors through a common effect on the development of fetal neuropil involving dendritic arborization.[78] In either case it would be wrong to control for head size, as this would diminish or negate true cocaine effects on development.[92] Moreover, an argument has been made for not controlling for factors that are in part caused by the exposure, such as cocaine's effects on fetal brain growth, as this may also introduce bias.[93] A case in point is the fetal alcohol syndrome, which would not exist as a separate entity if investigators were to control for head size prior to making this diagnosis. The practice of routinely controlling for head size should be reconsidered if we are to avoid overcontrolling cocaine's effects in future neurodevelopmental studies.

Neurological Effects. High scores on the Movement Assessment of Infants, indicating poor motor performance, were found among 4-month-old cocaine/polydrug prenatally exposed infants compared to unexposed infants.[94,95] As these instruments do not assess neurological status such as muscle tone, the cause of the impaired motor performance could not be determined. Two prospective studies that focused on neurological function yielded discrepant results.[87,88] One reported high rates of hypertonia associated with cocaine-positive urine toxicology among children at risk for HIV. Rates of hypertonia were maximal at age 6 months and resolved in most children by age 2

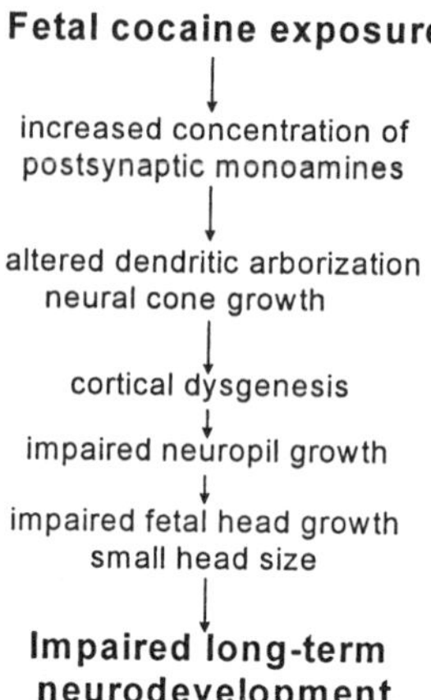

FIGURE 1. Possible mechanism by which small head size may lie in the causal pathway of cocaine effects on neurodevelopment.

years, arms first and legs last.[87] A diagnosis of hypertonic tetraparesis was more strongly associated with cocaine positivity than were all types of hypertonia combined: 27% of 51 cocaine-positive infants compared with 9% of 68 cocaine-negative infants (chi-square, $p = 0.006$; OR = 4.0, 95% CI = 1.5–10.8). Cocaine exposure remained significantly associated with hypertonia in logistic regression models that controlled for 11 variables, including gestational age, birth weight, head circumference, HIV infection, and opiate withdrawal, and interacted significantly with smallness for gestational age: cocaine-exposed infants who were small for their gestational age were less likely to show hypertonia than were infants in the normal range. The adjusted odds of hypertonia associated with cocaine was 3.4 at age 6 months, 5.4 at age 12 months, and 8.7 at age 18 months. Of note, these associations were not evident when the data were analyzed on the basis of maternal self-report irrespective of urine toxicology results, suggesting that heavier or more prolonged cocaine exposure is needed to perceive adverse neurological effects. Development quotients were similar between cocaine-exposed and unexposed children. However, cocaine-exposed children with hypertonic tetraparesis at age 6 months showed lower developmental quotients (mental and psychomotor) than did children without hypertonic tetraparesis, even at later ages when hypertonic tetraparesis had resolved. Thus, hypertonic tetraparesis would appear to be a marker for later developmental impairments. The other study reported no differences between cocaine-exposed and unexposed infants in assessment of tone and reflexes.[88] The discrepancy noted between these two studies might be explained by differences in the characteristics of the study population, the degree of cocaine exposure, and the sensitivity of the neurological instrument used.

In a prospective study of school-aged children Chiriboga *et al.*[91] found higher rates of microcephaly (OR = 2.3; 95% CI = 0.8–6.8) and pyramidal signs (OR = 2.8; 95% CI = 1.0–8.2) among cocaine-exposed children; however, findings did not reach statistical significance. Gross motor function was not impaired in children with pyramidal tract signs. Cerebellar function and microcephaly, but not pyramidal tract signs, were significantly associated with impaired cognitive function.

Cocaine and HIV. American cohorts of HIV-positive children show high rates of neurological abnormality, even among those who passively lose acquired maternal antibodies (HIV seroreverters). Although in part these high rates are attributable to cocaine exposure,[87,96] this does not explain why cocaine-positive HIV-positive children (including seroreverters) are at greater risk of exhibiting neurological abnormalities than are cocaine-positive HIV-negative children. Although a neurotoxic effect of HIV on the developing nervous system is theoretically possible independently of HIV infection (e.g., GP120 or cyotokin exposure),[97] this is unlikely to explain findings, for among cocaine-unexposed children rates of neurological impairments were similar for HIV seroreverters and HIV-negative children.[96] HIV would thus appear to act synergistically with cocaine exposure. For cocaine-addicted women who exchange sex for cocaine, their risk of contracting HIV parallels their level of cocaine use. The interaction between HIV and cocaine exposure may therefore reflect higher levels of cocaine-exposure among HIV-infected women.

Cocaine and Gender. Animal studies involving prenatal exposure reported that cocaine-exposed females showed greater neurobehavioral abnormalities and neurochemical abnormalities in dopaminergic systems than did males,[79] whereas males showed greater alteration in serotoninergic systems than did females.[83] Two clinical studies targeting neurological function in newborns[17] and in toddlers[87] found that males showed greater rates of neurological abnormalities than did females.

Behavioral Effects. Whether fetal cocaine exposure results in long-term behavioral abnormalities is not known. Anecdotally, cocaine-exposed children appear to show high rates of attention deficit disorder, but few, if any, studies focus on cocaine-related behaviors. Infants with polydrug exposure, including cocaine, exhibited significantly lower scores on the Fagan Test of Infant Intelligence (FTII), a structured test of visual memory.[98] Differences in attention and distractibility between groups were also noted. In a large controlled study by Jacobson *et al.*[36] a subset of infants were administered the FTII. Cocaine-exposed infants were found to have poor recognition memory and information-processing abilities as well as a faster reaction time to stimulus. Although the Fagan test is a good predictor of later intelligence, it is less apt at predicting subsequent behaviors. In a study that targeted habituation at age 3 months, cocaine-exposed infants were noted to be excessively irritable, resulting in a significantly larger proportion of cocaine-exposed infants who were unable to begin testing. Differences in psychomotor but not mental development were also noted; however, cocaine-related abnormalities in state regulation may have influenced these findings. Habituation, in those who were testable, was similar in cocaine-exposed and control infants.[99] Cocaine-exposed infants have also been described as excessively excitable[38] and exhibiting a preference for higher rates of stimuli.[100] Cocaine-induced abnormalities in modulation of attention have been invoked to explain these aberrant behaviors.

To date, most cohorts reported are much too young for behavioral estimates to be made reliably. However, a study of school-age children that recruited few ($n = 28$) low risk cocaine-exposed children found no differences in behavioral scores between cocaine-exposed and unexposed children using the Child Behavioral Checklist.[89] Because of its small number of exposed children, low statistical power to detect such abnormalities might have contributed to the negative results. Exposed children, however, performed less well on the Continuous Performance Test, a vigilance test that purportedly measures attention.

Before abnormal behaviors can be causally linked to fetal cocaine exposure, the influence of maternal psychopathology and adverse child-mother interactions on child behaviors should be carefully examined. The importance of taking maternal mental health into account cannot be overstated as it may be key to explaining possible behavioral differences.[101] Because pregnant cocaine-using women show greater depressive symptoms than unexposed women[102,103] and because depressive symptoms among cocaine users tend to result in a poor response to addiction treatment and higher relapse rates,[104] cocaine use could thus simply be a surrogate for maternal psychopathology. Maternal psychopathology could then adversely influence the child's behavior through two possible mechanisms: (1) its influence on the child's environment, in which behavior is altered by adverse maternal-child interactions or poor parenting skills; or (2) genetic factors that confer the offspring of women with mental illness with a greater biological susceptibility to behavioral problems.

SUMMARY

Of late a more realistic appraisal of the fate of cocaine-exposed children has emerged when, contrary to expectations, larger studies have found no cognitive deficits related to fetal cocaine exposure, except as mediated through cocaine effects on head size. Although fetal cocaine exposure has been linked to numerous abnormalities in arousal, attention, and neurological and neurophysiological function, with the exception of inattentiveness, such effects appear to be self-limited and restricted to early infancy and childhood. Whether these transient abnormalities place infants at greater risk of subsequent neurodevelopmental and behavioral problems, however, is not known. Despite these encouraging reports, the question of whether cocaine exerts long-term adverse effects on the developing human nervous system has not yet been resolved, largely because of the limitations of existing studies that rely on inadequate, mostly qualitative ascertainment of cocaine exposure. In addition, older child cocaine studies are few in number and suffer from attrition or limited statistical power.

The absence of tangible evidence of detrimental long-term cocaine effects may reflect limitations in the methods used to identify children at greatest risk for adverse outcome or difficulties in identifying the circumstances (e.g., stressful situations) under which cocaine-related differences may be elicited. Reminiscent of the relationship between alcohol and fetal alcohol syndrome, heavy cocaine exposure may be a necessary, but not a sufficient cause of cocaine-related impairment. Conceivably, in addition to a threshold of exposure, the fetus must also harbor a genetic susceptibility or the *in utero* or postnatal milieu must meet specific requirements. Future neurodevelopmental studies that are based on quantitative ascertainment of cocaine exposure may facilitate identifying children at greatest risk of impairment.

REFERENCES

1. O'Malley, P.M., L.D. Johnston & J.G. Bachman. 1991. Quantitative and qualitative changes in cocaine use among American high school senior, college students and young adults. NIDA Res. Monogr. **110:** 19–43.
2. Johanson, C.E. & M.W. Fischman. 1989. The pharmacology of cocaine related to its abuse. Pharmacol. Rev. **41:** 3–52.
3. Kurth, C.P., C. Monitto, M.L. Albuquerque, P. Feuer, E. Anday & L. Shaw. 1993. Cocaine and its metabolites constrict cerebral arterioles in newborn pigs. J. Pharmacol. Exp. Ther. **265:** 587–591.
4. Konkol, R.J., B.A. Erickson, J.K. Doerr, R.G. Hoffman & J.A. Madden. 1992. Seizures induced by cocaine metabolite benzoylecgonine in rats. Epilepsia **33:** 420–427.
5. Schenker, S., Y. Yang, R.F. Johnson *et al.* 1993. The transfer of cocaine and its metabolites across the term human placenta. Clin. Pharmacol. Ther. **53:** 329–339.
6. Woods, J.R., M.S. Plessinger & K.E. Clark. 1987. Effects of cocaine on uterine blood flow. JAMA **257:** 957–961.
7. Brust, J.C.M. 1993. Cocaine. *In* Neurological Aspects of Substance Abuse. (J.C.M. Brust, Ed.: 82–114. Butterworth-Heinemann. Boston.

8. Woolverton, W.L. & K.M. Johnson. 1992. Neurobiology of cocaine abuse. Trends Pharmacol. Sci. **13:** 193–200.
9. Dackis, C.A. & M.S. Gold. 1985. New concepts in cocaine addiction: The dopamine depletion hypothesis. Neurosci. Biobehav. Rev. **9:** 469–477.
10. Fischman, M.W. 1984. The behavioral pharmacology of cocaine in humans. NIDA Res. Monogr. **50:** 72–91.
11. Goederds, N.E. & J.E. Smith. 1986. Reinforcing properties of cocaine in the medical prefrontal cortex: Primary action of presynaptic dopaminergic terminals. Pharmacol. Biochem. Behav. **25:** 191–199.
12. Deneau, G.A., T. Yanagita & M.H. Seevers. 1969. Self administration of psychoactive substances by monkeys. Psychopharmacologia **16:** 30–48.
13. Hamilton, H.E., J.M. Wallace, L.P. Shimek, S.C. Harris & J.G. Christienson. 1977. Cocaine and benzoylecgonine excretion in humans. J. Forensic Med. **22:** 697–707.
14. Weiss, R.D. & F.H. Gawin. 1988. Protracted elimination of cocaine metabolites in long-term high-dose cocaine abuser. Am. J. Med. **85:** 879–880.
15. Graham, K., G. Koren, J. Klein, J. Schneiderman & M. Greenwald. 1989. Determination of gestational cocaine exposure by hair analysis. JAMA **262:** 3328–3330.
16. Ostrea, E.M.J., M.J. Brady, P.M. Parks, D.C. Asensio & A. Naluz. 1989. Drug screening of meconium in infants of drug-dependent mothers: An alternative to urine testing. J. Pediatr. **115:** 474–477.
17. Chiriboga, C.A., J.C.M. Brust, D.A. Bateman & W.A. Hauser. 1997. Dose-response effect of fetal cocaine exposure on newborn neurological function. Ann. Neurol. **42:** 492 (Abstr.).
18. Vaughn, A.J., R.P. Carzoli, L. Sanchez-Ramos, S. Murphy, N. Khan & T. Chiu. 1993. Community wide estimation of illicit drug use in delivering women: Prevalence, demographic and associated risk factors. Obstet. Gynecol. **82:** 92–96.
19. Bateman, D.A., S.K. Ng, C.A. Hansen & M.C. Heagarty. 1993. The effect of intrauterine cocaine exposure in newborns. Am. J. Public Health **83:** 190–193.
20. McCalla, S., H.L. Minkoff, J. Feldman *et al.* 1991. The biological and social consequences of perinatal cocaine use in an inner city population: Results of an anonymous cross-sectional study. Am. J. Obstet. Gynecol. **164:** 625–630.
21. Zuckerman, B., D.A. Frank, R. Hingson *et al.* 1989. Effects of maternal marijuana and cocaine on fetal growth. N. Engl. J. Med. **320:** 762–768.
22. Ostrea, E.M., M.J. Brady, S. Gause, A.L. Raymundo & M. Stevens. 1992. Drug screening of newborns by meconium analysis: A large scale, prospective, epidemiological study. Pediatrics **89:** 107–113.
23. Habel, L., K. Kaye & J. Lee. 1990. Trends in the reporting of drug use and infant mortality among drug-exposed infants in New York City. Women Health **16:** 41–58.
24. DiGregorio, G.J., A.P. Ferko, E.J. Barbieri *et al.* 1994. Detection of cocaine usage in pregnant women by urinary EMIT drug screen and GC-MS analyses. J. Anal. Toxicol. **18:** 247–250.
25. Lindsay, M.K., H.B. Peterson, J. Boring, J. Gramling, S. Willis & L. Klein. 1992. Crack/cocaine as a risk factor for Human Immunodeficiency Virus Infection type I among inner city parturients. Obstet. Gynecol. **80:** 981–984.
26. Greenburg, MSZ, Singh T, Htoo M. 1991. The association between congenital syphylis and cocaine/crack use in New York City: A case control study. Am J Public Health, **81:** 1316–1318.
27. Knight, E.M., H. James, C.H. Edwards *et al.* 1994. Relationship of illicit drug concentrations during pregnancy to maternal nutrition status. J. Nutr. **124:** 973S.
28. Picone, T.A., L.H. Allen, P.N. Olsen & M.E. Ferris. 1982. Pregnancy outcome in North American women. II. Effects of diet, cigarette smoking, stress and weight gain on placentas, and on neonatal physical and behavioral characteristics. Am. J. Clin. Nutr. **36:** 1214–1223.
29. Moro, J.O., B. de Paredes, M. Wagner *et al.* 1979. Nutritional supplementation and outcome of pregnancy. I Birth weight. Am. J. Clin. Nutr. **32:**
30. Drillien, C.M. 1972. Abnormal neurological signs in the first year of life in low-birth weight infants: Possible prognostic significance. Dev. Med. Child. Neurol. **14:** 575–584.

31. Villar, J., V. Smerigilio, R. Martorell, C.H. Brown & R.E. Klein. 1984. Heterogeneous growth and mental development of intrauterine growth-related infants during the first 3 years of life. Pediatrics **89:** 67–77.
32. Chiriboga, C.A. 1993. Fetal effects. *In* Neurological Complications of Drug and Alcohol Abuse. J.C.M. Brust Ed.: 707–728.
33. Acker, D., B.P. Sachs & K.J. Tracy. 1983. Abruptio placentae associated with cocaine use. Am. J. Obstet. Gynecol. **146:** 220–221.
34. Hadeed, A.J. & S.R. Siegal. 1989. Maternal cocaine use during pregnancy: Effects on the newborn infant. Pediatrics **84:** 205–210.
35. Kain, Z.N., L.C. Mayes, C.A. Ferris, J. Pakes & R. Schottenfeld. 1996. Cocaine-abusing parturients undergoing cesarean section. A cohort study. Anesthesiology **85:** 1028–1035.
36. Jacobson, S.W., J.L. Jacobson, R.I. Sokol, S.S. Martier & L.M. Chiodo. 1996. New evidence for neurobehavioral effects of in utero cocaine exposure. J. Pediatr. **129:** 581–590.
37. Chasnoff, I.J., D.R. Griffith & S.N. MacGregor. 1989. Temporal patterns of cocaine use in pregnancy. JAMA **261:** 171–174.
38. Tronick, E.Z., D.A. Frank, H. Cabral, M. Mirochnick & B. Zuckerman. 1996. Late dose response effects of prenatal cocaine exposure on newborn neurobehavioral performance. Pediatrics **98:** 76–83.
39. Chasnoff, I.J., W.J. Burns, S.H. Scholl & K.A. Burns. 1985. Cocaine use in pregnancy. N. Engl. J. Med. **313:** 666–669.
40. Oro, A.S. & S.D. Dixon. 1987. Perinatal cocaine and methamphetamine exposure: Maternal and neonatal correlates. J. Pediatr. **111:** 571–578.
41. Bingol, N., M. Fuchs, V. Diaz, R.K. Stone & D.S. Gromisch. 1987. Teratology of cocaine use. J. Pediatr. **110:** 93–96.
42. Chiriboga, C.A., D. Bateman, J.C.M. Brust & W.A. Hauser. 1993. Neurological findings in cocaine-exposed infants. Ped. Neurol. **9:** 115–119.
43. Scafidi, F.A., T.M. Field, A. Wheeden *et al.* 1996. Cocaine-exposed preterm neonates show behavioral and hormonal differences. Pediatrics **97:** 851–855.
44. Napriorkowski, B.S., B.M. Lester, C. Freier *et al.* 1996. Effects of in utero substance exposure on infant neurobehavior. Pediatrics **98:** 71–75.
45. Eisen, L.N., T.M. Field, E.S. Bandstra, J.P. Roberts, C. Morrow & S.K. Larson. 1991. Perinatal cocaine effects on neonatal stress behavior and performance on the Brazelton Scale. Pediatrics **88:** 477–480.
46. Neuspiel, D.R., C. Hamel, E. Hochberg, J. Greene & D. Campbell. 1990. Maternal cocaine use and infant behavior. Neurotoxicol. Teratol. **13:** 229–233.
47. Chiriboga, C.A. & D.M. Ferriero. 1996. Neurological complications of maternal drug abuse. *In* Principles of Child Neurology, B.O. Berg, Ed.: 1363–1374. McGraw-Hill. New York.
48. Konkol, R.J., L.J. Murphey, D.M. Ferriero, D.A. Demsey & G.D. Olsen. 1994. Cocaine metabolites in the neonate: Potential for toxicity. J. Child Neurol. **9:** 242–248.
49. Chasnoff, I.J., M.E. Bussey, R. Savich & C.M. Stack. 1986. Perinatal cerebral infarction and maternal cocaine use. J. Pediatr. **108:** 456–457.
50. Tenorio, G.M., M. Nazvi, G.H. Bickers & R.H. Hubbird. 1988. Intrauterine stroke and maternal polydrug use. Clin. Pediatr. (Phila.) **27:** 567.
51. Dominguez, R., A.A. Vila-Coro, J.M. Slopis & T.P. Bohan. 1991. Brain and ocular abnormalities in infants with in-utero exposure to cocaine and other street drugs. AJDC **145:** 688–695.
52. Bejar, R. & S.D. Dixon. 1989. Echoencephalographic findings in neonates associated with maternal and methamphetamine use: Incidence and clinical correlates. J. Pediatr. **115:** 770–778.
53. Singer, L.T., T.S. Yamashita, S. Hawkins, D. Cairns, J. Baley & R. Kliegman. 1994. Incresed incidence of intraventricular hemorrhage and developmental delay in cocaine-exposed infants. J. Pediatr. **124:** 765–771.
54. Frank, D.A. & K. McCarten. 1992. Cranial ultrasounds in term newborns: Failure to replicate excess abnormalities in cocaine-exposed. Ped. Res. **31:** 247a.2.
55. Dusick, A.M., R.F. Covert, M.D. Schreiber *et al.* 1993. Risk of intracranial hemorrhage

and other adverse outcomes after cocaine exposure in a cohort of 323 very low birth weight infants. J. Pediatr. **122:** 438–445.

56. DOBERCZAK, T.M., S. SHANZER, R.T. SENIE & S.R. KANDALL. 1988. Neonatal electroencephalographic effect of intrauterine cocaine exposure. J. Pediatr. **113:** 354–358.
57. LEGIDO, A., R.R. CLANCY, A.R. SPITZER & L.P. FINNEGAN. 1992. Electroencephalographic and behavioral-state studies in infants of cocaine-addicted mothers. Am. J. Dis. Child. **146:** 748–752.
58. KRAMER, L.D., G.E. LOCKE, A. OGUNYEMI & L. NELSON. 1990. Neonatal cocaine-related seizures. J. Child. Neurol. **5:** 60–64.
59. CHAVEZ, G.F., J. MULINARE & J.F. CORDERO. 1989. Maternal cocaine use during early pregnancy as a risk factor for congenital urogenital anomalies. JAMA **262:** 795–798.
60. ANONYMOUS. 1989. Urogenital anomalies in the offspring of women using cocaine during early pregnancy-Atlanta 1968–1980. Morbid. Mortal. Wkly Rep. **38:** 536, 541–542.
61. HOYME, H.E., J.K. LYONS & S.D. DIXON. 1990. Prenatal cocaine exposure and fetal vascular disruption. Pediatrics **85:** 743–747.
62. SHEPARD, T.H., A.G. FANTEL & R.P. KAPUR. 1991. Fetal coronary thrombosis as a cause for single ventricle. Teratology **43:** 113–117.
63. HEIER, L.A., C.R. CARPANZO, J. MAST, P.W. BRILL, P. WINCHESTER & M.D. DECK. 1991. Maternal cocaine abuse: The spectrum of radiologic abnormalities in the neonatal CNS. AJNR **12:** 951–956.
64. ISENBERG, S., A. SPIERRER & S. INEKELIS. 1987. Ocular signs of cocaine intoxication in neonates. Am. J. Ophthal. **103:** 350.
65. GOOD, W.V., D.M. FERRIERO, M. GOLABI & J.A. KOBORI. 1992. Abnormalities of the visual system in infants exposed to cocaine. Ophthalmology **99:** 341–346.
66. TESKE, M. & M. TRESE. 1987. Retinopathy of prematurity like fundus and persistent hyperplastic primary vitreous associated with maternal cocaine use. Am. J. Ophthal. **103:** 719–720.
67. MAHALIK, M., R. GAUTIERRI & D. MAUN. 1980. Teratogenic potential of cocaine hydrochloride in CF-12 mice. J. Pharmacol. Sci. **111:** 703–706.
68. KLEINBAUM, D.G., L.L. KUPPER & H. MORGENSTERN. 1982. Epidemiological Research. Principles and Quantitative Methods. Van Norstrand Reinhold. New York, NY.
69. KANDALL, S.R., J. GAINES, L. HABEL, G. DAVIDSON & D. JESSON. 1993. Relationship of maternal substance abuse to subsequent infant death syndrome in offspring. J. Pediatr. **123:** 120–126.
70. DURAND, D.J., A.M. ESPINOZA & B.G. NICKERSON. 1990. Association between prenatal cocaine exposure and sudden infant death syndrome. J. Pediatr. **117:** 909–911.
71. DAVIDSON, S.L., D. BAUTISTA, L. CHAN *et al.* 1990. Sudden infant death syndrome in infants of substance-abusing mothers. J. Pediatr. **17:** 876–881.
72. BAUCHNER, H., B. ZUCKERMAN, M. MCCLAIN, D. FRANK, L.E. FRIED & H. KAYNE. 1988. Risk of sudden infant death syndrome among infants with in utero cocaine exposure. J. Pediatr. **113:** 831–834.
73. SILVESTRI, J.M., J.M. LONG, D.E. WEESE-MAYER & G.A. BARKOV. 1991. Effects of prenatal cocaine on respiration, heart rate and sudden infant death syndrome. Pediatr. Pulmonol. **11:** 328–334.
74. GINGRAS, J.L. & D. WEESE-MAYER. 1990. Maternal cocaine addiction. II. An animal model for the study of brainstem mechanisms operative in sudden infant death syndrome. Med. Hypotheses **33:** 231–234.
75. SALAMY, A., L. ELDREDGE, J. ANDERSON & D. BULL. 1990. Brainstem transmission time in infants exposed to cocaine in-utero. J. Pediatr. **117:** 627–629.
76. SHI, L., B. CONE-WESSON & B. REDDIX. 1988. Effects of maternal cocaine use and the neonatal auditory system. Int. J. Pediatr. Otorrhinlaryngol. **15:** 245–251.
77. ANDAY, E.K., M.E. COHEN, N.E. KELLEY & D.S. LEITNER. 1989. Effects of in utero cocaine exposure on startle and its modification. Dev. Pharmacol. **12:** 137–145.
78. GRESSENS, P., B. KOSOFSKY & P. EVRARD. 1992. Cocaine-induced disturbances in corticogenesis in the developing murine brain. Neuroscience **140:** 113–116.
79. DOW-EDWARDS, D.L. 1989. Long term neurochemical and neurobehavioral consequences of cocaine use during pregnancy. Ann. N.Y. Acad. Sci. **562:** 280–289.

80. Spear, L.P., L.K. Kirstein & N.A. Frambes. 1989. Cocaine effects on the developing central nervous system: Behavioral, psychopharmacological, and neurochemical studies. Ann. N.Y. Acad. Sci. **562:** 290–307.
81. Frick, G.S. & D.L. Dow-Edwards. 1994. The effects of cocaine on cerebral metabolic function in periweanling rates: The roles of serotonergic and dopaminergic uptake blockade. Brain Res. 158–170.
82. Dow-Edwards, D.L. 1996. Modification of acoustic startle reactivity by cocaine administration during the postnatal period: Comparison with a specific serotonin reuptake inhibitor. Neurotoxicol. Teratol. **18:** 289–296.
83. Battaglia, G., T.M. Cabrera & L.D. Van de Kar. 1995. Prenatal cocaine exposure produces biochemical and functional changes in brain serotonin systems in rat progeny. NIDA Res. Monogr. **158:** 115–148.
84. Davis, E., I. Fenoy & D. Laraque. 1992. Autism and developmental abnormalities in children with perinatal cocaine exposure. J. Natl: Med. Assoc. **84:** 315–319.
85. Chasnoff, I.J., D.R. Griffith, C. Freier & J. Murray. 1992. Cocaine/polydrug use in pregnancy. Pediatrics **89:** 284–289.
86. Azuma, S. & I.J. Chasnoff. 1993. Outcome of children prenatally exposed to cocaine and other drugs: A path analysis of three year data. Pediatrics **92:** 396–402.
87. Chiriboga, C.A., M. Vibbert, R. Malouf *et al.* 1995. Neurological correlates of fetal cocaine exposure: Transient hypertonia of infancy and early childhood. Pediatrics **96:** 1070–1077.
88. Hurt, H., N.L. Brodsky, L. Betancourt, L.E. Braitman, E. Malmud & J.J. Giannetta. 1995. Cocaine-exposed children: Follow-up through 30 months. J. Dev. Behav. Pediatr. **16:** 29–35.
89. Richardson G.A., M.L. Conroy & N.L. Day. 1996. Prenatal cocaine exposure: Effects on the development of school-aged children. Neurotoxicol. Teratol. **18:** 627–634.
90. Wasserman, G., J. Kline, D. Bateman *et al.* 1998. Prenatal cocaine exposure and school-age intelligence. Drug Alcohol Dep. In press.
91. Chiriboga, C.A., G.A. Wasserman, D.A. Bateman *et al.* 1997. Fetal cocaine exposure and neurological outcome in school-aged children. Unpublished data.
92. Breslow, N.E. & N.E. Day. 1980. The analysis of case control studies. *In* Statistical Methods in Cancer Research. IARC Scientific publications No. 32. Lyon International Agency for Research in Cancer.
93. Weinberg, C.R. 1993. Towards a clearer definition of confounding. Am. J. Epidemiol. **137:** 1–8.
94. Schneider, J.W. & I.J. Chasnoff. 1992. Motor assessment of cocaine/polydrug exposed infants at age 4 months. Neurotoxicol. Teratol. **14:** 97–101.
95. Fetters, L. & E.Z. Tronick. 1996. Neuromotor development of cocaine-exposed and control infants from birth through 15 months: Poor and poorer performance. Pediatrics **98:** 938–943.
96. Chiriboga, C.A., M. Vibbert, R. Malouf *et al.* 1993. Children at risk for HIV infection: Neurological and developmental abnormalities (abstr.) Ann. Neurol. **34:** 500–501.
97. Lipton, S.A. 1997. Neuropathogenesis of acquired immunodeficiency syndrome. Curr. Opin. Neurol. **10:** 274–253.
98. Struthers, J.M. & R.L. Hansen. 1992. Visual recognition memory in drugs exposed in infants. J. Dev. Behav. Pediatr. **13:** 108–111.
99. Mayes, L.C., M.H. Bornstein, M.A. Chawarska & R.H. Granger. 1995. Information processing and developmental assessments in 3-month old infants exposed to cocaine. Pediatrics **95:** 539–545.
100. Karmel, B.Z. & J.M. Gardner. 1996. Prenatal cocaine exposure effects on arousal modulation attention during the neonatal period. Dev. Psychobiol. **29:** 463–480.
101. Stanger, C.M., S. McConaughy & T. Achenbach. 1992. Three-year course of a national sample of 4- to 16-year old. II. Predictors of syndromes. J. Am. Acad. Child. Adolesc. Psychiatry **31:** 941–950.
102. Strickland, T.L., R. James, H. Myers, W. Lawson, X. Bean & J. Mupps. 1993. Psychological characteristics related to cocaine use during pregnancy: A postpartum assessment. J. Natl. Med. Assoc. **85:** 758–760.

103. Zuckerman, B., H. Amaro, H. Bauchner & H. Cabral. 1989. Depressive symptoms during pregnancy: Relationship to poor health behaviors. Am. J. Obstet. Gynecol. **160:** 1107–1111.
104. Zeidonis, D.M. & T.R. Kosten. 1991. Depression as a prognostic factor for pharmacological treatment of cocaine dependence. Psychopharmacol. Bull. **27:** 337–343.
105. Miller, H.C. & K. Hassanein. 1971. Diagnosis of impaired fetal growth in newborn infants. Pediatrics **48:** 511–522.

Regulation of Arousal and Attention in Preschool Children Exposed to Cocaine Prenatally

LINDA C. MAYES,[a,c] CHRISTIAN GRILLON,[b] RICHARD GRANGER,[a] AND RICHARD SCHOTTENFELD[b]

[a]*Yale Child Study Center and* [b]*Department of Psychiatry, Yale School of Medicine, New Haven, Connecticut 06520, USA*

ABSTRACT: Four lines of evidence suggest a plausible link between prenatal cocaine exposure (CE) and specific effects on the mechanisms subserving arousal and attention regulation in infants and preschool-aged children. These are (1) the association of prenatal CE with alterations in monoaminergic system ontogeny; (2) neurobehavioral effects of prenatal CE in animals consistent with an enduring increased level of activity in response to novelty and inhibited exploration and altered responses to stress, suggesting overarousal in the face of novel/stressful situations and disrupted attention and exploration; (3) altered norepinephrine system function in cocaine-exposed human infants; and (4) neurobehavioral findings in infants and preschool-aged children suggestive of disrupted arousal regulation in the face of novelty, increased distractibility, and consequent impaired attention to novel, structured tasks. This paper summarizes findings on response to novel challenges from a cohort of prenatally cocaine-exposed infants and preschool-aged children followed longitudinally since birth. Arousal regulation in the face of novel challenges is operationalized behaviorally as state and emotional reactivity and neurophysiologically as the startle response and heart rate variability. Across different ages and tasks, behavioral and neurophysiological findings suggest that prenatally cocaine-exposed children are more likely to exhibit disrupted arousal regulation. Because the regulation of arousal serves as a gating mechanism to optimize orientation and attention, arousal regulation has important implications for ongoing information processing, learning, and memory. Furthermore, impaired arousal regulation predisposes children to a lower threshold for activation of "stress circuits" and may increase their vulnerability to the developmentally detrimental effects of stressful conditions particularly when such children are also exposed to the chaotic environmental conditions often characterizing substance-abusing families.

INTRODUCTION

Within the last decade, many investigators have focused on the potential physical, neurodevelopmental, and neuropsychological effects of prenatal cocaine exposure (CE) on infants and young children. These studies have utilized a variety of designs including longitudinal, cross-sectional, case-control, and retrospective cohorts, have defined in multiple ways the independent variable(s), that is, the amount and duration of cocaine as well as other drug exposure, and have emphasized a host of different outcomes. (For a review of central methodologic issues in studies of prenatal CE, see refs. 1–3). The oldest children in reported longitudinally maintained cohorts were between 8 and 10 years of age, but most children in these longitudinally followed cohorts are

[c] Address for correspondence: Linda C. Mayes, MD, Yale Child Study Center, 230 S. Frontage Road, New Haven, CT 06520. Phone, 203-785-7211; fax, 203-737-4197; e-mail, Linda.Mayes@yale.edu

now reaching preschool and early school age (3–6 years).[4–9] Although still scant, inconsistent, or inconclusive on many crucial issues and marked by a number of methodologic problems, published studies to date nonetheless reveal the beginnings of a profile of possible cocaine-related effects on neuropsychological functions subserving arousal and attention regulation and reactivity to stressful conditions. (For recent reviews, see refs. 10–13). That profile is further elaborated by findings from several animal models in which important factors such as duration and type of exposure as well as environmental conditions may be more adequately controlled.[14–17]

CONCEPT OF AROUSAL REGULATION

Arousal refers to the level of central nervous system activation that governs the facility with which attention can be directed towards and responses made to external events.[18–20] Schematically, an inverted U-shaped relation exists between arousal and responsiveness (FIG. 1) with optimal responsiveness, attention, or reactivity being at the apex of the curve. Behaviorally, shifts in arousal are manifest by changes in behavioral state, level of alertness and attention, and physiologically by changes in, for example, blood pressure, basal heart rate, and heart rate variability, skin conductance, serum or salivary cortisol, and catecholamine secretion.[21–23] External stimulation increases levels of arousal (FIG. 1). A marked increase in arousal in response to a new stimulus may overshoot optimal orienting and instead result in irritability, anxiety, and, for some individuals, avoidance—in short, the behavioral experience of being overwhelmed by an experience.

Individual differences in children's arousal or self-regulatory capacities may have

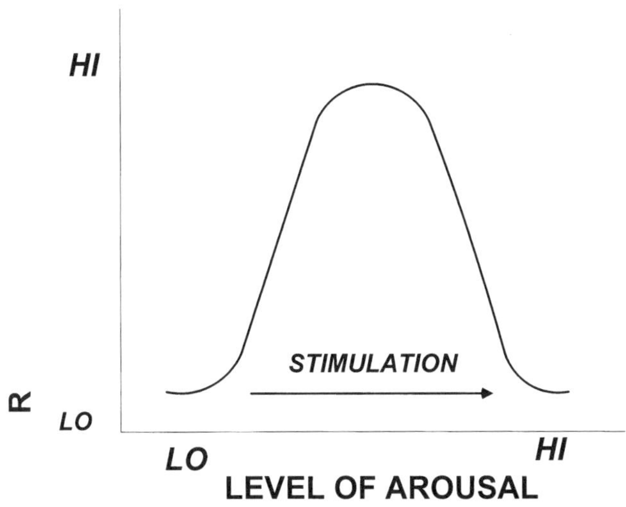

FIGURE 1. Schematic representation of relations among response, stimulation, and levels of arousal.

their origins in genetic, constitutional, and/or experiential factors.[19] Genetic factors are indicated in the increased incidence of affect regulation impairment among children of parents with anxiety disorders.[24,25] Constitutional factors are evidenced in differing rates of maturation of cortical and subcortical inhibitory systems and of the autonomic nervous system.[19,26,27] Prenatal experiential factors include specific gestational events such as cocaine exposure and less specific, more general perinatal risks such as intrauterine growth retardation. Postnatal experiences including characteristics of the parenting environment may also influence infant arousal regulation.[28] Because regulation of arousal serves as a gating mechanism to optimize orientation and attention, arousal regulation has important implications for ongoing information processing, learning, and memory.[18,19,29] Furthermore, impaired arousal regulation (or, in related domains of discourse, high reactivity to novel situations[30]) predisposes children to a lower threshold for activation of "stress circuits"[21] and may increase their vulnerability to the developmentally detrimental effects of stressful conditions particularly when such children are also exposed to the chaotic environmental conditions[31,32] often characterizing substance-abusing families.

LINES OF EVIDENCE RELATING AROUSAL REGULATION TO PRENATAL COCAINE EXPOSURE

Four lines of evidence suggest a plausible link between prenatal CE and specific effects on the mechanisms subserving arousal and attention regulation in infants and preschool-aged children. These are: (1) the association of prenatal CE with alterations in monoaminergic system ontogeny; (2) neurobehavioral effects of prenatal CE in animals consistent with altered responses to stress; (3) altered monoaminergic and glucocorticoid system function in cocaine-exposed human infants; and (4) neurobehavioral findings in infants and preschool-aged children suggestive of disrupted arousal regulation in the face of novelty, increased distractibility, and consequently impaired attention to novel, structured tasks.

COCAINE AND MONOAMINERGIC SYSTEM ONTOGENY

At pharmacologically active doses in mature animals, cocaine inhibits the reuptake of monoamines (norepinephrine [NE], dopamine [DA], and serotonin [5-HT] at the presynaptic junction. This leads to increased concentration of these neurotransmitters in the synaptic cleft and higher levels of activation in the central catecholaminergic systems.[33,34] The increase in postsynaptic transmitter levels is paralleled by presynaptic depletion and a compensatory increase in synthesis. Concomitant upregulation of postsynaptic receptors may also result in supersensitivity to catecholamines.[35]

Because monoaminergic-rich regions of the brain (e.g., amygdala, striatum, locus coeruleus, ventral tegmental area, and posterior parietal cortex) are involved in arousal and attention regulation,[36,37] exposure to cocaine *in utero* may adversely affect those developing regions of the brain regulating arousal and attention by potentially altering cortical morphology as well as monoaminergic ontogeny and function. Monoaminergic systems appear early in fetal brain development—NE, DA, and 5-HT neurons can be detected by the end of the second month of gestation[38]—and exert trophic influences on the ontogeny of other brain cells.[39,40] Because of this trophic influence, monoamines play a role in each phase of brain development including the earliest proliferative phase (2–4 months for neurons and 5 months' gestation to 1 year postnatal for glial cells), the neuronal migration phase (3–5 months' gestation), and an organizational phase with synaptogenesis and neuronal maturation and differentiation (6 months' gestation to several years postnatally).[41] Cocaine-related effects on monoaminergic ontogeny and metabolism may lead to mistimed radial gliogenesis with resultant changes in cortical morphology (early gestation effects) as well as alterations in synaptic connections and neuronal maturation in both cortex and monoaminergic-rich subcortical regions (late gestation effects) (e.g., refs. 40, 42–44).

Neuromorphologic Changes in Animal Models Associated with Prenatal Cocaine Exposure. Some evidence is available for cocaine-related effects on the earliest phases of brain cell proliferation and neuronal migration, and thus on cortical morphology. In rats, prenatal CE interferes with radial gliogenesis and thus disrupts neocortical architecture.[45–48] In rhesus monkeys, intermittent prenatal CE resulted in cerebral cortices with highly abnormal structural characteristics including disrupted cortical laminar architecture with an increased number of cells in the underlying white matter, suggesting markedly impaired neuronal migration.[49] Findings such as these may reflect disrupted monoaminergic system-regulated processes that control the genesis of radial glial cells necessary for proper neuronal migration to cortical layers.[40,50] Disruption of such processes is likely not compensated for later in gestation, inasmuch as neurogenesis is complete by day 120–125[51] and neuronal migration by the end of the second trimester. Fewer studies are available specifically examining the effects of cocaine on later gestation events such as continuing gliogenesis, synaptogenesis, and neuronal connectivity. At least one group has reported decreased striatal neurotrophic activity with cocaine that in turn limits the growth of DA neurons postnatally.[52] Prenatal CE also appears to affect 5-HT and NE connecting fiber density (to both increase and decrease) in different brain regions.[53,54]

In Vivo *and* In Vitro *Evidence for Cocaine-Related Effects on Monoaminergic System Development.* The specific effects of fetal exposure on enduring changes in monoaminergic function (e.g., concentration of monoamines and their precursors and metabolites, on receptor density and binding, on monoaminergic activity, and on monoaminergic-associated fiber density) will depend on the timing of exposure during gestation, and these timing issues are far from well studied. Furthermore, because specific monoaminergic systems are interactive, upregulation at one level of, for example, DA activity may be associated with compensatory downregulation at NE or 5-HT function or with another aspect of DA function. Although these types of interrelationships and the differential effects of exposure during different prenatal periods have not been examined in detail, several neurochemical effects have been reported in both *in vivo* and *in vitro* models, each pointing to prenatal CE-related effects on monoaminergic system development at the level of transmitter synthesis, activity, or receptor formation/function. These include reductions in brain 2-deoxyglucose uptake and neuronal electrophysiologic activity in DA-rich regions,[55–56] transiently reduced 5-HT immunoreactivity in the hippocampus and late-onset increased 5-HT immunoreactivity in the striatum,[53,54] increased striatal D_1 and D_2 receptor binding,[55,57] and decreased striatal DA concentration.[52] In cell culture, cocaine inhibits the development of reuptake mechanisms in 5-HT neurons.[58] Prenatal cocaine administration *increases* NE receptor density,[59] receptor binding, presynaptic synthesis of NE, NE activity, and NE concentration throughout NE-innervated regions.[60–62] It is important to note that with postnatal maturation, monoaminergic system development is ongoing, and further shifts in neurotransmitter synthesis and receptor function may occur with some neonatal effects apparently disappearing or reversing in the direction of effect from attenuation to upregulation or vice versa,[53,63] an area requiring far more investigation.

ANIMAL NEUROBEHAVIORAL MODELS

A number of neurobehavioral alterations have been observed concomitant with cocaine-associated changes in monoaminergic system function; however, the relations of the gestational exposure period to neurobehavioral outcomes have not been adequately defined. Most neurobehavioral findings come from rat models in which adult rodent offspring exposed to cocaine prenatally exhibit different apparently cocaine-related neurobehavioral sequelae in the following functional domains: cognition or learning, social, and arousal/stress regulation (for review, see refs. 15, 64–67). Deficits in cognitive functioning are suggested by deficits in classical conditioning,[68,69] impairments in active and passive avoidance tasks,[69] increased response perseveration,[70] diminished proximal cue learning,[65] and impaired habituation.[71] All of these effects are generally found at doses far less than those causing overt physical malformations.[72] Social dysfunctions appear in two different areas, sex-typical behaviors[73] and parenting,[74] and these behavioral alterations are paralleled by sex-differentiated effects on catecholamine levels in specific brain regions.[75] In terms of parenting behaviors, cocaine-exposed animals rearing their biologic pups appear significantly more aggressive towards intruders,[74] are slower to begin, and engage in fewer, species-expected parenting behaviors.[76] As infants, exposed offspring exhibit fewer socially directed play behaviors.[77]

Enduring alterations in arousal regulation and stress-related responses have also been documented. In contrast to non-cocaine-exposed animals, prenatally cocaine-exposed animals inhibit approaching novel conditions and open-field exploration,[78] and when they do engage in novel exploration after a delay, they do so with markedly increased activity suggesting overarousal.[59,79,80] Cocaine-exposed animals show atypical responses to standard stressful paradigms including footshock and swim tests.[68,70,81–84] In these situations, exposed animals exhibit markedly increased activity and efforts to avoid the aversive situation, a finding interpreted by some as indicative of impaired arousal regulation and increased fearfulness once the animal is stressed and overaroused.[82] Moreover, wall climbing, a monoaminergic-associated behavior, is attenuated with footshock in prenatally cocaine-exposed animals, a finding suggesting attenuation of monoaminergic system activity.[79] Related to dysfunctional arousal or stress regulation are alterations in state regulation as measured by altered sleep patterns and diminished REM sleep in cocaine-exposed fetal sheep[84] and attenuated startle responses in exposed offspring as infants.[85] As is also true of human studies, few data are available from animal models regarding the relation of neurobehavioral (or neurochemical) effects to critical periods and duration of exposure, but in the studies available there is a suggestion of differential neurobehavioral effects depending on the period of gestational exposure.[65]

NEUROCHEMISTRY IN HUMAN INFANTS

In human infants, neurochemical studies following prenatal CE are to date scant, but two areas of work point to effects on those neurochemical systems most related to arousal regulation and stress reactivity. Three studies examined metabolites, precursors, or levels of norepinephrine or dopamine in the serum or cerebrospinal fluid of newborns exposed to cocaine prenatally and found a significant increase in plasma NE[86] and catecholamine precursors in cerebrospinal fluid[87] and a decrease in the metabolites of dopamine,[88] findings suggesting an alteration in monoaminergic system function at least neonatally. Furthermore, for the cocaine-exposed infants norepinephrine levels were inversely related to features of the infant's neurobehavioral profile.[87] Second, cocaine-exposed infants exhibit an attenuated cortisol response to noninvasive (neurobehavioral examination) and invasive (heel-stick) manipulations despite no differences in baseline cortisol levels,[89] suggesting that glucocorticoid-mediated arousal regulatory systems are altered by *in utero* CE or the chronically stressful conditions associated with CE.[90] Stated another way, the infants do not respond in the usually expected ways to novel stimulation; they require more stimulation to reach levels of responsiveness equivalent to those of nonexposed infants, and their cortisol responses to such stimulation are attenuated.

NEUROBEHAVIORAL PROFILES IN HUMAN INFANTS AND YOUNG CHILDREN

Neurodevelopmentally, in the immediate perinatal period, findings are inconsistent and range from reports of no differences when compared to non-cocaine-exposed neonates[91] to impairments in neonatal habituation and state regulation.[92,93] Additionally, impairments in the distribution of sleep states, startle response, brainstem evoked potential, overall neurological maturity, and cry characteristics indicative of delays in neurological maturation have been described in cocaine-exposed neonates.[94–98] Postnatally, in terms of overall developmental competency measured by standardized assessment instruments (e.g., Bayley[99] and Stanford-Binet[100]), studies to date of human infants exposed prenatally to cocaine have failed to reveal consistent differences between cocaine-exposed and non-cocaine-exposed infants and young children.[5,6,9,101,102] Moreover, differences apparent in infancy in motor and/or mental development are not apparent later in the first or second year.[103] However, three caveats pertain. First, despite no apparent differences between cocaine and non-cocaine-exposed infants, cocaine-exposed groups reportedly show more variability and scatter in their performance on standardized assessments, suggesting minimally greater heterogeneity among cocaine-exposed samples and possibly more difficulty in meeting the attentional demands of a standardized testing situation.[4,9] Moreover, when domains such as persistence during developmental testing are also scored, cocaine-exposed children appear less persistent or attentive to the task, and persistence scores are highly correlated with IQ.[4] Second, significant differences have been reported between cocaine-exposed and non-cocaine-exposed groups on individual developmental domains, most notably speech and language for preschool-aged children[7,104] as well as motor delays at least during the first year.[105] Third, standardized developmental assessments do not directly measure the domains of arousal and impulse regulation and attention modulation or more specific executive functions or information-processing strategies,[106,107] areas for which there are conceptual reasons to hypothesize specific cocaine-related effects on development.[108,109]

In the areas of arousal, attention, and executive functioning (e.g., habituation, conditioned learning, and novelty recognition), differences were noted between cocaine-exposed and non-cocaine-exposed infants.[10] Struthers and Hansen[110,111] reported impaired recognition memory among cocaine- or amphetamine-exposed infants compared to a non-drug–exposed group between 7 and 8 months of age. Similarly, Alessandri and colleagues[112] reported delays in novelty responsiveness and conditioned responsiveness well into the second half of the first year of life. Mayes and colleagues[113,114] reported increased reactivity and irritability in response to novel stimulation among cocaine-exposed infants, and these differences occurred in the context of no differences on measures of infant information processing (e.g., rate of habituation). Azuma and Chasnoff[4] also reported poor task persistence and increased irritability and distractibility among cocaine-exposed 3-year olds participating in standardized testing. Ramsey and colleagues[115] showed an increased behavioral reactivity and attenuated cortisol response to stressful events (e.g., a routine inoculation) at 2 months. Reports of longer term follow-up of arousal and attention regulation or of executive function in cocaine-exposed young children are not yet available.

OVERALL STUDY DESIGN AND CHARACTERISTICS OF THE SAMPLE

In our laboratory, we have been studying a cohort of children from birth through age 7 years with biannual visits. Three exposure groups are defined by a combination of maternal history and prenatal/perinatal maternal and infant toxicology. These groups are: exposure to cocaine with or without other drugs including alcohol, marijuana, or tobacco (CE); exposure to other drugs but no cocaine (NC); and no prenatal exposure to any drug including tobacco (ND). Positive prenatal CE status was considered present if use was reported by the mother even if urine or meconium toxicologic results were negative. Conversely, if mothers reported that they did not use cocaine, but clinic or hospital urine toxicologic or meconium results were positive, infants were considered exposed. The demographic characteristics of the enrolled sample of 601 families enrolled at birth are shown in TABLE 1. As has been found in other groups, cocaine using women are usually older, have had more pregnancies and more prenatal complications, and their infants are smaller with reduced head circumference and an increased incidence of intrauterine growth retardation. TABLE 2 shows the amount of other drug use in the non-cocaine- and cocaine-using groups with, as has also been described before, cocaine-using women reporting more alcohol and tobacco use as well as on average 5 years of cocaine use before their child was born. We have been able to maintain contact with 82% of originally enrolled families, and no differences were noted in the demographic, perinatal, and drug use characteristics between those enrolled and those maintained in follow-up.

The overall study focuses on outcomes tapping into arousal and attention regulation with converging measures for children in the following domains: arousal and attention

TABLE 1. Demographic and Perinatal Characteristics of Follow-up Sample ($n = 601$)

	ND ($n = 136$)	NC ($n = 88$)	CE ($n = 377$)	F/X²
Maternal age (yr)	24.9 (4.6)	25.8 (5.4)	28.1 (4.5)	26.9***
% African-American	76.5	70.9	81.9	X² 8.3
Caucasian	12.5	17.4	12.4	
% High school diploma	82.4	68.4	46.1	X² 56.1***
Number of pregnancies	3.2 (1.8)	3.8 (1.8)	5.1 (2.5)	38.9***
OCS[a]	94.8 (22.6)	97.6 21.8)	81.4 (21.1)	30.3***
Infant gender (% m)	55.1	44.3	51.4	X² 2.5
Birth weight (gm)	3279 (531)	3074 (515)	2708 (661)	46.5***
Head circumference (cm)	33.6 (2.0)	33.2 (1.8)	32.2 (2.6)	20.9***
% Small-gestational age[b]	6.0	4.6	12.9	X² 8.6*

ABBREVIATIONS: ND = exposure to cocaine with or without other drugs including alcohol, marijuana, or tobacco; NC = exposure to other drugs but no cocaine; ND = no prenatal exposure to any drug including alcohol.

[a]Obstetric Complications Scale Score.

[b]Criteria were ≥ 2 SD expected birth weight for gestational age.

*$p < 0.05$; **$p < 0.01$; ***$p < 0.001$.

TABLE 2. Amount of Other Drug Use[a] in Cocaine-Using and Other Drug-Using Groups

Mean (Standard Error), Range	ND	CE
Alcohol—Years of Use	5.8 (0.80), 1–21	9.2 (0.44), 1–30
Days alcohol use per month[a]	2.8 (0.54), 1–15	6.5 (0.74), 1–30
Marijuana—Years of Use	1.9 (0.41), 1–15	5.1 (0.43), 1–23
Days marijuana use per month[a]	1.7 (0.42), 1–15	2.8 (0.46), 1–30
Tobacco—Years of Use	6.6 (0.91), 1–25	10.2 (0.41), 1–25
Average number per day[a]	1.9 (0.28), 1–10	1.8 (0.09), 1–8
Years of Cocaine Use	. . .	5.1 (0.24), 1–15

For abbreviations, see TABLE 1.
[a]All estimates of use are based on the 30 days before subject knew she was pregnant.

regulation, executive and cognitive function, adaptive and maladaptive behavior, and childhood psychiatric status. The study builds on an interactive model which proposes that children with developmental risks are more or less vulnerable to poor outcomes depending on the severity of their environmental disruption and stress. Data on arousal and attention regulation come from both behavioral observations and neurophysiologic/psychological measures.

Behavioral Data Regarding Arousal Systems

Behaviorally, arousal is operationalized as behavioral state in response to a novel situation or stimulus. We examined in detail patterns of change in the behavioral markers of arousal in response to the presentation of novel visual stimuli during a task in which novel stimuli presentations are followed by repeat presentation of the then familiar stimuli. Across the different assessment procedures, we have found increased irritability and overall negative affective and behavioral state, more so in the cocaine-exposed group than in either the NC or the ND groups. Additionally, cocaine-exposed infants have shown less sustained and selective attention to novel tasks.

- In a habituation procedure at 3 months, cocaine-exposed infants are significantly more likely than either NC or ND infants to become irritable and cry on stimulus presentation and to drop-out of the procedure.[113,114]
- In novel visual and tactual exploratory procedures at 12 and 18 months in which novel toys are presented to the child, cocaine-exposed infants explore novel items for proportionately less time than do either NC or ND children and spend proportionately more time in nonexploratory, non-task–related activities
- At 24 months of age, in a delayed response task, compared to ND or NC children, the cocaine-exposed group was more likely to show discordant responses between gaze and reaching, that is, to have a correct gaze response but reach incorrectly, suggesting at the least impulsive behavior

Neurophysiologic Measures of Arousal

The startle reflex is a ubiquitous, cross-species response to strong exteroceptive stimuli with abrupt onset in various sensory modalities (e.g., somatosensory, acoustic, or visual). Its plasticity to experimental manipulation, ease of recording, and short latency make it a useful index for investigating sensorimotor reactivity to different stimulus conditions. For the current study, startle is particularly relevant because it permits (1) testing of basic sensorimotor mechanisms that have been shown impaired at least early on in infants exposed to cocaine,[85,96,114] (2) study of the separate but related contributions of attentional (e.g., prepulse inhibition[117,118]) and emotional (e.g., fear-potentiation[119]) processes. Furthermore, the startle reflex in humans and animals shares a number of similar parametric characteristics and also displays different types of plasticity such as habituation, sensitization, and prepulse inhibition.[120] All of these characteristics suggest that modulation of startle in humans provides an important experimental paradigm that could be closely modeled in animals. Thus, if abnormalities in sensorimotor reactivity are detected in cocaine-exposed children, these could be further investigated in animal models.[121]

In humans, startle is measured using the eyeblink, the earliest and most reliable component of the startle reflex. The startle response is inhibited by brief (20 ms in duration or less), low intensity, nonstartling stimuli presented at short intervals (30–240 ms) prior to the startle stimulus.[117,118] The developmental significance of prepulse inhibition is the subject of considerable interest, and data are available regarding the developmental maturation of the prepulse response in 3–8-year-old children.[122] Several investigators have suggested that prepulse inhibition occurs as a result of preattentive processes triggered by the transient prestimulus.[123] The preattentive processes are assumed to protect encoding by gating out other stimulation that occurs in close temporal proximity to the initial stimulus, and thus diminished prepulse inhibition would suggest less efficient gating mechanisms. Whereas prepulses presented at short intervals before the start stimulus have inhibitory effects, discrete prepulses presented at long intervals (>1,400 ms) facilitate startle. This prepulse facilitation effect is due to an orienting-attentional process when variable prestimulation intervals are used.[124]

The startle response is also potentiated by heightened arousal in the face of fear, stress, or anxiety and can be diminished by anxiolytic drugs.[125–126] Lesions of the amygdala, a structure associated with fear and anxiety, block fear-potentiated startle in animals. Work on anticipatory anxiety[127,128] or aversive conditioning[129] in humans parallels findings from animal models. In cocaine-exposed animals, fear-potentiated startle appears accentuated, whereas nonpotentiated (baseline) startle response appears diminished.[130] Serotonergic and dopaminergic pathways particularly in the amygdala and connected regions appear critical to the modulation of the startle reflex in both fear- and prestimulus-potentiated or inhibited conditions.[119]

Startle Data

In our laboratory, we use a standard acoustic startle presentation procedure. Beginning at age 54 months, children are asked to wear a set of headphones and sit in a comfortable chair in front of a computer screen on which a screen saver displays images from popular science fiction/space travel programs. The startle pulse is a 40-ms white noise burst at 110 dB. Prepulse stimuli to inhibit or facilitate startle include 70-dB 1,000-Hz tones presented at 120 and 4,000 ms prior to the startle pulse. Skin conductance, basal heart rate, and heart rate variability are also assessed during the procedure.

Startle data from 47 children reveal the following findings. Because of small sample sizes, the two non-cocaine groups are combined for these analyses. Across the three trial types, cocaine-exposed children from 54–66 months of age show diminished EMG response to pulse alone and prepulse trials (TABLE 3). Cocaine-exposed children show less facilitation of the startle response with a prepulse trial than do the non-cocaine-

TABLE 3. Startle Response between Cocaine and Non-Cocaine-Exposed 54-Month-Olds ($n = 47$)

	Mean (SD) EMG Response (μV)				
Trial Type	Non-Cocaine ($n = 19$)	Cocaine ($n = 28$)	F (Exp)	F (Trial)	F (Exp X Tr)
Pulse	14.5 (15.6)	9.9 (13.8)	43.9***	30.7***	3.5*
Prepulse	14.2 (15.5)	8.6 (10.8)			
inhibition		27.1 (23.3)	15.8 (18.3)		
Prepulse facilitation					

*$p \leq 0.05$; ** $p \leq 0.01$; *** $p \leq 0.001$.

exposed group. Diminished response to a startle stimulus occurs in the context of other indicators of a lowered baseline arousal state including lower skin conductance both before and after the startle pulse across the three conditions and lower heart rate across the three conditions. Both suggest a lowered state of physiologic arousal even in the face of a novel situation.

Attention and Reaction Time Data

Prior to the startle procedure, children are administered a computerized attention task with three components: a standard continuous performance task (CPT), a CPT with distractors in which children are asked to select only a target stimulus as five distracting stimuli are presented randomly and serially, and a response inhibition task in which children are asked not to respond to a stimulus previously identified as a target. The stimuli are salient for preschool children and include attractive pictures of familiar objects (e.g., house, car, and dog). Reaction time data for 178 children aged 48–54 months are shown in TABLE 4. As the demands of the task become more difficult with the inclusion of distractors or with the requirement to inhibit a response, reaction times for all children increase, but cocaine-exposed children show less increase in reaction time and overall quicker responses.

SUMMARY OF FINDINGS

To summarize, based on findings from our and others' laboratories, cocaine-exposed children appear to show in various settings, diminished responsiveness to novel and/or stressful situations or stimuli, a possibly decreased baseline arousal state, but greater be-

TABLE 4. Mean Reaction Times (SD) among Three Exposure Groups

Trial Type	ND ($n = 32$)	NC ($n = 31$)	CE ($n = 115$)	F (Exp)	F (Trial)	F (Exp X Tr)
CPT	.74 (0.23)	0.77 (0.24)	0.73 (0.23)	6.02**	65.3***	1.01
Distractors	1.01 (0.27)	1.05 (0.28)	0.98 (0.27)			
Response inhibition	1.21 (0.46)	1.28 (0.55)	1.17 (0.39)			

*$p \leq 0.05$; **$p \leq 0.01$; ***$p \leq 0.001$.

havioral lability and increased impulsive responsiveness. These findings may suggest a pattern of altered stress responsiveness whereby usual patterns of increased arousal in the face of stress are blunted. The cortisol data from infancy also suggest such a pattern.[89,115,116] Furthermore, it may be that there is an association with prenatal cocaine-exposure and altered attention/arousal relations as shown schematically in FIGURE 2. Children exposed to cocaine require more stimulation to reach more optimal states of arousal for responsiveness but have less tolerance or range of acceptable arousal states and can quickly become overaroused and inattentive, poorly responsive. In short, they appear to require more stimulation to increase arousal and attention, but they modulate higher states of arousal much less well. Whether or not these patterns speak to altered monaminergic regulation of arousal states at the level of transmitter synthesis, receptor density, or function is not clear. Recall earlier findings regarding downregulation of aspects of monoamine function as well as decreased glucocorticoid response among cocaine-exposed neonates. It may be that usual monoaminergic-regulated pathways do not function in expected ways during CNS activation. Also, not clear is whether or not there may be alterations in subcortical/cortical connections and therefore in the link between stimulation, arousal, and responsiveness.

METHODOLOGIC CAVEATS

Several caveats are critical (see also refs. 1–3, 131), the first of which is that these data are clearly preliminary and do not address the following issues: (1) Amount of exposure to either cocaine or other drugs; (2) postnatal environment; and (3) postnatal environment. Several studies are now demonstrating a dose-related response whereby higher levels of cocaine exposure are associated with more clear group differences than are lower levels.[132] Similarly, it is important to consider the amount of exposure to al-

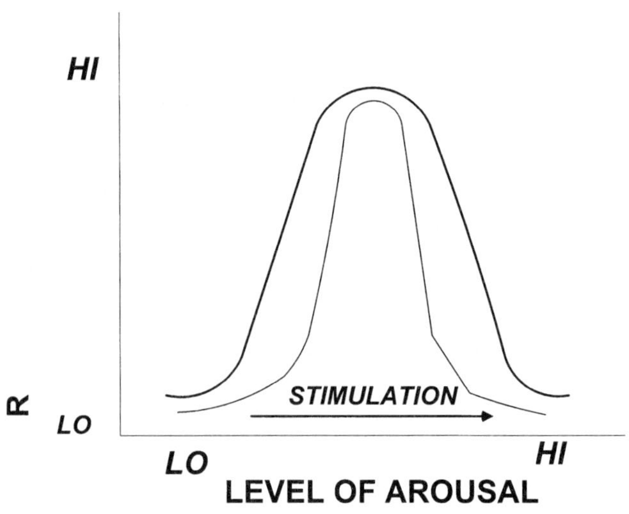

FIGURE 2. Schematic representation of different patterns of arousal regulation.

cohol and other drugs and not just their presence or absence. Most children exposed prenatally to cocaine continue to be exposed postnatally through passive inhalation of crack smoke. The magnitude and impact of postnatal, passive exposure have yet to be adequately estimated. The outcomes of interest in this and related studies—arousal, attention, and stress reactivity—are also quite sensitive to experience and environment. Children growing up in drug-using households are more likely to be exposed to violence and trauma, events that surely influence arousal and stress reactivity, and are more likely to be inconsistently if not inadequately cared for. These circumstances, while difficult to quantify, nonetheless do influence postnatal brain development and the elaboration of subcortical/cortical interconnections.

CONCLUSION AND FUTURE DIRECTIONS

Cocaine/crack use continues at moderate to high rates among certain groups of pregnant women. How early deficits in arousal and attention regulation may be expressed later in children's cognitive development, learning, school performance, social functioning, capacity to metabolize stressful conditions, and psychiatric/psychological dysfunctions of attention (e.g., ADHD), anxiety, and/or conduct disorders is a long-term implication of our ongoing work. The developmental trajectory of the relations among arousal, stimulation, and attention/responsiveness is a critical question. It is likely that these altered patterns of arousal/attention regulation do not stay the same as the child matures but are expressed in a variety of ways including potentially attentional difficulties as well as anxiety disorders. Tasks that use paradigms that increase levels of arousal such as fear-potentiated startle may prove fruitful based on both findings in animal models as well as the conceptual model proposed from the findings in human infants. Similarly, studies of stress-related neurochemistry (e.g., norepinephrine and cortisol) in older children as well as psychopharmalogic challenges using drugs such as clonidine that block anxiolytic responses may also prove revealing. Finally, as drug-exposed children reach school age, it will be important to examine in detail the incidence of childhood psychiatric disorders related to arousal/attention regulation including anxiety and attentional disorders.

REFERENCES

1. Neuspiel, D.R. 1995. The problem of confounding in research on prenatal cocaine effects on behavior and development. *In* Mothers, Babies, and Cocaine: The Role of Toxins in Development. M. Lewis *et al.*, Eds.: 95–110. Lawrence Erlbaum Associates. Hillsdale, NJ.
2. Lester, B.M., K. Freier & L. LaGasse. 1995. Prenatal cocaine exposure and child outcome: What do we really know? *In* Mothers, Babies, and Cocaine: The Role of Toxins in Development. M. Lewis *et al.*, Eds.: 19–40. Lawrence Erlbaum Associates. Hillsdale, N.J.
3. Brooks-Gunn, J., C. McCarton & T. Hawley. 1994. Effects of in utero drug exposure on children's development. Review and recommendations. Arch. Pediatr. Adolesc. Med. **148:** 33–39.
4. Azuma, S.D. & I.J. Chasnoff. 1993. Outcome of children prenatally exposed to cocaine and other drugs: A path analysis of three-year data, Pediatrics **92:** 396–402.
5. Hurt, H., N.L. Brodsky, L. Betancourt, L.E. Braitman, E. Malmud & J. Giannetta. 1995. Cocaine-exposed children: Follow-up through 30 months, J. Dev. Behav. Pediatr. **16:** 29–35.
6. Nulman, I., J. Rovet, D. Altmann, C. Bradley, T. Einarson & G. Koren. 1994. Neurodevelopment of adopted children exposed in utero to cocaine [see comments]. Can. Med. Assoc. J. **151:** 1591–1597.
7. Angelilli, M.L., H. Fischer, V. Delaney-Black, M. Rubinstein, J.W. Ager & R.J.

SOKOL. 1994. History of in utero cocaine exposure in language-delayed children. Clin. Pediatr. (Phil.) **33:** 514–516.

8. VAN BAAR, A. & B.M. DE GRAAFF. 1994. Cognitive development at preschool-age of infants of drug-dependent mothers. Dev. Med. Child. Neurol. **36:** 1063–1075.
9. GRIFFITH, D.R., S.D. AZUMA & I.J. CHASNOFF. 1994. Three-year outcome of children exposed prenatally to drugs. J. Am. Acad. Child. Adolesc. Psychiatry **33:** 20–27.
10. MAYES, L.C. & M.H. BORNSTEIN. 1995. Developmental dilemmas for cocaine-abusing parents and their children. *In* Mothers, Babies, and Cocaine: The Role of Toxins in Development. M Lewis *et al.*, Eds.: 251–272. Lawrence Erlbaum Associates. Hillsdale, N.J.
11. FRANK, D.A., K. BRESNAHAN & B.S. ZUCKERMAN. 1993. Maternal cocaine use: Impact on child health and development. Adv. Pediatr. **40:** 65–99.
12. RICHARDSON, G.A., N.L. DAY & P.J. MCGAUHEY. 1993. The impact of prenatal marijuana and cocaine use on the infant and child. Clin. Obstet. Gynecol. **36:** 302–318.
13. SINGER, L., K. FARKAS & R. KLIEGMAN. 1992. Childhood medical and behavioral consequences of maternal cocaine use. J. Pediatr. Psychol. **17:** 389–406.
14. DOW-EDWARDS, D.L. 1991. Cocaine effects on fetal development: A comparison of clinical and animal research findings. Neurotoxicol. Teratol. **13:** 347–352.
15. DOW-EDWARDS, D. 1993. The puzzle of cocaine's effects following maternal use during pregnancy: Still unsolved [comment]. Neurotoxicol. Teratol. **15:** 295–296 (discussion 311–2).
16. SPEAR, L.P. 1995. Alterations in cognitive function following prenatal cocaine exposure: Studies in an animal model. *In* Mothers, Babies, and Cocaine: The Role of Toxins in Development. M Lewis *et al.*, Eds.: 207–228. Lawrence Erlbaum Associates. Hillsdale, N.H.
17. NEEDLMAN, R., D.A. FRANK, M. AUGUSTYN & B. ZUCKERMAN. 1995. Neurophysiological effects of prenatal cocaine exposure: Comparison of human and animal investigations. *In* Mothers, Babies, and Cocaine: The Role of Toxins in Development. M Lewis *et al.*, Eds.: 229–250. Lawrence Erlbaum Associates. Hillsdale, N.J.
18. POSNER, M. & S. PETERSEN. 1988. Structures and functions of selected attention. *In* Master Lectures of Clinical Neuropsychology. T Boll *et al.*, Eds.: 173–202. American Psychological Association. Washington, DC.
19. ROTHBART, M. & M. POSNER. Temperament and the development of self-regulation. *In* Neuropsychology of Individual Differences: A Developmental Perspective. H Hartlage *et al.*, Eds.: 93–123. Plenum. New York.
20. THOMPSON, R. 1994. Emotion regulation: A theme in search of definition. *In* The Development of Emotion Regulation. N Fox, Ed.: 25–42. Monograph of the Society for the Research in Child Development.
21. STANSBURY, K. & M. GUNNAR. 1994. Adrenocortical activity and emotion regulation. Monographs of the Society for Research in Child Development **59:** 108–134.
22. PORGES, S., J. DOUSSARD-ROOSEVELT & A. MAITI. 1994. Vagal tone and the physiological regulation of emotion. Monographs for the Society for Research in Child Development **59:** 167–186.
23. JEMERIN, J. & T. BOYCE. 1992. Cardiovascular markers of biobehavioral reactivity. J. Dev. Behav. Pediatr. **13:** 46–49.
24. TURNER, S., D. BEIDEL & A. COSTELLO. 1987. Psychopathology in the offspring of children with anxiety disorders patients. J. Consult. Clin. Psychol. **55:** 229–235.
25. WEISSMAN, M., J. LECKMAN, K. MERIKANGAS *et al.* 1984. Depression and anxiety disorders in parents and children: Results from the Yale Family Study. Arch. Gen. Psychiatry **41:** 845–852.
26. DAWSON, G. 1994. Frontal encephalographic correlates of individual differences in emotion expression in infants: A brain systems perspective on emotion. *In* The Development of Emotion Regulation. N. Fox, Ed. Monographs of the Society for Research in Child Development, 135–151.
27. FOX, N. & H. FITZGERALD. 1990. Autonomic functions in infancy. *Merrill-Palmer Q.* **36:** 27–51.
28. GABLE, S. & R. ISABELLA. 1992. Maternal contributions to infant regulation of arousal. Infant Behav. Dev. **15:** 95–107.
29. POSNER, M. & PETERSEN, S. 1990. The attention system of the human brain. Ann. Rev. Neurosci. **13:** 25–42.

30. KAGAN, J., J. RESNICK & N. SNIDMAN. 1987. The physiology and psychology of behavioral inhibition in young children. Child Dev. **58:** 1459–1473.
31. BOYCE, W. & J. JEMERIN. 1990. Psychobiological differences in childhood stress response: I. Patterns of illness and susceptibility. Dev. Behav. Pediatr. **11:** 86–94.
32. BOYCE, W. & S. SOBOLEWSKI. 1989. Recurrent injuries in school-age children. Am. J. Dis. Child. **143:** 338–342.
33. GAWIN, F. & F. ELLINWOOD. 1988. Cocaine and other stimulants. N. Engl. J. Med. **318:** 1173–1182.
34. WISE, R. 1984. Neural mechanisms of the reinforcing action of cocaine. Natl. Inst. Drug Abuse Res. Monogr. **50:** 15–33.
35. NUNES, E. & J. ROSECAN. 1987. Human neurobiology of cocaine. *In* Cocaine Abuse: New Directions in Treatment and Research. H Spitz *et al.*, Ed.: 48–94. Brunner Mazel. New York.
36. LEDOUX, J. 1987. Emotion. *In* Handbook of Physiology. 1. The Nervous System: Vol. 5: Higher Functions of the Brain. E Plum, Ed. American Psychological Society. Bethesda, MD.
37. GONZALEZ-LIMA, F. 1989. Functional brain circuitry related to arousal and learning in rats. *In* Visuomotor Coordination. J Ewert *et al.*, Ed. Plenum. New York.
38. OLSEN, L., L. BOREUS & A. SEIGER. 1972. Histochemical demonstration and mapping of 5-hydroxytryptamine- and catecholamine-containing neuron systems in the human fetal brain. Z. Anat. Entwickl-Gesch. **139:** 259–282.
39. LAUDER, J. 1988. Neurotransmitters as morphogens. Prog. Brain Res. **73:** 365–387.
40. LIDOW, M. & P. RAKIC. 1994. Unique deployment of adrenergic receptor subtypes during development of the primate cerebral cortex including transient subplate and proliferative zones. J. Neuosci. **14:** 4064–4078.
41. VOLPE, J. 1987. Neurology of the Newborn. WB Saunders. Philadelphia.
42. MATTSON, M. 1988. Neurotransmitters in the regulation of neuronal cytoarchitecture. Brain Res. **472:** 179–212.
43. SWANN, A. 1990. Cocaine: Synaptic effects and adaptations. *In* Cocaine in the Brain. N. Volkow *et al.*, Eds.: 58–94. Rutgers University Press. New Brunswick.
44. LAUDER, J. 1991. Neuroteratology of cocaine: Relationship to developing monamine systems. NIDA Res. Monogr. **114:** 233–247.
45. AKBARI, H.M., P.M. WHITAKER-AZMITIA & E.C. AZMITIA. 1994. Prenatal cocaine decreases the trophic factor S-100 beta and induced microcephaly: Reversal by postnatal 5-HT1A receptor agonist [published erratum appears in Neurosci. Lett. 1994 4; 175:176]. Neurosci. Lett. **170:** 141–144.
46. GRESSENS, P., B.E. KOSOFSKY & P. EVRARD. 1992. Cocaine-induced disturbances of corticogenesis in the developing murine brain. Neurosci. Lett. **140:** 113–116.
47. GRESSENS, P., F. GOFFLOT, G. VAN MAELE-FABRY, J.P. MISSON, J.F. GADISSEUX, P. EVARD & J.J. PICARD. 1992. Early neurogenesis and teratogenesis in whole mouse embryo cultures. Histochemical, immunocytological, and ultrastructural study of the premigratory neuronal-glial units in mouse embryo influenced by cocaine and retinoic acid. J. Neuropathol. Ex. Neurol. **51:** 206–219.
48. YABLONSKY-ALTER, E., I. GLESER, C. CARTER & M. JUVAN. 1992. Effects of prenatal cocaine treatment on postnatal development of neocortex in white mice: Immunocytochemistry of calbindin- and paralbumin-positive populations of gabaergic neurons. Soc. Neurosci. Abstr. **18:** 367.
49. LIDOW, M. 1995. Prenatal cocaine exposure adversely affects development of the primate cerebral cortex. Synapse **21:** 332–341.
50. SEIDLER, F.J., S.W. TEMPLE, E.C. MCCOOK & T.A. SLOTKIN. 1995. Cocaine inhibits central noradrenergic and dopaminergic activity during the critical developmental period in which catecholamines influence cell development. Brain Res. Dev. Brain Res. **85:** 48–53.
51. RAKIC, P. 1988. Specification of cerebral cortical areas. Science **241:** 170–176.
52. WEESE-MAYER, D.E., J.M. SILVESTRI, D. LIN, C.M. BUHRFIEND, E.S. LO & P.M. CARVEY. 1993. Effect of cocaine in early gestation on striatal dopamine and neurotrophic activity. Pediatr. Res. **34:** 389–392.
53. AKBARI, H.M., H.K. KRAMER, P.M. WHITAKER-AZMITIA, L.P. SPEAR & E.C. AZMITIA. 1992. Prenatal cocaine exposure disrupts the development of the serotonergic system. Brain Res. **572:** 57–63.

54. Snyder-Keller, A.M. & R.W. Keller, Jr. 1993. Prenatal cocaine increases striatal serotonin innervation without altering the patch/matrix organization of intrinsic cell types. Dev. Brain Res. **74:** 261–267.
55. Dow-Edwards, D.L., L.A. Freed & T.A. Fico. 1990. Structural and functional effects of prenatal cocaine exposure in adult rat brain. Brain Res. Dev. Brain Res. **57:** 263–268.
56. Minabe, Y., C.R. Ashby, Jr., C. Heyser, L.P. Spear & R.Y. Wang. 1992. The effects of prenatal cocaine exposure on spontaneously active midbrain dopamine neurons in adult male offspring: An electrophysiological study. Brain Res. **586:** 152–156.
57. Scalzo, F.M., S.F. Ali, N.A. Frambes & L.P. Spear. 1990. Weanling rates exposed prenatally to cocaine exhibit an increase in striatal D2 dopamine binding associated with an increase in ligand affinity. Pharmacol. Biochem. Behav. **37:** 371–373.
58. DeGeorge, G., S. Hochberg, R. Murphy & E. Azmitia. 1989. Serotonin neurons may be a major target for the action of cocaine: Evidence from *in vitro* and tissue culture studies. Soc. Neurosci. Abstr. **15:** 418.
59. Henderson, M.G., M.M. McConnaughey & B.A. McMillen. 1991. Long-term consequences of prenatal exposure to cocaine or related drugs: Effects on rat brain monoaminergic receptors. Brain Res. Bull. **26:** 941–945.
60. Akbari, H. & E. Azmitia. 1992. Increased tyrosine hydroxylase immunoreactivity in the rat cortex following prenatal cocaine exposure. Dev. Brain Res. **66:** 277–281.
61. Seidler, F.J. & T.A. Slotkin. 1992. Fetal cocaine exposure causes persistent noradrenergic hyperactivity in rat brain regions: Effects on neurotransmitter turnover and receptors. J. Pharmacol. Exp. Ther. **263:** 413–421.
62. Hadfield, M.G. & C. Milio. 1992. Cocaine and regional brain monoamines in mice. Pharmacol. Biochem. Behav. **43:** 395–403.
63. Henderson, M.G. & B.A. McMillen. 1993. Changes in dopamine, serotonin and their metabolites in discrete brain areas of rat offspring after in utero exposure to cocaine or related drugs. Teratology **48:** 421–430.
64. Vorhees, C.V. 1995. A review of developmental exposure models for CNS stimulants: Cocaine. *In* Mothers, Babies, and Cocaine: The Role of Toxins in Development. M Lewis, *et al.,* Eds.: 71–94. Hillsdale, NJ. Lawrence Erlbaum Associates.
65. Vorhees, C.V., T.M. Reed, K.D. Acuff-Smith, M.A. Schilling, G.D. Cappon, J.E. Fisher & C. Pu. 1995. Long-term learning deficits and changes in unlearned behaviors following in utero exposure to multiple daily doses of cocaine during different exposure periods and maternal plasma cocaine concentrations. Neurotoxicol. Teratol. **17:** 253–264.
66. Spear, L. 1995. Neurobehavioral consequences of gestational cocaine exposure: A comparative analysis. *In* Advances in Infancy Research. L Lipsett *et al.,* Eds.: 55–106. Ablex. Norwood, NJ.
67. Church, M.W. 1993. Does cocaine cause birth defects? Neurotoxicol. Teratol. **15:** 289; discussion 311–312.
68. Spear, L.P., C.L. Kirstein, J. Bell, V. Yoottanasumpun, R. J. Greenbaum, H. Hoffmann & N.E. Spear. 1989. Effects of prenatal cocaine exposure on behavior during the early postnatal period. Neurotoxicol. Teratol. **11:** 57–63.
69. Heyser, C., W. Chen, J. Miller, N. Spear & L. Spear. 1990. Prenatal cocaine exposure induces deficits in Pavlovian conditioning and sensory preconditioning among infant rat pups. Behav. Neurosci. **104:** 955–963.
70. Smith, R.F., K.M. Mattran, M.F. Kurkjian & S.L. Kurtz. 1989. Alterations in offspring behavior induced by chronic prenatal cocaine dosing. Neurotoxicol. Teratol. **11:** 35–38.
71. Heyser, C.J., D.L. McKinzie, F. Athalie, N.E. Spear & L.P. Spear. 1994. Effects of prenatal exposure to cocaine on heart rate and nonassociative learning and retention in infant rats. Teratology **49:** 470–478.
72. Henderson, M.G. & B.A. McMillen. 1990. Effects of prenatal exposure to cocaine or related drugs on rat development and neurological indices. Brain Res. Bull. **24:** 207–212.
73. Vathy, I., L. Katay & K.N. Mini. 1993. Sexually dimorphic effects of prenatal cocaine on adult sexual behavior and brain catecholamines in rats. Brain Res. Dev. Brain Res. **73:** 115–122.

74. Heyser, C.J., V.A. Molina & L.P. Spear. 1992. A fostering study of the effects of prenatal cocaine exposure: I. Maternal behaviors. Neurotoxicol. Teratol. **14:** 415–421.
75. Maecker, H.L. 1993. Perinatal cocaine exposure inhibits the development of the male SDN. Brain Res. Dev. Brain Res. **76:** 288–292.
76. Kinsley, C.H., D. Turco, A. Bauer, M. Beverly *et al.* 1994. Cocaine alters the onset and maintenance of maternal behavior in lactating rats. Pharmacol. Biochem. Behav. **47:** 857–864.
77. Wood, R., M. Bannoura & I. Johanson. 1994. Prenatal cocaine exposure: Effects on play behavior in the juvenile rat. Neurotoxicol. Teratol. **16:** 139–144.
78. Johns, J.M., M.J. Means, D.R. Anderson, L.W. Means & B.A. McMillen. 1992. Prenatal exposure to cocaine. II. Effects on open-field activity and cognitive behavior in Sprague-Dawley rats. Neurotoxicol. Teratol. **14:** 343–349.
79. Spear, L., N. Frambes & C. Kirstein. 1989. Fetal and maternal brain and plasma levels of cocaine and benzoylecgonine following chronic SC administration of cocaine during gestation in rats. Psychopharmacology **97:** 427–431.
80. Hutchings, D.E., T.A. Fico & D.L. Dow-Edwards. 1989. Prenatal cocaine: Maternal toxicity, fetal effects and locomotor activity in rat offspring. Neurotoxicol. Teratol. **11:** 65–69.
81. Molina, V.A., J.M. Wagner & L.P. Spear. 1994. The behavioral response to stress is altered in adult rats exposed prenatally to cocaine. Physiol. Behav. **55:** 941–945.
82. Bilitzke, P.J. & M.W. Church. 1992. Prenatal cocaine and alcohol exposures affect rat behavior in a stress test (the Porsolt swim test). Neurotoxicol. Teratol. **14:** 359–364.
83. McMillen, B., J. Johns, E. Bass & L. Means. 1991. Learning and behavior of rats exposed to cocaine throughout gestation. Teratology **43:** 495.
84. Burchfield, D.J., A.J. Peters, R.M. Abrams & D. Phillips. 1995. Fetal behavioral state patterns during and after prolonged exposure to cocaine in sheep. Am. J. Obstet. Gynecol. **172:** 1223–1228.
85. Sobrian, S.K., L.E. Burton, N.L. Robinson, W.K. Ashe, H. James, D.L. Stokes & L.M. Turner. 1990. Neurobehavioral and immunological effects of prenatal cocaine exposure in rat. Pharmacol. Biochem. Behav. **35:** 617–629.
86. Davidson Ward, S., S. Schuetz, L. Wachsman, X. Bean, D. Bautista, S. Buckley, S. Sehgal & D. Warburton. 1991. Elevated plasma norepinephrine levels in infants of substance-abusing mothers. Am. J. Dis. Child. **145:** 44–48.
87. Mirochnick, M., J. Meyer, J. Cole, T. Herren & B. Zuckerman. 1991. Circulating catecholamine concentrations in cocaine-exposed neonates: A pilot study. Pediatrics **88:** 481–485.
88. Needlman, R., B. Zuckerman, G.M. Anderson, M. Mirochnick & D.J. Cohen. 1993. Cerebrospinal fluid monoamine precursors and metabolites in human neonates following in utero cocaine exposure: A preliminary study. Pediatrics **92:** 55–60.
89. Mangano, C., J. Gardner & B. Karmel. 1992. Differences in salivary cortisol levels in cocaine-exposed and noncocaine-exposed NICU infants. Dev. Psychobiol. **25:** 93–103.
90. Karmel, B.Z., J.M. Gardner & C.L. Magnano. 1991. Neurofunctional consequences of in utero cocaine exposure. NIDA Res. Monogr. **105:** 535–536.
91. Coles, C.D., K.A. Platzman, I. Smith, M.E. James & A. Falek. 1992. Effects of cocaine and alcohol use in pregnancy on neonatal growth and neurobehavioral status. Neurotoxicol. Teratol. **14:** 23–33.
92. Mayes, L.C., R.H. Granger, M.A. Frank, R. Schottenfeld & M.H. Bornstein. 1993. Neurobehavioral profiles of neonates exposed to cocaine prenatally. Pediatrics **91:** 778–783.
93. Eisen, L.N., T.M. Field, E.S. Bandstra, J.P. Roberts, C. Morrow, S.K. Larson & B.M. Steele. 1991. Perinatal cocaine effects on neonatal stress behavior and performance on the Brazelton Scale. Pediatrics **88:** 477–480.
94. Regaldo, M., V. Schechtman, A. Del Angel & X. Bean. 1995. Sleep disorganization in cocaine-exposed neonates. Infant Behav. Dev. **18:** 319–327.
95. Shih, L., B. Cone-Wesson & B. Reddix. 1988. Effects of maternal cocaine abuse on the neonatal auditory system. Int. J. Pediatr. Otorhinolaryngol. **15:** 245–251.
96. Anday, E.K., M.E. Cohen, N.E. Kelley & D.S. Leitner. 1989. Effect of *in utero* cocaine exposure on startle and its modification. Dev. Pharmacol. Ther. **12:** 137–145.

97. Chiriboga, C.A., D.A. Bateman, J.C. Brust & W.A. Hauser. 1993. Neurologic findings in neonates with intrauterine cocaine exposure. Pediatr. Neurol. **9:** 115–119.
98. Corwin, M.J., B.M. Lester, C. Sepkoski, S. McLaughlin, H. Kayne & H.L. Golub. 1992. Effects of in utero cocaine exposure on newborn acoustical cry characteristics. Pediatrics **89:** 1199–1203.
99. Bayley, N. 1993. The Bayley Scales of Infant Development. The Psychological Corporation. New York.
100. Thorndike, R., E. Hagen & J. Sattler. 1986. The Stanford-Binet Intelligence Scale: Fourth Edition. Riverside Publishing. Chicago.
101. Chasnoff, I.J., D.R. Griffith, C. Freier & J. Murray. 1992. Cocaine/polydrug use in pregnancy: Two-year follow-up [see comments] Pediatrics **89:** 284–289.
102. Graham, K., A. Feigenbaum, A. Pastuszak, I. Nulman, R. Weksberg, T. Einarson, S. Goldberg, S. Ashby & G. Koren. 1992. Pregnancy outcome and infant development following gestational cocaine use by social cocaine users in Toronto, Canada. Clin. Invest. Med. **15:** 384–394.
103. Chasnoff, I. & D. Griffith. 1989. Cocaine-exposed infants: Two-year follow-up. Pediatric Res. **25:** 429.
104. Malakoff, M.E., L.C. Mayes & R.S. Schottenfeld. 1994. Language abilities of preschool-age children living with cocaine-using mothers. Am. J. Addictions **3:** 346–354.
105. Schneider, J.W. & I.J. Chasnoff. 1992. Motor assessment of cocaine/polydrug exposed infants at age 4 months. Neurotoxicol. Teratol. **14:** 97–101.
106. Jacobson, J. & S. Jacobson. 1991. Assessment of teratogenic effects on cognitive and behavioral development in infancy and childhood. NIDA Res. Monogr. Series **114:** 248–261.
107. Bendersky, M., S. Alessandri, M.W. Sullivan & M. Lewis. 1995. Measuring the effects of prenatal cocaine exposure. *In* Mothers, Babies, and Cocaine: The Role of Toxins in Development. M Lewis *et al.,* Eds.: 163–178. Lawrence Erlbaum Associates. Hillsdale, NJ.
108. Porges, S. & S. Greenspan. 1991. Regulatory disorders. II. Psychophysiologic perspectives. NIDA Res. Monogr. Series **114:** 173–181.
109. Karmel, B.Z., J.M. Gardner & C.L. Magnano. 1991. Neurofunctional consequences of *in utero* cocaine exposure. NIDA Res. Monogr. **105:** 535–536.
110. Struthers, J.M. & R.L. Hansen. 1992. Visual recognition memory in drug-exposed infants. J. Dev. Behav. Pediatr. **13:** 108–111.
111. Hansen, R.L., J.M. Struthers & S.M. Gospe, Jr. 1993. Visual evoked potentials and visual processing in stimulant drug-exposed infants. Dev. Med. Child. Neurol. **35:** 798–805.
112. Alessandri, S., M. Sullivan, S. Maizumi & M. Lewis. 1993. Learning and emotional responsivity in cocaine-exposed infants. Dev. Psychol. **29:** 989–997.
113. Mayes, L.C., M.H. Bornstein, K. Chawarska & R.H. Granger. 1995. Information processing and developmental assessments in 3-month-old infants exposed prenatally to cocaine. Pediatrics **95:** 539–545.
114. Mayes, L.C., M.H. Bornstein, K. Chawarska, O.M. Haynes & R.H. Granger. 1996. Impaired regulation of arousal in three-month-old infants exposed prenatally to cocaine and other drugs. Dev. Psychopathol. **8:** 29–42.
115. Ramsay, D., M. Bendersky & M. Lewis. 1996. Effect of prenatal cocaine and other drug exposure on 2- and 6-month old infants' adrenocortical reactivity to stress. Presentation to International Conference on Infant Studies, Providence, RI.
116. Karmel, B. & J.M. Gardner. 1996. Prenatal cocaine exposure effects on arousal-modulated attention during the neonatal period. Dev. Psychol. **29:** 463–480.
117. Harbin, T. & W. Berg. 1983. The effects of age and prestimulus duration upon reflex inhibition. Psychophysiology **23:** 624–634.
118. Graham, F. & G.M. Murray. 1977. Discordant effects of weak prestimulation on magnitude and latency of the reflex blink. Physiol. Psychol. **5:** 108–114.
119. Davis, M., W.A. Falls, S. Campeau & M. Kim. 1993. Fear-potentiated startle: A neural and pharmacological analysis. Behav. Brain Res. **58:** 175–198.
120. Davis, M. 1984. The mammalian startle response. *In* Neural Mechanisms of Startle Behavior. R. Eaton, Ed.: 287–351. Plenum. New York.

121. Davis, M. 1985. Cocaine: Excitatory effects on sensorimotor reactivity measured with acoustic startle. Psychopharmacology **86:** 31–36.
122. Ornitz, E.M., D. Guthrie, A. Kaplan, S.L. Lane & R.J. Norman. 1986. Maturation of startle modulation. Psychophysiology **23:** 624–634.
123. Graham, F. 1992. Attention: The heartbeat, the blink, and the brain. *In* Attention and Information Processing in Infants and Adults: Perspective from Human and Animal Research. B.A. Campbell *et al.*, ed. Erlbaum. Hillsdale, NJ.
124. Anthony, B. 1985. In the blink of an eye: Implications of reflex modification for information processing. Adv. Psychophysiol.: 167–218. JAI Press. Greenwich, CT.
125. Davis, M. 1992. The role of the amygdala in fear-potentiated startle: Implications for animal models of anxiety. Trends Pharmacol. Sci. **13:** 35–41.
126. Grillon, C., R. Ameli, S.W. Woods, K. Merikangas & M. Davis. 1991. Fear-potentiated startle in humans: Effects of anticipatory anxiety on the acoustic blink reflex. Psychophysiology **28:** 588–595.
127. Grillon, C., R. Ameli, K. Merikangas, S.W. Woods & M. Davis. 1993. Measuring the time course of anticipatory anxiety using the fear-potentiated startle reflex. Psychophysiology **30:** 340–346.
128. Grillon, C., A.R. Ameli, M. Foot & M. Davis. 1993. Fear-potentiated startle: Relationship to the level of state/trait anxiety in healthy subjects. Biol. Psychiatry **33:** 566–574.
129. Hamm, A.O., M.K. Greenwald, M.M. Bradley, B.N. Cuthbert & P.J. Lang. 1991. The fear potentiated startle effect: Blink reflex modulation as a result of classic aversive conditioning. Integrative Physiol. Behav. Sci. **26:** 119–126.
130. Borowski, T.B. & L. Kokkinidis. 1994. Cocaine pre-exposure sensitizes conditioned fear in a potentiated acoustic startle paradigm. Pharacol. Biochem. Behav. **49:** 935–942.
131. Zuckerman, B. & D.A. Frank. 1994. Prenatal cocaine exposure: Nine years later [editorial; comment]. J. Pediatr. **124:** 731–733.
132. Jacobson, S.W., J.L. Jacobson & R.J. Sokol. 1994. Effects of fetal alcohol exposure on infant reaction time. Alcohol Clin. Exp. Res. **18:** 1125–1132.

Prenatal Cocaine Exposure

A Longitudinal Study of Development[a]

GALE A. RICHARDSON[b]

Western Psychiatric Institute & Clinic, University of Pittsburgh School of Medicine, 3811 O'Hara Street, Pittsburgh, Pennsylvania 15213, USA

ABSTRACT: The current study examines the effect of prenatal cocaine use on physical, cognitive, and behavioral development at birth, 1, 3, and 7 years, controlling for other factors that affect child development. Women who used cocaine during pregnancy were more likely to be single and to use alcohol, marijuana, and tobacco than were women who did not use cocaine. Prenatal cocaine use was associated with reduced gestational age, but not with birth weight, length, or head circumference. Neonatal neurobehavioral assessments were affected by prenatal cocaine exposure. Growth at 1 year was not affected by prenatal cocaine use. At 3 years, prenatal cocaine use was a significant predictor of head circumference and of the composite score on the Stanford-Binet Intelligence Scale (4th edition). Prenatal cocaine use was also associated with temperamental differences at 1 and 3 years and with behavior problems at 3 years. These findings represent a pattern of central nervous system effects, related to prenatal cocaine exposure, which is predicted by the teratologic model.

INTRODUCTION

The purported long-term effects of prenatal cocaine exposure on child development have received much media attention.[1–3] Those of us who conduct research in this area are concerned about the accuracy of these reports, especially given that follow-up of cocaine-exposed offspring beyond the infancy period has been reported by very few researchers. In one of the only published reports of the effects of prenatal cocaine use on preschoolers, Griffith *et al.*[4] reported on the effects of prenatal cocaine use on the physical, cognitive, and behavioral development of 3-year-old children. When regression analyses were used to control for covariates of cocaine use, there were no effects at 3 years on growth or on the Stanford-Binet Intelligence Scale (4th edition) composite score; however, cocaine use did predict lower scores on the verbal reasoning subscale of the Stanford-Binet. Cocaine use also predicted more externalizing problems on the Child Behavior Checklist, as rated by the primary caregiver. It remains to be seen whether other longitudinal studies will corroborate these findings.

Previous research on the effects of prenatal cocaine use has been characterized by a number of methodologic limitations, including lack of a control group and failure to control for correlates of cocaine use, such as demographic characteristics, prenatal care, and health and nutritional status, each of which can influence outcome.[5,6] In addition, cocaine users are generally polydrug users. They have different patterns of drug use than do women who do not use cocaine and this can also affect outcome. Analyses must control for other substance use such as alcohol, tobacco, and marijuana when evaluating the effects of cocaine.[6]

[a] This research was supported by National Institute on Drug Abuse Grants DA05460, DA06839, and DA08916 (G. Richardson, Principal Investigator).

[b] Phone, 412-681-3482; fax, 412-681-1261; e-mail, gar + @pitt.edu

Another methodologic issue is the ascertainment of drug use. Identification of exposed and nonexposed groups on the basis of medical records, enrollment in treatment programs, or urinalysis yields no information regarding quantity, frequency, pattern, or timing of substance use,[7–9] information that is critical when evaluating the effect of a teratogen. (See Richardson and Day[10] for a more detailed discussion of this issue.)

There is also the issue of recall bias in those studies that rely on retrospective reporting at delivery, or even later in the postpartum period, of cocaine and other substance use over the entire pregnancy.[11,12]

An additional methodologic difficulty is that women who use drugs are difficult to follow up. Neuspiel *et al.*[13] reported follow-up rates at 2 months of 31% for the cocaine-exposed group and 52% for the comparison group. Azuma and Chasnoff[14] had follow-up rates at 3 years of 44% and 50% of the original cohort for the drug-exposed and comparison groups, respectively. Thus, there can be both a high rate of subject loss and a greater rate of attrition in the exposed group. These factors limit the conclusions that can be drawn and may seriously bias the interpretation of the findings.

MATERIAL AND METHODS

This study was designed specifically to evaluate the effects of prenatal cocaine exposure with a carefully controlled schedule of data collection and measurement. Improvements over previous research include: (1) the women were recruited from a prenatal care clinic rather than a drug treatment program; (2) the quantity, frequency, and pattern of cocaine, crack, alcohol, marijuana, tobacco, and other drug use are assessed at each phase; (3) other risk factors such as demographic factors, medical history, life events, social support, psychological characteristics, and environmental factors are carefully measured; and (4) exceptional follow-up rates have been achieved.

We do not obtain biologic confirmation of cocaine use. When we originally designed this study in 1987, urine screening was the most reliable laboratory measure of cocaine use available. At best, urine screening covers a window of only 1 week from the most recent exposure.[15,16] This methodology would not have freed us from interviewing the women to obtain trimester-specific information. We would not have been able to estimate patterns of use or to obtain information about use early in pregnancy. In addition, we felt that asking the women for biologic specimens would dramatically increase both our refusal rate and the cost of the study.

However, to address this issue, we were able to obtain information from the women's medical charts regarding any screening that was conducted by the hospital staff. We compared the urine screen results to the use reported on our interview. In this prenatal care sample, 18% of the women were screened by the hospital. One hundred percent of the women who had cocaine-positive urine screens were identified as users by our interview. By contrast, 79% of the women who had a negative urine screen admitted cocaine use on the interview. Thus, these data support our decision not to conduct urine screens. In addition, our prevalence rate of cocaine use is comparable to the rates reported by other researchers.

We refer to this project as the Maternal Health Practices and Child Development Project. This is an ongoing, prospective study of women who attended a medical assistance prenatal clinic at Magee-Womens Hospital. These women were not in drug treatment during their pregnancies, but rather they are a representative group of women attending a prenatal clinic. Recruitment at Phase 1 occurred from 1988 to 1992. Women and their offspring were assessed at various time points through 7 years of age.

Women who were at least 18 years of age were initially interviewed during their fourth or fifth prenatal month. They were asked about their use of cocaine, crack, alcohol, marijuana, tobacco, and other drugs for the year prior to pregnancy and for the first trimester. All women who reported using any cocaine or crack during the first trimester were enrolled. The next woman interviewed who reported no cocaine or crack use was also enrolled. Ninety percent of those women eligible to be interviewed consented to participate in the study. Medical chart reviews of a random sample of women who refused to participate indicated that only 5% had a history of drug use during the current pregnancy. Information was also obtained on sociodemographic and life-style characteristics, social support, and psychiatric symptoms. This is referred to as the core dataset.

Of the women initially interviewed, 325 (18%) met the inclusion criteria and were enrolled in the study. Women selected for the study were interviewed at 7 months about their substance use during the second trimester and were interviewed with the rest of the core dataset. The women were also interviewed at 24–48 hours postpartum, when they were asked about third trimester substance use and the core dataset. All newborns received comprehensive physical examinations, generally within 24–48 hours of delivery, by our nurse clinicians who were unaware of prenatal exposure status. Subsets of full-term infants received further assessments such as the Brazelton Neonatal Behavioral Assessment Scale (BNBAS), an EEG-sleep study, and a feeding observation.

The infants were assessed again at 1 year, when the Bayley Scales of Infant Development were administered. Mothers were interviewed about their current substance use and completed self-report measures about the child's temperament and home environment. At 3 years, children were assessed with the Stanford-Binet Intelligence Scale (4th edition). Mothers were interviewed with the core dataset and were asked about the child's temperament, home environment, and behavior problems.

At the 7-year follow-up, mothers are interviewed again with the core dataset. They also report on the child's behavior problems, activity level, home environment, and temperament. The child's growth and medical history are assessed, and the Stanford-Binet, Wide Range Achievement Test, and a neuropsychological battery are administered.

TABLE 1 shows our follow-up rates, which are excellent at both our 1-year and 3-year phases. We have a completion rate of 93% of the eligible subjects at 1 year; for the 3-year phase, we have a 95% follow-up rate. These are exceptional follow-up rates for a longitudinal study of low-income women, some of whom used drugs during pregnancy.

Women were, on average, 25 years old, 52% were Caucasian, and 48% were African-American. Women were of lower socioeconomic status, with a mean family income of $650 per month and an average educational level of 12 years. Twenty percent were married and 41% worked and/or went to school during the first trimester. Twenty-four percent were primigravidous and 42% were primiparous. According to Kessner *et al.*'s[17] definition, 47% of the women had adequate prenatal care, 48% had an intermediate level of care, and 5% had inadequate prenatal care.

Fifty-four percent of the infants were male. The average gestational age was 39.7

TABLE 1. Study Follow-Up Rates

	1 Year	3 Years
Completions (*n*)	269	271
Refusals	3%	3%
Lost to follow-up	4%	2%
Completion rate[a]	93%	95%

[a]Of eligible subjects.

weeks and mean Apgar scores were 7.9 and 8.9 at 1 and 5 minutes, respectively. Mean birth weight was 3,254 g, mean length was 49.7 cm, and mean head circumference was 34.5 cm.

The mean age of the children at the 3-year assessment was 38.3 months. The average weight was 33.3 pounds, average height 38.2 inches, and average head circumference 50.1 cm. Twenty-four percent of the children attended preschool or day care and 6% were not in maternal custody. The mean Stanford-Binet composite score was 93 (range 67–118). This average is within the range expected for low socioeconomic status samples and is comparable to that obtained in our other studies.

The prevalence of cocaine use for the selected sample is shown in TABLE 2. Occasional users were defined as women who used less than one line of cocaine per day, and frequent users were women who used one or more lines of cocaine per day. During the year prior to pregnancy, 23% of the women were frequent users of cocaine. During the first trimester, 19% of the women were frequent users. The mean level of cocaine use for the women who used during the first trimester was approximately 14 lines per day. In the second and third trimesters, 5% and 6%, respectively, were frequent users, using one or more lines per day. During the second and third trimesters, mean use for the users was approximately 5 lines per day. The rate of frequent cocaine use at the 1- and 3-year follow-ups was 7%. The mean level of use for the women who used at the 1- and 3-year phases was approximately 9 and 8 lines per day, respectively.

Women who were frequent users of cocaine during the first trimester differed from women who did not use. Frequent first trimester users of cocaine were older (27 *vs* 24 years) and were more likely to be African-American (64% *vs* 43%) than were nonusers. They were less often married (10% *vs* 26%) and had lower family incomes ($459 *vs* $720/mo) than did women who were nonusers during the first trimester. Fewer frequent first trimester users had adequate prenatal care (29% *vs* 54%) than did nonusers.

Women who were frequent users of cocaine during the first trimester were significantly more likely than nonusers to use other substances as well. Eighty-five percent of the frequent cocaine users smoked tobacco compared with 45% of the cocaine nonusers. The frequent first trimester cocaine users also were more likely to use alcohol (88% *vs* 56%), marijuana (64% *vs* 18%), and illicit drugs (15% *vs* 3%), such as amphetamines and tranquilizers, during the first trimester than were nonusers.

Women who used cocaine during the third trimester were more likely to be African-American (84% *vs* 42%), to have lower family incomes ($443 *vs* $680/mo), and to have had more pregnancies (4.7 vs. 2.9), births (2.6 vs. 2.0), miscarriages (0.8 *vs* 0.3), and abortions (1.3 *vs* 0.6) than were women who did not use cocaine in the third trimester. No significant differences were noted in age, education, marital status, work/school status, weight gain during pregnancy, and labor or delivery conditions between groups. Third trimester users had significantly fewer prenatal visits (7.5 *vs* 10.4) and more pregnancy conditions (4.0 *vs* 2.3), and fewer received adequate prenatal care (28% *vs* 49%) than did women who did not use cocaine in the third trimester.

TABLE 2. Prevalence of Cocaine Use (%)

	Year Prior	1st Trimester	2nd Trimester	3rd Trimester	1 Year	3 Years
None	54	57	92	90	86	86
Occasional[a]	23	24	3	4	7	7
Frequent[b]	23	19	5	6	7	7

[a]Less than one line/day.
[b]One or more lines/day.

Women who used cocaine in the third trimester also used more of other substances than did women who did not use cocaine in the third trimester. During the third trimester, cocaine users smoked more cigarettes (10 *vs* 7 cigarettes/day), drank more alcohol (1.1 *vs* 0.2 drinks/day), used more marijuana (0.1 *vs* 0.04 joints/day) and other illicit drugs (9% *vs* 1% users) than did women who did not use cocaine in the third trimester.

Women who were frequent users of cocaine during the first trimester continued to be different at the 3-year follow-up. They were more likely to use cocaine (28% *vs* 3%), marijuana (24% *vs* 17%), and tobacco (76% *vs* 45%) at 3 years compared with women who did not use cocaine during the first trimester. Although the percentage who used alcohol did not differ, women who were frequent users of cocaine were more likely to be heavier users of alcohol than were nonusers of cocaine. In addition, women who used cocaine at 3 years provided less stimulating and organized home environments, as measured by the Home Screening Questionnaire, than did women who did not use currently. These findings highlight the importance of controlling for the environmental, demographic, and substance use characteristics associated with cocaine use.

Stepwise regressions were used for outcome analyses. Measures of cocaine use included the trimester-specific measures. Covariates were included in the regression model if they were significantly related to the outcome in a bivariate analysis.[18] The following variables were included in all of the analyses: child gender and age at assessment, maternal race and age, and prenatal and current alcohol, marijuana, and tobacco use. These additional variables were added to specific outcomes: maternal height for growth outcomes; environmental stimulation, as measured by the Home Screening Questionnaire,[19] and preschool attendance for the Stanford-Binet; one or two of the socioeconomic status variables depending on the outcome (income, education, marital status, and work status); and maternal depression, measured by the CES-D,[20] for temperament and behavior outcomes. Analyses presented here are preliminary. Model development and diagnostics have not yet been completed.

To illustrate the findings, we also conducted analyses of covariance with one group defined as women who used cocaine frequently in the first trimester and a second group defined as those who did not use cocaine in the first trimester. Variables that were significant predictors of outcome from the regression analyses were used as control variables in the analyses of covariance.

RESULTS

At birth, there were no significant relationships between cocaine use during any trimester and infant birth weight, length, or head circumference, when the covariates were considered and stepwise multiple regressions were used to evaluate the effect of prenatal cocaine use.[21] These results are consistent with preliminary findings reported by Richardson and Day.[22] Cocaine use was also not associated with an increased risk of minor physical anomalies, low birth weight, or being small-for-gestational age, after controlling for confounding variables. First trimester cocaine use was a significant predictor of reduced gestational age, with infants of frequent users being born about 1 week earlier than infants of nonusers.

At birth, the development of the central nervous system (CNS) in term infants was assessed with the Brazelton Neonatal Behavioral Assessment Scale (BNBAS)[23] and EEG-sleep studies. The Lester, Als, and Brazelton[24] clusters were the outcome variables for the BNBAS. Poorer autonomic stability was significantly predicted by cocaine exposure during each trimester of pregnancy. An increased number of abnormal reflexes was associated with cocaine exposure during the first and second trimesters, decreased scores on motor maturity were significantly associated with second and third trimester exposure, and decreased ability to regulate state was associated with third trimester exposure.[25]

Analyses of the EEG-sleep studies demonstrated that infants of women who used cocaine displayed less well developed spectral correlations between homologous brain regions.[26] These findings represent a different EEG-sleep pattern from that observed in non-cocaine-exposed infants or in infants exposed prenatally to alcohol or marijuana.[27]

At 1 year, prenatal and current cocaine use were not significant predictors of weight, length, or head circumference in the regression analyses. In addition, the Bayley Scales of Infant Development mental (MDI) and motor (PDI) scales were used to assess development. There was a significant effect of second trimester cocaine use on the PDI.[28] Women who used cocaine in the second trimester had infants with significantly lower motor scores than did women who did not use (adjusted $\bar{x}$ or mean PDI = 104 *vs* 114). There was no effect of first or third trimester use and no effect of prenatal or current cocaine use on performance on the MDI.

The Bates Infant Characteristics Scale[29] was used to assess temperament at 1 year. This instrument has four subscales: fussy/difficult, unadaptable, persistent, and unsociable. The fussy/difficult subscale was significantly predicted by cocaine use during the first, second, and third trimesters. Unadaptability and excessive persistence were both predicted by first and second trimester cocaine use.[30] Current cocaine use was not a significant predictor of the mother's rating of the infant's temperament.

To provide a measure of the infant's behavior that was independent of the mother's report, we analyzed the examiner ratings of the BSID Infant Behavior Record. Examiners, who were blind to maternal substance use, rated infants of women who used cocaine in the first trimester as less responsive, less reactive to test materials, and as having shorter attention spans than infants of women who did not use cocaine in the first trimester.

At 3 years, prenatal cocaine use was not a significant predictor of child weight or height. However, first trimester cocaine use was a significant predictor of 3-year head circumference. Analysis of covariance illustrated that children of women who used frequently during the first trimester had significantly smaller adjusted mean head circumferences than did the offspring of women who did not use cocaine in the first trimester (adjusted $\bar{x}$ or mean = 49.7 *vs* 50.2 cm).

First trimester cocaine use also significantly predicted the performance of children on the Stanford-Binet at age 3. Women who used cocaine frequently in the first trimester had children with significantly lower adjusted composite (adjusted $\bar{x}$ or mean = 90 *vs* 93) and short-term memory scores (adjusted $\bar{x}$ or mean = 97 *vs* 100) than those of women who did not use first trimester.

First trimester cocaine use was a significant predictor of the mother's rating of the child's temperament, as measured by the Bates Scale. Children of women who used frequently in the first trimester were rated as more fussy and difficult and as more unadaptable than were those of women who did not use.

First trimester cocaine use was also related to the mother's rating of behavior problems on the Child Behavior Checklist.[31] Children who were exposed to cocaine in the first trimester were rated by their mothers as having more total behavior problems and more internalizing problems than did those whose mothers did not use in the first trimester. In a further analysis, a logistic regression was used to analyze the scores on the CBCL that were above the borderline clinical cutoff score.[31] First and third trimester use were significant predictors of meeting clinical criteria for internalizing behaviors. Current cocaine use did not predict the mother's rating of the child's behavior problems.

For independent corroboration of the child's behavior, we analyzed the examiner ratings of the child's behavior during the Stanford-Binet assessment. Examiners, unaware of maternal substance use, rated children of women who used cocaine first trimester as having shorter attention spans, less focused attention, more restlessness, and as making more attempts to distract the examiner than children of women who did not use cocaine.

DISCUSSION

Thus, at 3 years we found that first trimester cocaine use is associated with decreased head circumference and IQ and with increased fussiness/difficultness and behavior problems. We carefully assessed cocaine and all other drug use for each trimester of pregnancy and were able to control for the covariates of cocaine use.

Our findings across phases indicate a consistent pattern of CNS effects. In analyses of our BNBAS examinations at birth, cocaine exposure was related to poorer autonomic stability and an increased number of abnormal reflexes.[25] At our 1-year follow-up, effects were noted on the Bates Scale, as the children were reported by their mothers to be more fussy and difficult. These findings were confirmed at 3 years of age. Independent observations from the examiners also substantiated these findings, as at 3 years, Stanford-Binet examiners reported that the children who were prenatally exposed to cocaine had decreased attention span, more difficulty focusing, and were more restless during testing. At 3 years, we found indications of cognitive deficits on the Stanford-Binet composite and short-term memory scores. Prenatal cocaine exposure was also associated with increased behavior problems. In addition, at 3 years of age, we identified a significant effect of prenatal cocaine exposure during the first trimester on head circumference, a growth parameter, but one that is correlated with CNS functioning.

Therefore, we consistently found that CNS deficits result from prenatal cocaine exposure. We found the same pattern of CNS deficits in our earlier studies of prenatal alcohol and marijuana use where exposure during the first trimester significantly predicted a decrease in IQ and an increase in behavior problems. Other researchers have reported a similar pattern of effects. In the Seattle Longitudinal Study, exposure to alcohol during the period prior to pregnancy recognition was associated with decreased IQ scores[32] and increased attentional errors and reaction time at 4 years.[33] These CNS effects were found in the absence of growth and morphologic changes.[34] These findings are also consistent with Spear's[35] review of the animal research literature, in which neurobehavioral effects of cocaine were found in the absence of growth or morphologic anomalies at lower dose exposures.

Thus, we found signs of subtle CNS effects. This pattern is predicted by the teratologic model, which states that low levels of exposure to a toxin should lead to CNS effects in the absence of morphologic effects. Although CNS effects were more difficult to detect at the youngest ages, as the children have aged, the effects of cocaine exposure have become more detectable. This pattern, of effects becoming more apparent as the child develops, has been noted in studies of other teratogens as well, particularly in samples that are not heavily exposed, for example, Fried's[36] study of prenatal marijuana exposure and our own studies of prenatal alcohol and marijuana use. Because of this, it is important to continue to study the effects of prenatal cocaine use in samples that are exposed to light and moderate levels of use.

Our next step is to study this cohort at 7 years of age. We will continue to assess the domains we have previously assessed such as growth, intelligence, temperament, and behavior. In addition, we have added a neuropsychological assessment to the 7-year phase to obtain more detailed information regarding CNS functioning. Our neuropsychological battery at age 7 was designed to target the areas of learning and memory, psychomotor speed and eye-hand coordination, mental flexibility, and attention and impulsivity. We will be able to obtain a better estimate of CNS effects as the children develop and as more demands are made on their cognitive abilities. We believe that the image of the "crack baby" as portrayed by the media is not accurate. However, there are subtle effects on the CNS of exposure to low doses of cocaine, which serve as a marker that a teratogen has had an effect.

REFERENCES

1. ELLIOTT, K.T. & D.R. COKER. 1991. Crack babies: Here they come, ready or not. J. Instructional Psych. **18:** 60–64.
2. GREGORCHIK, L.A. 1992. The cocaine-exposed children are here. Phi Delta Kappan **May:** 709–711.
3. RIST, M.C. 1990. The shadow children. Am. School Board J. **177:** 19–24.
4. GRIFFITH, D.R., S.D. AZUMA & I.J. CHASNOFF. 1994. Three-year outcome of children exposed prenatally to drugs. J. Am. Acad. Child Adolesc. Psychiatry **33:** 20–27.
5. LUTIGER, B., K. GRAHAM, T.R. EINARSON & G. KOREN. 1991. Relationship between gestational cocaine use and pregnancy outcome: A meta-analysis. Teratology. **44:** 405–414.
6. RICHARDSON, G.A., N.L. DAY & P.J. MCGAUHEY. 1993. The impact of prenatal marijuana and cocaine use on the infant and child. Clin. Obstet. Gynecol. **36:** 302–318.
7. HADEED, A. & S. SIEGEL. 1989. Maternal cocaine use during pregnancy: Effect on the newborn infant. Pediatrics **84:** 205–210.
8. KAYE, D., L. ELKIND, D. GOLDBERG & A. TYTUN. 1989. Birth outcomes for infants of drug abusing mothers. N.Y. State J. Med. **89:** 256–261.
9. LITTLE, B., L. SNELL, V. KLEIN & L. GILSTRAP. 1989. Cocaine abuse during pregnancy: Maternal and fetal implications. Obstet. Gynecol. **73:** 157–160.
10. RICHARDSON, G.A. & N.L. DAY. 1998. Epidemiological studies of the effects of prenatal cocaine exposure on child development and behavior. *In* Handbook of Developmental Neurotoxicology. W. Slikker & L. Chang, Eds. Academic Press, Inc., San Diego, CA. In press.
11. BINGOL, N., M. FUCHS, V. DIAZ, R. STONE & D. GROMISCH. 1987. Teratogenicity of cocaine in humans. J. Pediatr. **110:** 93–96.
12. CHERUKURI, R., H. MINKOFF, J. FELDMAN, A. PAREKH & L. GLASS. 1988. A cohort study of alkaloidal cocaine ("crack") in pregnancy. Obstet. Gynecol. **72:** 147–151.
13. NEUSPIEL, D.R., S.C. HAMEL, E. HOCHBERG, J. GREENE & D. CAMPBELL. 1991. Maternal cocaine use and infant behavior. Neurotoxicol. Teratol. **13:** 229–233.
14. AZUMA, S.D. & I.J. CHASNOFF. 1993. Outcome of children prenatally exposed to cocaine and other drugs: A path analysis of three-year data. Pediatrics **92:** 396–402.
15. JULIEN, R. 1995. A Primer of Drug Action, 7th Ed. W. H. Freeman. New York.
16. VEREBY, K. 1987. Cocaine abuse detection by laboratory methods. *In* Cocaine: A Clinician's Handbook. A.M. Washton & M.S. Gold, Eds. Guilford Press. New York.
17. KESSNER, D., J. SINGER, C. KALK & E. SCHLESINGER. 1973. Infant death: An analysis by maternal risk and health care. *In* Contrasts in Health Status, Vol. 1. Institute of Medicine. Washington, D.C.
18. KLEINBAUM, D., L. KUPPER & K. MULLER. 1988. Applied Regression Analysis and Other Multivariable Methods, 2nd Ed. PWS-Kent Publishing Co. Boston, MA.
19. FRANKENBURG, W. & C. COONS. 1986. Home Screening Questionnaire: Its validity in assessing home environment. J. Pediatr. **108:** 624–626.
20. RADLOFF, L. 1977. The CES-D scale: A self-report depression scale for research in the general population. Applied Psych. Measurement **1:** 385–401.
21. RICHARDSON, G.A., S.C. HAMEL, L. GOLDSCHMIDT & N.L. DAY. 1998. Growth and morphology of infants prenatally exposed to cocaine: A comparison of prenatal care and no prenatal care samples. In preparation.
22. RICHARDSON, G.A. & N.L. DAY. 1994. Detrimental effects of prenatal cocaine exposure: Illusion or reality? J. Am. Acad. Child Adolesc. Psychiatry **33:** 28–34.
23. BRAZELTON, T.B. 1984. Neonatal Behavioral Assessment Scale, 2nd Ed. Lippincott. Philadelphia, PA.

24. LESTER, B.M., H. ALS & T.B. BRAZELTON. 1982. Regional obstetric anesthesia and newborn behavior: A reanalysis toward synergistic effects. Child Dev. **53:** 687–692.
25. RICHARDSON, G.A., S.C. HAMEL, L. GOLDSCHMIDT & N.L. DAY. 1996. The effects of prenatal cocaine use on neonatal neurobehavioral status. Neurotoxicol. Teratol. **18:** 519–528.
26. SCHER, M.S., G.A. RICHARDSON & N.L. DAY. 1998. Effects of prenatal cocaine/crack exposure on EEG-sleep studies at birth and one year. In preparation.
27. SCHER, M.S., G.A. RICHARDSON, P. COBLE, N.L. DAY & D. STOFFER. 1988. The effects of prenatal alcohol and marijuana exposure: Disturbances in neonatal sleep cycling and arousal. Pediatr. Res. **24:** 101–105.
28. RICHARDSON, G.A., N.L. DAY & L. GOLDSCHMIDT. 1995. A longitudinal study of prenatal cocaine exposure: Infant development at 12 months. Paper presented at the Society for Research in Child Development, Indianapolis, IN, March 1995.
29. BATES, J., C. FREELAND & M. LOUNSBURY. 1979. Measurement of infant difficultness. Child Dev. **50:** 794–803.
30. RICHARDSON, G.A., S.C. HAMEL, N.L. DAY & L. GOLDSCHMIDT. 1994. Maternal rating of temperament of cocaine-exposed infants. Paper presented at the Society for Behavioral Pediatrics, Minneapolis, MN, September 1994.
31. ACHENBACH, T. 1992. Manual for the Child Behavior Checklist/2–3 and 1992 Profile. University of Vermont Department of Psychiatry. Burlington, VT.
32. STREISSGUTH, A.P., H. BARR, P. SAMPSON, B. DARBY & D. MARTIN. 1989. IQ at age 4 in relation to maternal alcohol use and smoking during pregnancy. Dev. Psychol. **25:** 3–11.
33. STREISSGUTH, A.P., D. MARTIN, H. BARR, B. SANDMAN, G. KIRCHNER & B. DARBY. 1984. Intrauterine alcohol and nicotine exposure: Attention and reaction time in 4-year-old children. Dev. Psychol. **20:** 533–541.
34. STREISSGUTH, A.P. 1992. Fetal alcohol syndrome and fetal alcohol effects: A clinical perspective of later developmental consequences. *In* Maternal Substance Abuse and the Developing Nervous System. I. Zagon & T. Slotkin, Eds.: 5–25. Academic Press. San Diego, CA.
35. SPEAR, L. 1995. Neurobehavioral consequences of gestational cocaine exposure: A comparative analysis. *In* Advances in Infancy Research. C. Rovee-Collier & L. Lipsitt, Eds.: 55–105. Ablex Publishing Co. Norwood, NJ.
36. FRIED, P.A. 1996. Behavioral outcomes in preschool and school-age children exposed prenatally to marijuana: A review and speculative interpretation. *In* Behavioral Studies of Drug-Exposed Offspring: Methodological Issues in Human and Animal Research. NIDA Research Monograph **164:** 242–250. Rockville, MD.

Round Table 2. Consensus on Postnatal Deficits: Comparability of Human and Animal Findings

Moderator: THEODORE SLOTKIN
Panelists: LINDA SPEAR, JOHN A. HARVEY, CLAUDIA A. CHIRIBOGA, LINDA MAYES, GALE RICHARDSON
Discussants: BARRY LESTER (*Brown*), ROBIN BLITZ (*Arizona*), GIDEON KOREN (*Toronto*), DONNA FERREIRO (*UCSF*), CHARLIE BAUER (*U Miami*), BARRY E. KOSOFSKY (*MGH*)

THEODORE SLOTKIN: I'd like to start off by discussing the swing of the pendulum of Crack Baby Syndrome. Initially, Crack Baby Syndrome was described as the worst thing to hit America in recent years. Then, as longitudinal studies came out, people started to say well maybe there isn't any Crack Baby Syndrome. Now we're settling back into knowing what variables we need to look at in order to really define this. What we have just heard is that there really is such a syndrome. It's just that the effects are a lot more subtle than we originally thought, and it becomes a question of what tools we need to handle this. Two important points regarding study design came from today's presentation: (1) Studying baseline behavior is not enough; to demonstrate changes requires that the system be put under stress. There may be sufficient adaptations to normalize the essential behaviors that you need to survive as a human being, but it may be adaptability that's comprised. (2) It has now become realistic to start to factor out significant covariables so that we can distinguish what the components are that might mask Crack Baby Syndrome.

The general question that I would like to see addressed is: Let's assume that everybody is successful and defines the neurobehavioral correlates of cocaine abuse. What do we do with this information?

JOHN HARVEY: Anything we learn about neuropathology, especially if it is placed within the context of understanding how various neurotransmitter systems may be interrupted or enhanced, what the behavioral consequences are, and what neuroanatomic systems are involved, can provide a better mechanistic understanding of the clinical problem.

THEODORE SLOTKIN: In a sense that's using cocaine as a probe for neurodevelopment.

JOHN HARVEY: I think it is. In fact, Pat Levitt wrote an article for Trends in Neuroscience (**20:** 269–274, 1997) with exactly that title. You can look at cocaine exposure as a situation in which you have interfered with the dopamine system during a time when it's not a transmitter system in the usual sense of the term, but rather a morphogen that directs certain aspects of neuronal development. By interfering with that, you interfere eventually with certain kinds of function. Since these are monoamine systems, it's going to be subtle. The very early talk by Dr. Hyman (not reproduced here) was a statement that the brain is infinitely capable of compensating for whatever we try to do to it, but only so much. Your point is well taken: for the survival of the species, or for doing certain normal things, such insults may be "silent." All of us know that we can bring a brain-damaged individual here and under the right circumstances we wouldn't know that they were brain damaged unless we were to probe in some way.

THEODORE SLOTKIN: I'm reminded of a report that appeared, I think, in *Nature* about 20 years ago, called "Is Your Brain Necessary?" (Lorber, J. 1980. Science **210:** 1232–1234). It was written by an English clinician who was struck by the fact that he had many medical students come through who had hydrocephalus (individuals with spina bifida and associated hydrocephalus, who presumably had normal or above normal intelligence). One of the students agreed to have a CAT scan and demonstrated only about a 2-mm mantle of cortical cells along the inside of the head. Then they subjected him to the kinds of tests that you do to detect cryptic multiple sclerosis, such as a heat stress test, and then all the compensatory mechanisms broke down. This may be one way to look at plasticity during development, and its limitations, that we can adapt from classical neurology and learn about alterations in more subtle neurobehaviors. Will knowing these mechanisms permit us to design proper therapeutic interventions as kids get older?

SPEAKER: I agree with the use of perturbed systems as a way of understanding normal development, but remember that these children come with a host of other difficulties including family problems, developmental problems, and psychiatric problems. For example, these data raise the question of whether our usual psychopharmacologic interventions for attention deficit disorder will work. We typically use stimulants to modulate attention deficits in preschool-age or school-age children. Will such drugs be effective in this population? Do we need to prescribe drugs that act on the same neurochemical pathway? Should we even think about cocaine- or alcohol-induced inattention as we do attention deficit disorder? Is it the same kind of deficit neurochemically or behaviorally?

THEODORE SLOTKIN: Presumably if there are dopamine receptor response defects, it's not going to work.

LINDA MAYES: The other clinical point is to ask questions about the usual ways of intervening in school programs for children with various arousal and attentional problems. We have very standard ways of doing that, but if some of these data are right, then they really demand a new way of thinking about educational interventions.

SPEAKER: Exactly. All of the data that we were looking at in animal models, which apply even more to the human situation, is that the animals were able to do things; they were finally able to solve the problems. What might happen with special programs of education and training and attention to these things? Just as with attentional disorders, there may be a big argument about whether or not we should be giving drugs to affected children. If you don't have a lot of family supports around, you may have to try medication.

THEODORE SLOTKIN: One of the nice things about a conference like this is it gets everyone up to snuff as to where the field is headed, and maybe 5 years from now we'll have people showing us, at least in animal models, about appropriate interventions that might be translatable to the clinical population.

ROBIN BLITZ: There are a lot of confounding variables that everyone talks about and looks at such as alcohol, cigarettes, and malnutrition, and I'm wondering if anybody's looked at the mother's comorbidities. You've talked about depression, but what about the mother's history of attention deficit disorder, learning disabilities, difficulties with arousal, difficulties with neurobehavioral differences, and neuroanatomical differences? Can those be looked at?

SPEAKER: We don't get that detailed when taking the mother's history; we conduct a 4-hour assessment of her current psychological status.

SPEAKER: We have some data, though not consistent and not across the whole cohort, and, again, even these data have their caveats, suggesting that cocaine-using women more often report a history of school-related problems manifest presumably before the onset of their drug use and manifest as attentional problems, learning difficulties, and sometimes specific reading disabilities. So the suggestion is that it's an extraordinarily multigenerational, high-risk group.

THEODORE SLOTKIN: That doesn't necessarily mean that the effect is genetic, because you may actually have people who are cocaine abusers or smokers who are self-medicating and thereby by nongenetic means passing on the same problems to their kids.

SPEAKER: This is something that we see in Fetal Alcohol Syndrome; we get generation after generation of drug-abusing women. The kid has Fetal Alcohol Syndrome; so does the mom. It turns out that the grandmother is an alcoholic too. Drug abuse may actually be multigenerational. Why not this with the cocaine-abusing women as well? She may not be functionally normal because maybe she was an alcohol-exposed baby herself, or a drug-exposed baby, or a malnourished baby.

THEODORE SLOTKIN: The counter to that, though, is that since there are real homologies between the results of animal models of neurobehavioral deficits and the human ones, it would argue that even if that component is there, there is a direct drug effect component superimposed on it. I don't know if everyone else would agree with that, but I have to say that the overlap of the animal and the human results are surprisingly consistent, given the history of this field or any other area of maternal drug abuse.

SPEAKER: Yes, there is good animal data with both alcohol and now with cocaine (Keller, R. W. *et al.* 1996. Neurosci. Lett. **205:** 153–156) and in our lab we have shown increased self-administration of cocaine and alcohol after prenatal exposure to those drugs (Spear, L. P. 1996. NIDA Research Monograph **164:** 125–145).

SPEAKER: I just wanted to remind people that humans usually come from fathers and mothers. It's not all mitochondrial and maternal inheritance of genes that we're talking about here.

SPEAKER: I just wanted to go back to something that's been a continuing theme. We've just spent a whole session on longitudinal studies, and I think that the studies that have just been described are extraordinarily elegant and incredibly hard to perform and offer us unique opportunities to get at some of the human data. But I would like to put in a plug for continuing to observe what we see in the clinic and for observational cohort studies, especially when we are at the beginning of learning about something. That's how we learned about multiple sclerosis, most of the neurodegenerative diseases, and many other things that we've just talked about. I would like to hear what the panel feels about observational cohort versus longitudinal studies in relationship to all that we've said about caveats.

SPEAKER: As a clinician, I agree with you in the value of clinical observation for generating hypotheses. That's been a standard of clinical work. The other side, though, after all that came out about the problems of cocaine-exposed children in schools, is that they were different and so forth. Whether or not that story turns out to have some validity, it nonetheless was born out of observations made without control groups, without blindness, and the like. So I think that there always has to be that caution.

SPEAKER: Observational studies do not necessarily need to be unblinded; they can be controlled. The whole science of observational studies is a very important one. From what we have heard, this is probably one of the most difficult clinical research problems in medicine. It's a high risk population, with addiction, a moving population; the methodologies we have for observational studies can be performed well or poorly. Each of us in different areas tries to "meta-analyze," but from what I have just heard for the first time, I think there is more truth here than any meta-analysis would bring. If some of the people who did the meta-design studies sat together, they could probably combine their data on at least some aspects in a way that would bring an even higher level of truth. That may be one of the advantages of a meeting such as this.

THEODORE SLOTKIN: One of the problems, though, is that because this is such a politically visible issue, individual bad studies tend to get picked up and magnified and distorted in the press before we have the opportunity to sit down together and combine bad studies into a good meta-analysis.

CHARLIE BAUER: We've seen a lot of statistical significance, but I'm wondering if the panel would comment on clinical significance. I'm concerned that with the large number of studies that we're now seeing, which are very sophisticated and very nicely done, you're going to see statistical significance. However, with the kind of numbers that you're talking about, is a 3-point difference (97 versus 100 on the Stanford-Binet IQ test that Dr. Richardson just reported on) that was statistically significant at $p < 0.05$ clinically significant?

I just wonder that we're not going back with the pendulum towards looking at clinical significance—not looking at clinical significance, which may lead us falsely to worry more than we should. Obviously, all the trends and all of the values taken together make us concerned that something's going on, but I just think that we need to look at clinical significance.

I also wonder what role environment plays, and not many people have looked at its impact. It's a very difficult thing to do. Is environment playing an equal role or a greater role in producing the kinds of outcomes and the kinds of findings that you are reporting? Certainly things like arousal, which Linda Mayes was talking about, are influenced by the environment. Many of these babies live in very violent, very stimulating environments, and they may shut down just for survival. Is it the environment that's causing the altered behaviors or is it the cocaine?

GALE RICHARDSON: When we designed the study, our focus was to have a large epidemiologic study, with a large number of women allowing for good control statistically. Taking that approach, the cocaine effects that we see are small. You wouldn't notice them in any one child; a child wouldn't stand out to you in a clinic. But after controlling for the other environmental variables, the other substance use variables, we are still seeing consistent cocaine effects. And, as I said, we think that that's a marker for the fact that this teratogen had an effect.

The other point about the environmental factors: we looked at maternal IQ, we looked at the mother's rating of the home environment, at the 3-year phase. They have a stronger effect on the child's current development than the prenatal cocaine use does. But even after controlling for those, we still see the prenatal effect.

THEODORE SLOTKIN: I want to add two points about the IQ issue. I don't think anyone would argue that elevated lead in a kid's blood stream is bad for the brain and that costs you 5 IQ points. Secondly, just do the following calculation: it's very easy to do with a Gaussian curve such as IQ distribution. A 5 IQ point shift doesn't change very much the area under the curve of the so-called normal people—people between –3 SDs and +3 SDs on the IQ scale—but it costs you two thirds of the people who have genius IQ's and it triples the number of people who have IQ's below 55. So don't think that a small shift in the mean doesn't mean anything to society when it's amortized over a very large population. The real action is what happens in the tails of the distribution and a 3 IQ point shift in the mean makes a tremendous change out in the tails.

LINDA MAYES: I just want to discuss the maternal variables. There are distal maternal variables and there are proximal maternal variables in terms of what happens on a day-to-day, moment-to-moment interaction between parents and their children. Surely those kinds of proximal variables do influence things like attention and arousal. For example, we've looked at mother-baby interaction among the women in our study, and there's a pattern of increased withdrawal. Drug-abusing mothers more often withdraw from the interactions with their babies, more often turning away and tuning out, and, when the baby cries, not responding. If that goes on a day-to-day basis, we presume that it would have a remarkable effect on these very things that we're looking at.

SPEAKER: I'm not very aware of what goes on in drug treatment programs, but is there any therapeutic use of stimulant medications such as Ritalin in the possibility that there is a subsegment of cocaine-abusing women that is self-medicating?

THEODORE SLOTKIN: The whole concept of a self-medicating subpopulation, at this point, is hypothetical and based primarily on the issue of why people smoke cigarettes. The extension to other drugs of abuse is by analogy to that. About half the people in the United States who smoke are essentially self-medicators, because if you treat them with the nicotine patch, you take away their desire to smoke, whereas people who are smoking, who are using other cues for reward, still want those cues. The whole self-medication hypothesis right now is a hypothesis. I don't think there is any really hard data to support that, although it's an attractive hypothesis to explain substance abuse in general.

SPEAKER: There are data showing that women who use cocaine are more likely to be depressed and those who are more depressed are more likely to relapse and use cocaine. So you can postulate that in that regard, they are self-medicating for their underlying problem.

THEODORE SLOTKIN: In a great leap of faith, by the way, this is already being applied in therapeutics. The whole principle of Buproprion (Wellbutrin) as a "stop-smoking drug," as it has just been approved for, is the idea that there is a subpopulation of smokers who are treating their own depression with nicotine.

BARRY KOSOFSKY: This afternoon's discussion was spectacular; the "second generation" of studies that you've heard about and that you'll hear more about over the next few days, both at the preclinical and at the clinical levels, have made tremendous progress. In some ways the human studies are doing better than the animal studies in terms of identifying the gestational timing and quantity of drug exposure and the independent contribution of particular patterns of *in utero* cocaine exposure in altering outcomes. The human studies have identified that there is not one cocaine-exposed phenotype, but many cocaine-exposed phenotypes, which may be partially determined by the pattern of maternal cocaine use. Animal researchers are always asked, "What you're saying is probably true, but is it relevant?" Human studies researchers are often asked, "What you're studying is relevant, but is it true?" For the first time we are seeing a convergence of clinical and preclinical findings, which strongly supports that the findings observed are relevant and true with profound implications for clinicians, scientists, educators, parents, and children. We want to thank our speakers and our moderator for emphasizing these points, and we look forward to our next session for making additional progress in our understanding.

Role of the Neurotrophic Properties of Serotonin in the Delay of Brain Maturation Induced by Cocaine[a]

PATRICIA M. WHITAKER-AZMITIA[b]

Department of Psychology, State University of New York at Stony Brook, Stony Brook, New York 11794-2500, USA

INTRODUCTION

Cocaine exerts its action in the adult central nervous system (CNS) through interactions with monoamine transporter molecules. This interaction results principally in inhibition of reuptake of the neurotransmitters serotonin and dopamine. Overall, this results in an increase in these neurotransmitters in the synaptic cleft. The developing mammalian brain also contains these transporter molecules, and cocaine will bind to these sites as well, but there are some important differences. In the developing brain, cocaine binding can be pharmacologically characterized as binding predominantly to the serotonin transporter, whereas in the adult brain, it is predominantly to the dopamine transporter.[1] Cocaine's effects on the fetal serotonin transporter are different as well. At low concentrations, cocaine specifically releases serotonin much in the same way as does the classic serotonin releaser, fenfluramine.[2] Thus, the fetal brain may respond to cocaine primarily through actions on the serotonin system.

In the developing brain, serotonin does not act like a classic neurotransmitter. Although many of the same receptors, enzymes, and uptake mechanisms are present, serotonin instead plays a role in developing and maturing the CNS.[3–7] Any change in the levels of serotonin during development, as through maternal drug use, could thus seriously affect the development of the brain. With these facts in mind, we tested the hypothesis that the toxic effects of cocaine on brain development are mediated through its interference with the developmental properties of serotonin.

Like all developmental factors, serotonin has critical periods during development when specific actions are evident. There are three apparent critical periods for serotonin: autoregulation of serotonin neurons, astroglial maturation, and neuronal maturation. In our model, we chose the earliest period of serotonin's actions, autoregulation, largely because it corresponds approximately to the first trimester of human pregnancy, a time when a mother may not be aware of pregnancy and the risk of drug abuse may be greater.

Autoregulation of serotonin neurons begins almost as soon as the serotonin neuron is differentiated. In the rat, this occurs at approximately gestational day (GD) 13, and therefore our studies used cocaine treatments from GD 13 until birth. In these studies, cocaine hydrochloride was given subcutaneously (sc) into the nape of the neck of pregnant Sprague-Dawley rats at a dose of 40 mg/kg once daily. To test our hypothesis of the role of serotonin, we examined the brain at the three critical periods for changes that we knew could be brought about by changes in serotonin. The results are therefore discussed under each critical period.

[a] This work was supported by a grant from the National Institute on Aging.

[b] Phone, 516/632-9899; e-mail, whitaker@psych1.psy.sunysb.edu

Autoregulation. During development, serotonin neurons use what could be referred to as a negative feedback mechanism for regulating their own growth. Using both tissue culture[8] and whole animal studies,[9,10] it was shown that increased extracellular serotonin at this critical time causes a decreased outgrowth of serotonin neurons. In some cases, for example if the increased serotonin is caused by inhibition of monoamine oxidase, the decreased growth leaves the serotonin system permanently lacking.[11] In other cases, if receptor agonists are used to mimic the effects of increased serotonin, the effects are temporary.[9] If cocaine's effects on brain development are mediated though the serotonin system, then treating with cocaine during the critical period referred to as autoregulation should cause a decrease in outgrowth of serotonin terminals. Using our model of cocaine treatment, this is what we have found.[12]

At 1 day after birth, rat pups treated prenatally with cocaine showed decreased serotonin terminal density in hippocampus, but no decrease in brainstem. This decrease is still observed 1 week postnatally, but the terminal density is normal at 4 weeks. The distribution of serotonin fibers at 4 weeks is comparable to that of control animals. This observation, plus the fact that the terminal density was normalized so rapidly (i.e., 3 weeks), suggests that the serotonin terminals were not damaged and re-grew, but rather that their growth was delayed.

Although we did not specifically examine the striatum, others have. Using a comparable treatment paradigm, Snyder-Keller and Keller[13] and their collaborators found that serotonin terminals show hyperinnervation of this region, beginning at birth. This may be an example of a developmental process whereby reciprocal growth takes place within a neurotransmitter system. That is, if growth is decreased in one area, it is increased elsewhere.

This return to normal of serotonin terminals by 4 weeks should not be interpreted as the end of the problem. In previous studies, we showed that delaying serotonin terminal development, even briefly, causes behavioral deficits in the adult.[9] This may be because serotonin levels were reduced during the two subsequent critical periods of serotonin's developmental role. In particular, in the immediate postnatal period (PND 1–7), serotonin is required for astroglial maturation, and in the later developmental stages (PND 10–20) serotonin plays an important role in neuronal maturation. Thus, assuming that serotonin is lacking at these times, the developing brain should show changes during these critical periods as well.

At this point, it is important to emphasize the role of these critical periods in the effects of exposure to cocaine. If, as in our model, exposure occurred during the first critical period, then serotonin levels would be decreased in the two subsequent periods. However, if exposure took place later (for example, from birth to PND 20 in the rat or from midgestation to 2 years of life in the human), then serotonin levels would be increased, and the resulting effects on brain development would be different. In preliminary studies, we found that exposure to serotonin agonists at these later times may accelerate brain maturation and cause significant behavioral changes, such as increased anxiety and hypereactivity.[14]

Astroglial Maturation. Astroglial cells play an important role in brain development in both guidance and production of growth factors. In the mammalian brain, the 5-HT1A receptor peaks in number early in development.[15,16] This peak number appears to be largely on astroglial cells[17,18] and plays a dual function. One function is maturation of the astroglial cell. This maturation is principally observed morphologically; the cells become more stellate, that is, they have smaller cell bodies and more and shorter processes. The longer process needed for guidance of neuronal migration (that is, the radial glial cell) is lost and the cell no longer stains for vimentin. In addition, the cells lose a significant amount of their 5-HT1A receptors. The second function of the 5-HT1A receptor on astroglial cells is to release the growth factor S-100β.[19–22]

In our hypothesis, delaying maturation of the serotonin system with prenatal cocaine would interfere with the role of serotonin in glial proliferation and maturation and in the release of S-100β. Thus, if cocaine interferes with brain development via a serotonin mechanism, the brain of cocaine-exposed animals should show delayed glial maturation (such as a prolonged radial glial cell stage) and decreased glial proliferation. To test for these changes, we used an immunocytochemical marker for radial glial cells (vimentin). To study astroglial proliferation, we injected rat pups with bromodeoxyuridine (BrdU) 1 hour before sacrifice. Once incorporated into dividing cells, the cells could be stained with an antibody against BrdU. Prenatally exposed rat pups examined at PND 6 did show the changes in astroglial cells that we had anticipated.[23]

As expected, few astroglial cells of the control pups stained positively for vimentin, that is, they were no longer radial glial cells and were acquiring the stellate morphology of a mature astroglial cell. Conversely, the astroglial cells in the brains of pups exposed to cocaine were still vimentin positive. In fact, the presence of radial glial cells was still very much in evidence, as many positively stained processes extended from the ventricle to the cortical surface.

Using the BrdU technique for proliferating cells, the cocaine-exposed pups had fewer astroglial cells both in the primary germinative area of the subventricular zone and in the hippocampal germinative zones. In addition, there were fewer astroglial cells in the cortex, and the cortex itself was much thinner. In a primate model of fetal cocaine exposure, loss of astroglial cells was also observed in the cortex, at 2 months of age.[24] Unfortunately, older animals were not studied in either of these models, and it is not known if the decreased number of astroglial cells is permanent. Clearly, lack of these cells in the mature brain could have severe consequences to normal brain functioning. This lack could also be important in the developing brain, as these cells are important sources of growth factors, such as S-100β. In fact, immunochemical staining for S-100β in the brain of the cocaine pups was significantly reduced.[23,25] Thus, even if serotonin levels return to normal, and even if astroglial cells return to normal, this important growth factor may not have been at a sufficient level during its critical period.

Neuronal Maturation. Role of S-100β: Serotonin also plays a role in maturation of the target regions that it innervates. The earliest studies on serotonin and target maturation were by Lauder who, using the tryptophan hydroxylase inhibitor *p*-chlorophenylalanine (PCPA), showed that prenatal depletion of serotonin in the rat caused delayed maturation and prolonged proliferation of target regions.[3] Using hippocampal slice cultures, Chubakov *et al.*[7,26] have further suggested that serotonin plays a role in neurite outgrowth in the target region, increases electrical interconnections, and promotes synaptogenesis. In developing chicks, serotonin depletion (with PCPA) delays hippocampal neuronal differentiation and decreases the number of synapses in the cerebral cortex and hippocampus.[27] In rats, depletion of serotonin at PND 3 (with the selective neurotoxin 5,7 DHT) results in a decreased density of granule cell dendritic spines, which worsens as the animals grow into adolescence.[28] Depletion in rats at PND 10–20, with the tryptophan hydroxyalse PCPA, causes loss of dendrites, as seen in changes of the dendritic marker MAP-2, in the animals up to 1 year of age. Moreover, there are severe deficits in a variety of learning models.[29] Many of these effects of serotonin on neuronal maturation may be direct (for example, see refs. 30 and 31), but others may in fact be due to serotonin-mediated release of S-100β.

S-100β is a highly important trophic factor, the gene for which is located on chromosome 21 and thus may be involved in such developmental disorders as Down's syndrome and the resultant Alzheimer's disease. S-100β causes neurite outgrowth[20,32,33] and promotes neuronal plasticity.[34,35] In a mutant mouse model, the polydactyl Nagoya mouse, cortical levels of S-100β[36] are decreased and there is little development of cortex.[37] In the mature animal, S-100β is important in the long-term potentiation model of learning.[38] If S-100β is decreased in the cocaine animals, all of these aspects of its function will be lacking, that is, the animals should show decreased or delayed neurite outgrowth, smaller cortices, decreased dendritic development, and deficits in learning and memory.

To assess the effects of prenatal cocaine on neurite outgrowth, we examined rat brains at PND 6 for the presence of the growth-associated protein GAP-43. This protein is present in actively growing growth cones and diminishes or is absent when the growth cone reaches its target. In rats, GAP-43 is largely diminished by PND 6. However, GAP-43 staining was increased in the cocaine-exposed pups.[23] This increased staining was seen in fiber tracts, such as the corpus callosum, the fornix, cingulum bundle, and hippocampal commissure as well as within the CA fields of the hippocampus. If the GAP-43 staining had been increased only in the hippocampus, it might indicate an increase in neuronal plasticity; however, the increase in fiber tracts indicates that neurite outgrowth had been delayed.

More detailed morphologic studies of brain development, which have been done by others, may support our hypothesis. In a primate model, cocaine-exposed offspring show deficits in neuronal migration into cortex, possibly as a consequence of the astroglial deficits.[24] In the cocaine-exposed rabbit model, changes in MAP-2–stained dendrites are observed.[39] However, this study looked principally at cortical regions rich in dopamine innervation, and the rabbit does not appear to show the glial changes observed in the rat or primate model. Nonetheless, it is important that persistent MAP-2–labeled dendritic changes have been shown.

Finally, the numerous studies showing learning and memory deficits in the cocaine-exposed fetus, both human[40–42] and nonhuman,[43–45] could be expected from our hypothesis, because our studies show that serotonin depletion during neuronal maturation decreases S-100β and induces learning and memory deficits.

CONCLUSION AND RELEVANCE TO THE HUMAN FETUS EXPOSED TO COCAINE

Using an animal model of cocaine exposure, we have examined the effects of this drug on brain development and how many of these effects may be mediated through the serotonin system. The studies have supported our hypothesis that increased extracellular serotonin in the fetus causes delayed outgrowth of serotonin terminals through autoregulation. Furthermore, this delay in serotonin outgrowth causes delay in astroglial maturation, delay in release of S-100β, and subsequent loss of neuronal maturation. This loss may also lead to a loss of synapses in the mature animal and thus to deficits in learning and memory. Recently, the model was also used to test a potential therapeutic strategy.

According to our hypothesis, much of the detrimental effect of fetal cocaine exposure is ultimately caused by decreased release of the trophic factor S-100β. This factor is released by the actions of serotonin on the astroglial 5-HT_{1A} receptor. Thus, 5-HT_{1A} agonists, such as 8-OH-DPAT, ipsaperone, or buspirone, at the critical time should cause release of S-100β and restore normal development. In cocaine-exposed pups, we found this to be the case.[25] Using our usual paradigm of cocaine exposure *in utero,* we examined the effects of treatment with a 5-HT_{1A} agonist on postnatal days 1–5. The exposed animals treated with the agonist showed increases in S-100β in both cortex and hippocampus compared to the cocaine alone group. Moreover, there was a significant increase in brain size.

Thus, in our preliminary animal studies, at least some of the detrimental effects of cocaine on the brain of a developing fetus apparently can be reversed by treatment with a serotonin 5-HT$_{1A}$ agonist at the appropriate time. This approach also reversed the effects of serotonin depletion on dendritic development and restored normal serotonin levels in a model of fetal alcohol syndrome.[46,47] If human studies show morphological, neurochemical, and/or behavioral changes comparable to those we found in the animal model, it may be worthwhile to consider the use of a 5-HT$_{1A}$ agonist in preventing the detrimental effects to the brain of cocaine exposure *in utero.*

ACKNOWLEDGMENTS

The author wishes to express gratitude to her colleagues, Drs. E. Azmitia, H. Akbari, H. K. Kramer, and C. Clarke.

REFERENCES

1. Shearman, L.P., L.M. Collins & J.S. Meyer. 1996. Characterization and localization of 125-I-RTI-55-labeled cocaine binding sites in fetal and adult rat brain. JPET **277:** 1770–1783.
2. Kramer, K., E.C. Azmitia & P.M. Whitaker-Azmitia. 1994. *In vitro* release of [3H]5-hydroxytryptamine from fetal and maternal brain by drugs of abuse. Dev. Brain Res. **78:** 142–146.
3. Lauder, J.M. & H. Krebs. 1978. Serotonin as a differentiation signal in early neurogenesis. Dev. Neurosci. **1:** 15–20.
4. Lauder, J.M. & H. Krebs. 1976. Effects of *p*-chlorophenylalanine on time of neuronal origin during embyrogenesis in the rat. Brain Res. **107:** 638–644.
5. Lauder, J.M. 1990. Ontogeny of the serotonergic system in the rat: Serotonin as a developmental signal, Ann. N.Y. Acad. Sci. **600:** 297–314.
6. Whitaker-Azmitia, P.M. 1991. Role of serotonin and other neurotransmitter receptors in brain development: Basis for developmental pharmacology. Pharmacol. Rev. **43:** 553–561.
7. Chubakov, A.R., E.A. Gromova, G.V. Konovalov, E.I. Chumasov & E.F. Sarkisova. 1986. Effects of serotonin on the development of a rat cerebral cortex tissue culture. Neurosci. Behav. Physiol. **16:** 490–497.
8. Whitaker-Azmitia, P.M. & E.C. Azmitia. 1986. Autoregulation of fetal serotonergic neuronal development: Role of high affinity serotonin receptors. Neurosci. Lett. **67:** 307–312.
9. Shemer, A.V., E.C. Azmitia & P.M. Whitaker-Azmitia. 1991. Dose-related effects of prenatal 5-methoxytryptamine (5-MT) on development of serotonin terminal density and behavior. Brain Res. **59:** 59–63.
10. Diefenbach, T.J., B.D. Sloley & J.I. Goldberg. 1995. Neurite branch development of an identified serotonergic neuron from embryonic Helisoma: Evidence for autoregulation by serotonin. Dev. Biol. **167:** 282–293.
11. Whitaker-Azmitia, P.M., X. Zhang & D. Raio. 1994. Gestational exposure to monoamine oxidase inhibitors in rats: Preliminary behavioral and neurochemical studies. Neuropsychopharmacology **11:** 125–130.
12. Akbari, H.M., H.K. Kramer, P.M. Whitaker-Azmitia, L.P. Spear & E.C. Azmitia. 1992. Prenatal cocaine exposure disrupts the development of the serotonergic system. Brain Res. **572:** 57–63.
13. Snyder-Keller, A.M. & R.W. Keller. 1993. Prenatal cocaine increases striatal serotonin innervation without altering the patch/matrix organization of intrinsic cell types. Dev. Brain Res. **74:** 261–267.
14. Borella, A., M. Bindra & P.M. Whitaker-Azmitia. 1997. Role of the 5-HT1A receptor in development of the neonatal rat brain: Preliminary behavioral studies. Neuropharmacology **36:** 445–450.

15. Bar-Peled, O., R. Gross-Isseroff, H. Ben-Hur, I. Hoskins, Y. Groner & A. Biegon. 1991. Fetal human brain exhibits a prenatal peak in the density of serotonin 5-HT1A receptors. Neurosci. Lett. **127:** 173–176.
16. Daval, G., D. Verge, A. Becerril, H. Gozlan, U. Spampinato & M. Hamon. 1987. Transient expression of 5-HT1A receptor binding sites in some areas of the rat CNS during postnatal development. Int. J. Dev. Neurosci. **5:** 171–80.
17. Hellendall, R.P., U. Schambra, J. Liu, G.R. Breese, D.E. Millhorn & J.M. Lauder. 1992. Detection of serotonin receptor transcripts in the developing nervous system. J. Chem. Neuroanat. **5:** 299–310.
18. Whitaker-Azmitia, P.M. & E.C. Azmitia. 1986. 5-Hydroxytryptamine binding to brain astroglial cells: Differences between intact and homogenized preparations and mature and immature cultures. J. Neurochem. **46:** 1186–1189.
19. Whitaker-Azmitia, P.M. & E.C. Azmitia. 1989. Stimulation of astroglial serotonin receptors produces media which regulates development of serotonergic neurons. Brain Res. **497:** 80–85.
20. Whitaker-Azmitia, P.M., R. Murphy & E.C. Azmitia. 1990. S-100 protein is released from astroglial cells by stimulation of 5-HT1a receptors and regulates development of serotonin neurons. Brain Res. **528:** 155–160.
21. Whitaker-Azmitia, P.M. & E.C. Azmitia. 1994. Astroglial 5-HT1a receptors and S-100 beta in development and plasticity. Perspect. Dev. Neurobiol. **2:** 233–238.
22. Lauder, J.M. & J. Liu. 1994. Glial heterogeneity and developing neurotransmitter systems. Perspect. Dev. Neurobiol. **2:** 239–250.
23. Clarke, C., K. Clarke, J. Muneyyirci, E. Azmitia & P.M. Whitaker-Azmitia. 1996. Prenatal cocaine delays astroglial maturation: Immunodensitometry shows increased markers of immaturity (vimentin and GAP-43) and decreased proliferation and production of the growth factor S-100. Dev. Brain Res. **91:** 268–273.
24. Lidow, M.S. 1995. Prenatal cocaine exposure adversely affects development of the primate cerebral cortex. Synapse **21:** 332–341.
25. Akbari, H.M., P.M. Whitaker-Azmitia & E.C. Azmitia. 1994. Prenatal cocaine decreases the trophic factor S-100β and induces microcephaly: Reversal by postnatal 5-HT1a agonist. Neurosci. Lett. **170:** 141–144.
26. Chubakov, A.R., V.G. Tsyganova & E.F. Sarkisova. 1993. The stimulating influence of the raphe nuclei on the morphofunctional development of the hippocampus during their combined cultivation. Neurosci. Behav. Physiol. **23:** 271–276.
27. Cheng, L., K. Hamaguchi, M. Ogawa, S. Hamada & N. Okado. 1993. PCPA reduces both monoaminergic afferents and nonmonoaminergic synapses in the cerebral cortex. Neurosci. Res. **19:** 111–116.
28. Yan, W., C.C. Wilson & J.H. Haring. 1997. Effects of neonatal serotonin depletion on the development of rat dentate granule cells. Dev. Brain Res. **98:** 177–184.
29. Mazer, C., J. Muneyyirci, K. Taheny, N. Raio, A. Borella & P.M. Whitaker-Azmitia. 1997. Serotonin depletion during synaptogenesis leads to decreased synaptic density and learning deficits in the adult rat. A model of neurodevelopmental disorders with cognitive deficits. Brain Res. **760:** 68–74.
30. Sikich, L., J.M. Hickok & R.D. Todd. 1990. 5-HT1A receptors control neurite branching during development. Dev. Brain Res. **56:** 269–274.
31. Riad, M., M.B. Emerit & M. Hamon. 1994. Neurotrophic effects of ipsapirone and other 5-HT1A receptor agonists on septal cholinergic neurons in culture. Dev. Brain Res. **82:** 245–258.
32. Lui, J.P. & J.M. Lauder. 1992. S-100 beta and insulin-like growth factor-II differentially regulate growth of developing serotonin and dopamine neurons in vitro. J. Neurosci. Res. **33:** 248–254.
32. Kligman, D. & D. Marshak. 1985. Purification and characterization of a neurite extension factor from bovine brain. Proc. Natl. Acad. Sci. USA **82:** 7136–7142.
34. Muller, C.M., A.C. Akhavan & M. Bette. 1993. Possible role of S-100 in glia-neuronal signalling involved in activity dependent plasticity in the developing mammalian cortex. J. Chem. Neuroanat. **6:** 215–220.
35. Gerlai, R., J.M. Wojtowicz, A. Marks & J. Roder. 1995. Overexpression of a calcium

binding protein, S-100β, in astrocytes impairs synaptic plasticity and spatial learning in transgenic mice. Learning Memory **2:** 26–34.
36. NARUSE, I., K. KATO, T. ASANO, F. SUZUKI & Y. KAMEYAMA. 1990. Developmental brain abnormalities accompanied with the retarded production of S-100 beta protein in genetic polydactyly mice. Dev. Brain Res. **51:** 253–259.
36. UEDA, S., X.F. GU, I. NARUSE, P.M. WHITAKER-AZMITIA & E.C. AZMITIA. 1993. Neuroglia neurotrophic interactions in the S-100 beta retarded mutant mouse (polydactylyl Nagoya). Brain Res. **633:** 275–282.
38. LEWIS, D. & T.J. TEYLER. 1986. Anti-S-100 serum blocks long-term potentiation in the hippocampal slice. Brain Res. **383:** 159–167.
39. JONES, L., I. FISCHER & P. LEVITT. 1996. Nonuniform alteration of dendritic development in the cerebral cortex following prenatal cocaine exposure. Cereb. Cortex **6:** 431–445.
40. AZUMA, S.D. & I.J. CHASNOFF. 1993. Outcome of children prenatally exposed to cocaine or other drugs: A path analysis of three-year data. Pediatrics **92:** 396–402.
41. VAN BAAR, A. & B.M. DE GRAAFF. 1994. Cognitive development at preschool-age of infants of drug-dependent mothers. Dev. Med. Child Neurol. **36:** 1063–75.
42. RICHARDSON, G.A., M.L. CONROY & N.L. DAY. 1996. Prenatal cocaine exposure: Effects on the development of school-age children. Neurotoxicol. Teratol. **18:** 627–634.
43. CUTLER, A.R., A.E. WILKERSON, J.L. GINGRAS & E.D. LEVIN. 1996. Prenatal cocaine and/or nicotine exposure in rats: Preliminary findings on long-term cognitive outcome and genital development at birth. Neurotoxicol. Teratol. **18:** 635–643.
44. ROMANO, A.G. & J.A. HARVEY. 1996. Prenatal exposure to cocaine disrupts discrimination learning in adult rabbits. Pharmacol. Biochem. Behav. **53:** 617–621.
45. HUGHES, H.E., L.M. DONOHUE & D.L. DOW-EDWARDS. 1994. Prenatal cocaine exposure affects the acoustic startle response in adult rat. Behav. Brain Res. **75:** 83–90.
46. TAJUDDIN, N. & M.J. DRUSE. 1993. Treatment of pregnant alcohol-consuming rats with buspirone/Effects on serotonin and 5-HIAA content in offspring. Alcohol Clin. Exp. Res. **17:** 110–115.
47. YAN, W., C.C. WILSON & J.H. HARING. 1997. 5-HT1a receptors mediate the neurotrophic effect of serotonin on developing dentate granule cells. Dev. Brain Res. **98:** 185–190.

Changes in the Midbrain-Rostral Forebrain Dopamine Circuitry in the Cocaine-Exposed Primate Fetal Brain[a]

OLINE K. RØNNEKLEIV,[b] YUAN FANG, WAN S. CHOI,[c] AND LIN CHAI[d]

Department of Physiology and Pharmacology, Oregon Health Sciences University, Portland, Oregon 97201, USA

Division of Neuroscience, Oregon Regional Primate Research Center, Beaverton, Oregon 97006, USA

ABSTRACT: To ascertain cocaine's effects in the fetus, we developed a nonhuman primate model in which pregnant monkeys were administered cocaine (3 mg/kg im) or saline four times a day from day 20 through days 40–70 of a 165-day gestation. At the time of cesarean section, plasma levels of cocaine in fetal blood were 231 ± 70 ng/ml. Fetal brains were examined using immunocytochemistry, *in situ* hybridization, receptor autoradiography, and nuclease protection assay analysis. No differences were found in the expression of tyrosine hydroxylase and dopamine receptor mRNAs by days 40–45 of gestation. However, by day 60 the midbrain of monkeys exposed to cocaine had significantly reduced expression of tyrosine hydroxylase, the rate-limiting enzyme in dopamine synthesis. Moreover, dopamine D_1 and D_2 receptor mRNAs were significantly elevated in the rostral forebrain as were D_1 and D_2 receptor binding sites in days 60–70 cocaine-exposed fetuses. Cocaine treatment from day 20 to days 60 and 70 of gestation also significantly increased the mRNA concentrations of dynorphin and enkephalin in the rostral forebrain. These findings suggest that *in utero* cocaine exposure has profound effects on the developing dopamine neurocircuitry.

INTRODUCTION

Cocaine use alone or in combination with other drugs during pregnancy may have adverse effects on the development of the fetus, which is reflected in the various behavioral problems observed postnatally.[1–5] Such observations are further substantiated by the more rigorous experiments performed in animals.[6–11] These studies have demonstrated cocaine-induced deficits in cognitive functions, disturbances in corticogenesis, and alterations in dopamine neural circuits.[6,7,9–16] Brain dopamine systems play a central role in the control of movement, hormone release, and many complex behaviors.[17] Two major dopamine systems originate in the ventral midbrain: the nigrostriatal

[a] This work was supported by DA 07165, Medical Research Foundation of Oregon, T32 HD 01733, HD 18185, RR 00163.

[b] Address for correspondence: Dr. Oline K. Rønnekleiv, Department of Physiology and Pharmacology, L334, Oregon Health Sciences University, 3181 SW Sam Jackson Park Road, Portland, OR 97201–3098.

[c] Present address: Department of Anatomy, School of Medicine, Gyeongsang National University, Chinju, Korea.

[d] Present address: Veterans Administration Medical Center, Portland, OR 97201.

dopamine system and the mesocorticolimbic dopamine system. The nigrostriatal dopamine system is important for motor control.[18] The mesocorticolimbic dopamine system is thought to be critical for psychomotor stimulant reward and is believed to be the most important pathway for drug reinforcement.[19,20] The neurons of this system originate in the ventral tegmental area (VTA) and project to the nucleus accumbens (nAcb), ventral striatum, septal area, olfactory tubercle, frontal cortex, and amygdala.[18]

Dopamine (DA) acts at specific dopamine receptor sites, and the molecular cloning of multiple subtypes of the DA receptor gene family has revealed at least five distinct receptors that cluster into D_1-like (D_1 and D_5) and D_2-like (D_2, D_3, and D_4) subfamilies.[21] Dopamine D_2 receptor mRNA and binding sites that are located in the pars compacta of the substantial nigra (SN) and in the VTA show similar distribution to that of the DA neurons in this region.[22,23] Therefore, the D_2 receptor is believed to be the main autoreceptor on DA neurons, which directly modulates the excitability of DA cells and the synthesis of DA.[23,24] Dopamine D_1 receptors in the midbrain are located on striatal GABA projection neurons to the SN and VTA and modulate transmitter release from GABA afferents and thus indirectly affect DA neuronal activity.[25]

Dynorphin- and enkephalin-containing neurons in the rostral forebrain express dopamine D_1 and D_2 receptors and are regulated by dopaminergic neurons.[18,26–29] For example, in Parkinson's and Huntington's disease in which the nigrostriatal dopaminergic system is disrupted, there are alterations in the expression of enkephalin mRNA.[30,31] Thus, experimentally induced Parkinson's disease in various animal models including nonhuman primates results in increased expression of enkephalin mRNA.[18,26,32–34] Additionally, expression of dynorphin mRNA is elevated in rostral forebrain regions of cocaine-addicted animals.[35–38]

In our studies, we examined the effects of chronic treatment of pregnant rhesus monkeys with cocaine on the development of dopamine neurons, their receptors, and the dopamine target neurons enkephalin and dynorphin in their fetuses. The studies focused primarily on fetal days 40–70 because this is a critical period for the development of dopamine neurons.[14]

ANIMAL MODEL AND TREATMENT PARADIGM

Animal Model. To analyze the consequences of prenatal cocaine exposure on dopamine neural circuits, we used the rhesus monkey as the experimental subject because the monkey has a long gestation period (165 days) and the development of its fetus is similar to that of the human.[39] Also, in contrast to many other studies, we have been exploring cocaine's action in the fetal brain to better understand the consequences of cocaine as the brain is being formed versus the effects of gestational cocaine that are found later in development or in the mature central nervous system.

Cocaine Treatment. Our initial experiments to determine the dose regimen of cocaine have been described in detail.[14] On the basis of reports of cocaine use in pregnant women (average 500 mg with each use)[1] and our initial observation of cocaine concentrations in monkey maternal and fetal plasma, a dose of 3 mg/kg was used in subsequent studies.[14] Cocaine (3 mg dissolved in 50 μl 0.9% saline/kg) or saline solution was injected im four times daily at 8 A.M., 12 noon, 4 P.M., and 8 P.M. beginning at approximately day 20 of pregnancy. After a cocaine injection, plasma levels of cocaine reached maximum levels of ≈ 800 ng/ml 10–15 minutes later.[14]

Cocaine Levels in Body Fluids at the Time of Cesarean Section. Fetuses were delivered by cesarean section. On the day of cesarean section, each animal received the final injection of cocaine or saline solution at 8:40 A.M.. Shortly thereafter, the animal was sedated with Ketamine, transported to the surgical area, and anesthetized with halothane. Twenty to thirty minutes after the last cocaine injection, average maternal plasma cocaine levels were 408 ± 72 ng/ml, which is about half the maximum plasma cocaine levels found in these animals.[14] Only one blood sample was obtained from each fetus at approximately 45 minutes after maternal cocaine injection. At that time, the fetal plasma sample and a second maternal blood sample contained approximately the same cocaine content, 231 ± 70 and 220 ± 47 ng/ml, respectively (FIG. 1).

Maternal Effects of Cocaine. Pregnant females treated with cocaine did not show any long-term overt signs of cocaine intolerance. No difference in body weight was found between animals treated with cocaine and those treated with saline solution. Both groups of animals received a special fruit snack following each injection. With this reinforcement both groups appeared eager to get their injection, and no obvious behavioral indicators of stress were observed.

Fetal Growth. Body weight, crown-rump length, head circumference, and brain weight were recorded prior to fetal dissections. Moreover, on days 60 and 70 of gestation the fetuses were separated according to sex. Maternal cocaine treatment did not significantly affect body weight or crown-rump length on days 40, 60, or 70 of gestation or head circumference and brain weight on days 60 and 70. However, within the

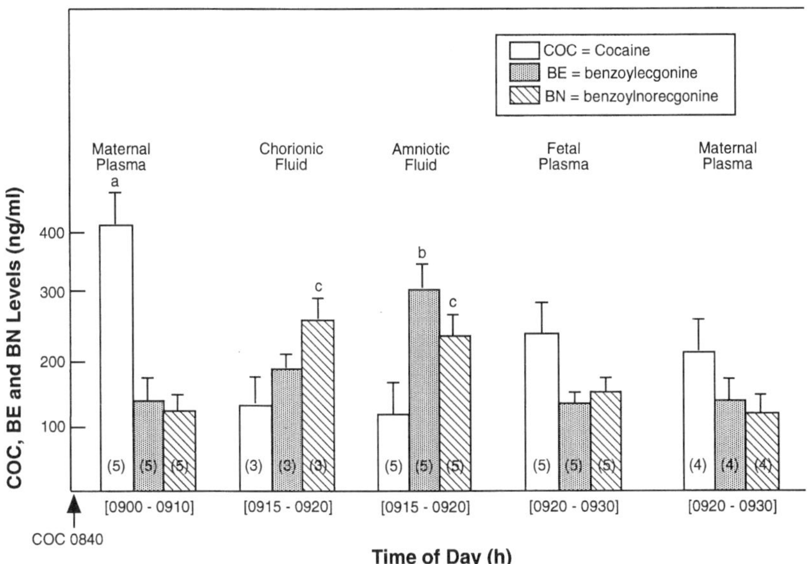

FIGURE 1. Levels of cocaine (COC), benzoylecgonine (BE), and benzoylnorecgonine (BN) in maternal and fetal plasma, and amniotic and chorionic fluids at the time of cesarean section on day 60 of pregnancy. Data are presented as means *(bars)* ± SEM *(vertical lines)*. Number of animals per group is indicated at the base of each bar. The final cocaine injection was given at 8:40 AM designated by (↑), and the samples were obtained at the time-interval indicated along the abscissa. Lower case letters a–c indicate significantly different values from those of COC, BE, and BN, respectively, at other time points; $p < 0.05$. From Rønnekleiv and Naylor.[14] Reprinted with permission from the *Journal of Neuroscience.*

latter two age groups, fetal males were significantly heavier than the corresponding females (FIG. 2).

EFFECTS OF COCAINE ON DOPAMINE NEURONS

The purpose of initial experiments was to elucidate the effects of cocaine on the developing dopamine neurons of the rhesus monkey and to determine the earliest time in fetal development when the actions of cocaine are manifested. In the rhesus monkey, which has a gestation period of approximately 165 days, all mesencephalic dopamine neurons are born in a short time span between embryonic days 36 and 43.[40] Initially, we determined the effects of cocaine on tyrosine hydroxylase (TH), the rate-limiting enzyme in dopamine synthesis,[41] in the rhesus macaque fetus at days 40–60 of gestation which is a critical period of development.[14]

Ontogeny of Neurons Containing Tyrosine Hydroxylase. In control and cocaine-treated fetal brains, adjacent sections were either stained immunocytochemically for TH or subjected to *in situ* hybridization for TH mRNA as previously described.[14] TH immunoreactive (TH-IR) cells and fibers were present in the mesencephalic area and the diencephalon of day-40 fetuses. TH mRNA was detected in the same regions and showed a distribution similar to that of TH-IR cells.[14] By day 60 of gestation the fetal monkey brain was much larger than that of the day-40 fetus; consequently, the area occupied by TH-IR cell groups within the mesencephalon and the diencephalon was greatly increased in size.[14]

Consequences of Cocaine Exposure. At day 40 no differences were noted in the location or content of immunoreactive TH and TH mRNA in control versus cocaine-

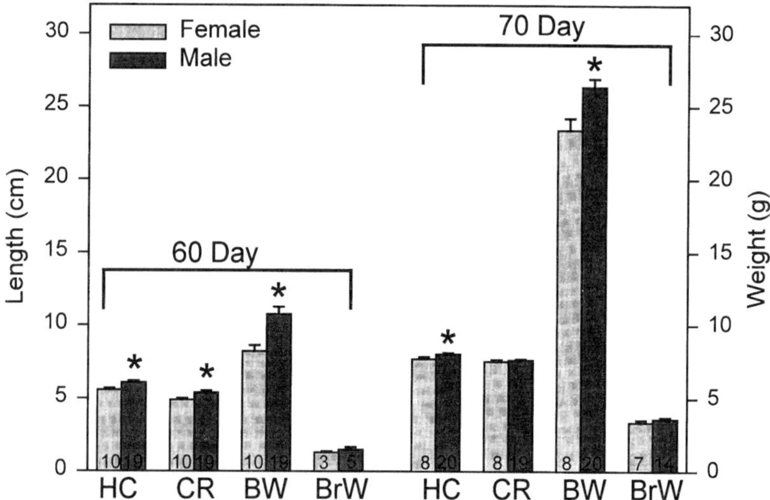

FIGURE 2. Head circumference (HC), crown-rump length (CR), body weight (BW), and brain weight (Br.W) of day-60 and day-70 female and male rhesus macaque fetuses. Data are presented as means *(bars)* ± SEM *(vertical lines)*. Number of animals per group is indicated at the base of each bar. ★ $p < 0.05$, males versus females.

exposed animals.[14] Also in day 60 fetuses, the distribution and staining intensity of the various TH cell types were similar in control and cocaine-treated fetuses. Due to difficulties in quantifying the immunocytochemical data in fetal tissues, all quantifications were performed on the *in situ* hybridization materials. The major finding was that TH mRNA levels were significantly reduced in the SN/VTA area as a consequence of cocaine exposure from day 20 to day 60 of gestation. Overall, the density of TH mRNA was significantly reduced in the cocaine-treated group as compared to controls ($p < 0.05$). Moreover, the area covered by grains (indicative of TH mRNA) in the midbrain was significantly reduced in cocaine-treated fetal brains as compared to saline-treated controls (TABLE 1; $p < 0.01$). Also, the number of cells expressing TH mRNA per unit area was significantly reduced in the cocaine-treated animals; however, the total number of cells in the SN/VTA area was not different (FIG. 3).

Distribution of TH-Containing Fibers in the Rostral Forebrain. The TH fiber distribution to the rostral forebrain was investigated in day-60 and day-70 fetuses. In day-60 animals, scattered TH-IR fibers were observed in the intermediate layer of the frontal cortex, while dense fiber stain was found in the striatal area. Within the striatum the TH-IR fibers appeared slightly patchy. In day-70 fetuses the TH-IR fiber distribution to the frontal cortex was greater than that observed at day 60. At this stage in development, TH-IR fibers were found primarily in the intermediate layer of the frontal cortex, but were also observed traversing the subplate and reaching the cortical plate. Within the striatum, the distribution of TH-IR fibers was clearly patchy. Our preliminary observations indicate that the overall TH fiber distribution was similar in control and cocaine-exposed day-60 and day-70 fetuses; however, the effects of cocaine on the TH fiber input to the rostral forebrain have not yet been evaluated.

EFFECTS OF COCAINE ON DOPAMINE RECEPTORS

Expression of mRNAs Encoding the Dopamine Transporter and the D_1, D_2, and D_5 Dopamine Receptor Subtypes

We found that in day-60 cocaine-treated fetal monkeys TH mRNA expression is significantly reduced in the SN/VTA as compared to that in saline-treated controls.[14] Since TH is the rate-limiting enzyme in dopamine synthesis, we hypothesized that the rate of dopamine synthesis and perhaps dopamine release is reduced as a result of chronic gestational cocaine exposure in the fetal monkey.[14] It is known that reduction in dopamine input to the rostral forebrain may lead to dopamine receptor supersensitivity and per-

TABLE 1. Expression of TH mRNA in the Fetal Midbrain[a]

		Areas from Rostral to Caudal (mm^2)			
Group	Animals (*n*)	I	II	III	IV
Control	4	2.96 ± 0.20	3.42 ± 0.23	3.70 ± 0.40	3.75 ± 0.43
Cocaine	4	2.25 ± 0.08*	2.56 ± 0.33*	2.76 ± 0.35*	2.82 ± 0.36*

Areas covered by silver grains in four matched sections from rostral (I) to caudal (IV) regions of the midbrain in control and cocaine-treated day-60 fetal monkeys were quantified. This analysis revealed that the area covered by grains, indicative of TH mRNA, was significantly reduced in cocaine-treated animals. I, II, III, IV: Areas through the midbrain from rostral (I) to caudal (IV) approximately 10–15 sections apart (150–225 μm). Numbers are expressed as mean ± SEM.

*$p < 0.01$ ANOVA for repeated measures.

[a]Adapted from Rønnekleiv and Naylor, 1995.

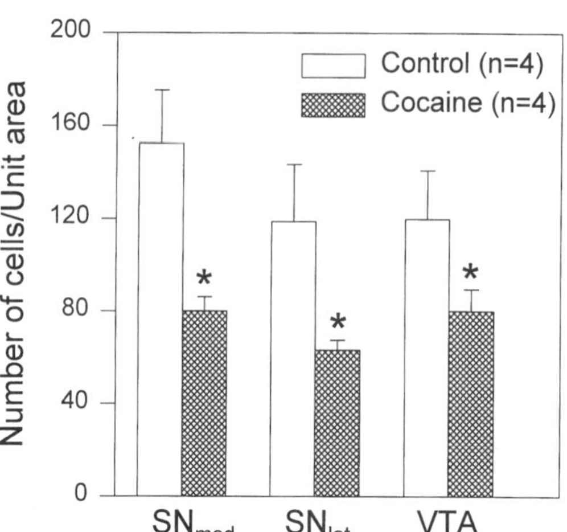

FIGURE 3. Number of cells expressing TH mRNA in the ventral tegmental area (VTA), medial substantia nigra (SN_{med}), and lateral SN (SN_{lat}) of controls and cocaine-exposed fetuses. Unit area is $(150\ \mu m)^2$. ★ $p < 0.05$ cocaine versus control. Adapted from Ronnekleiv and Naylor.[14]

haps receptor proliferation.[42] Therefore, we studied the development of dopamine receptor subtypes and of the dopamine transporter in day-45 and day-60 fetal monkey brains and explored the effects of *in utero* cocaine exposure on this development using nuclease protection assay analysis.[15] Each brain was dissected into three (day 45) or six (day 60) regions, and total RNAs from these tissues were isolated as described previously.[15,43]

Dopamine Receptors and Dopamine Transporter mRNAs. Dopamine transporter mRNA was expressed, albeit in low quantities, in day-45 fetal monkey brain, and D_1 and D_2 receptor subtype mRNAs were also present; however, D_5 receptor mRNA was not detected.[15] Moreover, there appeared to be no effects of cocaine at this stage of gestation. In day-60 fetal brains the concentration of D_1 and D_2 receptor subtype mRNAs and dopamine transporter mRNA was much greater than day-45 levels, and D_5 receptor mRNA was also expressed. The highest concentration of dopamine D_1 receptor mRNA was found in the frontal cortex/striatal area and in the rostral temporal lobe (Fig. 4A). The other brain areas had low levels of dopamine D_1 receptor mRNA (Fig. 4A). Dopamine D_2 receptor mRNA was found in relatively high levels in the rostral forebrain regions, the diencephalon and the midbrain (Fig. 4B). Dopamine D_5 receptor mRNA was lightly expressed in the six different brain areas, whereas dopamine transporter mRNA was found in the midbrain only.[15]

Fetal monkeys exposed to cocaine during days 20–60 of gestation exhibited a significant increase in the concentration of D_1 ($p < 0.003$) and D_2 ($p < 0.03$) receptor mRNA subtypes in the rostral brain area, which contains the frontal cortex and striatum (Fig. 4A and B). Cocaine had no significant effect on dopamine D_1 and D_2 receptor mRNA subtypes in any other brain regions. Dopamine transporter mRNA was not significantly altered in brain tissues from cocaine-treated fetal monkeys as compared to controls.

Dopamine Receptor Binding Densities in Fetal Brain

Our findings that fetal exposure to cocaine causes increased expression of dopamine D_1 and D_2 receptor mRNAs in the fetal forebrain would suggest that re-

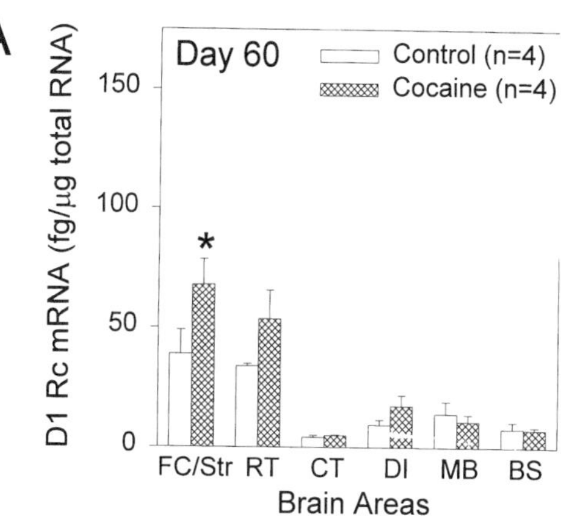

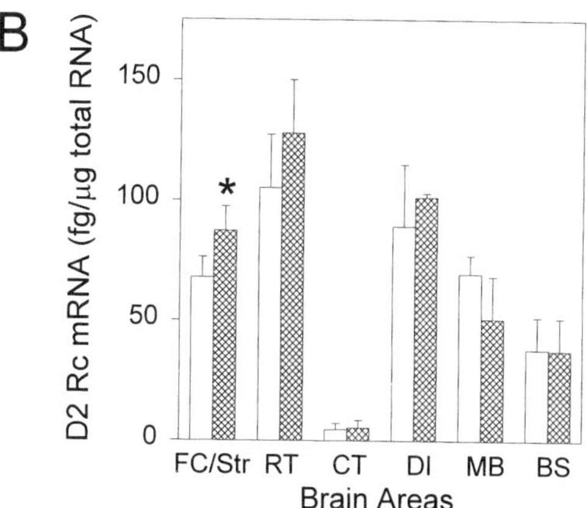

FIGURE 4. Distribution and quantitative analysis of dopamine D_1 **(A)** and D_2 **(B)** receptor mRNA subtypes in brain tissue obtained from saline-treated controls and cocaine-treated fetal monkeys. mRNA was quantified using ribonuclease protection assay analysis. The content of both D_1 and D_2 receptor mRNA subtypes was significantly increased in the frontal cortex/striatal area (FC/Str) in cocaine-exposed animals. $^*p < 0.003$ **(A)** and 0.03 **(B)**. RT = rostral part of the temporal lobe; CT = caudal part of the temporal lobe; DI = diencephalon; MB = midbrain; BS = brainstem. Adapted from Choi and Ronnekleiv.[15]

ceptor protein was also affected by cocaine. Therefore, we measured the effects of *in utero* cocaine on receptor binding densities in the fetal brain. The animals were treated as just described except that cocaine treatment was continued until day 70 of gestation to assure that dopamine receptor protein was present in large enough quantities to be measured. All fetuses used in this study were male. We used [^{3}H]SCH23390 (2 nM, 71.3 Ci/mmol, NEN, Boston, Massachusetts), which binds D_1 and D_5 receptors,[44] and [^{3}H]spiperone (0.6 nM, 96 Ci/mmol, Amersham, Arlington Heights, Illinois), which at this low concentration binds specifically D_2, D_3, and D_4 receptors,[44,45] to characterize cocaine-induced changes. Receptor autoradiography was performed as previously described.[46]

Distribution of D_1- and D_2-Like Receptors in Day-70 Fetal Monkey Brain. Dense D_1-like dopamine receptor binding was found in the striatum, nucleus accumbens, globus pallidus, and SN (TABLE 2). Dopamine D_1-like receptor binding was also observed in the cortical plate of the frontal cortex and the habenula (TABLE 2). However, in these regions D_1-like receptor binding density was low. Within the striatum, D_1-like receptor binding had a characteristic patchy appearance with the highest densities in the striosomes (FIG. 5). The overall distribution and density of D_2-like receptor binding sites were similar to those described for D_1-like receptors, except that D_2-like receptor binding was not found in the habenula or the SN at this stage of gestation (TABLES 2 and 3).

Effect of Cocaine on D_1-Like and D_2-Like Dopamine Receptor Binding Site Density. The distribution of dopamine D_1-like and D_2-like binding sites was similar in control and cocaine-treated fetal brains. However, fetal monkeys exposed to cocaine from day 22 to day 70 of gestation exhibited a significant increase in the density of D_1-like receptor binding sites in the striatum ($p < 0.05$) and the SN ($p < 0.01$), with an accompanying increase in the density of D_2-like receptor binding sites in the striatum ($p < 0.01$), compared to that in controls (TABLES 2 and 3 and FIG. 5).

Our current findings suggest that D_1- and D_2-like receptors are expressed in neurons receiving dopamine input, whereas D_2-like autoreceptors cannot be detected in dopamine neurons of the day-70 fetal monkey midbrain. Cocaine treatment of moth-

TABLE 2. Binding Densities (nCi/g) of Dopamine D_1-Like Receptors in Day 70 Fetal Monkey Brains

	D_1-Like	
Brain Area	Control	Cocaine
Frontal cortex	356.67 ± 152.15	424.67 ± 88.97
Nucleus accumbens	1,334.33 ± 364.33	1,458.33 ± 406.43
Striatum	1,864.70 ± 181.09	2,558.30 ± 266.47*
Globus pallidus	1,268.67 ± 189.44	1,304.67 ± 335.88
Habenula	281.67 ± 54.27	357.67 ± 154.61
Substantia nigra	3,457.07 ± 204.15	4,210.74 ± 237.06**

Ligand binding of dopamine D_1-like receptors was determined in day-70 control ($n = 3$) and cocaine-treated ($n = 3$) fetuses. This analysis revealed that gestational cocaine exposure caused increased binding density of D_1 receptors in the striatum and the substantia nigra. Values are expressed as mean ± SEM.

*,**$p < 0.05$, and 0.01, respectively, control group versus cocaine group. Adapted from Fang and Rønnekleiv, 1997.

TABLE 3. Binding Densities (nCi/g) of Dopamine D_2-Like Receptors in Day-70 Fetal Monkey Brains[a]

	D2-Like	
Brain Area	Control	Cocaine
Frontal cortex	546.67 ± 198.65	494.33 ± 191.98
Nucleus accumbens	2,104.00 ± 174.63	2,054.33 ± 313.35
Striatum	2,257.18 ± 96.78	3,085.66 ± 150.95[a]
Globus pallidus	1,546.33 ± 173.10	1,548.00 ± 348.93
Habenula	ND	ND
Substantia nigra	ND	ND

Ligand binding of dopamine D_2-like receptors was determined in day-70 control ($n = 3$) and cocaine-treated ($n = 3$) fetuses. This analysis revealed that gestational cocaine exposure caused increased binding sites of dopamine D_2-like receptors in the striatum. ND = nondetectable. Values are expressed as mean ± SEM.

**$p < 0.01$ control group versus cocaine group.

[a]Adapted from Fang and Rønnekleiv, 1997.

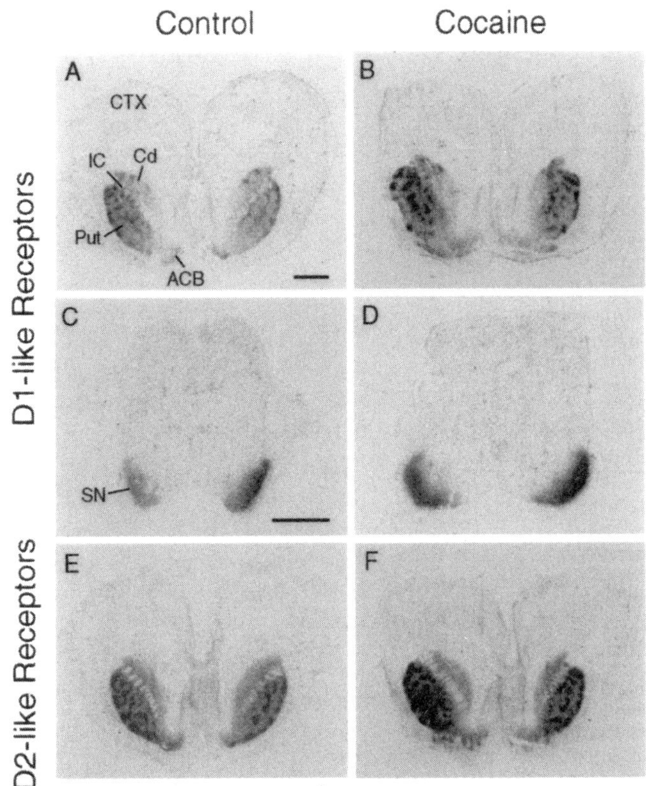

FIGURE 5. Computer images of autoradiograms illustrating the binding sites of [^{3}H]SCH23390 to dopamine D_1-like receptors in fetal monkey striatum (**A**, **B**) and substantia nigra (**C**, **D**), and [^{3}H]spiperone to dopamine D_2-like receptors in the fetal striatum (**E**, **F**). Each shade represents a range of receptor binding densities; the darker the shade, the higher the density. The *left panel* is from a representative saline-treated control and the *right panel* from a cocaine-treated animal at day 70 of gestation. Cocaine treatment increased the densities of D_1-like receptors in the striatum (**B** *vs* **A**) and substantia nigra (**D** *vs* **C**), and D_2-like receptors in the striatum (**F** *vs* **E**). Abbreviations: ACB = nucleus accumbens; Cd = the caudate; CTX = the frontal cortex; IC = internal capsule; Put = putamen; SN = the substantia nigra. Scale bars: 2 mm.

ers from days 22 to 70 of pregnancy resulted in increased expression of both dopamine D_1- and D_2-like receptors in the striatum and D_1-like receptors in the SN of their fetuses.

EFFECTS OF COCAINE ON DYNORPHIN AND ENKEPHALIN GENE EXPRESSION

Dynorphin- and enkephalin-containing neurons in the striatum express dopamine D_1 and D_2 receptors and are regulated by dopaminergic input.[18,27] Based on our findings that dopamine D_1 and D_2 receptor binding densities are increased in the striatal area as a result of cocaine exposure, we examined the effects of chronic cocaine treat-

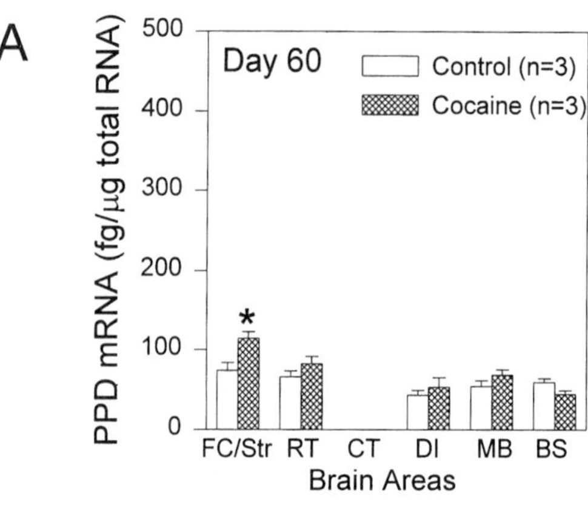

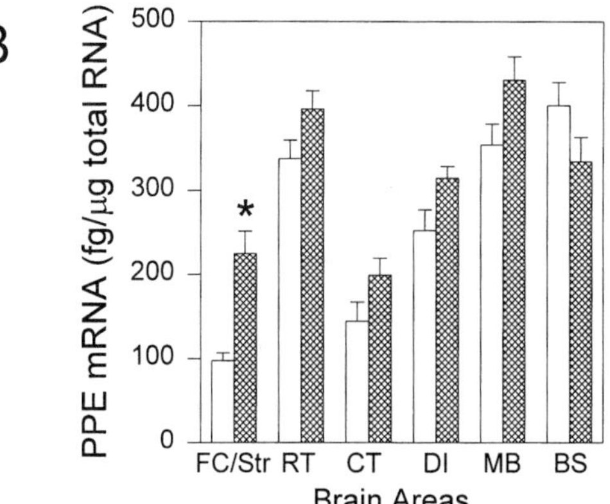

FIGURE 6. Distribution and quantitative analysis of **(A)** preprodynorphin (PPD) and **(B)** preproenkephalin (PPE) mRNA in brain tissue obtained from control and cocaine-treated fetal monkeys at day 60 of gestation. The mRNA was quantified using ribonuclease protection assay analysis. The content of both PPD and PPE mRNA was significantly increased in the frontal cortex/striatal area (FC/Str) in cocaine-exposed animals. $*p < 0.05$. RT = rostral part of the temporal lobe; CT = caudal part of the temporal lobe; DI = diencephalon; MB = midbrain; BS = brainstem. Adapted from Chai *et al.*[16]

ment of pregnant monkeys on the development of enkephalin and dynorphin mRNAs in their fetuses. We used a sensitive ribonuclease protection assay to quantify the levels of preprodynorphin (PPD) and preproenkephalin (PPE) mRNAs in the fetal monkey brain as described previously.[16]

Distribution of PPD and PPE mRNA. In day-60 control fetuses, all brain regions showed approximately equal amounts of PPD mRNA, with the exception of the caudal temporal lobe, where PPD mRNA was not found (FIG. 6A). Gene expression for PPE was higher than that for PPD in all brain regions; in particular, PPE mRNA was highly expressed in the rostral temporal lobe, the midbrain, and the brainstem (FIG. 6). PPE mRNA was moderately expressed in the diencephalon and was found in lower concentrations in the frontal cortex/striatal area (FIG. 6B). On day 70, the highest concentrations of PPD mRNA were found in the striatum, the diencephalon, and the midbrain, whereas PPD mRNA was not expressed in the frontal cortex (FIG. 7). PPE mRNA was found in high concentrations in the rostral temporal lobe, the diencephalon, and the midbrain (FIG. 7B). Relatively high concentrations were found in the frontal cortex and the striatum (FIG. 7B).

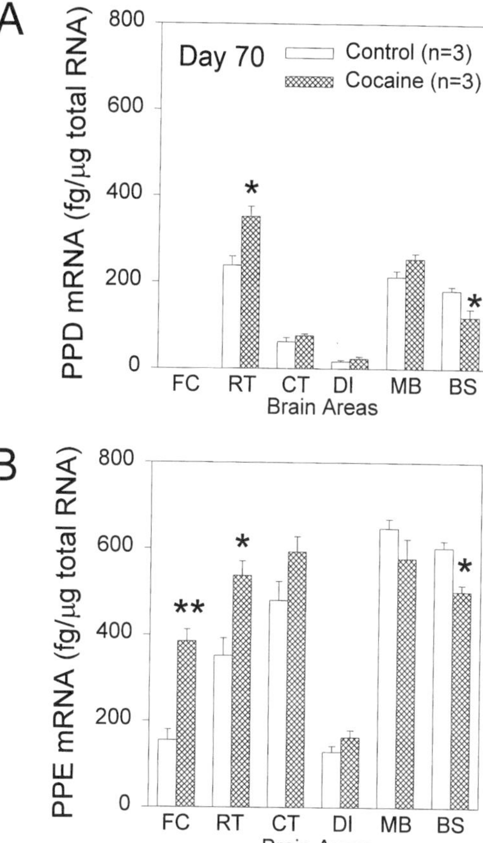

FIGURE 7. Distribution and quantitative analysis of PPD **(A)** and PPE **(B)** mRNA in brain tissue obtained from control and cocaine-treated fetal monkeys at day 70 of gestation. The mRNA was quantified using ribonuclease protection assay analysis. The content of PPD mRNA was significantly increased in the striatal area (ST) and significantly decreased in the midbrain (MB) of cocaine-exposed fetuses. PPE mRNA was significantly increased in both the frontal cortex (FC) and the ST, and significantly decreased in the MB as a result of cocaine exposure. *$p < 0.05$; **$p < 0.005$. Adapted from Chai *et al.*[16]

Effects of Cocaine on PPD and PPE mRNAs. On day 60 of gestation, chronic cocaine treatment of the mother caused a significant increase in the mRNA expression of both PPD ($p < 0.05$) and PPE ($p < 0.05$) in the frontal cortex/striatal area of the fetus (FIG. 6). On day 70, fetal PPD mRNA was significantly increased in the striatum ($p < 0.05$) and significantly decreased in the midbrain ($p < 0.05$) of cocaine-treated animals (FIG. 7A). In day-70 fetuses, cocaine treatment significantly increased PPE gene expression in both the developing frontal cortex ($p < 0.005$) and the striatal area ($p < 0.05$) as compared to that in saline-treated fetuses (FIG. 7B). Similar to PPD mRNA, PPE mRNA levels declined significantly in the midbrain region after cocaine ($p < 0.05$) (FIG. 7B).

Anatomic Distribution of PPD and PPE in the Rostral Forebrain. We used *in situ* hybridization to determine the cellular distribution of PPD and PPE mRNA in the rostral forebrain of day-70 fetuses and evaluated the effects of cocaine exposure during gestation. These experiments indicated that PPE mRNA is widely expressed in several forebrain regions such as the prelimbic area of the frontal cortex, the medial septum, the olfactory bulbs, the striatum, and the nucleus accumbens (ACB). By contrast, PPD mRNA is only expressed in the striatum and the nucleus accumbens at this stage in gestation. A similar distribution is also observed in cocaine-treated fetuses; however, our preliminary analysis suggests that PPE and PPD mRNA expression is increased in the striatal area of cocaine-exposed animals, thus supporting the ribonuclease protection assay findings.

DISCUSSION

Using a fetal monkey model we found that the midbrain of monkeys exposed to cocaine early in gestation exhibits reduced expression of TH, the rate-limiting enzyme in dopamine synthesis. In the same animal model, dopamine D_1 and D_2 receptor-subtype mRNAs are elevated in the rostral forebrain regions as well as in dopamine D_1 and D_2 receptor binding sites in cocaine-exposed fetuses. *In utero* cocaine exposure from day 20 to day 60 of gestation also significantly increased the mRNA concentrations of the opioid peptides PPD and PPE in the rostral forebrain region. By day 70 of gestation, PPD mRNA expression increased in the striatal area and decreased in the midbrain of cocaine-exposed subjects. In comparison, PPE mRNA expression on day 70 increased in both the frontal cortex and the striatum and declined in the midbrain in fetuses from cocaine-treated mothers.

In these studies we evaluated the effects of cocaine on the expression of TH, dopamine receptor subtypes, dopamine transporter, and opioids at days 40/45 to days 60 and 70 of gestation. In day-40/45 fetal monkeys, expression of TH and dopamine receptors appeared to be the same in the two treatment groups. We attribute these findings to the immaturity of the dopamine transporter system in day-40/45 fetal monkeys. Because fetal monkey dopamine transporter mRNA expression is very low in day-45 animals and significantly increased in day-60 animals, we hypothesize that the dopamine transporter is not yet functional by days 40–45. Therefore, cocaine, which binds to the dopamine transporter, is unable to affect the dopamine neurocircuitry at this early stage in gestation.[14]

In contrast, by day 60 of gestation, TH mRNA levels in the substantia nigra-ventral tegmental area were significantly reduced in cocaine-treated fetal monkeys.[14] Because TH is the rate-limiting enzyme in dopamine synthesis,[41] we hypothesize that the reduction in TH mRNA is a direct result of cocaine binding to functional dopamine transporter binding sites causing a reduction in dopamine synthesis.[14] As predicted from this model, dopamine D_1 and D_2 receptor subtype mRNAs increase in the rostral forebrain after cocaine treatment. In addition, we found that the density of dopamine D_1 and D_2 receptors is increased in the fetal striatum after *in utero* cocaine exposure from day 20 to day 70 of gestation. The increase in receptor binding was not due to an increased number of striatal cells, because cell density was not significantly different in the two fetal groups. Receptor mRNA and protein are apparently both impacted by cocaine treatment and show covariation.[15,46]

We also found that [^{3}H]SCH23390 binding to D_1-like receptors was increased in the SN of cocaine-treated fetuses. Low levels of dopamine D_1 receptor mRNA are present in the midbrain of day-60 monkey fetuses but appear not to be influenced by cocaine exposure.[15] The D_1 receptor mRNA measured in the midbrain is most likely located in areas other than the SN.[15,43] The most parsimonious explanation for the upregulation of dopamine D_1 receptor binding sites in the substantia nigra is that it is a consequence of cocaine-induced alterations in dopamine D_1 receptors located on striatonigral nerve terminals. Therefore, D_1 receptor mRNA and receptor protein are increased in dopamine target neurons in the striatal area, and receptor protein is also increased in their terminals in the SN following cocaine treatment. The increased densities of D_1 receptors on GABA terminals could act to inhibit the cellular activity of dopamine neurons via the increase in GABA release.[25] Consistent with this interpretation is our observation that the level of TH mRNA is significantly decreased in the SN/VTA area of fetuses exposed to cocaine.[14] In the adult, it is known that reduced stimulation of dopamine receptors as a result of lesions or neuroleptic drug treatment leads to receptor supersensitivity accompanied by receptor upregulation in the brain.[42] Also in the developing brain, reduction of dopaminergic input to the rostral forebrain region results in dopamine receptor supersensitivity, but often without changes in the number of dopamine receptors.[42] It is apparent that a very complex, age-dependent interaction between dopamine and the many dopamine receptor subtypes participates in the regulation of dopamine homeostasis.[42,44,47]

To our knowledge, no other studies have examined the effects of chronic cocaine exposure on dopamine receptors in fetal brain. However, a number of studies have examined the effects of *in utero* cocaine exposure on rat and rabbit dopamine receptor mRNAs and binding sites at various postnatal developmental stages after cocaine withdrawal late in gestation.[7,13,48–50] These studies reported inconsistent results with either a decrease, no change, or an increase in the expression of D_1 and D_2 receptor mRNAs and ligand binding to the respective receptors.[13,48–50] These varied results may be due to methodologic differences between studies. However, the ability to dopamine to stimulate the binding of [^{35}S]GTPyS to G proteins in the striatum of *in utero* cocaine-exposed rabbits is reduced at 10, 50, and 100 days postnatally,[50] suggesting that prenatal cocaine may have long-term effects on dopaminergic functions. In addition, adult male monkeys that received a similar cocaine-treatment regimen as our pregnant monkeys were found to exhibit decreased D_1, but not D_2 receptor binding sites in the caudate nucleus when measured 2 weeks after the last cocaine injection.[51] Cocaine treatment apparently has different effects in the adult versus fetal brain and that withdrawal from cocaine may induce compensatory alterations of dopamine neural transmission, which has been found in adult animals.[52]

Chronic prenatal cocaine treatment increased PPD gene expression in the rostral forebrain region of day-60 and day-70 fetal monkeys. These results agree with earlier findings that chronic cocaine treatment increases PPD mRNA expression and peptide levels in the striatal region in adult animals.[35–38] Elevation in PPD mRNA and peptide expression following chronic cocaine treatment is probably mediated by dopamine D_1 receptors, because PPD gene expression in the striatum appears to be regulated primarily by D_1 receptors through activation of G_S and adenylyl cyclase.[18,29,35] The D_1 receptor activation of adenylyl cyclase causes phosphorylation of cAMP response elements (CREs) binding proteins (CREB) which bind to CREs in the PPD promotor and stimulate PPD synthesis.[29] Consistent with these observations, we found that dopamine D_1 receptor mRNA and binding sites in the fetal monkey increased significantly in the striatal area after chronic cocaine treatment. These data indicate that cocaine exposure upregulates dopamine receptors in the fetus. Collectively, these observations suggest that PPD gene expression in the macaque fetus is increased due to cocaine-induced activation of the D_1-receptor/adenylylcyclase/protein kinase A (PKA) cascade. However, the specific mechanism by which PPD gene expression is regulated in cocaine-exposed fetal primates remains to be elucidated.

Our findings that PPE mRNA levels increase significantly in the rostral forebrain of day-60 and day-70 cocaine-exposed fetal monkeys appears to be contradictory to findings in adult animals. Most reports suggest that cocaine treatment causes increased PPD mRNA levels, but has no effect on the expression of enkephalin in adult rats.[35,53] However, adult rats that have variable free access to cocaine self-administration for 24 hours exhibit increased levels of both PPD and PPE mRNA in the nucleus accumbens,[36] suggesting that these peptides covary in response to certain cocaine treatment paradigms.

The mechanism through which PPE gene expression is affected by cocaine *in utero* is not known. Enkephalin-containing neurons are known to express dopamine D_2 receptors.[18,54] Thus, lesions of dopamine input to the striatal area in rodents and primates are associated with elevated PPE mRNA levels.[18,26,33,34,55] Similarly, lesions of midbrain dopamine neurons or depletion of dopamine by reserpine results in increases in D_2 receptor binding and mRNA levels in the striatal area.[55–57] Therefore, our results showing increased PPE mRNA coupled with our findings that D_2 receptor mRNA and binding increase in the striatal area suggest that dopamine input to the striatal area is reduced in cocaine-exposed fetal monkeys. The increased expression of dopamine D_2 receptors, which inhibits adenylyl cyclase,[21] concurrent with increased PPE gene expression suggests that the D_2 receptor is uncoupled from its effector system in the rostral forebrain of the fetal primate. In this respect, chronic cocaine treatment decreases G_i and G_o in the nucleus accumbens of the adult rat.[58]

Enkephalin neurons in the striatum are also regulated by dopamine D_1 receptors. Dopamine D_1- and D_2-receptor agonist treatment increases and decreases the levels of PPE mRNA, respectively, presumably through activation (D_1) and inhibition (D_2) of adenylyl cyclase and PKA. These data suggest that D_1 and D_2 receptor activation differentially regulates striatal PPE mRNA levels.[54,59] Similar to the PPD gene, promoter regions of the PPE gene contain CREs, and activation of the adenylyl cyclase/PKA pathway leads to phosphorylation of CREB, which then induces PPE transcription.[60] Prolonged cocaine treatment increases levels of adenylyl cyclase and PKA in the rat nucleus accumbens, and it has been postulated that such adaptations may be partly responsible for drug reinforcement and addiction.[58] Therefore, we hypothesize that in the fetal monkey, chronic, intermittent exposure to cocaine upregulates adenylyl cyclase/PKA in the frontal cortex and striatal neurons, which in turn stimulate PPE (and PPD) synthesis. However, we do not know the cellular mechanism of interaction between the upregulated dopamine D_1 and D_2 receptors in the fetal forebrain and the increased PPD and PPE gene expression.

We have observed that the body weight, crown-rump length, head circumference, and brain weight remained unchanged after cocaine exposure in fetal monkeys. Therefore, cocaine exposure from day 20 to day 70 of gestation apparently does not compromise fetal growth. An interesting observation, however, is that the rhesus macaque male is significantly heavier than the age-matched female fetus already by day 60 of gestation.

In conclusion, we have found that cocaine exposure during early gestation in the nonhuman primate alters several components of the midbrain-rostral forebrain dopamine neurocircuitry. Moreover, these changes occur during a critical period of development, and we have preliminary evidence that some of the effects of cocaine may be long lasting. The mechanisms through which these changes occur in the fetal brain are currently unknown. However, alterations in dopamine circuitry that mediate motivation and reward, as well as motor control, provide further evidence for profound consequences of *in utero* cocaine exposure on the developing fetal monkey brain. Future studies should examine in more detail the long-term effects of gestational cocaine and potential functional consequences.

REFERENCES

1. Chasnoff, I.J., D.R. Griffith, S. MacGregor, K. Drikes & K.A. Burns. 1989. Temporal patterns of cocaine use in pregnancy. JAMA **261:** 1741–1744.
2. Struthers, J.M. & R.L. Hansen. 1992. Visual recognition memory in drug-exposed infants. Dev. Behav. Pediatr. **13:** 108–111.
3. Azuma, S.D. & I.J. Chasnoff. 1993. Outcome of children prenatally exposed to cocaine and other drugs: A path analysis of three-year data. Pediatrics **92:** 396–402.

4. FRIES, M.H., J.A. KULLER, M.E. NORTON, J. YANKOWITZ, J. KOBORI, W.V. GOOD, D. FERRIERO, V. COX, S.S. DONLIN & M. GOLABI. 1993. Facial features of infants exposed prenatally to cocaine. Teratology **48:** 413–420.
5. MAYES, L.C., M.H. BORNSTEIN, K. CHAWARSKA & R.H. GRANGER. 1995. Information processing and developmental assessment in 3-month-old infants exposed prenatally to cocaine. Pediatrics **95:** 539–545.
6. GRESSENS, P., B.E. KOSOFSKY & P. EVRARD. 1992. Cocaine-induced disturbances of corticogenesis in the developing murine brain. Neurosci. Lett. **140:** 113–116.
7. DOW-EDWARDS, D.L., L.A. FREED & T. FICO. 1990. Structural and functional effects of prenatal cocaine exposure in adult rat brain. Dev. Brain Res. **57:** 263–268.
8. PERIS, J., M. COLEMAN-HARDEE & W.J. MILLARD. 1992. Cocaine *in utero* enhances the behavioral response to cocaine in adult rats. Pharmacol. Biochem. Behav. **42:** 509–515.
9. HEYSER, C.J., W.-J. CHEN, J. MILLER, N.E. SPEAR & L.P. SPEAR. 1990. Prenatal cocaine exposure induces deficits in Pavlovian conditioning and sensory preconditioning among infant rat pups. Behav. Neurosci. **104:** 955–963.
10. HEYSER, C.J., N.E. SPEAR & L.P. SPEAR. 1992. Effects of prenatal exposure to cocaine on conditional discrimination learning in adult rats. Behav. Neurosci. **106:** 837–845.
11. WANG, L. & D.K. PITTS. 1994. Perinatal cocaine exposure decreases the number of spontaneously active midbrain dopamine neurons in neonatal rats. Synapse **17:** 275–277.
12. KELLER, R.W., JR., I.M. MAISONNEUVE, D.M. NUCCIO, J.N. CARLSON & S.D. GLICK. 1994. Effects of prenatal cocaine exposure on the nigrostriatal dopamine system: An *in vivo* microdialysis study in the rat. Brain Res. **643:** 266–274.
13. LESLIE, C.A., M.W. ROBERTSON, A.B. JUNG, J. LIEBERMANN & J.P. BENNETT, JR. 1994. Effects of prenatal cocaine exposure upon postnatal development of neostriatal dopaminergic function. Synapse **17:** 210–215.
14. RØNNEKLEIV, O.K. & B.R. NAYLOR. 1995. Chronic cocaine exposure in the fetal rhesus monkey: Consequences for early development of dopamine neurons. J. Neurosci. **15:** 7330–7343.
15. CHOI, W.S. & O.K. RÖNNEKLEIV. 1996. Effects of *in utero* cocaine exposure on the expression of mRNAs encoding the dopamine transporter and the D1, D2 and D5 dopamine receptor subtypes in fetal rhesus monkey. Dev. Brain Res. **96:** 249–260.
16. CHAI, L., W.S. CHOI & O.K. RÖNNEKLEIV. 1997. Matenal cocaine treatment alters dynorphin and enkephalin mRNA expression in brains of fetal rhesus macaques. J. Neurosci. **17:** 1112–1121.
17. MOAL, L.M. & H. SIMON. 1991. Mesocorticolimbic dopaminergic network: Functional and regulatory roles. Physiol. Rev. **71:** 155–233.
18. GERFEN, C.R. & C.J. WILSON. 1996. The basal ganglia. *In* Handbook of Chemical Neuroanatomy, Vol. 12: Integrated systems of the CNS, Part III. L.W. Swanson, A. Björklund & T. Hökfelt, Eds.: 371–468. Elsevier Science, B.V.
19. KUHAR, M.J., M.C. RITZ & J.W. BOJA. 1991. The dopamine hypothesis of the reinforcing properties of cocaine. Trends Neurosci. **14:** 299–302.
20. KOOB, G.F. 1992. Drugs of abuse: Anatomy, pharmacology and function of reward pathways. Trends Pharmacol. Sci. **13:** 177–184.
21. CIVELLI, O., J.R. BUNZOW & D.K. GRANDY. 1993. Molecular diversity of the dopamine receptors. Annu. Rev. Pharmacol. Toxicol. **33:** 281–307.
22. MANSOUR, A., J.H. MEADOR-WOODRUFF, Q.-Y. ZHOU, O. CIVELLI, H. AKIL & S.J. WATSON. 1991. A comparison of D_1 receptor binding and mRNA in rat brain using receptor autoradiographic and *in situ* hybridization techniques. Neuroscience **45:** 359–371.
23. KALIVAS, P.W. 1993. Neurotransmitter regulation of dopamine neurons in the ventral tegmental area. Brain Res. Rev. **18:** 75–113.
24. LACEY, M.G., N.B. MERCURI & R.A. NORTH. 1987. Dopamine acts on D2 receptors to increase potassium conductance in neurones of the rat substantia nigra zona compacta. J. Physiol. (Lond.) **392:** 397–416.
25. CAMERON, D.L. & J.T. WILLIAMS. 1993. Dopamine D1 receptors facilitate transmitter release. Nature **366:** 344–347.
26. LI, S.J., S.P. SIVAM, J.F. MCGINTY, H.K. JIANG, J. DOUGLASS, L. CALAVETTA & J.S. HONG.

1988. Regulation of the metabolism of striatal dynorphin by the dopaminergic system. J. Pharm. Exp. Ther. **246:** 403–408.

27. SURMEIER, D.J., J. EBERWINE, C.J. WILSON, Y. CAO, A. STEFANI & S.T. KITAI. 1992. Dopamine receptor subtypes colocalize in rat striatonigral neurons. Proc. Natl. Acad. Sci. USA **89:** 10178–10182.
28. HYMAN, S.E., C. KONRADI, L. ROBIERSKI, R. COLE, P. SENATUS & D. GREEN. 1994. Pharmacologic regulation of striatal proenkephalin gene expression via transcription factor CREB. Prog. Clin. Biol. Res. **390:** 155–171.
29. COLE, R.L., C. KONRADI, J. DOUGLASS & S.E. HYMAN. 1995. Neuronal adaptation to amphetamine and dopamine: Molecular mechanisms of prodynorphin gene regulation in rat striatum. Neuron **14:** 813–823.
30. NISBET, A.P., O.J.F. FOSTER, A. KINGSBURY, D.J. EVE, S.E. DANIEL, C.D. MARSDEN & A.J. LEES. 1995. Preproenkephalin and preprotachykinin messenger RNA expression in normal human basal ganglia and in Parkinson's disease. Neuroscience **66:** 361–376.
31. RICHFIELD, E.K., K.A. MAGUIRE-ZEISS, C. COX, J. GILMORE & P. VOORN. 1995. Reduced expression of preproenkephalin in striatal neurons from Huntington's disease patients. Ann. Neurol. **37:** 335–343.
32. YOUNG, W.S., III, T.I. BONNER & M.R. BRANN. 1986. Mesencephalic dopamine neurons regulate the expression of neuropeptide mRNAs in the rat forebrain. Proc. Natl. Acad. Sci. USA **83:** 9827–9831.
33. AUGOOD, S.J., P.C. EMSON, I.J. MITCHELL, S. BOYCE, C.E. CLARKE & A.R. CROSSMAN. 1989. Cellular localization of enkephalin gene expression in MPTP-treated cynomolgus monkeys. Mol. Brain Res. **6:** 8592.
34. ASSELIN, M.-C., J. SOGHOMONIAN, P. CÔTÉ & A. PARENT. 1994. Striatal changes in preproenkephalin mRNA levels in parkinsonian monkeys. NeuroReport **5:** 2137–2140.
35. SIVAM, S.P. 1989. Cocaine selectively increases striatonigral dynorphin levels by a dopaminergic mechanism. J. Pharm. Exp. Ther. **250:** 818–824.
36. HURD, Y.L., E.E. BROWN, J.M. FINLAY, H.C. FIBIGER & C.R. GERFEN. 1992. Cocaine self-administration differentially alter mRNA expression of striatal peptides. Mol. Brain Res. **13:** 165–170.
37. DAUNAIS, J.B. & J.F. MCGINTY. 1995. Cocaine binges differentially alter striatal preprodynorphin and zif/268 mRNAs. Mol. Brain Res. **29:** 201–210.
38. SPANGLER, R., E.M. UNTERWALD & M.J. KREEK. 1993. 'Binge' cocaine administration induces a sustained increase of prodynorphin mRNA in rat caudate-putamen. Mol. Brain Res. **19:** 323–327.
39. GRIBNAU, A.A.M. & L.G.M. GEIJSBERTS. 1981. Developmental stages in the rhesus monkey (macaca mulatta). *In* Advances in Anatomy, Embryology and Cell Biology. A. Brodal, W. Hild, J.V. Limborgh, R. Ortmann, J.E. Pauly, T.H. Schiebler & E. Wolff, Eds.: 1–84. Springer-Verlag. New York.
40. LEVITT, P. & P. RAKIC. 1982. The time of genesis, embryonic origin and differentiation of the brain stem monoamine neurons in the Rhesus monkey. Dev. Brain Res. **4:** 35–57.
41. AXELROD, J. 1972. Catecholamines. N. Engl. J. Med. **287:** 237–242.
42. KOSTRZEWA, R.M. 1995. Dopamine receptor supersensitivity. Neurosci. Biobehav. Rev. **19:** 1–17.
43. CHOI, W.S., C.A. MACHIDA & O.K. RÖNNEKLEIV. 1995. Distribution of dopamine D_1, D_2, and D_5 receptor mRNAs in the monkey brain: Ribonuclease protection assay analysis. Mol. Brain Res. **31:** 86–94.
44. SEEMAN, P. & H.H.M. VAN TOL. 1994. Dopamine receptor pharmacology. Trends Pharmacol. Sci. **15:** 264–270.
45. MALMBERG, A., E. JERNING & N. MOHELL. 1996. Critical reevaluation of spiperone and benzamide binding to dopamine D_2 receptors: Evidence for identical binding sites. Eur. J. Pharmacol. **303:** 123–128.
46. FANG, Y., A. JANOWSKY & O.K. RÖNNEKLEIV. 1997. Cocaine exposure in fetal rhesus monkey: Consequences for dopamine D1- and D2-like receptor binding densities. Dev. Brain Res. **104:** 163–174.
47. GRACE, A.A. 1995. The tonic/phasic model for dopamine system regulation: Its relevance for

understanding how stimulant abuse can alter basal ganglia function. Drug Alc. Depend. **37:** 111–129.

48. SCALZO, F.M., S.F. ALI, N.A. FRAMBES & L.P. SPEAR. 1990. Weanling rats exposed prenatally to cocaine exhibit an increase in striatal D2 dopamine binding associated with an increase in ligand affinity. Pharmacol. Biochem. Behav. **37:** 371–373.
49. DE BARTOLOMEIS, A., M.C. AUSTIN, G.A. GOODWIN, L.P. SPEAR, D. PICKAR & J.N. CRAWLEY. 1994. Dopaminergic and peptidergic mRNA levels in juvenile rat brain after prenatal cocaine treatment. Mol. Brain Res. **21:** 321–330.
50. WANG, H., E. RUNYAN, E. YADIN & E. FRIEDMAN. 1995. Prenatal exposure to cocaine selectively reduces D1 dopamine receptor-mediated activation of striatal Gs proteins. J. Pharm. Exp. Ther. **273:** 492–498.
51. FARFEL, G.M., M.S. KLEVEN, W.L. WOOLVERTON, L.S. SEIDEN & B.D. PERRY. 1992. Effects of repeated injections of cocaine on catecholamine receptor binding sites, dopamine transporter binding sites and behavior in rhesus monkey. Brain Res. **578:** 235–243.
52. BONCI, A. & J.T. WILLIAMS. 1996. A common mechanism mediates long-term changes in synaptic transmission after chronic cocaine and morphine. Neuron **16:** 631–639.
53. BRANCH, A.D., E.M. UNTERWALD, S.E. LEE & M.J. KREEK. 1994. Quantitation of preproenkephalin mRNA levels in brain regions from male Fischer rats following chronic cocaine treatment using a recently developed solution hybridization assay. Mol. Brain Res. **14:** 231–238.
54. POLLACK, A.E. & G.F. WOOTEN. 1992. Differential regulation of striatal preproenkephalin mRNA by D_1 and D_2 dopamine receptors. Mol. Brain Res. **12:** 111–119.
55. SOGHOMONIAN, J. 1993. Effects of neonatal 6-hydroxydopamine injections on glutamate decarboxylase, preproenkephalin and dopamine D_2 receptor mRNAs in the adult rat striatum. Brain Res. **621:** 249–259.
56. JABER, M., M.C. FOURNIER & B. BLOCH. 1992. Reserpine treatment stimulates enkephalin and D_2 dopamine receptor gene expression in the rat striatum. Mol. Brain Res. **15:** 189–194.
57. RADJA, F., M. EL MANSARI, J.-J. SOGHOMONIAN, K.M. DEWAR, A. FERRON, T.A. READER & L. DESCARRIES. 1993. Changes of D_1 and D_2 receptors in adult rat neostriatum after neonatal dopamine denervation: Quantitative data from ligand binding, *in situ* hybridization and iontophoresis. Neuroscience **57:** 635–648.
58. SELF, D.W. & E.J. NESTLER. 1995. Molecular mechanisms of drug reinforcement and addiction. Annu. Rev. Neurosci. **18:** 463–495.
59. ANGULO, J.A. 1992. Involvement of dopamine D_1 and D_2 receptors in the regulation of proenkephalin mRNA abundance in the striatum and accumbens of the rat brain. J. Neurochem. **58:** 1104–1109.
60. KONRADI, C., L.A. KOBIERSKI, T.V. NGUYEN, S. HECKERS & S.E. HYMAN. 1993. The cAMP-response-element-binding protein interacts, but Fos protein does not interact, with the proenkephalin enhancer in rat striatum. Proc. Natl. Acad. Sci. USA **90:** 7005–7009.

Nonhuman Primate Model of the Effect of Prenatal Cocaine Exposure on Cerebral Cortical Development

MICHAEL S. LIDOW[a]

Department of Oral and Craniofacial Biological Sciences, University of Maryland, Baltimore, Maryland 21201, USA

ABSTRACT: To investigate the effects of prenatal cocaine exposure on the corticogenesis in primates we developed a monkey model in which pregnant animals received 10 mg/kg cocaine orally twice a day from the 40th to the 102nd day of pregnancy. The animals gave birth at term, and brains of the 2-month and 1.5-year-old infants were examined. Examination revealed the structural abnormalities throughout the cerebral cortex that would be expected from modulation of the nonselectively diffusing circulation-derived monoamines. They include: (1) reduction in the number of cortical cells, which most likely reflects abnormal cell proliferation; (2) inappropriate positioning of cortical neurons, which resulted from alterations in migration of cortical cells; and (3) altered glial morphology. The structural alterations were accompanied by abnormalities in animal temperament reminiscent of those seen in human infants of drug-abusing mothers. As predicted by the morphologic studies, we found that cocaine treatment produced significant changes in the levels of monoamines and their receptors in all laminae of the frontal, parietal, temporal, and occipital regions of the fetal cerebral wall. This indicates that cocaine abuse by pregnant human mothers may affect the global levels of monoamines in the fetal brain and, in doing so, interfere with a broad range of developmental events regulated by these chemicals.

INTRODUCTION

The epidemic of cocaine abuse in women of child-bearing age has led to a remarkable increase in the incidence of fetal cocaine exposure,[1–3] creating a significant interest in understanding the consequences of such exposure for offsprings of drug-abusing mothers. Unfortunately, human studies have provided only limited information because of the inability to stage controlled experiments.[4] Consequently, several animal models of *in utero* cocaine exposure have been introduced aimed at evaluating the effects of cocaine on brain development.[5–12] Among these models, several focused on interference of cocaine with corticogenesis.[7,9,10,12] They revealed two modes of cocaine action. In one mode, exemplified by the rabbit model,[12] low doses of cocaine interfere with certain aspects of cortical development, such as growth of the pyramidal cell dendrites and maturation of the interneuronal GABA synthetic machinery, in the cortical areas rich in dopaminergic innervation. In the second mode, associated with higher dosages of cocaine, the drug produces much more global negative effects on cerebral cortical development. This mode is exemplified by the monkey model of prenatal cocaine exposure which is the subject of the present review.

[a] Address for correspondence: Michael S. Lidow, Ph.D., Department of OCBS, University of Maryland, Baltimore, 5-A-12, HHH, 666 West Baltimore Street, Baltimore, MD 21201. Phone, 410/706-4435; fax, 410/706-0865; e-mail, mlidow@umaryland.edu

PRENATAL COCAINE EXPOSURE ADVERSELY AFFECTS DEVELOPMENT OF THE MONKEY CEREBRAL CORTEX

To investigate the effect of cocaine on cerebral cortical development, pregnant rhesus monkeys were treated with 10 mg/kg cocaine administered orally in fruit treats twice a day, at 8:00 AM and 8:00 PM. This dose of the drug, while higher than the one chosen for the aforementioned rabbit model, still produced blood concentrations of cocaine (peak plasma levels 670–980 mg/ml) that were well within the range characteristic of human abusers.[10] In the original experiment,[10] three pregnant animals received cocaine for 62 days, from the 40th to the 102nd day of pregnancy (E40-E102). This is the period during which cortical neurons destined for cerebral cortical layers VI-II are generated in the ventricular and subventricular proliferative zones of the fetal cerebral wall.[13] The three age-matched pregnant control animals received fruit treats without cocaine. All monkeys were fed High Protein Monkey Chow (Ralston Purina Co.) and were given fresh fruit twice a day, with control animals being on pair-feeding regimen. However, there was no significant reduction in food intake by drug-treated animals. The monkeys were allowed to give birth at term (E165). To eliminate possible differences in rearing, all newborn monkeys were separated from their mothers and raised in the primate nursery. At 2 months after birth (P60), their brains were processed for histologic analysis.

Examination of brain sections of *in utero* cocaine-exposed animals showed significant abnormalities in all areas of the cerebral cortex. In contrast to the cortex of the control monkeys, which showed clear laminar organization (FIG. 1A), the cocaine-exposed animals displayed practically no lamination of this structure (FIG. 1C). The distinct cortical layers were substituted by a homogeneous mass of cells. Only cell-poor layer I remained clearly recognizable. The cocaine affected not only the cortical gray matter, but also the white matter underlying the disorganized cortex. It contained an unusually large number of cells, most with large pale nuclei characteristic of neurons. Furthermore, examination of the distribution of cells labeled by two injections of [^{3}H]thymidine, at E64 and E65, revealed that in contrast to the localization of these cells in a narrow band within the cerebral cortex of control monkeys (FIG. 1B), the labeled cells in drug-exposed animals were dispersed within the cerebral cortex and the white matter (FIG. 1C). The counting of the labeled cells on the slides under 1 mm of cortical surface conducted in the occipital cerebral wall (primary visual area) revealed close to a 35% decrease in the number of such cells in cocaine-exposed animals compared to controls. Finally, whereas in control animals the protoplasmic astrocytes of layer I (stained with antisera directed towards glial fibrillary acidic protein [GFAP] formed multiple processes descending through layers II and III (FIG. 2A), in the cocaine-exposed animals such astrocytes produced very few descending processes (FIG. 2B).

Additional studies in three monkeys that were allowed to survive 1.5 years after birth showed that the cocaine-induced changes in cortical morphology were permanent with no amelioration of abnormalities during postnatal cortical development.

The *in utero* cocaine-exposed monkey infants were also tested to assess their temperament because it was shown that this assessment has value in predicting later personality and cognitive competence.[14] For this purpose, we (in collaboration with the laboratory of Dr. Stephen Suomi at the National Institute of Child Health and Human Development) used the Brazelton National Behavioral Assessment Scale (BNBAS) modified for evaluation of temperament in nonhuman primates.[15] The test, conducted in four cocaine-exposed and six control animals at 2 weeks, 4 weeks, and 2 months after birth, showed that cocaine-exposed monkey infants displayed two distinct behavioral styles neither of which was observed in drug-naive animals. The first style was characterized by poor performance on those items that require attention to stimuli or inhibition of movement. The infants displaying this behavioral style tended to look around

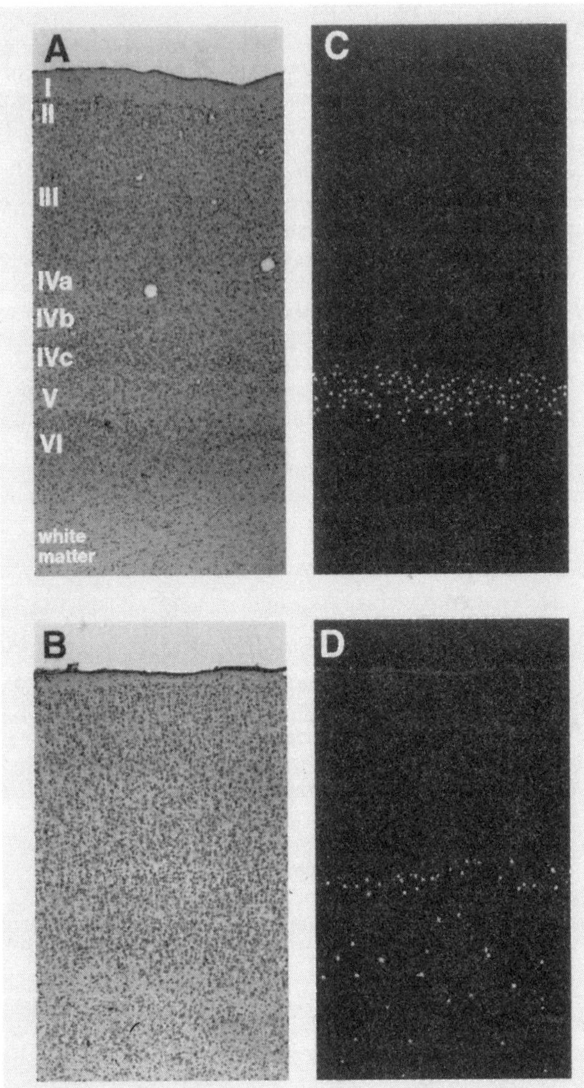

FIGURE 1. Micrographs of the typical primary visual cortex of a 2-month-old cocaine-naive (**A** and **C**) and *in utero* cocaine-exposed (**B** and **D**) rhesus monkeys. (**A** and **B**) Cresyl violet-stained coronal sections. Note that whereas the cortex of a drug-naive monkey has a well-defined laminar structure, the cortex of the drug-exposed animal appears homogeneous with increased number of cells in the white matter. (**C** and **D**) Dark-field images of the same sections. They show the distribution of cells labeled by two [^{3}H]thymidine injections carried out at E64 and E65. Note that in the control monkey all labeled cells occupy a narrow band corresponding to cortical layer V. By contrast, labeled cells are dispersed in the white matter as well as in cortical layers VI and V of the drug-exposed animal. (From Lidow[10] with permission.)

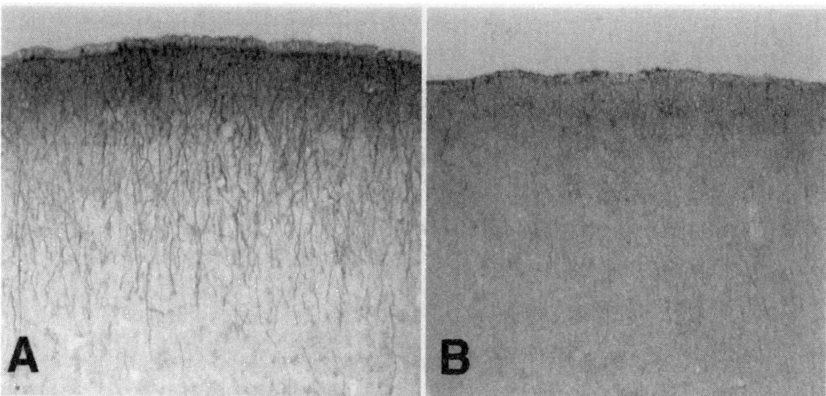

FIGURE 2. Typical distribution of GFAP-specific immunocytochemical staining (antibodies were purchased from DACO, Co.; DAB reaction) in the upper layers of the visual cortex of drug-naive **(A)** and cocaine-exposed **(B)** 2-month-old monkeys. Note that the upper cortical layers of drug-naive cortex **(A)** contain a large number of GFAP-positive glial processes. By contrast, cocaine-exposed cortex shows much fewer GFAP-positive fibers **(B)**. (From Lidow[10] with permission.)

the room rather than watch the experimenter or the visual stimuli being presented. During testing, these animals were overactive, struggled frequently, exhibited agitation, and were difficult to console. The second behavioral style was totally opposite to the first one. The infants exhibiting this style appeared overstimulated by the examination as manifested by their attempts to sleep during the test. We found no improvement in the test performance of both overexcitable and overdepressed infants during the entire 2-month period of testing. All this closely mirrors the excitable and depressed patterns of behavior characteristic of human infants born of cocaine-abusing mothers as reported in published BNBAS assessment studies.[16]

POSSIBLE MECHANISM OF COCAINE INTERFERENCE WITH CEREBRAL CORTICAL DEVELOPMENT

Cocaine can exert its effects on the organism through multiple mechanisms. For example, it blocks Na^+ channels, elevates intracellular free Ca^{2+} as well as binds to σ-opioid, 5-HT_3-serotonergic, and muscarinic cholinergic receptors.[17–21] However, the main action of cocaine is to block uptake of the monoaminergic neurotransmitters dopamine, noradrenaline, and serotonin and thus interfere with the extracellular levels of these chemicals.[22] One source of monoamines in the fetal cerebral wall is specific cortical afferents.[23] As demonstrated in fetal rabbits,[12] low doses of cocaine (due to its ability to concentrate preferentially in the embryonic brain[24]) can interfere with the levels of monoamines released by the local cortical afferents and influence the developmental processes regulated by these afferents in selected (monoamine fiber-rich) regions and laminae.

Role of Circulation-Derived Monoamines in Regulation of Corticogenesis

It is now widely accepted that monoaminergic afferents do not represent the major source of monoamines present in the embryonic cerebral wall during cortical formation. This is clearly evident from the disparity between the adult-like levels of monoaminergic neurotransmitters (with the concentration of serotonin being even higher than that in adults) in the primate cerebral wall during the second trimester[25] (the embryonic period when cerebral cortex is being formed) and a very immature state of monoamine synthesizing machinery characteristic for cortical afferents even after the third trimester.[26] Some amount of monoamines in the fetal cerebral wall may diffuse there from the cerebrospinal fluid which receives these neurotransmitters from monoamine-secreting brain cells at some distance away. For example, many serotonergic neurons of the raphe nucleus in the fetal brain send thick processes directly to the ventricular surface.[27] However, the bulk of monoamines in the developing cerebral wall most likely originates outside the fetal brain and pass there through blood circulation. Such passage should be easy because of the absence of the brain-blood barrier and the presence of large intracellular spaces in the embryonic brain.[28] This proposition is strongly supported by our recent observation (FIG. 5) that the levels of noradrenaline and dopamine throughout the monkey embryonic cerebral wall prior to formation of the brain-blood barrier (E70, E90, and E120) are 70–80 times higher than those shortly after the establishment of this barrier (P1).

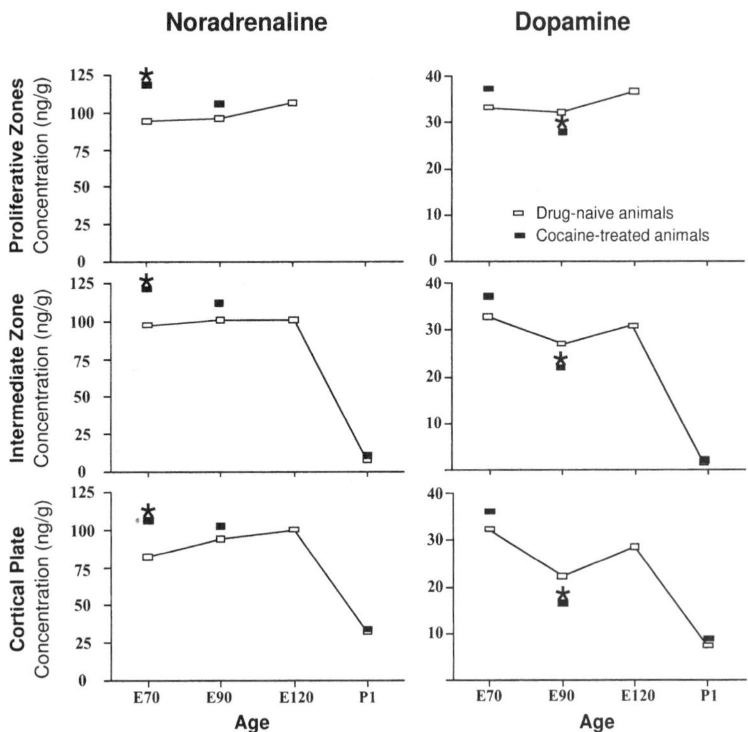

FIGURE 5. Levels of noradrenaline and dopamine in the laminae of the occipital cerebral wall in the developing drug-naive and cocaine-exposed monkeys. Cocaine (20 mg/kg/day) was administered orally in fruit treats from E40 to E102. Control animals received fruit treats only. Statistically significant differences (two-tailed Student t test; $p < 0.05$) were marked by an *asterisk* on the top of the *black square.*

The mother is probably one of the main sources of monoaminergic neurotransmitters in the fetal circulation because these chemicals can easily cross the placental barrier.[29–31] The importance of the mother as a source of monoamines is supported by the observation that embryonic mice unable to synthesize noradrenaline because of dopamine-β-hydroxylase knockout have a greater chance of survival if their mothers can synthesize this neurotransmitter.[32] Significant quantities of monoamines can also be synthesized in the peripheral tissue of the fetus itself. For example, noradrenaline is so important for normal development that it is produced in a special transient paraganglionic organ of Zuckerkandl found only in the embryos.[33]

The presence of significant levels of monoamines diffusing throughout the entire cerebral wall resolves the problem of a much wider distribution of monoaminergic receptors compared to the neurotransmitter-specific innervation.[12] In particular, recent immunocytochemical and *in situ* hybridization studies of the embryonic cerebral wall demonstrated that specific subtypes of monoaminergic receptors are present on multiple cellular elements not associated with neurotransmitter-specific innervation.[34,35] They include dividing cells in the ventricular and subventricular proliferative zones, migrating cortical neurons in the intermediate zone as well as radial- and astroglial cells (FIG. 3). These receptors are most likely activated by the nonselectively diffusing monoaminergic neurotransmitters that are therefore in a position to influence proliferation and migration of cortical cells as well as glial structural development during corticogenesis. The ability of monoaminergic neurotransmitters to regulate such developmental activities was demonstrated previously *in vitro* as well as *in vivo,* although in the latter case it was largely outside of the cerebral wall.[34–36] Of particular significance in this respect is our recent finding (in collaboration with Dr. Brian Kobilka from Stanford University) that genetic disruption of α_2B adrenergic receptors in mice[37] interferes with normal positioning of the neurons in the cerebral cortex reminiscent of that seen in animals prenatally exposed to cocaine (FIG. 4). It is also important to understand that the role of monoaminergic neurotransmitters in regulating developmental events is to assure certain speed of execution rather than to provide a signal for their initiation or cessation.[34,35] Therefore, the effectiveness of the nonselectively diffusing neurotransmitters in the fetal cerebral wall is not compromised by an apparent lack of large laminar gradients in their distribution. One can argue that the major feature of the nonselectively diffusing monoaminergic neurotransmitters and their receptors is the presence in nearly every lamina throughout the entire embryonic cerebral wall which allows them to influence multiple aspects of development in all cortical areas.

Cocaine May Interfere with Development of the Primate Cerebral Cortex by Altering Global Levels of Monoamines in Mother and Fetus

The cocaine treatment employed in the monkey model of the deleterious action of cocaine on cerebral cortical development showed precisely the types of effects that would be expected from modulation of the nonselectively diffusing monoamines not associated with neurotransmitter-specific innervation. They are seen throughout the entire cerebral cortex and include: (1) reduction in the number of cortical cells, which most likely reflects abnormal cell proliferation; (2) inappropriate positioning of cortical neurons resulting from alterations in migration of cortical cells; and (3) altered glial morphology. Therefore, it is reasonable to propose that cocaine at large doses affects the global levels of monoamines in both mother and fetus and, by doing this, interfere with the regulatory effects of the nonselectively diffusing fraction of these chemicals. If this hypothesis is true, then the cocaine treatment employed in the monkey model of prenatal cocaine exposure should affect monoamines and their receptors in

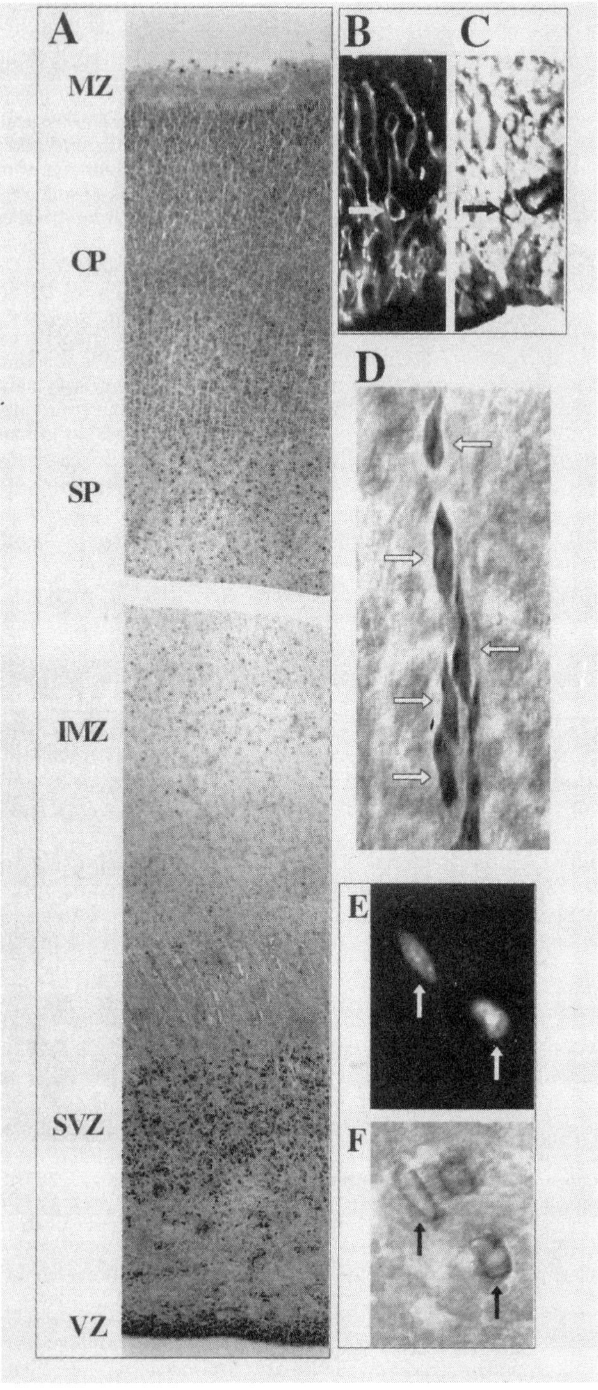

FIGURE 3. *See legend on facing page.*

←

FIGURE 3. Examples of the presence of monoaminergic receptors in the fetal cerebral wall. **(A)** Micrographs of the coronal section through the E90 monkey occipital cerebral wall containing developing primary visual cortex processed for immunocytochemistry with α_2B receptor-specific antibodies (antibodies were provided by Dr. Robert Lefkowitz, Duke University; visualized by DAB reaction). Note that α_2B receptor immunolabeling is present in all laminae of the fetal cerebral wall including the marginal zone **(MZ)**, cortical plate **(CP)**, subplate zone **(SP)**, intermediate zone **(IZ)**, subventricular zone **(SV)**, and ventricular zone **(VZ)**. **(B** and **C)** Micrographs of the section through the intermediate zone of the E70 embryonic cerebral wall simultaneously stained with GFAP-specific antibodies (**B**; monoclonal antibodies G-A-5 monoclonal antibodies from Sigma Co; visualized by rhodamine) and antisera for D_1 dopaminergic receptors (**C**; D_1-specific antisera were provided by Dr. Clare Bergson, Pennsylvania State University; visualized by DAB reaction). *(Arrow)* Double-labeled radial glial cell (identified by the long radial process). **(D)** Spindle-shaped migrating cortical neurons in the E90 monkey occipital cerebral wall labeled with D5 receptor-specific antibodies (D5-specific antisera were provided by Dr. Clare Bergson, Pennsylvania State University; visualized by DAB reaction). **(E** and **F)** Micrographs of the section through the proliferative subventricular zone in the E70 occipital cerebral wall simultaneously stained with antisera for proliferation-associated nuclear antigen Ki-67 (**E**; antibodies were purchased from AMAC, Inc; visualized by rhodamine) and D5 receptor-specific antibodies (**F**; visualized by DAB reaction). *(Arrow)* Double-labeled cells.

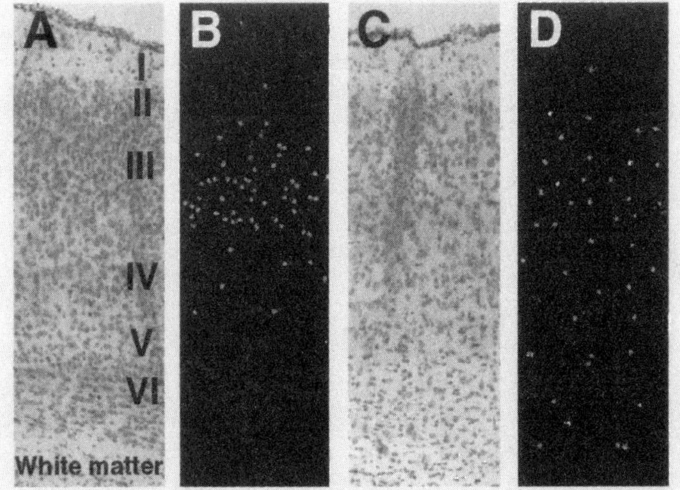

FIGURE 4. Micrographs of typical primary somatosensory cortex of P9 mice with normal α_2B adrenergic receptors (**A** and **B**) and their littermates with genetic disruption of these receptors (**C** and **D**). (**A** and **C**) Cresyl violet-stained coronal sections. Note that although the cortex of the normal mouse has laminar structure and clear demarcation from the white matter, the cortex of the mutant animal has a much more homogeneous appearance with a large number of cells in the white matter. (**B** and **D**) Dark-field images of the same sections showing the distribution of cells labeled on E14 by [^{3}H]thymidine injections. Note that labeled cells are more widely dispersed in the mutant mouse than in the control animal.

multiple laminae across the fetal cerebral wall. To test the aforementioned assumption we examined the effect of cocaine treatment on the concentration of noradrenaline and dopamine as well as the density of α_2 adrenergic and D_1 dopaminergic receptors in the proliferative zones, intermediate zone, and cortical plate of the frontal, parietal, temporal, and occipital regions of the fetal cerebral wall. The regiment of cocaine treatment was similar to that just described, 20 mg/kg/day po, starting at E40. In two animal groups, treatment continued until cesarean section at E70 (2 animals; 1 hour after the morning cocaine injection) and E90 (2 animals; 1 hour after the morning cocaine injection). In the third group (2 animals) treatment continued until E102. In this group, monkeys were allowed to give birth at term. The brain of the newborn animals was removed for analysis. The drug-naive monkeys included four groups (2 animals each): E70, E90, E120, and P1. The levels of noradrenaline and dopamine were measured using high pressure liquid chromatography with electrochemical detection,[38] whereas the densities of α_2 adrenergic and D_1 dopaminergic receptors were evaluated using [^{3}H]yohimbine and [^{3}H]SCH23390 autoradiography (nonspecific binding was deter-

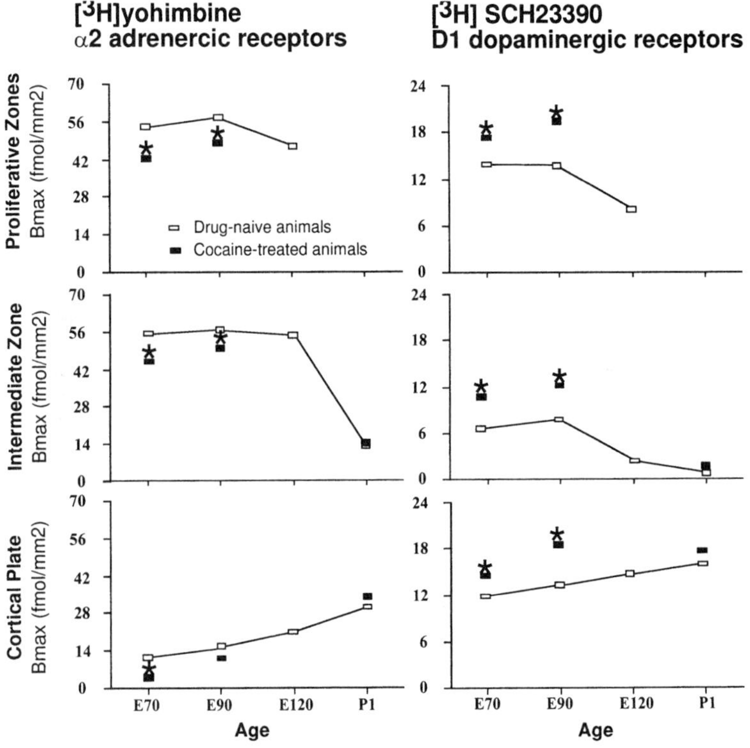

FIGURE 6. Density of α_2 adrenergic and D_1 dopaminergic receptors (determined by specific binding of [^{3}H]yohimbine and [^{3}H]SCH23390, respectively) in the laminae of the occipital cerebral wall in the developing drug-naive and cocaine-exposed monkeys. Cocaine (20 mg/kg/day) was administered orally in fruit treats from E40 to E102. Control animals received fruit treats only. Statistically significant differences (two-tailed Student t test; $p < 0.05$) were marked by an *asterisk* on the top of the *black square.*

mined in the presence of 100 μM noradrenaline and 2 μM *cis*-flupentixol, respectively).[39]

As predicted, the drug treatment employed in the monkey model of the effect of prenatal cocaine exposure on cerebral cortical development altered levels of noradrenaline and dopamine and their receptors in the proliferative and intermediate zones and cortical plate throughout the fetal cerebral wall (FIGS. 5 and 6). In particular, statistically significant differences between concentrations of noradrenaline in the cerebral wall of control and drug-exposed fetuses were seen at E70. For dopamine, statistically significant differences were present at E90. In the proliferative and intermediate zones, statistically significant differences in the density of α_2 adrenergic and D_1 dopaminergic receptors were observed at E70 and E90. In the cortical plate, such differences were detectable at E70 for α_2 receptors and at E70 and E90 for D_1 receptors. We also found that 50 days of cocaine treatment (from E40 to E90) resulted in uncoupling of the D_1 receptors in the fetal cerebral wall from their Gi-proteins. This was indicated[40] by the fact the cocaine-exposed tissue produced a much smaller guanylimidodiphosphate (GppNHp)-dependent shift to the right of the displacement curve of [^{3}H]SCH23390 by agonist SKF-82958 (FIG. 7).

CONCLUDING REMARKS

An obvious question is what can we learn from these studies, particularly since the cocaine administration regimen and route employed are very different from those used by most human drug abusers. We believe that our data provide several important conclusions:

1. While the level of abnormalities described here is much more severe than those present in most cocaine-exposed infants, our studies clearly demonstrate the danger posed by prenatal cocaine exposure.

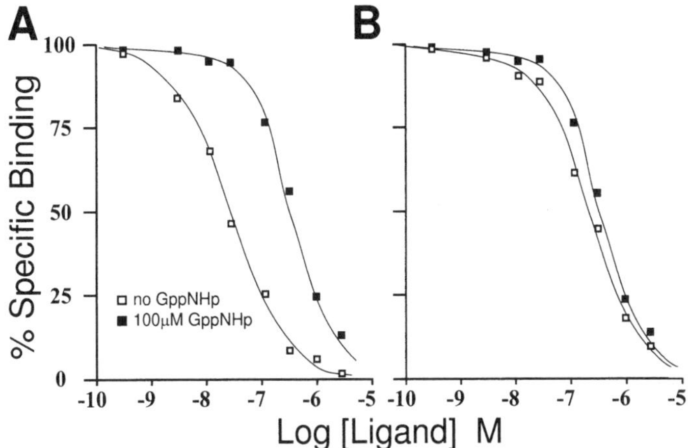

FIGURE 7. Effect of GppNHp on SKF-82958 competition for [^{3}H]SCH23390 in homogenates of tissue from the E90 cerebral wall of drug-naive **(A)** and cocaine-exposed **(B)** fetuses. Note that addition of GppNHp to the drug-exposed tissue produced a smaller shift of the displacement curve than that in the control tissue. This suggests that cocaine treatment causes uncoupling of D_1 dopaminergic receptors from their Gi-proteins.

2. The fact that the dopaminergic system is involved in addictive properties of cocaine does not mean that it is involved in teratologic effects of this drug. The latter can result from disturbances in multiple monoaminergic and other systems.

3. Teratologic effects of cocaine are related to its actions not only within the fetus but also within the mother. Therefore, to understand the effect of cocaine on fetal development in any given case consideration must be given to the previous history of drug abuse by the mother which may modulate responses of the mother's monoaminergic systems to cocaine during pregnancy.

4. The fact that cocaine may produce certain teratogenic effects through specific monoaminergic sites does not mean that postnatal treatment should be directed at the same sites because they may not be there after birth.

REFERENCES

1. Singer, L., K. Franks & R. Kleiegman. 1992. Childhood medical and behavioral consequences of maternal cocaine use. J. Pediatr. Psychol. **17:** 389–406.
2. Gonzales, N.M. & M. Campbell. 1994. Cocaine babies: Does prenatal exposure to cocaine affect development? J. Am. Child Adolesc. Psychiatry **33:** 16–19.
3. Scherling, D. 1994. Prenatal cocaine exposure and childhood psychopathology: A developmental analysis. Am. J. Orthopsychiatry **64:** 9–19.
4. Lewis, M. & M. Bendersky. 1995. Mothers, Babies, and Cocaine. Lawrence Erlbaum Associates. Hilsdale, NJ.
5. Spear, L.P., C.L. Kristein, J. Bell, V. Yoottanasumpun, R. Greenbaum, O.J. Shea, H. Hoffman & N.E. Spear. 1989. Effects of prenatal cocaine exposure on behavior during the early postnatal period. Neurotoxicol. Teratol. **11:** 57–63.
6. Henderson, M.G., M.M. McConnaughey & B.A. McMillen. 1991. Long-term consequences of prenatal exposure to cocaine or related drugs: Effects on rat brain monoaminergic receptors. Brain Res. Bull. **26:** 941–945.
7. Gressens, P., B.E. Kosofky & P. Evrad. 1992. Cocaine-induced disturbances of corticogenesis in the developing Murine brain. Neurosci. Lett. **140:** 113–116.
8. Seidler, F.J. & T.A. Slotkin. 1992. Fetal cocaine exposure causes persistent noradrenergic hyperactivity in rat brain regions: Effects on neurotransmitter turnover and receptors. J. Pharm. Exp. Ther. **263:** 413–421.
9. Akbari, H.M., P.M. Whitaker-Azmitia & E.C. Azmitia. 1994. Prenatal cocaine decreases the trophic factor S-100β and induces microcephaly: Reversal by postnatal 5-HT1A receptor agonist. Neurosci. Lett. **170:** 141–144.
10. Lidow, M.S. 1995. Prenatal cocaine exposure adversely affects development of the primate cerebral cortex. Synapse **21:** 332–341.
11. Ronnekleiv, O.K. & B.R. Naylor. 1995. Chronic cocaine exposure in the fetal rhesus monkey: Consequences for early development of dopamine neurons. J. Neurosci. **15:** 7330–7343.
12. Levitt, P., J.A. Harvey, E. Friedman, K. Simansky & E.H. Murphy, 1997. New evidence for neurotransmitter influences on brain development. Trends Neurosci. **20:** 269–274.
13. Rakic, P. 1982. Early developmental events: Cell lineages, acquisition of neuronal position and areal and laminar development. Neurosci. Res. Progr. Bull. **20:** 439–451.
14. Schneider, M.L., C.F. Moore, S.J. Suomi & M. Champoux. 1991. Laboratory assessment of temperament and environmental enrichment in rhesus monkey infants *(Macaca mulatta).* Am. J. Primatol. **25:** 137–155.
15. Schneider, M.L. & S.J. Suomi. 1992. Neurobehavioral assesment in rhesus monkey neonates *(Macaca mulatta):* Developmental changes, behavioral stability, and early experience. Infant Behav. Dev. **15:** 155–177.
16. Lester, B.M., K. Freier & L. LaGasse. 1995. Prenatal cocaine exposure and child outcome: What do we really know? *In* Mothers, Babies, and Cocaine. M. Lewis & M. Bendersky, Eds.: 19–39. Lawrence Erlbaum Associates. Hillsdale, NJ.

17. SHARKEY, J., K.A. GLEN, S. WOLFE & M.J. KUHAR. 1988. Cocaine binding at σ receptors. Eur. J. Pharmacol. **149:** 171–174.
18. FRANK, D.B., B.S. ZUCKERMAN, H. AMARO, K. ABOAGYE, H. BUCHNER, H. CABRAL, L. FRIED, R. HINGSON, H. KAYNE, S. M. LEVENSON, S. PARKER, S. H. REECE & R. VINCI. 1988. Cocaine use during pregnancy: Prevalence and correlates. Pediatrics **82:** 888–895.
19. RITZ, M.C., M.J. KUHAR & F.R. GEORGE. 1992. Molecular mechanisms associated with cocaine effects. Possible relationship with effects of ethanol. *In* Alcohol and Cocaine: Similarities and Differences. M. Galanter, Ed.: 273–302. Plenum Press. New York.
20. WANG, G.K. 1988. Cocaine-induced closures of single batrachotoxin-activated Na^+ channels in planar lipid bilayers. J. Gen. Physiol. **92:** 747–765.
21. HE, G-Q., A. ZANG, B.T. ALTURA & B.M. ALTURA. 1994. Cocaine-induced cerebrovasospasms and its possible mechanism of action. J. Pharm. Exp. Ther. **268:** 1532–1539.
22. HAMMER, R.P. 1995. The Neurobiology of Cocaine. CRC Press. New York.
23. JOHNSTON, M.V. 1988. Biochemistry of neurotransmitters in cortical development. *In* Cerebral Cortex, Vol. 7. A. Peters & E.G. Jones, Eds.: 211–236. Plenum Press. New York.
24. MITTLEMAN, R.E., J.C. COFINO & W.L. HEARN. 1989. Tissue distribution of cocaine in a pregnant woman. J. Forens. Sci. **34:** 481–486.
25. MASUDI, N.A. & D.P. GILMORE. 1983. Biogenic amine levels in the mid-term human fetus. Dev. Brain Res. **7:** 9–12.
26. GOLDMAN-RAKIC, P.S. & R.M. BROWN. 1982. Postnatal development of monoamine content and synthesis in the cerebral cortex of rhesus monkeys. Dev. Brain Res. **4:** 339–349.
27. LAUDER, J.M. 1983. Hormonal and humoral influences on brain development. Psychopharmacology **8:** 121–155.
28. NICHOLSON, G. & M.E. RICE. 1991. Diffusion of ions and transmitters in the brain cell microenvironment. *In* Volume Transmission in the Brain. K. Fuxe & L.F. Agnati, Eds.: 279–294. Raven Press. New York.
29. MORGAN, G.D., M. SANDER & M. PANIGLE. 1972. Placental transfer of catecholamines *in vitro* and *in vivo.* J. Obstet. Gynecol. **112:** 1068–1075.
30. PARVEZ, S. & H. PARVEZ. 1974. Placental transfer of ^{3}H-epinephrine and its metabolites in the fetal heart during variable hormonal treatments. Horm. Res. **5:** 321–330.
31. SANDLER, M., C.R. RUTHVEN & C. WOOD. 1974. Metabolism of C^{14}-norepinephrine and C^{14}-epinephrine and their transmission across the human placenta. Int. J. Neuropharmacol. **3:** 123–128.
32. THOMAS, S.A., A.M. MATSUMOTO & R.D. PALMITER. 1995. Noradrenaline is essential for mouse fetal development. Nature (Lond.) **374:** 643–646.
33. WEST, G.B., D.M. SHEPHERD, R.B. HUNTER & A.R. MACGREGOR. 1953. The function of the organ of Zuckerkandl. Clin. Sci. **12:** 317–325.
34. WANG, F. & M.S. LIDOW. 1997. α_2A-Adrenergic receptors are expressed by diverse cell types in the fetal primate cerebral wall. J. Comp. Neurol. **378:** 493–507.
35. WANG, F., C. BERGSON, R.L. HOWARD & M.S. LIDOW. 1997. Differential expression of D1 and D5 dopamine receptors in the fetal primate cerebral wall. Cerebral Cortex **7:** 711–721.
36. LIDOW, M.S. & F. WANG. 1995. Neurotransmitter receptors in the developing cerebral cortex. Crit. Rev. Neurobiol. **9:** 395–418.
37. MACDONALD, E., B.K. KOBILKA & M. SCHEININ. 1997. Gene targeting-homing in on α2-adrenoceptor-subtype function. Trends Pharm. Sci. **18:** 211–219.
38. LIDOW, M.S., J.D. ELSWORTH & P.S. GOLDMAN-RAKIC. 1997. Down-regulation of the D1 and D5 dopamine receptors in the primate prefrontal cortex by chronic treatment with antipsychotic drugs. J. Pharm. Exp. Ther. **281:** 597–603.
39. LIDOW, M.S. & P. RAKIC. 1995. Neurotransmitter receptors in the proliferative zones of the developing primate occipital lobe. J. Comp. Neurol. **360:** 393–402.
40. POYNER, D. 1990. Receptor-G-protein complex in solution. *In* Receptor-Effector Coupling. E.C. Hulme, Ed.: 31–58. Oxford University Press. New York.

Prenatal Exposure to Cocaine Impairs Neuronal Coding of Attention and Discriminative Learning[a]

MICHAEL GABRIEL[b] AND CARRIE TAYLOR

Department of Psychology, Beckman Institute for Advanced Science and Technology, 405 N. Mathews Avenue, Urbana, Illinois 61801, USA

ABSTRACT: Cingulate cortex and related areas of the thalamus are critically involved in the mediation of discriminative avoidance learning, wherein rabbits step in response to an acoustic conditional stimulus (CS+) to avoid foot shock and they learn to ignore a different acoustic stimulus (CS–) not followed by shock. Studies of multi-unit neuronal activity recorded simultaneously in many cingulothalamic areas have documented massive learning-related neuronal firing changes during the course of behavioral acquisition. Stimulated by findings (this volume) of neurobiological changes in anterior cingulate cortex in rabbits exposed *in utero* to cocaine, we investigated behavioral learning and correlated neuronal activity in several cingulothalamic areas in cocaine-exposed rabbits. In an initial study, training-induced enhancement of cingulate cortical neuronal firing in response to the CS+ and CS– was abolished in rabbits exposed to cocaine *in utero.* Yet discriminative neuronal activity (greater firing in response to the CS+ than to the CS–) did develop during training, and behavioral learning was normal in the cocaine-exposed rabbits. In a second study, we reduced the salience of the CS+ and CS– by employing 200 msec CSs rather than standard 500 msec CSs. Early training-stage development of anterior cingulate cortical discriminative neuronal activity was abolished, the elicited neuronal discharge profiles were altered, and behavioral learning was impaired in rabbits exposed to cocaine, relative to saline-exposed controls. The specificity of these changes to low-salience CSs suggested that prenatal cocaine results in disturbed associative attentional processes of anterior cingulate cortex in adult rabbits. Consideration of the neuronal response profile alterations together with other reported neurobiological changes suggested that the cocaine-related attentional deficit is due to impaired dopaminergic afferent activation of GABA neurons in anterior cingulate cortex.

INTRODUCTION

Background. Substantial progress has been made recently in documenting the neurocognitive changes that occur in children born of mothers who abused cocaine during pregnancy.[1–4] Research with animal subjects has an important role to play in relation to this issue. Animal models allow assessment of the effects of controlled drug doses administered by various routes in various gestational stages, in the absence of confounding effects of other drug and lifestyle variables.[5–10] The immediate effects of cocaine on the neurobiology of the fetus as well as possible sequelae that extend over time through the postnatal period and into adulthood can be directly and invasively studied at all levels, from molecular and genetic to behavioral and cognitive.

Rabbits and Prenatal Exposure to Cocaine. The studies described in this chapter were stimulated by other work reported in this volume, which showed that rabbits exposed to cocaine *in utero* exhibited alterations in brain areas which receive dopaminergic fiber projections. These included the striatum,[11] hippocampus,[12,13] and anterior cin-

[a] This research was supported by grants from the National Institute on Drug Abuse (DA11164), National Institutes of Health Grant NS36591, and National Science Foundation Grant BIR95-04842.

[b]Phone, 217/244-3463; fax, 217/244-5180; e-mail, mgabriel@s.psych.uiuc.edu.

gulate cortex.[14] Changes found in the anterior cingulate cortex of the cocaine-exposed rabbits included: a) a decrease in depolarization-evoked [^{3}H]dopamine release[15]; (b) an uncoupling of the D1 dopamine receptor from its associated G-protein[16]; (c) an increased number of GABA-immunoreactive neurons[17]; (d) an increase in the number of dendrites exhibiting immunoreactivity to parvalbumin[18]; and (e) pyramidal cells with elongated, "wavy" apical dendrites and bent synaptic spines.[19] These effects were measured in relation to corresponding indices in saline-exposed controls.

***Rationale: Studies of the Neural Mediation of Discriminative Avoidance Learning in Rabbits Exposed to Cocaine* in Utero.** We were intrigued by the changes found in cingulate cortex in rabbits exposed to cocaine *in utero,* especially because of our previous findings concerning the involvement of cingulate cortex and related areas in the mediation of discriminative avoidance learning in rabbits. Our findings were based on the use of discrete brain lesions in concert with multi-site recording technology, whereby multi-unit neuronal activity is monitored during behavioral acquisition simultaneously in six areas of the learning-relevant circuitry.

The rabbits in these studies learn to step in response to a tone (CS+) in order to avoid a foot shock unconditional stimulus (US) and they learn to ignore a different tone (CS–) not predictive of the US. As discriminative responding develops, cingulate cortical neurons exhibit training-induced activity (TIA), including discriminative TIA (a greater firing frequency in response to the CS+ than to the CS–) and excitatory TIA (increased firing in response to the CS+ during training, relative to activity elicited in stressful conditions before training). Similar changes occur in areas of the thalamus, the anterior and medial dorsal nuclei, which reciprocate fiber projections with the cingulate cortex.[20]

Discriminative avoidance learning was severely impaired in rabbits given combined anterior and posterior cingulate cortical lesions, or combined lesions of the anterior and medial dorsal thalamic nuclei. The learning deficits were correlated with lesion magnitude and were not attributable to a disturbance of sensory or motor function.[21] In addition, lesions of the amygdala and lesions of the medial geniculate nucleus of the thalamus completely blocked the development of TIA in the cingulothalamic areas and they produced, as did the aforementioned cingulothalamic lesions, a severe deficit in behavioral acquisition.[22,23]

It occurred to us that the application of our analysis to rabbits exposed to cocaine *in utero* might help to elucidate the functional consequences of the cocaine-related neurobiological changes in the rabbit anterior cingulate cortex. An understanding of the functional consequences of the cocaine-induced alterations in animals could shed light on the neural etiology of the attentional and cognitive deficits reported to occur in humans exposed to cocaine *in utero.*

PRENATAL COCAINE AND CINGULOTHALAMIC NEURONAL ACTIVITY DURING DISCRIMINATIVE AVOIDANCE LEARNING

Prologue. Our initial goal was to document the activity of cingulate cortical neurons and related thalamic neurons during discriminative avoidance learning in rabbits that were exposed to cocaine *in utero.* Cocaine and saline were given to pregnant Dutch-belted rabbits at Allegheny University, as described by Murphy *et al.*[24] Two daily intravenous injections of cocaine (4 mg/kg) or physiological saline, were given to Dutch-belted rabbit does during gestation. These doses of cocaine yielded the aforementioned neural changes in the offspring of the injected does, but did not affect the body weight of the does or rabbit kits, litter size, survival rate, brain size or general brain development of the kits.

Offspring of the cocaine- and saline-exposed rabbits were shipped after weaning to the University of Illinois Beckman Institute Vivarium in cohorts of 3–8. After a minimum period of seven days for quarantine, the rabbits were prepared for surgical implantation of fixed-position electrodes suitable for the recording of multi-unit neuronal activity. Electrodes were positioned while the rabbits were under full surgical anesthesia in each of the following regions of the anterior cingulate cortex (Brodmann's area 24b): (a) a supra-genual region 1 mm anterior to bregma; (b) a pre-genual region 3.8 mm anterior to bregma; and (c) a far anterior region 5.2 mm anterior to bregma. In addition, one electrode each was positioned in the posterior cingulate cortex (Brodmann's area 29c/d), the anterior ventral (AV) thalamic nucleus, and the medial dorsal (MD) thalamic nucleus.

Behavioral Training and Neuronal Recording. Following recovery from surgery the rabbits received discriminative avoidance training. The minimum age of the rabbits at the onset of testing was 90 days. The training procedure is illustrated in FIGURE 1. Training was administered while the rabbits occupied a Brogden-Culler rotating wheel apparatus designed for the conditioning of small animals.[25] The CS+ and CS– were 1–, or 8-kHz pure tones, the assigned values being counterbalanced. The duration of the CS+ and CS– was 500 ms. The CS+ was followed after 5 seconds by a footshock US, an alternating current of 1.5–2.5 mA administered through the grid floor of the wheel. The foot shock US was terminated by locomotion-induced wheel rotation, and locomotion during the 5 sec CS–US interval prevented the scheduled US. The CS– was never followed by the US.

The rabbits experienced a single training session each day, consisting of 60 presentations each of the CS+ and CS–, in an irregular sequence. Daily sessions were given until a criterion of performance was attained, wherein the percentage of avoidance responses to the CS+ exceeded the percentage of responses to the CS– by 60% or more, in two consecutive training sessions. Criterion attainment was followed by ten sessions of reversal training, in which the original CS+ served as the CS–, and the original CS– served as the CS+. Before acquisition, the rabbits received a preliminary training session in which the tones to be used as CS+ and CS–, and the foot shock US were presented in an explicitly unpaired manner.

The neuronal records from the six implanted electrodes were amplified and recorded online throughout behavioral training, as detailed by Gabriel.[21] Two recording methods were employed: (1) the overall discharge frequency of the largest three or four spikes detected with window discriminators was counted every 10 ms; (2) the records were integrated electronically and the output of the integrators was digitized every 10 ms. Sampling occurred for 1.0 second, including 0.3 second before and 0.7 second after CS onset. The two sampling methods are usefully complementary. Due to the smoothing effect of time constants, the integrated unit activity yields less precise temporal profiles of the elicited neuronal discharges than the profiles yielded by the spike frequency data. However, because the spike frequency method samples the activity of relatively few neurons, it is less sensitive to experimental manipulations than the more inclusive integrated activity measure, which occasionally reveals significant relationships not found or found only as nonsignificant trends in the analysis of spike frequency. Several stringent controls were employed to reject and repeat occasional trials in which the onset of movement (e.g., locomotion, grooming, sneezing) was coincident with CS presentation and resulted in movement-triggered electrical artifacts.

Dutch-Belted and New Zealand White Rabbits. An important initial question concerned whether discriminative avoidance learning and cingulothalamic training-induced neuronal activity, documented previously in male New Zealand White (NZW) rabbits, would be comparable in Dutch-belted male and female rabbits. The results showed essential similarity in both the neuronal and behavioral measures. The rate of learning, the asymptotic avoidance rate, and the levels of discriminative performance

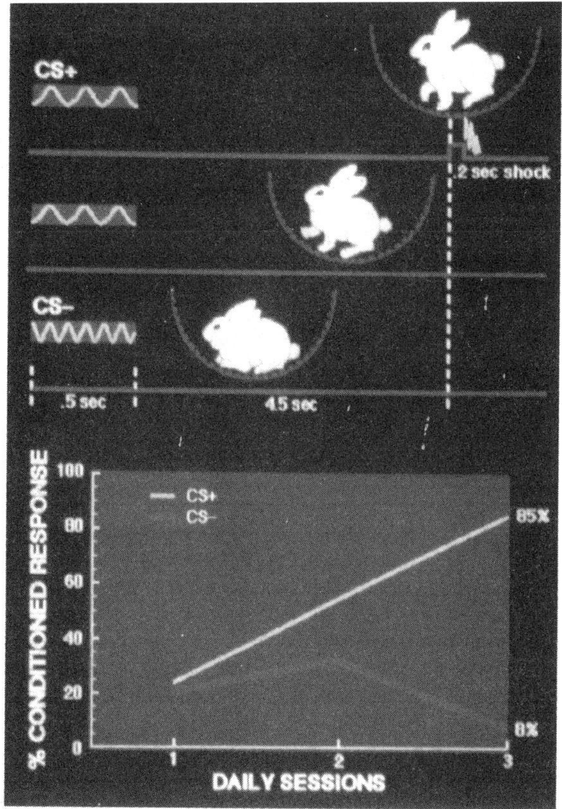

FIGURE 1. *Upper portion:* the stimulus relations employed for discriminative avoidance conditioning (details in text). *Lower portion*: the approximate modal rate and asymptote of discriminative avoidance learning in rabbits.

attained by Dutch-belted rabbits were essentially identical to the values found previously for NZW rabbits. Moreover, cingulothalamic neuronal populations exhibited area-specific temporal discharge profiles in response to the conditional stimuli, training-induced excitation (excitatory TIA) and training-induced discrimination (discriminative TIA), that were remarkably similar to these features of the neuronal activity in the NZW rabbits.

In Utero ***Cocaine and the Anterior Cingulate Cortex.*** All of the following effects of prenatal cocaine were supported by statistically significant individual comparisons following significant main effects and interactions in the analysis of variance.[26]

Exposure to cocaine *in utero* significantly reduced the magnitude of the tone-elicited neuronal discharges in the anterior cingulate cortex of Dutch-belted rabbits. In addition, excitatory TIA was eliminated in rabbits exposed to cocaine. That is, the rabbits exposed to cocaine *in utero* lacked completely the robust training-related increases of multi-unit discharge amplitude in response to CS+ and CS– during discriminative

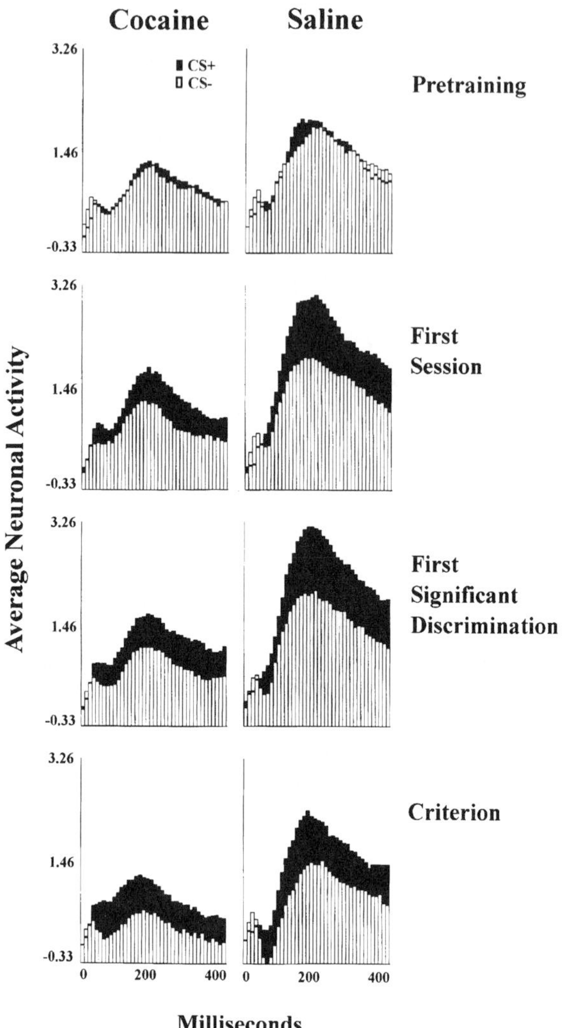

FIGURE 2. Average integrated multi-unit neuronal activity recorded during behavioral acquisition, in anterior cingulate cortex in response to the CS+ *(solid bars)* and CS– *(open bars)* in rabbits (male and female) exposed to cocaine *(left column)* or saline *(right column) in utero.* Each panel shows the unit activity during the first 40 consecutive 10-ms intervals following CS onset. The onset of the CS+ or CS– occurred at the leftmost position on the horizontal axis of each panel. The plotted values are difference scores: the results of subtracting the response magnitude in each 10-ms interval following CS onset from the mean score of 30 pre-CS intervals. Records were obtained during the pretraining session *(first row),* the first session of training *(second row),* the session of first significant discrimination *(third row),* and the criterial session *(fourth row),* as described in the text.

avoidance learning, measured relative to the discharge magnitudes found before training when the CS and US were unpaired (FIG. 2).

The foregoing effects were based on a significant interaction of the Exposure Treatment (cocaine and saline), Sex (male and female), Training Stage (pretraining, first session, first significant discrimination, and criterion), Stimulus (CS+ and CS–) and Post-CS Interval (40 10-msec intervals after CS onset) factors of the analysis of variance ($p < 0.001$).

Follow-up analysis of this interaction showed, remarkably, that the effects of prenatal cocaine exposure on anterior cingulate cortical neuronal activity during behavioral acquisition were specific to female rabbits. No significant loss of excitatory TIA was found in male rabbits. Full elaboration of this and other sex differences found in this study is given in a report by Taylor *et al.*[26]

The tone-elicited discharges recorded during reversal learning were significantly attenuated in rabbits exposed to cocaine, relative to saline-exposed controls, and this effect was found in both male and female rabbits (FIG. 3).

Despite the loss of excitatory TIA in the anterior cingulate cortex in rabbits exposed to cocaine, the temporal profile of the average neuronal response to the tones was preserved, as was discriminative TIA (i.e., development during training of a significantly greater neuronal response to the CS+ than to the CS–). The discriminative effect can be seen by comparing the light to the dark histogram profiles of trained rabbits in FIGURE 2.

In Utero *Cocaine and the Posterior Cingulate Cortex.* As in the anterior cingulate cortex, the magnitude of the average tone-elicited neuronal discharges during original acquisition was reduced and excitatory TIA was abolished in the posterior cingulate cortex (Brodmann's area 29c/d) in rabbits exposed to cocaine *in utero* (FIG. 4). Unexpectedly, a "reverse" sex difference was found in relation to the activity in this area, relative to the effect found in the anterior cingulate cortex: the cocaine-related attenuation of the neuronal response in the posterior cingulate cortex was significantly more pronounced in males than in females. Nevertheless, the cocaine-related attenuation occurred significantly in both sexes. There were no significant effects of prenatal cocaine on posterior cingulate cortical activity during reversal learning.

As in the anterior cingulate cortex, the tone-elicited excitation and excitatory TIA in posterior cingulate cortex were attenuated by exposure to cocaine, but discriminative TIA was not. The individual comparisons following a significant interaction of the Exposure Treatment, Training Stage, Stimulus, and Post-CS Interval factors of the analysis ($p < 0.001$) indicated that discriminative TIA in the posterior cingulate cortex was actually enhanced in rabbits exposed to cocaine *in utero* relative to the saline-exposed controls. This enhancement can be visualized as the greater difference (indicated by the dark areas) between CS+ and CS– related histograms during all training stages in FIGURE 4.

In Utero *Cocaine and the Limbic Thalamic Nuclei.* Exposure of rabbits to cocaine *in utero* was associated with a general decrease in the overall magnitude of the average elicited neuronal discharges recorded in the AV thalamic nucleus. This effect was significant in the analysis of the data of acquisition ($p < 0.002$) and during reversal training ($p < 0.001$). Although there was a trend in the same direction, no significant effect of prenatal cocaine exposure was found in the neuronal data of the MD nucleus. Unlike the changes found in cingulate cortex, the effect of cocaine in the AV thalamic nucleus did not interact with the Training Stage or the Stimulus factor and therefore did not constitute an effect of cocaine on processes of associative learning.

In Utero *Cocaine and Behavior.* Despite the aforementioned robust effects of cocaine on the learning-related neuronal activity in the cingulate cortex, there were no effects

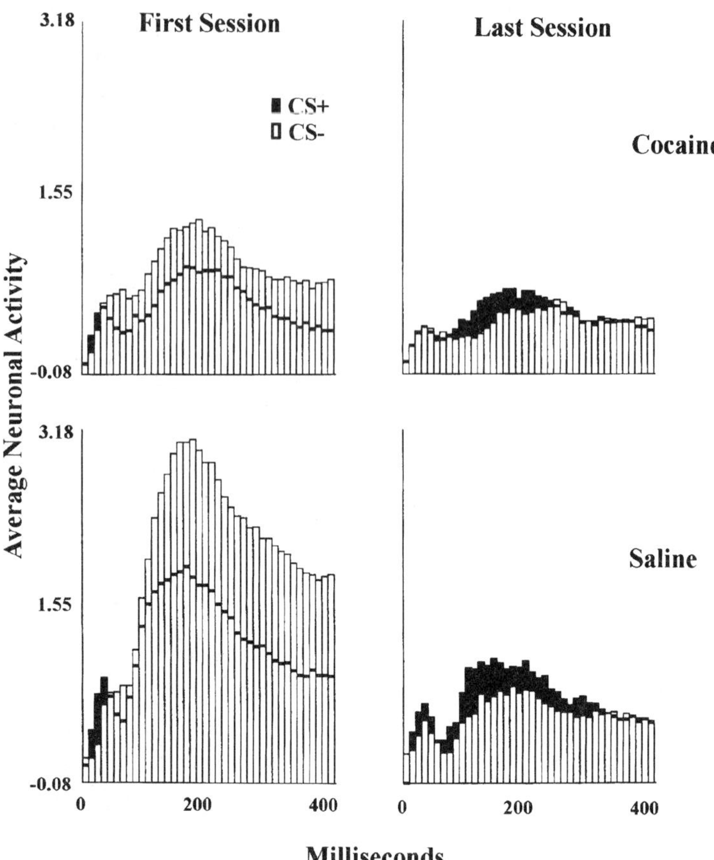

FIGURE 3. Average integrated multi-unit neuronal activity in anterior cingulate cortex during reversal training in response to the CS+ *(solid bars)* and CS– *(open bars)* in rabbits (male and female) exposed to cocaine or saline *in utero.* The details of format are described in the caption of FIGURE 2 with the following exception. In this figure, data are shown for the first and final sessions of reversal training, not acquisition. Note the "old habit effect" in the first reversal training session, wherein the neurons exhibited a greater discharge in response to the *original* CS+ than to the CS+ used for reversal training. Note also that this discrimination, appropriate to original learning, was replaced by a discrimination appropriate to the reversal task in the final session of reversal training.

of prenatal cocaine on discriminative avoidance learning. The rabbits exposed to cocaine exhibited normal rates of discriminative learning and asymptotic levels of responding. Moreover, no significant effects of the exposure treatment were found for the latency of the conditioned response or the unconditioned response.

The only significant behavioral effects of cocaine *in utero* were as follows: The locomotory conditioned avoidance responses to the CS+ during original acquisition in rabbits exposed to cocaine were of a significantly greater duration than were the responses of the saline-exposed rabbits. In addition, rabbits exposed to cocaine made

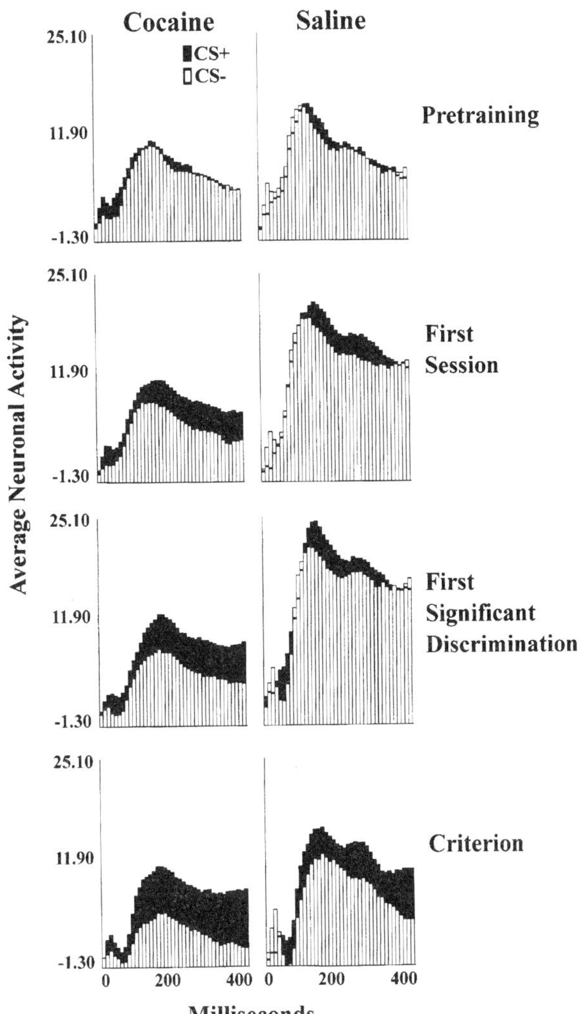

FIGURE 4. Average integrated multi-unit neuronal activity of posterior cingulate cortex during acquisition in response to the CS+ *(solid bars)* and CS– *(open bars)* in rabbits (males and females) exposed to cocaine or saline *in utero.* The details of format are described in the caption of FIGURE 2.

more inter-trial responses than did rabbits exposed to saline. The increased locomotory tendency is similar to results of other studies indicating an association of prenatal exposure to cocaine with increased activity levels[5,27,28] and lessened immobility in stressful situations.[29–31] Given the abundant evidence that striatal circuitry is involved in the priming and execution of locomotion,[32] we offer the suggestion that the changes of the striatal neurons reported to occur in cocaine-exposed rabbits[11] may underlie the locomotory changes exhibited by the rabbits in this study.

INTERPRETATION AND A HYPOTHESIS

Summary and Import of the Main Finding. The foregoing results represent the first demonstration that moderate, experimentally controlled levels of cocaine *in utero,* which did not produce any gross teratologic effects, nevertheless significantly altered cingulate cortical learning-relevant neuronal activity recorded *in vivo* during behavioral acquisition. These results thus afford new avenues towards understanding the etiology of learning impairments in subjects exposed to cocaine *in utero.*

Is Cingulothalamic Neuronal Activity Truly Relevant to Avoidance Learning? The claim that the neuronal activity that was attenuated in rabbits exposed to cocaine was learning-relevant neuronal activity may seem overstated. After all, behavioral learning in rabbits exposed to cocaine was the same in all respects as was the learning exhibited by saline-exposed controls.

On this point, it is important to note the sources of the claim of learning relevance. First, the discriminative training-induced activity is, de facto, learning-relevant activity because it meets the traditionally accepted criteria of associativity: the activity was specific to a stimulus that was paired with the reinforcer; it did not occur in response to a stimulus that was not paired with the reinforcer. Second, the activity was recorded in brain areas that are essential for learning, as known from lesion studies (reviewed above). These studies indicate that it is necessary to make large cingulothalamic lesions in order to produce a behavioral deficit. Thus, for example, lesions confined to the anterior cingulate cortex or to the posterior cingulate cortex produce only mild deficits, which occur in restricted stages of learning, early in the case of anterior cingulate cortical lesions and later in the case of posterior cingulate cortical lesions. Very similar, mild deficits were also found when lesions were confined to either the MD nucleus or the anterior nuclei. Also, lesions of the mamillothalamic tract (MTT) only produced behavioral impairment if the tract was completely transected.[33] Complete transection resulted in complete abolition of AV thalamic discriminative TIA. Incomplete transection of the MTT was associated with residual discriminative TIA and no significant behavioral deficit. Thus, the cingulothalamic circuitry exhibits "equipotentiality" in the sense that near-normative behavioral acquisition can be mediated by residual circuit elements that survive variously placed partial lesions. Lesions that allow residual TIA to develop do not result in measurably disturbed discriminative avoidance learning. Applying this principle to the foregoing results, substantial residual TIA was found in the anterior and posterior cingulate cortices in rabbits exposed to cocaine *in utero,* and this residual TIA may have allowed these rabbits to learn and perform at control levels.

Beyond these considerations, it is important to consider the possibility that training procedures more stringent than the discriminative avoidance training procedure, which place greater demand on the specific functional resources afforded by the neurons of cingulate cortex, may yield behavioral deficits in rabbits exposed to cocaine *in utero.* This possibility, confirmed by our second study (see below), raises an important question: What is the specific function subserved by cingulothalamic neuronal activity?

Function of Cingulate Cortical TIA: Associative Attention. Several observations have led us to propose that cingulate cortical TIA subserves *associative attention.* That is, the massive brief-latency CS+-specific cingulate cortical neuronal activity is necessary to allow the CS+, or more generally, any discrete phasic cue, to capture the subject's attention and thus to gain associative control of behavior. The attentional response of anterior cingulate cortical neurons is termed "associative" because it is a product of associative conditioning. It develops in response to conditional stimuli that predict the occurrence of reinforcement. It does not develop in response to stimuli that predict nonsignificant outcomes.

The hypothesis that cingulothalamic circuitry is involved in mediating associative attention is based on several findings. First, the discriminative TIA is clearly "cue-oriented," that is, elicited in a time-locked fashion by the CS+. It is not generalized background activity or activity that is directly predictive of the performance of the learned response. Moreover, as already noted, if the neural substrates that yield this activity are massively damaged, the rabbits are unable to use the CS+ as a cue for behavior, for example, rabbits fail to develop conditioned avoidance responses to the CS+, whereas they have no general locomotory impairment.

It could be argued that the inability of rabbits with large cingulothalamic lesions to produce a locomotory response on cue for shock avoidance is a subtle motoric deficit, such as a response initiation deficit, rather than an attentional deficit. However, recent observations argue against this possibility. Rabbits were trained in a discriminative approach task, wherein they learned to extend forward to drink from an inserted spout. Water was obtained when spout insertion followed the CS+ but not when the spout was inserted after the CS–. In this case, the response of extending forward and drinking from the spout was highly overlearned, as the rabbits had been drinking from spouts in their living cages for months prior to training. Thus, learning in the approach task did not involve acquisition of the spout response to the CS+. Rather, it was entirely a matter of suppressing the response to the spout when it was inserted into the testing chamber after presentation of the CS–. Rabbits with combined lesions of the anterior and MD thalamic nuclei, which abolish all cingulothalamic TIA, were substantially impaired in this learning.[34]

The key point is that rabbits with cingulothalamic damage were impaired in their ability to learn to use cues, whether the task required the subject to initiate a behavioral response to a cue or to suppress a well-established response on cue. In showing that the lesions impaired the subjects' ability to base their behavior on a discrete cue, for the widely divergent behavioral requirements of response initiation and response suppression, these data favor an attentional interpretation of cingulate cortical function.

Cue Salience and Associative Attention. Additional results that support the hypothesis that cingulothalamic circuitry mediates associative attention were obtained in a study by Sparenborg and Gabriel,[35] in which rabbits received discriminative avoidance training with the standard 500-ms CS+ and CS–. After criterion attainment, each rabbit received nine additional training sessions. In a given set of three consecutive sessions they received either the standard 500-ms CSs, 200-ms CSs, or long (5.0 s) "delay" CSs which bridged the full interval from CS onset to US onset. The sets of three consecutive sessions with a given CS duration were administered in a counterbalanced order.

The results showed that excitatory TIA magnitude in cingulate cortex was inversely proportional to the CS duration. The largest discharges were elicited by the briefest (i.e., the 200-ms) CS, whereas significantly lesser discharges were elicited by the more enduring CSs. This occurred in the anterior cingulate cortex (FIG. 5). A similar relationship was revealed by analysis of the posterior cingulate cortical neuronal data, but in this case the magnitude of the *discriminative* response, not the absolute discharge magnitude, was inversely proportional to CS duration, and this occurred in a restricted population of "late discriminating" posterior cingulate cortical neurons.[36] These findings suggested that cingulate cortical discharges in response to associatively significant cues are amplified as the duration of the cue is reduced.

It is important to note that the onset of the enhanced discharges in response to the brief CS in this study occurred 100–200 ms after CS onset, that is, prior to termination of the 200-ms CS+. Thus, the duration-related enhancement of the neuronal response was not a *direct* response to cue duration. Had it been a direct response to cue dura-

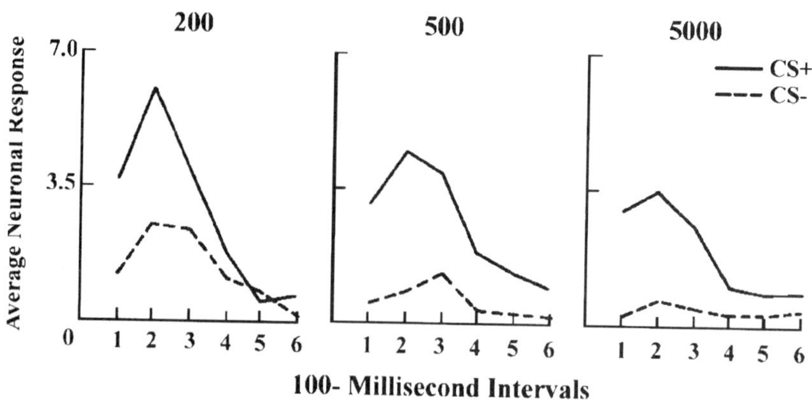

FIGURE 5. Average anterior cingulate cortical multi-unit spike frequency in six consecutive intervals of 100 ms each following the onset of the CS+ and CS–. Data were obtained during a series of counterbalanced sessions of discriminative avoidance training in which one of three CS durations was employed (200, 500, or 5,000 ms) following training to criterion with 500-ms CSs. Note the inverse relationship between CS duration and the anterior cingulate cortical neuronal response to the CS+.

tion, the duration-related discharge could not have occurred until after the offset of the cue. It follows that the responding neurons were "set" in advance of CS presentation to respond with a situation-appropriate discharge, that is, a discharge predicated on "foreknowledge" of CS duration.

In summary, these data support the notion that cingulate cortical coding of associative attention is amplified *in proportion to the salience of expected cues,* thus to promote the likelihood that cues of low salience, which are nonetheless significant, will capture the subject's attention.

We have tentatively proposed that the information that sets cingulate cortical neurons in advance to produce an appropriate attentional discharge is information projected from the subicular complex of the hippocampal formation to cingulate cortex. The studies documenting these projections were recently summarized.[37] This hypothesis is based on the finding that cingulate cortical TIA is significantly attenuated in rabbits with subicular complex lesions.[38]

The present interpretation of cingulate cortical function suggests that the importance of the associative attentional processes of the cingulate cortex increases as the salience of the stimuli to be processed decreases. This line of reasoning suggests that behavioral deficits as well as disturbed cingulate cortical processes are particularly likely to occur in subjects exposed to cocaine *in utero,* when task-relevant cues are of low salience. Results compatible with this view were found in recent studies in which rabbits exposed to cocaine *in utero* underwent Pavlovian conditioning of the nictitating membrane response. The results showed that rabbits exposed to cocaine *in utero* were able to acquire the conditioned nictitating membrane response as rapidly as control rabbits when a salient CS+ and a nonsalient CS– were used. However, acquisition was significantly retarded in cocaine-exposed rabbits when a nonsalient CS+ and a salient CS– were used. These results were found when the CSs were of different modalities (a tone and a flashing light) and when the CSs were of the same modality (a loud and a soft tone).[39]

SECOND EXPERIMENT: A TEST OF THE HYPOTHESIS

Prologue. The foregoing findings and theoretical development led to the prediction that rabbits exposed to cocaine *in utero* would show impaired cingulate cortical TIA and impaired behavioral acquisition when trained with less salient conditional stimuli than those used in our standard training paradigm. To test this hypothesis Dutch-belted rabbits exposed to cocaine *in utero* and saline-exposed controls received discriminative avoidance training with 200-ms CSs rather than the standard 500-ms CSs. The selection of the 200-ms CSs was based on the aforementioned finding that the 200-ms CS duration is associated with a significantly enhanced cingulate cortical coding response relative to the 500-ms and 5.0-second CS durations. Recordings were obtained in the areas monitored in the previous study. In addition, recordings were made in the "medial prefrontal" cortex (Brodmann's area 32) and the basolateral amygdala. However, as this experiment is presently in progress, not all data have been collected and analyzed. We report here results of preliminary analyses of the behavioral data and the neuronal activity of the anterior cingulate cortex.

***Early Behavioral Learning Impaired in Rabbits Exposed to Cocaine* in Utero.** Analysis of the behavioral data supported the hypothesis that a learning deficit would emerge in rabbits exposed to cocaine *in utero* when discriminative avoidance training was conducted with CSs of low salience. The cocaine-exposed rabbits made significantly fewer conditioned avoidance responses than did the saline-exposed rabbits during the first session of avoidance training, as indicated by simple effect tests following a significant interaction of the Exposure Condition and Training Session factors of the analysis of variance ($p < 0.021$) (FIG. 6). Nevertheless, learning to a normative asymptote of discriminative performance did occur in the rabbits exposed to cocaine, and the number of sessions required for the attainment of the behavioral criterion by rabbits exposed to cocaine was not significantly different from the number of sessions required by controls. This early-stage learning deficit is similar in certain respects to deficits found previously in rabbits subjected to experimental lesions of the anterior cingulate cortex or the MD thalamic nucleus.[21] Rabbits with these lesions required more sesions than did controls to attain the acquisition criterion, but they exhibited normative asymptotic levels of performance when the criterion was reached.

***Anterior Cingulate Cortical Early Training Stage Discriminative Neuronal Activity Was Abolished and Sustained Neuronal Firing Was Attenuated in Rabbits Exposed to Cocaine* in Utero.** The rabbits exposed to cocaine *in utero* and trained with the brief, 200-ms, CSs exhibited significantly altered anterior cingulate cortical neuronal activity. The alterations found in the previous study with 500-ms CSs occurred in this study, and additional alterations not seen before were also found.

Just as found for discriminative behavior, discriminative TIA during the first session of training was abolished in the rabbits exposed to cocaine, whereas significant discriminative TIA did occur in the controls during the first session, and both saline- and cocaine-exposed rabbits exhibited significant discriminative TIA during attainment of the criterion of behavioral acquisition (FIG. 7). These effects were indicated by simple effect tests carried out after a significant interaction of the Exposure Condition, Training Stage, Stimulus, and Post-CS Interval factors of the analysis ($p < 0.001$).

Anterior cingulate cortical neurons in rabbits exposed to cocaine exhibited less sustained firing than did neurons in controls after cessation of the 200-ms CS. This effect is evident from comparison of the levels of neuronal firing exhibited by saline- and cocaine-exposed rabbits from 200 ms to 400 ms after CS onset (FIG. 8).

***The Post-Stimulus Inhibitory Firing Pause in Anterior Cingulate Cortex Was Eliminated in Rabbits Exposed to Cocaine* in Utero.** The average CS-related post-stimulus histograms in rabbits exposed to cocaine had a different "wave-shape" than did the histograms of the saline-exposed rabbits. Specifically, the histograms of the

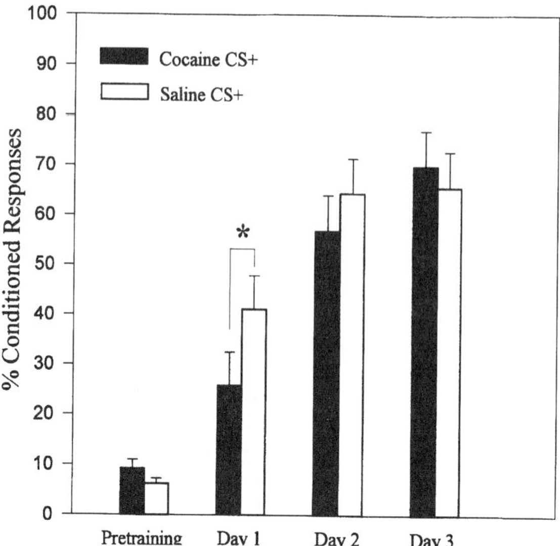

FIGURE 6. Average percentage of conditioned avoidance responses elicited by the CS+ in rabbits (male and female) exposed to cocaine or saline *in utero.* The percentage of trials in which avoidance responses were made was significantly reduced in cocaine-exposed rabbits during the first conditioning session (Day 1) as compared to the percentage of avoidance responses shown by controls. No significant between-group differences were noted in the incidence of avoidance responses in later sessions of training.

cocaine-exposed rabbits lacked the expected inhibitory pause, which occurred dramatically in controls from 40–80 ms after CS onset (FIG. 8) and which is a consistent feature of the CS-elicited temporal discharge profiles of neurons in the cingulate cortex and in the AV thalamic nucleus.[21]

Both the effects of prenatal cocaine on the inhibitory firing pause and sustained activity in the anterior cingulate cortex were based on the results of simple effect tests following a significant interaction of the Exposure Condition and Post-CS Interval factors of the analysis of variance ($p < 0.001$).

Finally, the previous finding of significantly reduced anterior cingulate cortical neuronal excitation in female rabbits exposed to cocaine relative to male rabbits exposed to cocaine was suggested by the occurrence of a significant interaction of the Exposure Condition, Sex, and Post-CS Interval factors ($p < 0.001$).

DISCUSSION

Hypothesis Supported. Rabbits exposed to cocaine *in utero* did not exhibit significant discriminative behavior in the initial session of discriminative avoidance training with 200-ms CSs, whereas similarly trained rabbits exposed to saline *in utero* did perform discriminative behavior in the initial session. By contrast, rabbits exposed to cocaine *in utero* and trained with 500-ms CSs learned to produce discriminative behavior in the first avoidance training session just as did saline-exposed controls. These results supported the hypothesis that behavioral acquisition would be impaired in rabbits exposed

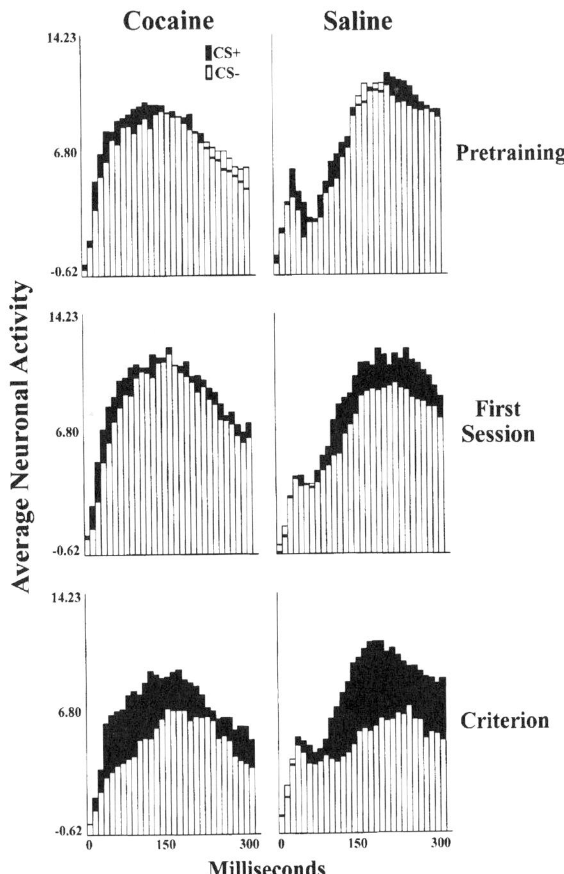

FIGURE 7. Average anterior cingulate cortical integrated multi-unit neuronal activity in 30 consecutive, 10-ms intervals after onset of brief (200-ms) conditional stimuli in rabbits (male and female) exposed to cocaine *in utero* and in saline-exposed controls. The onset of the CS+ and CS– occurred at the leftmost position on the horizontal axis of each panel. *Dark bars* indicate the neuronal response to the CS+ and *light bars* portray the neuronal response to the CS–. Data are shown for pretraining in which tones and unpaired footshock presentations were given, the first session of conditioning and the session of criterion attainment. Note the absence of training-induced discriminative neuronal activity in the first session of training *(left panel, second row)* in rabbits exposed to cocaine *in utero,* in contrast to the occurrence of significant discriminative activity present in saline-exposed controls *(right panel, second row).*

to cocaine if the attentional demands of the learning task were increased relative to the demands placed on attentional processing by standard training with 500-ms CSs.

These findings are also consistent with the more general hypothesis that cingulate cortex is importantly involved in the mediation of associative attention and that attention-relevant processes of cingulate cortex are disturbed in rabbits exposed to cocaine *in utero.* The fact that both the discriminative neuronal and behavioral deficits associated with prenatal cocaine exposure occurred in the first training session is consis-

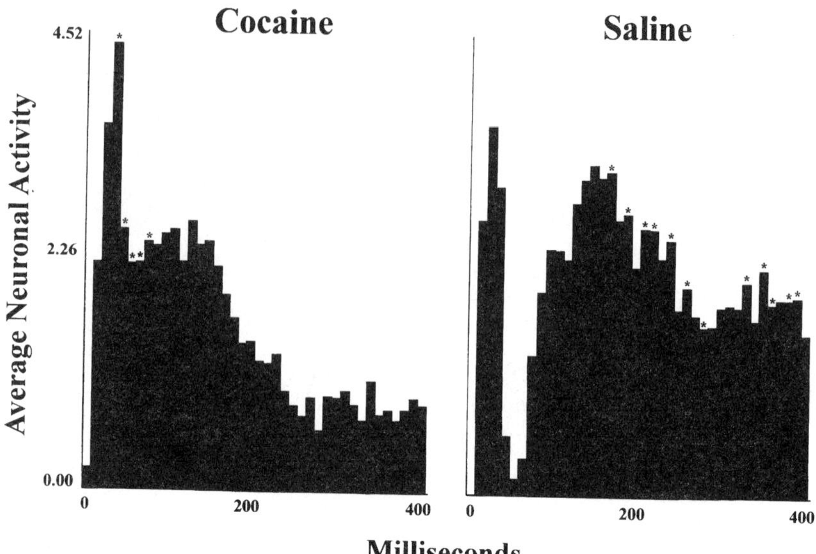

FIGURE 8. Average anterior cingulate cortical multi-unit spike frequency in 40 consecutive, 10-ms intervals after onset of brief (200-ms) conditional stimuli in rabbits (male and female) exposed to cocaine *in utero* and in saline-exposed controls. Data in each histogram are averages for all rabbits and training stages from pretraining to the session of criterion attainment. The onset of the conditional stimuli (CSs) occurred at the leftmost position on the horizontal axis of each panel. *Asterisks* indicate the occurrence of a significantly greater discharges in the indicated condition (prenatal exposure to saline or cocaine) than in the corresponding interval in the other condition.

tent with past results[21] indicating that anterior cingulate cortical processing is of particular importance for the early stages of behavioral acquisition.

***Behavioral Relevance of the Neuronal Changes Associated with Exposure to Cocaine* in Utero.** Rabbits exposed to cocaine *in utero* and trained with brief CSs showed a reduced amplitude of cingulate cortical CS-elicited neuronal activity, an absence of training-induced excitation, a loss of training-induced discrimination in the initial session of training, and abolition of the brief latency inhibitory neuronal firing pause. It is not possible with the present information to determine which, if any, of these changes are relevant to the first-session deficit of behavioral learning in the cocaine-exposed rabbits, as the neuronal data were correlative and not demonstrated as causal to the behavior. Yet, consideration of the specific findings can suggest which changes are of possible relevance to the behavioral effect.

Because the general loss of excitation associated with prenatal cocaine exposure in our experiment with 500-ms CSs was not associated with impaired behavioral learning, this phenomenon would not seem a compelling candidate for the substrate of the behavioral deficit. By contrast, the loss of discriminative firing in rabbits exposed to cocaine occurred in the very same session as did the loss of the behavior, and in both instances what was lost was discrimination between CS+ and CS–. Moreover, when behavioral discrimination did occur in later stages of training, so also did discriminative neuronal activity in the anterior cingulate cortex in rabbits exposed to cocaine. Thus, the loss of neuronal discrimination in the anterior cingulate cortex could have contributed to the impairment of the discriminative behavior, a possibility that receives further support from other studies which show that anterior cingulate cortical lesions produced learning impairment in the early stages of behavioral acquisition.

Loss of the brief-latency inhibitory "pause" component of the CS-elicited neuronal response in the anterior cingulate cortex was a most robust cocaine-related neuronal phenomenon in this study. Indeed, the magnitude of the inhibitory pause was larger in the saline-exposed rabbits trained with 200-ms CSs than in saline-exposed rabbits trained with 500-ms CSs. Thus, the magnitude of the inhibitory pause is a dynamic feature which may reflect directly the cue-related attentional "demand" made by a given conditioning paradigm. It is thus possible that the absence of the inhibitory pause in rabbits exposed to cocaine may be a direct neurologic indicant of impaired attention. The impaired attention could be related to the retardation of the discriminative neuronal activity and behavior during training in the rabbits exposed to cocaine *in utero* and trained with the brief CSs.

Resetting: Possible Functional Significance of the Cingulate Cortical Neuronal Firing Pause. Assume that different neurons in the anterior cingulate cortex fire at various rates and with various temporal patterns. It follows that some neurons would be engaged in bursting or rapid firing, whereas other neurons would be inactive at the moment of CS onset. Perhaps the momentary firing pause exhibited at CS onset by a large number of neurons in the population *resets* these neurons, thereby making them available for processing the CS. In the absence of resetting, many neurons already engaged in ongoing, rapid firing would not participate in processing the CS.

A putative dearth of neurons available for processing of the CSs due to resetting failure could have adverse consequences in the circuitry, such as failure to recruit existing modified synapses involved in classifying the incoming signal or retardation of synaptic plasticity development needed for the production of discriminative TIA.

Cellular Substrates of the Resetting Mechanism. It seems likely that the inhibitory pause of neuronal firing in the anterior cingulate cortex depends on the operation of GABA neurons in the cingulothalamic circuitry. For example, the arrival of the initial CS-triggered excitatory volley in anterior cingulate cortex could activate GABA neurons to rapidly and momentarily depress (reset) the firing of many neighboring cortical cells. It is noteworthy in this connection that the number of GABA-immunoreactive neurons in the anterior cingulate cortex was increased in rabbits exposed to cocaine *in utero.*[17] Perhaps disturbed activation of GABA neurons due to prenatal exposure to cocaine leads to a compensatory increase in the production of GABA neurons.

GABA Neurons and Dopamine Afferents. If the increased numbers of GABA neurons found in the anterior cingulate cortex in rabbits exposed to cocaine *in utero* were indeed the result of compensatory process, one can ask why the putative compensation did not work, that is, why did the increased GABA function presumably conferred by the increased numbers of GABA neurons fail to result in a restoration of the damaged resetting mechanism in anterior cingulate cortex?

A tentative answer is suggested by two additional findings. The first is the finding that dopamine-immunoreactive varicosities in anterior cingulate cortex interact abundantly with GABA neurons in anterior cingulate cortex.[40–42] This finding suggests that DA afferents represent an important source of afferent activation of cortical GABA neurons. The second finding is that of Friedman and colleagues[16] who demonstrated that the dopamine D_1 receptor is uncoupled from its G protein in rabbits exposed to cocaine *in utero.* This finding suggests a selective loss of D_1 related neurotransmission in the anterior cingulate cortex in cocaine-exposed subjects. Similarly, Little and Teyler[12] have shown that D_1-related modulation of hippocampal synaptic plasticity is significantly diminished in rabbits exposed to cocaine *in utero.*

Loss of D_1-related neurotransmission could induce the aforementioned compensatory increase in GABA neurons, yet if the basic defect in the circuit were a defect of D_1 neurotransmission, the increase in GABA neuron number would be without functional consequence.

These considerations suggest that the uncoupling of the D_1 receptor from its G protein may be the fundamental problem in rabbits exposed to cocaine *in utero.* As a result, the involvement of dopamine in the cue-triggered activation of GABA neurons would be disabled, thereby blocking key processes of associative attention in the anterior cingulate cortex.

REFERENCES

1. Mayes, L.C., R.H. Granger, M.A. Frank, R. Schottenfeld & M.H. Bornstein. 1993. Neurobehavioral profiles of neonates exposed to cocaine prenatally. Pediatrics **91:** 778–783.
2. Mayes, L.C., M.H. Bornstein, K. Chawarska & R.H. Granger. 1995. Information processing and developmental assessments in 3-month-old infants exposed prenatally to cocaine. Pediatrics **95:** 539–545.
3. Richardson, G.A., M.L. Conroy & N.L. Day. 1996. Prenatal cocaine exposure: Effects on the development of school-age children. Neurotoxicol. Teratol. **18:** 627–634.
4. Tronick, E.Z., D.A. Frank, H. Cabral, M. Mirochnick & B. Zuckerman. 1996. Late dose-response effects of prenatal cocaine exposure on newborn neurobehavioral performance. Pediatrics **98:** 76–83.
5. Barron, S. & J. Irvine. 1994. Behavioral effects of neonatal cocaine exposure using a rodent model. Pharmacol. Biochem. Behav. **50:** 107–114.
6. Church, M.W. & G.W. Overbeck. 1990. Prenatal cocaine exposure in the long-evans rat. II. Dose-dependent effects on offspring behavior. Neurotoxicol. Teratol. **12:** 335–343.
7. Heyser, C.J., N.E. Spear & L.P. Spear. 1992. Effects of prenatal exposure to cocaine on conditional discrimination learning in adult rats. Behav. Neurosci. **106:** 837–845.
8. Heyser, C.J., N.E. Spear & L.P. Spear. 1995. Effects of prenatal exposure to cocaine on Morris water maze performance in adult rats. Behav. Neurosci. **109:** 734–743.
9. Kosofsky, B.E., A.S. Wilkins, P. Gressens & P. Evrard. 1994. Transplacental cocaine exposure: A mouse model demonstrating neuroanatomic and behavioral abnormalities. J. Child Neurol. **9:** 234–241.
10. Vorhees, C.V., T.M. Reed, K.D. Acuff-Smith, M.A. Schilling, G.D. Cappon, J.E. Fisher & P. Cunfeng. 1995. Long-term learning deficits and changes in unlearned behaviors following in utero exposure to multiple daily doses of cocaine during different exposure periods and maternal plasma cocaine concentrations. Neurotoxicol. Teratol. **17:** 253–264.
11. Wang, H.-Y., S. Runyan, E. Yadin & E. Friedman. 1995. Prenatal exposure to cocaine selectively reduces D_1 dopamine receptor-mediated activation of striatal Gs proteins. J. Pharmacol. Exp. Ther. **273:** 492–498.
12. Little, J.Z. & T.J. Teyler. 1996. In utero exposure decreases dopamine D_1 receptor modulation of hippocampal long-term potentiation in the rabbit. Neurosci. Lett. **215:** 157–160.
13. Little, J.Z. & T.J. Teyler. 1996. Prenatal cocaine exposure leads to enhanced long-term potentiation in region CA1 of hippocampus. Dev. Brain Res. **92:** 117–119.
14. Levitt, P., J.A. Harvey, E. Friedman, K. Simansky & E.H. Murphy. 1997. New evidence for neurotransmitter influences on brain development. Trends Neurosci. **20:** 269–274.
15. Wang, H.-Y., J.M. Yeung & E. Friedman. 1995. Prenatal cocaine exposure selectively reduces mesocortical dopamine release. J. Pharmacol. Exp. Ther. **273:** 1211–1215.
16. Friedman, E., E. Yadin & H.-Y. Wang. 1996. Effects of prenatal cocaine on dopamine receptor-G protein coupling in mesocortical regions of rabbit brain. Neuroscience **70:** 739–747.
17. Wang, X.-H., P. Levitt, D.R. Grayson & E.H. Murphy. 1995. Intrauterine cocaine exposure of rabbits: Persistent elevation of GABA-immunoreactive neurons in anterior cingulate cortex but not visual cortex. Brain Res. **689:** 32–46.

18. Wang, X.-H., A.O. Jenkins, L. Choi & E.H. Murphy. 1996. Altered neuronal distribution of parvalbumin in anterior cingulate cortex of rabbits exposed in utero to cocaine. Exp. Brain Res. **112:** 359–371.
19. Jones, L., I. Fischer & P. Levitt. 1996. Nonuniform alteration of dendritic development in the cerebral cortex following prenatal cocaine exposure. Cereb. Cortex **6:** 431–445.
20. Vogt, B.A. & M. Gabriel. 1993. Neurobiology of Cingulate Cortex and Limbic Thalamus: A Comprehensive Handbook. Birkhäuser. Boston, MA.
21. Gabriel, M. 1993. Discriminative avoidance learning: A model system. *In* Neurobiology of Cingulate Cortex and Limbic Thalamus: A Comprehensive Handbook. B. Vogt & M. Gabriel, Eds.: 478–523. Birkhäuser. Boston, MA.
22. Poremba, A. & M. Gabriel. 1997. Amygdalar lesions block discriminative avoidance learning and limbic system training-induced neuronal activity in rabbits. J. Neurosci. **17:** 5237–5244.
23. Poremba, A. & M. Gabriel. 1997. Medial geniculate lesions block amygdalar and cingulothalamic learning-related neuronal activity. J. Neurosci. **17:** 8645–8655.
24. Murphy, E.H., J.G. Hammer, M.D. Schumann, M.Y. Groce, X.-H. Wang, L. Jones, A.G. Romano & J.H. Harvey. 1995. The rabbit as a model for studies of cocaine exposure in utero. Lab. Anim. Sci. **45:** 163–168.
25. Brogden, W.J. & F.A. Culler. 1936. A device for motor conditioning of small animals. Science **83:** 269.
26. Taylor, C., J. H. Freeman, Jr., W. Holt & M. Gabriel. 1998. Impairment of cingulothalamic learning-related coding in rabbits exposed to cocaine in utero: General and sex-specific effects. Submitted.
27. Hutching, D.E., T.A. Fico & D.L. Dow-Edwards. 1989. Prenatal Cocaine: Maternal toxicity, fetal effects and locomotor activity in rat offspring. Neurotoxicol. Teratol. **11:** 65–69.
28. Spear, L.P., C.L. Kirstein, J. Bell, V. Yoottanasumpun, R. Greenbaum, J. O'Shea, H. Hoffmann & N.E. Spear. 1989. Effects of prenatal cocaine exposure on behavior during the early postnatal period. Neurotoxicol. Teratol. **11:** 57–63.
29. Blitzke, P.J. & M.W. Church. 1992. Prenatal cocaine and alcohol exposures affect rat behavior in a stress test (the porsolt swim test). Neurotoxicol. Teratol. **14:** 359–364.
30. Molina, V.A., J.M. Wagner & L.P. Spear. 1994. The behavioral response to stress is altered in adult rats exposed prenatally to cocaine. Physiol. Behav. **55:** 941–945.
31. Wood, R.D., V.A. Molina, J.M. Wagner & L.P. Spear. 1995. Play behavior and stress responsivity in periadolescent offspring exposed prenatally to cocaine. Pharmacol. Biochem. Behav. **52:** 367–374.
32. Mogenson, G.J., S.M. Brudzynski, M. Wu, C.R. Yang & C.Y. Yim. 1993. From motivation to action: A review of dopaminergic regulation of limbic, nucleus accumbens, ventral pallidum, peduculopontine nucleus circuitries involved in limbic-motor integration. *In* Limbic Motor Circuits and Neuropsychiatry. P.W. Kalivas & C.D. Barnes, Eds.: 193–236. CRC Press. Boca Raton.
33. Gabriel, M., C. Cuppernell, J.I. Shenker, Y. Kubota, V. Henzi & D. Swanson. 1995. Mammillothalamic tract transection blocks anterior thalamic training-induced neuronal plasticity and impairs discriminative avoidance behavior in rabbits. J. Neurosci. **15:** 1437–1445.
34. Smith, D.M., J.H. Freeman, Jr., D. Nicholson, M. boule & M. Gabriel. 1997. Limbic thalamic lesions, approach learning, and cingulate cortical neuronal activity in rabbits (abstr.). Soc. Neuro. Abstr. **23:** 1617.
35. Sparenborg, S. & M. Gabriel. 1990. Neuronal encoding of conditional stimulus duration in the cingulate cortex and the limbic thalamus of rabbits. Behav. Neurosci. **104:** 919–933.
36. Gabriel, M., K. Foster & E. Orona. 1980. Interaction of the laminae of cingulate cortex and the anteroventral thalamus during behavioral learning. Science **208:** 1050–1052.
37. Amaral, D.G. & M.P. Witter. 1995. Hippocampal formation. *In* The Rat Nervous System. G. Paxinos, Ed.: 443–493 Academic Press. San Diego, CA.
38. Gabriel, M., S. Sparenborg & N. Stolar. 1987. Hippocampal control of cingulate cortical and anterior thalamic information processing during learning in rabbits. Exp. Brain Res. **67:** 131–152.

39. WILKINS, A.S., B.E. KOSOFSKY, A.G. ROMANO & J.A. HARVEY. 1996. Transplacental cocaine exposure: Behavioral consequences. *In* Prenatal Cocaine Exposure. R.J. Konkol & G.D. Olsen, Eds.: 149–165. CRC Press. Boca Raton.

40. BERGER, B. & C. VERNEY. 1984. Development of the catecholamine innervation in rat neocortex. Morphological features. *In* Monoamine Innervation of Cerebral Cortex. L. Descarries, T.R. Reader & H. H. Jasper, Eds.: 95–121. Alan R. Liss. New York, NY.

41. BENES, F.M., S.L. VINCENT & R. MOLLOY. 1993. Dopamine-immunoreactive axon varicosities form nonrandom contacts with GABA-immunoreactive neurons in rat medial prefrontal cortex. Synapse **15:** 285–295.

42. BENES, F.M., S.L. VINCENT, R. MOLLOY & Y. KHAN. 1996. Increased interaction of dopamine-immunoreactive varicosities with GABA neurons of rat medial prefrontal cortex occurs during the postweanling period. Synapse **23:** 237–245.

Round Table 3. Specificity of Developmental Effects in the CNS

Moderator: DONNA FERRIERO
Panelists: PATRICIA WHITAKER-AZMITIA, PAT LEVITT, OLINE K. RØNNEKLEIV, MICHAEL LIDOW
Discussants: KEN SIMANSKY (*Allegheny*), MERLE PAULE (*Arkansas*), TREVOR ROBBINS (*Cambridge*), HAZEL MURPHY (*Allegheny*), JEROME MEYER (*UMass*), EITAN FRIEDMAN (*Allegheny*), LINDA SPEAR (*Binghampton*), JAMES R. WOODS (*Rochester*), JOHN HARVEY (*Allegheny*)
Addendum: DONNA FERRIERO

KEN SIMANSKY: Dr. Lidow, I was struck by that fact that on P1, differences in receptor density that you reported disappeared. This relates to Dr. Ronnekleiv's monkey study also, because the D_1 receptors were elevated in both embryonically. That raises an issue about how important the changes that you see embryonically are for the development and subsequent behavior of the animal. the differences you described were very small, even those statistically significant differences in alpha-binding, and that was normalized on the basis of areas. So you're saying that there is a slight sparsity of those receptors, but a higher level of monoamine transmitter is available. The specific question is: Do you think there is any functional effect of that small change in alpha-receptors?

MICHAEL LIDOW: You have to remember that the dopaminergic receptors or adrenergic receptors that we are effecting are present in development in the cells that are no longer like in dividing cells. Migrating cells, which are no longer present in adulthood, may have a normal dopaminergic system. The dopamine effect may be gone, but there are some structural abnormalities that have to be treated maybe in a totally different way, maybe not even as dopamine or noradrenaline abnormalities, so something else has to be devised.

As far as levels of changes, it's really difficult to draw conclusions regarding statistical significance. With two selected timepoints, you don't know what's in between, so it is difficult to say what the implication of it is. Going back to a previous discussion, it is difficult to say whether such changes are clinically relevant or not. For this initial study I just wanted to see if there is a change. In the next study I am hoping to look at the actual mechanisms: Is there a change in addition to receptors? Is there a second messenger change? Is there some structural property change. I believe there is.

MERLE PAULE: The plasma levels you got were actually about the same as those reported by the previous presenter who gave 0.3 mg or 3 mg/kg IM. My question is: Since the plasma levels are not that high, what made you think that you couldn't go higher with an oral administration, if you really wanted to go to toxic levels? Your animals were still eating and everything seemed fine.

MICHAEL LIDOW: As I said, it's slightly higher. As far as I understand in this model, they last longer.

MERLE PAULE: Right, they do last a lot longer, but the maximal levels are about the same.

MICHAEL LIDOW: I know that it's a maximal level because when I actually did the experiment, I killed the monkey before I came up with the dosage. In the first animal I was giving a dosage. Then I said, fine, let's go higher and higher, until at 15 mg/kg, the animal died.

MERLE PAULE: The other question I had, with respect to the changing in dopamine receptor system functionality or any of the other biogenic amines, we have data (see our poster paper in this volume) showing that the response of living animals to challenges by cocaine and amphetamine are clearly developmentally dependent in that young animals are very insensitive to the behavioral effects of cocaine or amphetamine and get more sensitive as they get older.

TREVOR ROBBINS: I've got a question for Pat Levitt. I was struck by the changes in GABAergic neuron circuitry in the anterior cingulate consequent to D_1 receptor uncoupling. It was reminiscent of what I've read about Francine Bennes's results on the postmortem schizophrenic brain. Is that an informative parallel for either the fetal syndrome or schizophrenia?

PAT LEVITT: Why don't you answer that, Hazel.

HAZEL MURPHY: Francine Bennes has been looking at postmortem material from schizophrenic brains, and there are interesting parallels. The two major effects that she described which are specific for the anterior cingulate cortex, which is the area that we found to be targeted, are a change in the number of GABAergic neurons (and she finds it's predominately in the super granular layers, especially in lamina 2) and an 80% increase in innervation of glutamatergic fibers innervating the cortex. What she postulated is that there is this imbalance with excess excitation and a breakdown of the inhibitory system which is characteristic of the anterior cingulate cortex in schizophrenia. Although obviously we are not saying that the symptoms of schizophrenia and prenatal cocaine exposure are the same, there are some similarities in terms of effects of selective attention and so on.

The other interesting thing, which we haven't published yet, we found looking at subunits for GABA receptors. The changes we find there are predominately in lamina 2 which is where Dr. Bennes found her effects. Although we haven't looked at glutamate innervation, quantitative electron microscopy indicated a huge increase in excitatory synapses in this area. So the parallels are very similar, and there is increasing evidence that schizophrenia may well have its origins at the time of fetal development. The two studies at least give an indication of maybe some generality in terms of specificity of target and some of the basic mechanisms.

PATRICIA WHITAKER-AZMITIA: I'd just like to add to the comments about schizophrenia. There are now several studies showing that GAP43 is overexpressed in the hippocampus in schizophrenics, so there may be other markers of brain immaturity that could be seen in the cocaine model that we also see in the schizophrenic one.

JERRY MEYER: First, I have a question for Dr. Lidow and then a comment for the whole panel to take up. The cortical data are very interesting, but I have to raise questions about your rather interesting hypothesis about the neurotransmitter transfer from the mother to the fetus. I am aware of the *Nature* paper on the DBH knockout that you're talking about. The only problem with applying that to this situation is that earlier work, which you're probably aware of, in which there actually were studies of transport of radiolabeled norepinephrine from mother rodents to fetus, showed only small amounts of transport. There was some, but not a lot. I question then is whether there would be enough of such transport to produce high levels of these substances in the brain of the fetus. Second, in relating this to cocaine, the transport that does occur may well require, at least in substantial part, the neurotransmitter transporters in the placenta which would presumably be blocked by the cocaine. So there are two points: first, is there enough getting across, and second, what's happening when cocaine is there on board to block the placental transporters?

MICHAEL LIDOW: The majority of previous work, much of it done in the 1970s, suggests that no significant "barrier" is represented by the placenta. There were also several studies, similar to what I presented, in which they looked at the levels of monoaminergic neurotransmitters in the fetal brain before and after birth, which showed that the levels, for example, of serotonin and its metabolites are higher in the developing fetal cortex than in the adult animal.

PAT LEVITT: There's still evidence that it comes from the maternal side. In fact, there are fibers there very early on, and it's likely that a large amount of that is **not** produced locally in the cortex.

MICHAEL LIDOW: But again, there are data specifically in the monkey presented by Pat Goldman-Rakic and Roger Brown which show that at birth the activity level of the synthetic machinery is not that well developed at the time of birth in monkey than it is in the first year or two of life. With time, the level of neurotransmitter and the synthetic enzymes actually increase tremendously. The hypothesis that I am presenting is just a hypothesis. It's just one of the views, and I'm not trying to say that everything else is wrong.

JERRY MEYER: I also had a comment for the panel as a whole. One of the questions that was raised earlier, a comment, was that in Dr. Levitt's model system he was finding some interesting effects on the dopamine system and also in GABA. In Dr. Whitaker-Azmitia's work we saw some very interesting changes in the serotonergic system and the question was raised about how you reconcile those things. The fact, at least as far as I know, is that as far as what you've presented, you haven't really looked at what each other has looked for. It's great that we have different models and different species, using different routes of administration and different timings, because we have so much heterogeneity in the human situation in terms of when women take cocaine, how much, and by what route. However, it would really be tremendously valuable if some investigators who have well worked-out models could exchange tissues, perhaps, and look at some of the things using their tools in a different species and in a different model of administration, to see if some of these things, in fact, can be replicated and found to be generalizable. If we can get that sort of thing going, it would be very powerful.

PAT LEVITT: Hazel Murphy and I published a paper 1 or 2 years ago on the rabbit model, looking at TH and 5-HT innervation of the cortex. We did not find, given the IV route of administration in the model we used, was a delayed development of those systems as reported in the rat model. So there are the identical methodologies used to assay the same systems. In one case we were giving low dose IV versus a higher dose IP. In two different species you don't see the same change to those neurotransmitter systems. We also looked at astroglial development in the rabbit model and didn't see the same changes as in the rodent model. It's not necessarily surprising given the differences in the amount of the drug and how many sites it can bind in terms of the qualitative and quantitative differences in the duration of binding to the targeted neurotransmitter systems that may be affected differently depending on the route.

They did a simple experiment of giving tritiated-WIN-**35,428** IP and IV in the adult monkey. When they looked at binding in the adult monkey brain, they saw very different patterns of binding with two different routes of administration. They did really careful anatomic analysis. That's enough for me to think that it's very complicated and that with different models, even when you go back and try to look at the same system as we've done and compare it to the rodent, we just don't see the same things.

MICHAEL LIDOW: While what I have just shown seems a little out of whack with the rest of the models, it actually replicated very well the mouse model which Barry Kosofsky is going to present later.

SPEAKER: If I could just add something on differences between serotonin and dopamine. We've concentrated on the dopamine system, but one of the members of our group, Tim Tyler, who has been doing slice recordings from the hippocampus in the rabbits, has found significant changes in LTP and LTD in hippocampal neurons and also has data implicating the serotonergic system in that model. Despite their differences in route of administration and dose, there does seem, comparability and similarity. Eitan Friedman will probably describe that the changes that he's going to talk about were also found in the mouse model. It is important to compare data across models, and we've certainly been trying to do that with mouse and rat in terms of data that we have accumulated with the rabbit model.

EITAN FRIEDMAN: I want to emphasize some uniformity across some studies. We received some mouse brains that were treated by Barry Kosofsky and we found similar changes in uncoupling of D_1 receptors in these mice as we did in our rabbits. Next slide which he didn't I wonder if Michael wants to add something regarding his findings on uncoupling.

MICHAEL LIDOW: Basically when I heard about your findings in the rabbit, I happened to be doing receptor binding. I tried to replicate those findings, and I did see that after 50 days of cocaine treatment there was uncoupling of D_1 receptors throughout the cortex.

EITAN FRIEDMAN: I have another comment. Dr. Ronnekleiv, you mentioned a decrease in TH in the midbrain. Since this is the site of synthesis of these proteins, wouldn't a decrease suggest that later you might find decreases or changes in those and other structures.

OLINE K. RØNNEKLEIV: We did see a decrease in TH mRNA just in the substantia nigra and ventral tegmental area, but we have not looked later in gestation. We're starting those studies now to see if this holds up.

EITAN FRIEDMAN: Wouldn't that suggest that if you looked later on, you'd find decreases, because this is where protein synthesis takes place, right in the cell body.

OLINE K. RØNNEKLEIV: You have to remember that in our studies we treated with cocaine throughout gestation, and when we killed the animals, we took the fetuses about 50 minutes after last cocaine injection. We think it is a specific effect of cocaine. Now if we looked later in gestation and after a time of withdrawal, we might not see these changes. Based on studies in the rat, the steady-state level might be similar in controls versus cocaine-exposed animals. what I think is happening is what has been emphasized in rodent studies, that if you challenge the system, you will see these changes which I believe happen to this intracellular transduction system in these fetuses that were exposed to cocaine just as their systems are developing.

EITAN FRIEDMAN: Yes, I had another suggestion. Many studies in various animals showed that turnover of dopamine is either increased or unchanged. My suggestion would be that since measuring protein levels or mRNA may not reflect the activity of the enzyme, perhaps it would be worthwhile to look and measure actual enzymatic activity because tyrosine hydroxylase is an extremely regulated enzyme.

OLINE K. RØNNEKLEIV: Yes, I totally agree with that. If I was working in a different species where I had unlimited access to material, those would be the first studies I would do. Working with monkeys, with limited animals, and difficulties in getting funding, I just have to set priorities.

LINDA SPEAR: I wanted to comment on one other thing that may help us sort out some of the differences that we are seeing across models. This is something that we really have no idea about. Are the teratogenic effects observed attributable to the peak amount of cocaine that is reached or is it area under the curve? These different models are producing different levels, and we don't understand it. That has never been worked out for cocaine as far as I know, although it has been for alcohol. It's really area under the curve that is critical, and it isn't peak levels that are reached, whereas with other model systems, it's very much the peak amount that gets into the system. It may well be that whether it is peak levels or area under the curve could depend on what system and what independent measure you're looking at, as to whether what is the most critical factor affecting which is happening with the cocaine levels. So with these different models across species and also across routes, you're talking about big differences in area under the curve vs. peak levels.

MICHAEL LIDOW: On behalf of me and Oline, I could say that we are in real difficulty, because monkeys are very expensive. Moreover, at a certain point, you invest in designing your model and you are stuck with it, because whatever changes you go through, that enormous amount of money just gets you a couple of animals anyway. A single monkey for me is at least is $3,000 without housing. So how much could I actually go and check changes in concentrations, levels and so on. That's unfortunately the limitation for us.

JAMES R. WOODS: I have a question for Michael on the animals that died. This is a very interesting and seldom examined question, that is, how do people really get into trouble in pregnancy when they are using high-dose cocaine? In sheep, when you give it intravenously, you get cardiac arrhythmias first and then a strychnine-type seizure pattern just before death. When June Morheimo infused cocaine in the rat at very high levels, there were neurologic, neurotoxic effects first and only cardiovascular effects last. I've never heard of anybody giving it orally. How did these animals die? Did they have cardiac problems first and then have seizure? Did they seize and is that what you saw as the single event?

MICHAEL LIDOW: We started with 3 mg the first day, then we went to 4 mg, then everyday we were going higher, higher, and higher. Then one morning we gave 15 mg and the animal seemed to be dazed, but okay. I stayed with the animal for about half an hour. There was nothing that I could think of as abnormal, but when I came back 1 hour later, it was dead. So, I really wasn't there to see what happened.

JOHN HARVEY: I just wanted to comment about what one sees and what one doesn't see. Ten or perhaps 15 years ago nobody would have seen anything in these cocaine-treated animals because we didn't have the tools. God knows what we don't see today that we might see with some other probes.

There is another issue. If you are affecting any part of the brain, whether you're seeing a serotonin effect but not a dopamine effect or vice versa, it doesn't mean that the serotonin system isn't affected. The function can be very different because these systems aren't just sitting there by themselves. They're all talking to other systems, and they're going to have effects downstream that could result in large changes in the animal's response to drugs or whatever event might occur where you're going to have to activate a particular system, whether it's dopamine and you're activating the thalamus, and the cortex and the cerebellum. You're dealing with systems and what you're showing us, which is very important, is where those systems can be very vulnerable.

There is no question that there is a big difference in the route of administration. Sensitization and distribution of drugs change even on the second or third injection. At some point all of us have to a bite the bullet and see what we can find out about where these drugs really are at the times that we think are important.

BARRY KOSOFSKY: What is commonly seen is the response of the nervous system to achieve homeostasis. That balance of signaling whether it's a growth factor signaling system or a neurotransmitter signaling system appears to be very important for the nervous system to achieve, and when it's jarred in any particular way, it goes to great lengths to try to rebalance itself. It appears that what we're seeing reflected in each of these systems that is being discussed is basically what Steve Hyman talked about at the molecular level. It's basically trying to balance excitation/inhibition to achieve homeostasis. When I say excitation/inhibition I mean systems that are integrating information over a period of time, and developmentally that may mean something a little different than in the adult brain. When it tries to achieve that in development, it has significant consequences.

JOHN HARVEY: I guess I'm trying to put in a word for functional studies that try to relate themselves specifically to the anatomic system.

SPEAKER: The serotonin and dopamine systems, in particular, are well known to be interactive in development, and with 6-hydroxy-dopamine lesions in the neonate, you get sprouting of the serotonin system. We have shown decreased outgrowth of serotonin terminals in animals treated with the D_1 agonist SKF38393. There's a lot of interplay between those systems in particular.

DONNA FERRIERO: This has been a wonderful session and we have seen how difficult a task it is to study a system, especially the developing nervous system, which is on an incredibly steep slope and differs from model to model, and to apply principles learned from one system to another is extraordinarily difficult. I see the makings of a multicenter, research center, funded by all of our colleagues at NIH, just right around the corner, after this session, as soon as we go home and write the grants.

BARRY KOSOFSKY: I want to thank all of the speakers and Donna Ferriero for doing such a marvelous job. This is the state-of-the-art in terms of developmental mechanisms that underlie some of the toxic effects of gestational cocaine exposure. As John alluded to, we will consider functional deficits, and whether certain brain systems may be dysfunctional as a consequence of that exposure.

* * * * *

Addendum

DONNA M. FERRIERO

Departments of Neurology and Pediatrics, University of California San Francisco, San Francisco, California 94143-0114

In the first presentation, "Altered Brain Maturation in Rodents," Dr. Patricia Whitaker-Azmitia describes elegant studies in a rat model which suggest that cocaine might interact with developing astroglial cells at the level of the synapse. Using the trophic factor S100b as a marker for stabilized synapses, she has shown decreased S100 and serotonin immunoreactive terminals at P7 in the forebrain, suggesting that cocaine, through release of serotonin and depletion at the synapse, may modulate synaptogenesis.[1] In addition, she shows stunted growth of dissociated raphe neurons taken from E14 fetal rat brain in the presence of cocaine but not coca-ethylene, a metabolite of cocaine and alcohol. Using vimentin as a marker for radial glial cells, she demonstrates a delay in immunoreactive staining in cortical white matter.[2] These data are intriguing in light of preliminary observations in children exposed to cocaine *in utero* whose only remarkable MRI finding is delay in white matter myelination.[3] Could the delay in myelination in humans be analogous to that seen in the developing rodent as illustrated here? Dr. Whitaker-Azmitia also describes microcephaly in these cocaine-exposed rodents, as evidenced by decreased cell proliferation by BrdU staining and retarded neurite outgrowth by GAP-43 immunoreactivity.[2] One consistent observation from the human studies, both retrospective and prospective in design, has been decreased head circumference in the offspring of cocaine-abusing mothers.[4]

Dr. Pat Levitt, in his chapter entitled "*In utero* Cocaine Exposure Causes Targeted Changes in Cortical Development," presents data showing that apical dendrites of the anterior cingulate cortex course abnormally through the cortical layers of the rabbit brain prenatally exposed to cocaine.[5] Perhaps more importantly, this abnormality appears to be selective for this area of cortex, which is a dopamine-rich region. Drs. Murphy and Levitt also show that in addition to the structural changes in pyramidal neurons, the distribution of parvalbumin is increased in dendrites of gaba-ergic neurons and that coupling of the D1-like receptor and G proteins is decreased.[6] Although structural changes in the apical dendrites are unaffected by dose of cocaine, the distribution of the calcium-binding protein and the coupling changes are lost at lower doses. There are no data yet in humans to relate dose-effect and response, but these findings are particularly exciting because lesions of the cingulate cortex can result in changes in behavior such as attention and aggressivity.[7] In children born after *in utero* cocaine exposure, consistent changes in attention, impulsivity, and aggressivity cannot be accounted for by other confounding variables.[8–10]

Dr. Oline Rønnekleiv, in her chapter entitled "Changes in the Dopamine Circuitry in the Cocaine-Exposed Primate Fetal Brain," shows changes in dopamine precursor and receptor regulation as well as effects on enkephalin and dynorphin gene expression. Using a rhesus monkey model of *in utero* cocaine exposure, she found decreased tyrosine hydroxylase mRNA at E60 in substantia nigra and ventral tegmental areas, with increases in D1, D2, and D5 receptor expression in frontal cortex and striatum.[11,12] She also demonstrates an interaction with opioid expression in these areas. Cocaine-exposed brains have increased enkephalin mRNA in D2 receptor-rich areas of frontal cortex and striatum, whereas dynorphin mRNA is increased in the striatum and nucleus accumbens regions, areas rich in D1 receptors.[13] Normally, dopamine inhibits opioid gene expression through D2 receptor coupling to Gi/Go and inhibition of adenylyl cyclase. The increased expression of these opioid peptides may implicate signaling through G protein-coupled receptor kinases and protein kinase A pathways. Can we speculate on these data and relate these findings to developmental changes in human brain? The neurobehavioral correlates of *in utero* cocaine exposure are still mysterious, but preliminary data from investigators studying neonatal intoxication and withdrawal suggest that parallels might exist. Perhaps the early depression seen after cocaine intoxication in the neonate[14] is related to a cocaine-driven imbalance in the expression of the opioids in regions related to arousal. The neurotransmitter signaling abnormalities seen in the midbrain in both rodent and primate models may relate to the observed finding of hypertonia found in cocaine-exposed children neonatally and through the first few years of life.[15] Data showing that brain stem auditory responses in the neonatal period are predictive of poor neurological outcome may be strengthened by the animal findings of midbrain neurotransmitter disturbances.[16]

Finally, Dr. Michael Lidow, in his paper entitled "Effect of Cocaine Exposure on Cerebral Cortical Development in Non-Human Primates," describes, in another rhesus monkey model using a different route of administration of cocaine, data that are reminiscent of those shown by Dr. Whitaker-Azmitia in the rat model. Dr. Lidow demonstrates blurring of cortical layers and white matter zones at 2 months postnatally.[17] Altered lamination is evidenced by a decreased number of (^{3}H) thymidine-labeled cells in layers IV and V, as well as the presence of labeled cells in white matter regions and layer VI. Dr. Lidow also observes decreased GFAP-positive fibers in upper cortical layers. These anatomical similarities between monkey and rodent brain strengthen the correlations of human findings of delayed white matter myelination and microcephaly seen

TABLE 1. Correlations in Animal Models and Human after Gestational Cocaine Exposure

Observation	Nonhuman Species	Human Correlates
Microcephaly	Mouse, rat, rhesus monkey	Present through early childhood
Cortical astroglial delay	Rat, rhesus monkey	Myelination delay by MRI
Cingulate cortex abnormalities	Rabbit	Behavioral changes
Midbrain serotonin abnormalities	Rat	Neonatal ABR abnormalities
		Dysomnia
		Hypertonia
Midbrain and striatal dopamine-opioid interactions	Rhesus monkey	Neonatal depression and ABR abnormalities
	Hypertonia	

in children after cocaine exposure. These observations might allow for the development of subsequent behavioral animal models to relate structural abnormalities to later functional disturbances. In addition to these findings, Dr. Lidow shows that in cocaine-exposed monkey brain, blood vessels in the subventricular zone are positive for D1 receptors at E90. This finding raises the possibility of vasogenic regulation of CNS development by cocaine. If there is vasoreactivity in these developing progenitor zones, would this explain the increase in injury manifested by the presence of periventricular leucomalacia and deep gray matter abnormalities in term infants exposed to cocaine and amphetamines?[18] Are developing oligodendrocytes sensitive to changes in the vascular environment? Many questions raised by these findings will need to be answered by the combination of functional neuroimaging and neurobehavioral studies in monkeys surviving into maturity after gestational exposure.

Are we able then, at this point in our research endeavors, to claim specificity of effects of developmental exposure to cocaine? The data presented here certainly provide a fertile beginning for the study of neurobehavioral effects of gestational drug exposure in humans (TABLE 1). However, the problems of confounding variables, dealt with in human studies, must be addressed in our animal models as well. Now that findings have substantiated a role of disturbed central nervous system development after pure cocaine exposure, models must be developed that can mimic the effects of variables confounding the human condition. Is this feasible? Can research dollars be allocated for the development of animal models of polydrug exposure? There are relatively few women who abuse cocaine during their pregnancy who do not smoke cigarettes, drink alcohol and coffee, and eat poorly. Obviously, nicotine, carbon monoxide, ethanol, caffeine, and malnourishment have all been implicated in various model systems as causing or affecting central nervous system processes. How can we best dissect out the multiplicity and variability of these interactions at the level of the synapse? Are we studying biological phenomena that will lead us to correct assumptions? And ultimately, will these assumptions provide avenues for therapy, not only for the drug-exposed neonate and child, but also for the pregnant woman who needs intervention to stop the vicious cycle? Only collaborative research by investigators who work hand in hand, bench to bedside, will lead us to our goal.

REFERENCES

1. AKBARI, H.M., PM WHITAKER-AZMITIA & EC AZMITIA. 1994. Prenatal cocaine decreases the trophic factor S-100b and induces micorcephaly: Reversal by postnatal 5HT1alpha receptor agonist. Neurosci. Lett. **170:** 141–144.

2. Clarke, C., K. Clarke, J. Muneyyirci, E. Azmitia & P.M. Whitaker-Azmitia. 1996. Prenatal cocaine delays astroglial maturity: Immunodensitometry shows prolieration and production of the growth factor S-100. Brain Res. Dev. Brain Res. **91:** 268–273.
3. Latal Hajnal, B., J.C. Partridge, W.V. Good, C.H. Tsay & D.M. Ferriero. 1995. Neurologic and ophthalmologic abnormalities in infants with prenatal cocaine exposure. Ann. Neurol. **38:** 542A.
4. Zuckerman, B., D. A. Frank, R. Hingson *et al.* 1989. Effects of maternal marijuana and cocaine on fetal growth. New Engl. J. Med. **320:** 762–767.
5. Jones, L., I. Fischer & P. Levitt. 1996. Nonuniform alteration of dendritic development in the cerebral cortex following prenatal cocaine exposure. Cereb. Cortex **6:** 431–445.
6. Murphy, E. H., I. Fischer, E. Friedman, D. Grayson, L. Jones, P. Levitt, *et al.* 1997. Cocaine administration in pregnant rabbits alters cortical structure and function in their progeny in the absence of maternal seizures. Exp. Brain Res. **114:** 433–441.
7. Vogt, B.A., D.M. Finch & C.R. Olson. 1992. Functional heterogeneity in cingulate cortex: The anterior executive and posterior evaluative regions. Cereb. Cortex **1:** 434–443.
8. Bendersky, M. & M. Lewis. 1997. Prenatal cocaine exposure and impulse control at two years. Ann. N. Y. Acad. Sci., this volume.
9. Richardson, G.A. 1997. Prenatal cocaine exposure: A longitudinal study of development. Ann. N.Y. Acad. Sci., this volume.
10. Chasnoff, I.J. 1997. Prenatal cocaine exposure: Cognitive and behavioral development at six years of age. Ann. N.Y. Acad. Sci., this volume.
11. Choi, W.S. & O. Ronnekleiv. 1996. Effects of *in utero* cocaine exposure on expression of mRNAs encoding dopamine transporters and D1, D2 and D5 receptor subtypes in fetal rhesus monkeys. Brain Res. Dev. Brain Res. **96:** 249–260.
12. Ronnekleiv, O.K. & B.R. Naylor. 1995. Chronic cocaine exposure in fetal rhesus monkeys: Consequence for early development of dopamine neurons. J. Neurosci. **15:** 7330–7343.
13. Chai, L., W.S. Choi & O.K. Ronnekleiv. 1997. Maternal cocaine treatment alters dynoprhin and enkephalin mRNA expression in fetal rehesus macaques. J. Neurosci. **17:** 1112–1121.
14. Dempsey, D.A., D.M. Ferriero & S.N. Jacobson. 1996. Critical review of evidence for neonatal cocaine intoxication and withdrawal. *In* Prenatal Cocaine Exposure. R.J. Konkol & G.D. Olsen, Eds. : 115–141. CRC Press. New York, NY.
15. Chiraboga, C.A., M. Vibbert, R. Malouf *et al.* 1995. Neurological correlates of fetal cocaine exposure: Transient hypertonia of infancy and childhood. Pediatrics **96:** 1070–1077.
16. Karmel, B.Z., J.M. Gardner & R.L. Freedland. 1997. Neonatal neurobehavioral assessment and Bayley I & II scores of CNS-injured and cocaine-exposed infants. Ann. N.Y. Acad. Sci., this volume.
17. Lidow, M. S. 1995. Prenatal cocaine exposure adversely affects development of the primate cerebral cortex. Synapse **21:** 332–341.
18. Dixon, S.D. & R. Bejar. 1989. Echoencephalographic findings in neonates associated with maternal cocaine and methamphetamine use: Incidence and clinical correlates. J. Pediatr **115:** 770–775.

Neural Systems Underlying Arousal and Attention

Implications for Drug Abuse[a]

T. W. ROBBINS,[b] S. GRANON, J. L. MUIR, F. DURANTOU, A. HARRISON, AND B. J. EVERITT

Department of Experimental Psychology, University of Cambridge, Cambridge, UK

ABSTRACT: The monoaminergic and cholinergic systems are implicated in different forms of behavioral arousal that can be dissected in terms of their forebrain targets and the nature of the behavioral processes they modulate in distinct regions. Thus, evidence in rats with selective neurochemical manipulations tested behaviorally using an analog of an attentional task developed for human subjects indicates that the coeruleo-cortical noradrenergic system is implicated in divided and selective attention, the basal forebrain cholinergic system in stimulus detection, the mesostriatal and mesolimbic dopaminergic systems in response speed and vigor, and the mesencephalic serotoninergic or 5-HT systems in response inhibition. Our recent studies have focused on fractionating, in the same task, the differential contributions of the dorsal and median raphé 5-HT systems as well as elucidating the functions of the mesocortical dopaminergic system, each of which may be relevant to understanding the behavioral and cognitive sequelae of cocaine administration in human subjects as well as in experimental animals.

INTRODUCTION

Research into the neuronal and neural mechanisms of the action of cocaine and other psychomotor stimulant drugs, as well as their actions in behavioral contexts as reinforcers, has burgeoned in recent years, largely because of the problems for society they pose as drugs of abuse. There has also been considerable interest in the effects of chronic cocaine treatment, especially in neonates, because of evidence that this form of exposure can produce lasting behavioral and neural sequelae in experimental animals[1–6] and humans.[7] As the initial site of action of cocaine, via its interaction with transporter molecules, is to affect the reuptake and regulation of the monoamine neurotransmitters, dopamine (DA), noradrenaline (NA), and serotonin (or 5-hydroxytryptamine, 5-HT),[8] it is logical to investigate, in the first instance, the functions of these systems in order to assess the possible psychopathological effects of prior cocaine exposure. It is now becoming clear that these chemically defined systems of the reticular core of the brain (FIG. 1) are involved in many, probably distinct, aspects of behavioral and physiological functioning through their interactions with their diverse terminal domains, for example, in the forebrain. Although there is, as yet, no consensus about their roles in precise, behaviorally defined processes, there is common ground in believing that these

[a] This work was supported by a Wellcome Trust Programme Grant, a Wellcome Trust Travelling Award (to S.G.), Fyssen Fondation Fellowships (to F.D. and S.G.), and a BBSRC studentship (to A.H.)

[b] Address for correspondence: Department of Experimental Psychology, Downing St. Cambridge, CB2 3EB, UK. Fax, 44+1223 314547; phone, 44 1223 333558; e-mail, TWR2@cus.cam.ac.uk

systems have crucial roles in energetic behavioral processes such as the mediation of the effects of stressors, motivation, and general aspects of arousal and attention.[9–14] In this article we summarize some of our previous and new work comparing the functions of these systems, focusing in particular on their likely distinct roles in modulating cognitive function in corticostriatal systems, particularly within the prefrontal cortex.

FRACTIONATING NEUROTRANSMITTER AROUSAL SYSTEMS

A productive approach has been to use multidisciplinary investigations which attempt to synthesize information about these systems from a variety of neurobiological perspectives, including, for example, single cell recording in anesthetized or freely moving animals, anatomical investigations of the distribution of their complex and sometimes widely ramifying connections, identification of their main receptors using the techniques of molecular cloning, as well as classical neuropharmacological approaches,

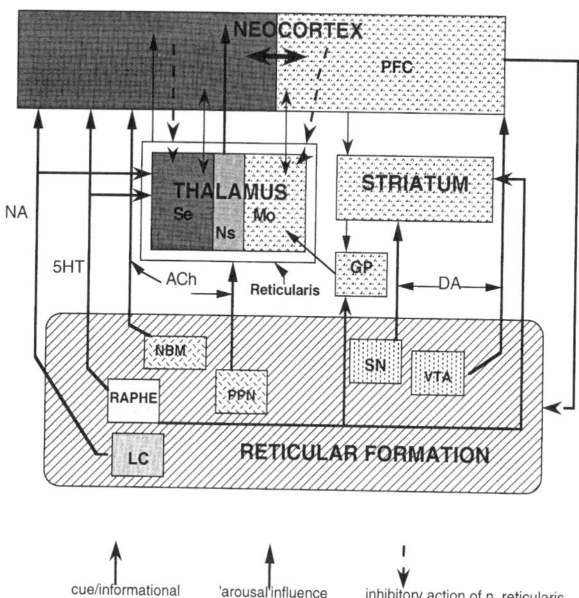

FIGURE 1. Schematic form of the main arousal systems of the forebrain. Both thalamic (e.g., nucleus reticularis) and reticular systems (i.e., ascending monoaminergic and cholinergic systems; for convenience, the histaminergic system has been omitted) are represented, the latter systems being most relevant to this chapter. Only main connections are depicted. *Abbreviations:* PFC = prefrontal cortex; Se = sensory thalamus; Ns = nonspecific thalamic nuclei; Mo = motor thalamus; GP = globus pallidus; NBM = nucleus basalis magnocellularis; PPN = pedunculopontine nuclei; SN = substantia nigra, pars compacta; VTA = ventral tegmental area; ACh = acetylcholine; DA = dopamine; NA = noradrenaline; 5-HT = 5-hydroxytryptamine; LC = locus coeruleus. Omitted for clarity are projections *between* the main neurotransmitter cell groups (e.g., dorsal raphé and ventral tegmental DA cell group to locus coeruleus; pedunculopontine nuclei to VTA etc). Note the descending, possibly regulatory influence of descending prefrontal cortical projections.

and *ex vivo,* as well as increasingly, *in vivo* neurochemical monitoring. These neurobiological methods promise most however when combined with sensitive behavioral paradigms that test predictions about the likely functions of these neural systems. While there is growing interest in the forms of functional interaction between the monoamine systems and the nature of the mutual regulation they appear to impose on one another, relatively few attempts have been made directly to compare the functioning of these systems in a common functional context, probably because of the ambitious and inevitably long-term nature of such a program.

In previous work, we attempted to utilize specific, though quite profound, manipulations of the monoamine and cholinergic systems, while studying rats in a test of visual attentional function based on a task that has been used to assess sustained attention under various environmental conditions in humans. In brief, this test requires rats to monitor five distinct locations in order to detect and respond to brief visual stimuli, presented randomly in space, on a continual basis. This "five choice serial reaction time" paradigm includes measures of accuracy and latency to respond, as well as errors of omission and inappropriate, premature responses. Several "behavioral challenges" can also be utilized, including manipulations of the temporal predictability, duration, and intensity of the target stimuli, as well as the interpolation of distracting bursts of white noise. The conditions in the original paradigm used for humans included exposure to noise, alcohol and other drugs, fluctuations in temperature, sleep deprivation, and the provision of incentives.[15] The fact that these various environmental manipulations failed to interact so as to affect behavioral performance in a way that could be understood in a unidimensional manner obviously poses problems for unitary theories of arousal. This is consistent with the notion that arousal processes are not, in fact, unitary, but can be fractionated, probably consistent with the multiplicity of monoaminergic and nonspecific thalamic influences on forebrain structures. It is also consistent

TABLE 1. Summary of the Main Effects of Manipulations of Monoaminergic and Cholinergic Systems on the Five-Choice Serial Reaction Task

Structure Lesioned	Main Behavioral Effects	References
Dorsal NA bundle	Impaired accuracy following:	
	Interpolated bursts of white noise	29,30
	Central or systemic D-amphetamine	39
	Temporal unpredictability of targets	29,30
Basal forebrain (cholinergic)	Impaired baseline accuracy	16, 17, 50
Dorsal raphé (5-HT)	Increased premature responding	21
Median raphé (5-HT)	Speeded latency to collect reward	21
Mesolimbic and mesostriatal DA systems	Slowed latencies to respond; increased omissions; reduced premature responses	19 and Baunez and Robbins (unpublished data)

FIGURE 2. Comparative effects of excitotoxic lesions of different portions of the frontal cortex (ADL = anterior dorsal lateral cortex; Mpfc = medial prefrontal cortex), catecholamine-depleting lesions of the frontal cortex (6-OHDA) on choice accuracy and latency in the first five sessions postsurgery. Note the lack of effect of 6-OHDA compared to the large effects of Mpfc and basal forebrain (BF) cholinergic lesions. Based, in part, on refs. 25 and 50.

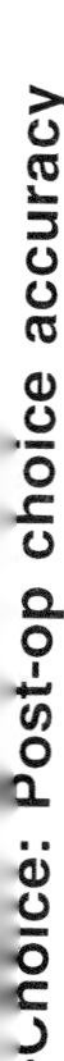

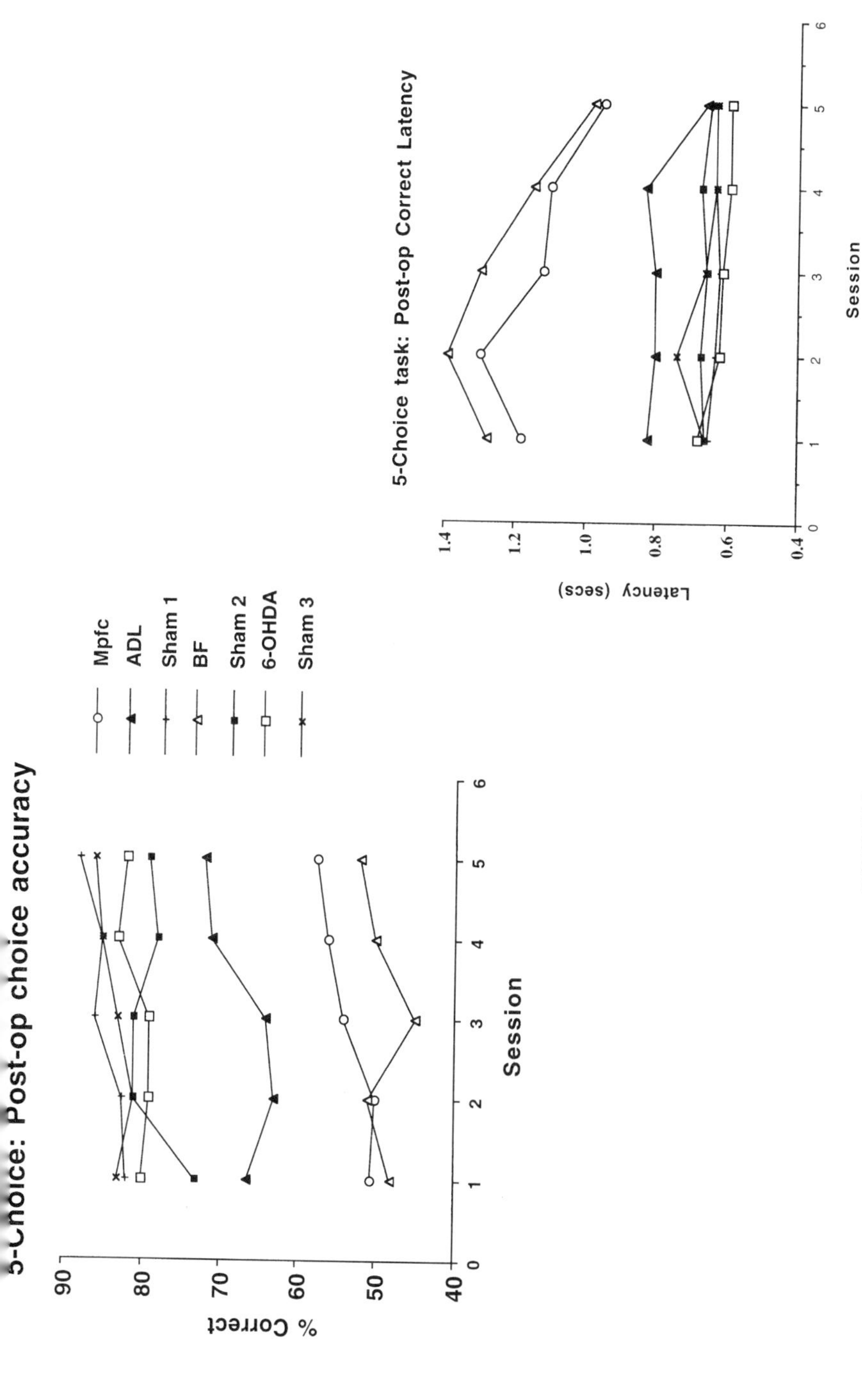

FIGURE 2. *See legend on facing page.*

with our own initial analyses of the effects of manipulations of the coeruleocortical noradrenergic system, the basalocortical cholinergic system, the mesolimbic DA system, and the mesencephalic 5-HT systems, summarized in TABLE 1. It should be made clear that the use of the five-choice task provides only a point of comparison between the effects of these manipulations of the different system, while helping to generate further hypotheses about their functions. The latter, however, usually have to be analyzed further using other specific behavioral test paradigms, so that the analysis is not dependent on a single type of test.[13]

The manipulations have included the use of neurotoxins such as 6-hydroxydopamine (6-OHDA) and 5,7 dihydroxytryptamine (5,7-DHT) that were infused into specific brain regions or, intracerebroventricularly, at appropriate parameters to produce permanent and profound depletions of forebrain NA, DA, and 5-HT.[13] These manipulations were supplemented by the use of systemic and intracerebral infusions of such agents as the indirectly acting catecholamine agonist D-amphetamine or the GABA-ergic agonist muscimol. In the case of the cholinergic system, infusions of the excitotoxic amino acid AMPA were used to induce relatively specific destruction of the cholinergic neurons of the nucleus basalis magnocellularis that project to the anterior cortex.[16] Pharmacological specificity has been established by the use of cholinergic agents such as nicotine or physostigmine.[17] Although some commonalities of effect existed across the different task variables, there was also a surprisingly distinct profile of deficits that were relatively specific for each of the main neurotransmitter systems studied. In brief, basal forebrain cholinergic lesions mainly affected the accuracy of responding, especially when the target stimuli were made very brief (FIG. 2). This deficit was ameliorated by systemic infusions of the anticholinesterase physostigmine or nicotine. Cholinergic lesions also increased the latency to respond and affected accuracy when distracting white noise was used, but these effects were less consistent sequelae of the lesion. Profound depletion of cortical NA produced by lesions of the dorsal noradrenergic ascending bundle only had effects under specially defined circumstances, mainly on indices of accuracy of responding, when the visual targets were presented in a temporally unpredictable manner, when bursts of distracting noise were interpolated just prior to the visual discriminanda or when the rats were challenged with systemic or intracerebral infusions of D-amphetamine into the nucleus accumbens (reviewed in ref. 18).

In normal rats, intra-accumbens D-amphetamine mainly induced changes in the overall speed and probability of responding, rather than its accuracy, effects that were blocked by the depletion of mesolimbic DA within the ventral striatum using 6-hydroxydopamine.[19] Bursts of white noise had similar effects on performance to those of D-amphetamine, that were also blocked by mesolimbic DA depletion. Such DA depletion by itself mainly reduced the speed and probability of responding, without affecting its accuracy.[19] Finally, profound depletion of 5-HT produced behavioral effects that resembled in many aspects those of systemic D-amphetamine. A recent study has shown that the most prominent effect of such depletion, across a range of conditions, is to produce large and long-lasting increases in premature responding, largely without effects on accuracy (except for some minor *improvements* following the 5-HT lesion).[20,21] The increases in premature responding produced by 5-HT depletion are of special interest because of their superficial resemblance to "impulsive" behaviors that have been linked with reductions in central 5-HT in human studies.[22,23]

A global interpretation of this complex pattern of data would be that these different systems are all implicated in this complex task, but in modulating separate aspects of performance, sometimes under special conditions. In theoretical terms the data are consistent with the idea that a broad distinction can be made between "arousal," which is especially associated with cortical mechanisms of stimulus processing, and "response activation." Although the data certainly cannot all be fitted into such a simple dichotomy, it is apparent that the manipulations of the subcortical DA systems, as well as the 5-HT system, mainly affect mechanisms controlling the overall level of response output, whereas manipulation of the cortical noradrenergic or cholinergic systems influences those mechanisms of choice or response selection that control the animals' accuracy. The broad distinction can be maintained using a variety of other sources of evidence; however, it is evident that the characterization of the individual processes requires further refinement. Whereas profound mesostriatal DA depletion (C. Baunez and T.W. Robbins, unpublished data), again produced using 6-hydroxydopamine, produces a similar profile of effects in the five-choice task to those of mesolimbic DA loss, there is little doubt, based on analyses of performance in other test situations, that the mesolimbic and nigrostriatal DA systems are involved in different aspects of activation, probably linked with incentive-motivational or reward processes (including those engaged by drugs of abuse) in the case of the mesolimbic (ventral striatal) system and response preparatory mechanisms in the case of the mesostriatal (dorsal striatal) system. (See ref. 24 for further discussion.)

A parallel series of studies has tried to identify some of the main cortical and striatal regions that contribute to performance on the five-choice task. The most important results have been that lesions of the prefrontal cortex mainly affect response accuracy and response latency (FIG. 2), whereas anterior cingulate cortex lesions have few lasting effects other than to increase premature responding.[25] Preliminary results indicate that excitotoxic lesions to the lateral and medial striatum also have major effects on task performance.[26] Lateral lesions greatly reduce the number of trials completed, perhaps because of impairments in the capacity to initiate responding, whereas medial lesions produce a combination of the effects of medial prefrontal cortex lesions, namely, reduced accuracy and increases in premature responding. A working hypothesis to account for these data is that the mechanisms governing the accuracy of response choice and the inhibition of inappropriate premature responding are at least partly dissociable. Premature responding seems to depend on an anterior cingulate system and medial as well as probably ventral regions of the striatum, whereas response accuracy depends rather more on the prefrontal cortex and those parts of the striatum to which it projects. The similarity of the effects of forebrain 5-HT depletion to the effects of anterior cingulate and striatal manipulations is consistent with recent observations of the effects of selective lesions of the dorsal raphé nuclei using 5,7-DHT.[21] Such lesions produce 80 and 60% reductions in cortical and striatal levels of 5-HT, respectively, with smaller depletions in the hippocampus, and they lead to consistent increases in premature responding. By contrast, similar 5,7-DHT lesions of the median raphé nuclei largely spare the striatum, but deplete the hippocampus by 96%, and produce only transient effects on premature responding, while significantly increasing the speed to collect earned food pellets. These results are consistent with the view that the two 5-HT systems modulate different types of processes related to incentive motivation (medial) and response preparation (dorsal). Circuitry including the cingulate cortex and the striatum is implicated in the production of premature responding; however, it is not clear from these data whether 5-HT depletion within the cingulate cortex is sufficient for this behavioral change to occur.

NEUROMODULATORY MECHANISMS WITHIN THE PREFRONTAL CORTEX

Effects of Selective Catecholaminergic Depletion

The finding that several regions of the frontal cortex (rather than, for example, the parietal cortex) in the rat were implicated in the control of performance on the five-choice task[25] has focused attention on this structure in the further analysis of the role of the ascending modulatory systems. The results are consistent with evidence that neurotoxic lesions of the cholinergic nucleus basalis magnocellularis produce qualitatively similar effects, as a major part of this cholinergic projection is to the frontal cortex. However, to date, there has been little analysis of the effects of other modulatory systems projecting to the same region. This is relevant to understanding the effects of cocaine, which certainly produces some of its effects, perhaps even some of its reinforcing action, in the prefontal cortex.[27] Such a comparison would obviously also be of theoretical interest, as it would enable a functional analysis of the possibly distinct roles of these neurotransmitter systems within common neural domains.

Our first attempts suggested that the cholinergic deficits had a high degree of neurochemical specificity. The catecholamine neurotoxin 6-OHDA was used to deplete both NA and DA from the anterior neocortex in the rat. Groups of rats were pretreated with pargyline (40 mg/kg, ip) 2 hours before surgery to increase the efficacy of the neurotoxin. Under anesthesia, rats were implanted with bilateral stainless steel cannulas in the prefrontal cortex, and all received intracerebral infusions of the 5-HT reuptake blocker talsupram (20 μg/μl; 1 μl/site) 2 hours prior to surgery, to protect 5-HT–containing neurons. Half the rats ($n = 10$) then received infusions of 6-OHDA (0.5 μl/site; 6 μg/μl) to deplete the catecholamines DA and NA, the other half receiving vehicle injections as a control. Infusions were made bilaterally at four sites in the medial prefrontal cortex: (coordinates AP, +3.0; L ±0.5; DV, –1.5, –3.0 mm; and also AP, +3.6, L ±0.5; DV –1.5, –3.0 mm). At the end of the experiment, depletion of the three monoamines was determined using high performance liquid chromatography, with electrochemical detection. Regional depletions relative to control values were: medial prefrontal cortex: 96% NA, 86% DA; cingulate cortex: 87% NA, 62% DA; anterodorsal frontal cortex: 85% NA, 60% DA. Cortical depletions of 5-HT were minimal, as were striatal depletions of all three monoamines.

Although the cortical catecholamines were profoundly depleted, there were no significant effects on any aspects of baseline performance of the five-choice task. The lack of effect on the accuracy measure is shown in FIGURE 2 for the first 5 days of testing after recovery from surgery (7–10 days postoperative), relative to the effects of other prefrontal cortex manipulations. Unfortunately, such negative effects cannot be conclusive for several reasons. First, the lack of behavioral effects following such lesions can always be attributed to the redundancy and potential for functional compensation through a number of mechanisms. Second, evidence indicates that simultaneous depletion of both DA and NA in the prefrontal cortex (which is difficult to avoid because of the functional dynamics of the regulatory systems in this region) has a surprising tendency mutually to oppose one another's effects.[28] On the other hand, it is of considerable interest that when the rats were behaviorally challenged, deficits did emerge in the 6-OHDA–lesioned group. Specifically, when the intertrial intervals (ITIs) were varied to make the target stimuli less predictable in temporal terms, the lesioned group exhibited a deficit in accuracy ($F(2,36) = 3.3$; $p < 0.05$: FIG. 3), probably as a consequence of impaired orienting to the locations of the stimuli. This result is reminiscent of the effects of depletion of NA from the dorsal noradrenergic bundle just described,[29,30] suggesting that some of the effects of that lesion did in fact depend on depletion of NA from the frontal cortex. However, the 6-OHDA–lesioned rats were not impaired in other challenges sensitive to the dorsal bundle lesions, including the use of a variable set of longer ITIs.

Although the local 6-OHDA lesion thus produced some results of interest, in view of the need to differentiate the roles of DA and NA more easily as well as of the other ascending neurotransmitter pathways, we have turned to the use of intracerebral infusions of specific agonists and antagonists in the rat prefrontal cortex.

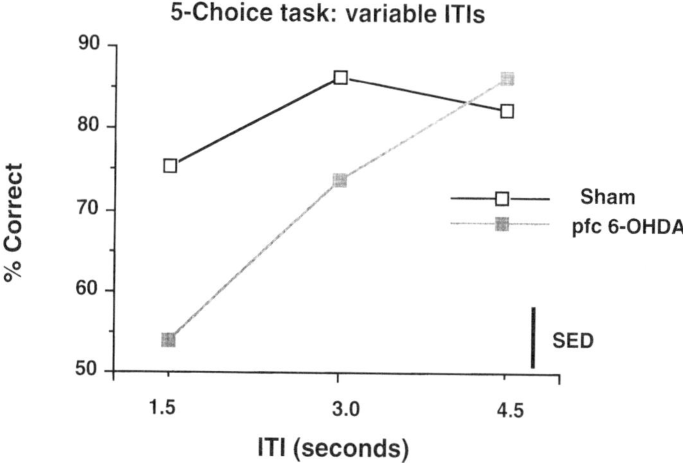

FIGURE 3. Significant deficit in accuracy of performance following 6-OHDA lesions of the medial frontal cortex in the variable, short intertrial intervals (ITI) condition of the five-choice task. The standard error of the difference (SED) between the means provides a visual index of variance taken from the analysis of variance that can be used directly for assessing statistical differences between pairs of mean values.

Effects of Intracortical Drug Infusions

Scopolamine. To validate further those effects of excitotoxic lesions of the rat nucleus basalis which indicated that impairments on the five-choice task resulted from a dysfunction of frontal cholinergic mechanisms, we tested the effects of the muscarinic receptor antagonist scopolamine infused into those medial prefrontal or anterodorsal frontal cortical sites exhibiting large reductions in choline acetyltransferase activity consequent to the basal forebrain lesions. In separate groups, rats were implanted with chronic bilateral stainless steel cannulas to receive infusions of vehicle or scopolamine in volumes of 0.5 µl at each site. The stereotactic coordinates for the guide cannulas within the medial prefrontal cortex were: AP, +3.5; L, ± 0.8; DV, −1.0 mm (with the acutely inserted infusion cannula extended 1.2 mm beyond). For the anterodorsal lateral (ADL) cortex, infusions were made at each of two sites, bilaterally (AP, +3.5 and 2.0; L, ± 3.0; DV, −0.5 mm, infusion cannulas extending 0.5 mm beyond). Slightly different dose ranges were employed for the two sites: medial prefrontal cortex: 3.0, 6.0, and 10.0 µg/site: ADL cortex: 2.5 and 5.0 µg/site. However, it should be remembered that the dual infusions employed for the ADL cortex would produce total doses of 5 and 10 µg for the region as a whole, thus being more comparable to the single doses infused into the medial prefrontal cortex.

The main findings are shown in FIGURE 4A and B. Scopolamine infusions into both areas produced deficits that qualitatively resembled the effects of the nucleus basalis lesions, but in order to reveal deficits it was not necessary to make the task any more difficult by reducing the visual targets from their usual 0.5-second duration (as had been the case when the rats with basal forebrain lesions were recovering from the initial effects of cholinergic loss). Significant effects were noted on both the latency to respond correctly as well as choice accuracy. A major difference between the two sites was that omissions were significantly increased for the ADL cortex at a dose of 2.5 µg/site with no significant effect on any other variable. However, in the medial prefrontal cortical site no significant increases in omissions were found at any dose tested. This might suggest that the anterodorsal lateral site is implicated in sensorimotor, as distinct from the attentional, aspects of the task. It was also interesting that variables related to response control (premature and perseverative responses) were not significantly altered, perhaps reflecting instead the likely role of the cingulate cortex in the control of premature, "impulsive" responding.

D_1 and D_2 Dopamine Receptor Agents

A second line of investigation examined the effects of DA receptor antagonists (D_1; SCH-23390: D_2; sulpiride) or the D_1 agonist SKF-38393, infused into similar sites in

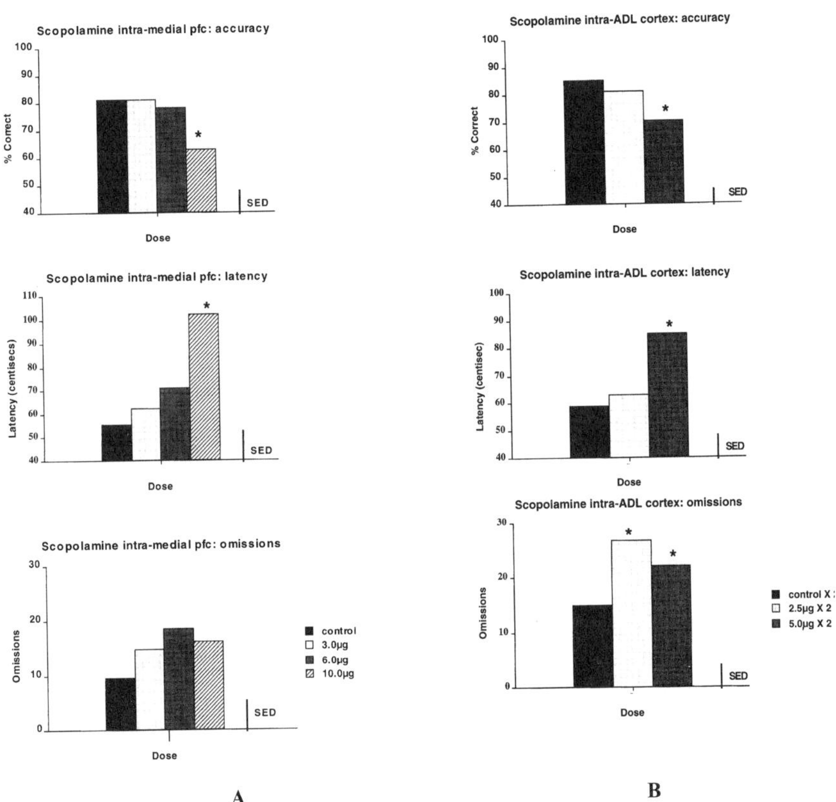

FIGURE 4. Effects of infusions of scopolamine into the medial prefrontal cortex (pfc) (**A**) or anterodorsal lateral cortex (ADL) (**B**) on aspects of performance on the five-choice task. *Asterisks* indicate significant effects compared with controls. Note the significant effect of ADL but not medial pfc infusions on errors of omission. SED refers to 1 standard error of the differences between the means. This provides a visual index of variance taken from the analysis of variance that can be used directly for assessing statistical differences between pairs of mean values.

the medial prefrontal cortex. Previous work, mainly in primates, has indicated that infusions of D_1 receptor antagonists into the dorsolateral prefrontal cortex impair the accuracy of performance on a delayed saccade, working memory task. (See ref. 31 for a review.) However, effects of the D_1 agents infused in the present five-choice task for rats were more subtle than those for scopolamine, although reliable under defined conditions. The D_1 receptor antagonist SCH-23390 produced deficits in discrimination, especially during the first quarter block of trials completed (normally 100 in total) and when the stimulus duration had been reduced from 0.5 to 0.25 second. Effects on other variables, including latency to respond, were much smaller. Even more convincing were the effects of the D_1 receptor agonist SKF-38393, which actually improved performance when it was titrated to a lower baseline of accuracy in the control conditions, at low and intermediate doses (FIG. 5). The D_2 receptor antagonist sulpiride had no effect on any task variable when infused into the same region.

These novel data are theoretically interesting for a variety of reasons. First, it is clear that manipulations of DA function can both impair and improve the accuracy of performance on this task when made within the prefrontal cortex. This is perhaps one of the first demonstrations of the possible facilitatory effects of cortical D_1 receptor activation on cognitive performance. The deficits produced by the intracortical infusions of the D_1 receptor antagonist SCH-23390 are also consistent with a role for D_1 cortical receptors in attentional performance. It is interesting that systemic injections of SCH-23390 fail to affect the accuracy of performance even at moderately high doses, although the speed and overall probability of responding are affected in ways similar to those following mesolimbic and mesostriatal DA depletion[19] (TABLE 1). This implies that the predominant effects observed with the systemically administered drug are due to actions within the striatum, which may also occlude any additional effects resulting from the blockade of cortical D_1 receptors. By contrast, striatal D_2 receptors may be implicated in response selection mechanisms, because systemic (but not intracortical) sulpiride does impair accuracy, but only at doses that are already slowing responding.

The data are also relevant to recent developments in our understanding of the more general role of prefrontal dopaminergic mechanisms. Electrophysiological findings using single unit recording have complemented behavioral results in demonstrating a neuromodulatory role for prefrontal DA in working memory.[32] However, under certain circumstances, activity in the mesocortical DA system apparently can impair performance on spatial working memory tasks such as delayed response and delayed alternation.[33,34] Moreover, the effects of prefrontal dopamine loss appear to depend on which type of behavior or cognitive processing is involved. Whereas spatial delayed response performance in monkeys can be impaired by prefrontal DA loss, the same study found parallel facilitatory effects on performance on an analog of the Wisconsin Card Sorting Test.[35]

A central requirement of both the Wisconsin Card Sorting Test and its analog is an "extra-dimensional shift" in which attention has to be shifted from one visual aspect or dimension of a compound stimulus to another. Prefrontal DA depletion was shown to facilitate such shifting relative to controls, while also upregulating striatal DA function.[35] Excitotoxic lesions of the prefrontal cortex region had the opposite pattern of effects.[36] The relationship of these tests for primates, not only to one another but also to the five-choice task for rodents, is not exactly clear. Performance on the five-choice task probably has aspects of both shifting spatial attention and maintaining "on-line" representations of visual targets over very short delays for the guidance of responses, as in the case of classic "working memory" tasks. However, the facilitatory effects on accuracy of performance of the five-choice task by the D_1 agonist SKF-38393 described here suggest that increasing dopaminergic transmission can boost as well as impair aspects of cognitive performance, depending on the test setting.

These findings imply that dopaminergic activation of the prefrontal cortex produces a hypothetical state that functions adaptively to optimize only certain types of cognitive function. A plausible notion is that this system provides a form of "corollary discharge" that signals to the prefrontal cortex the degree of subcortical activation delivered to the entire group of mesencephalic DA neurons. This would allow the prefrontal cortex to mediate not only decisional mechanisms of response choice, but also the speed or vigor of the behavior, by controlling striatal output mechanisms. In

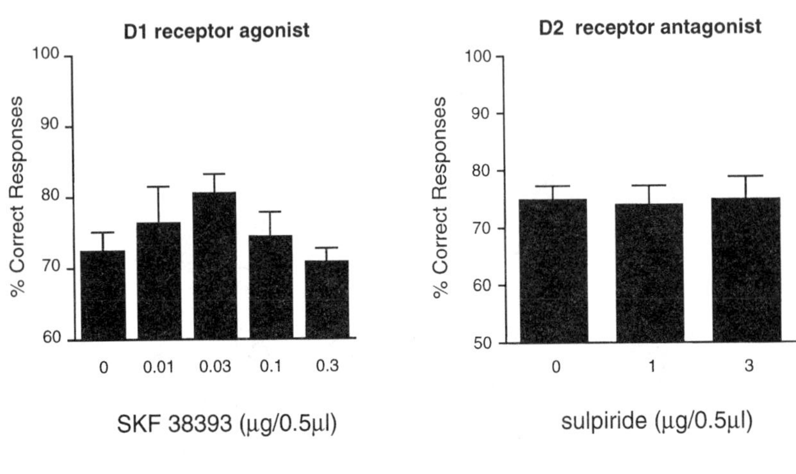

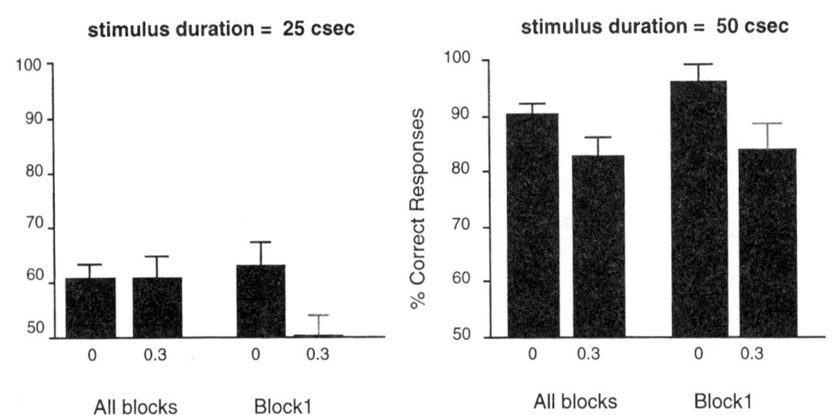

FIGURE 5. Comparative effects of D_1 receptor agonist SKF-38393 and D_1 (SCH-23390) and D_2 (sulpiride) receptor antagonists, infused intra-medial prefrontal cortex, on the accuracy of performance on the five-choice task. Note that data are provided for all four blocks of the task, but the effects are largely confined to the first block for SCH-23390. Values are presented as mean + SEM.

this way, monitoring mechanisms that trade speed for accuracy could be adjusted so as to optimize performance in situations such as the five-choice serial reaction time task.

POSSIBLE RELEVANCE TO HUMAN DRUG ABUSE AND ITS SEQUELAE

Drugs such as cocaine, which affect all of the main monoamine "arousal" systems, can potentially alter many different behavioral and cognitive processes. If it is postulated that optimal levels of activity exist within each of these systems, then the self-administration of cocaine by human subjects as well as experimental animals can be seen almost as a "homeostatic" need to maintain effective functioning. This makes predictions about the types of individual likely to self-administer the drug, for example, that they would have relatively low levels of activity or, in human terms, exhibit "dysphoria." Activity in the mesolimbic DA system generally can be thought of as magnifying the behavioral responsiveness to environmental stimuli,[37] and the slowed responding observed after mesolimbic DA depletion probably reflects reduced incentive motivation of these rats in the presence of food. If chronic exposure to cocaine produces downregulation of the 5-HT system, this would also lead to the occurrence of impaired mechanisms of response control, leading to possibly maladaptive, "impulsive" responding, which could further augment drug-seeking and drug-taking behavior or have psychopathological effects on social behavior and cognition.[23] There are important interactions between the DA and 5-HT systems as revealed in a variety of studies that are too complex to be summarized here.[38] It is of interest that many of the behavioral effects of intra-accumbens amphetamine in the five-choice task resemble the effects of central 5-HT depletion.[19,20] Moreover, systemic administration of a D_1 DA receptor antagonist blocked the increases in premature responding produced by 5-HT depletion, which, in turn, antagonized the increases in errors of commission produced by D_2 receptor blockade on the five-choice task.[20] The possible impact of altered functioning in the noradrenergic and cholinergic systems is less clear. Some evidence for dopaminergic-noradrenergic interactions in the five-choice task was summarized above.[39] It has been proposed that impaired mesolimbic DA function may impact on cortical functioning indirectly via effects on the basal forebrain cholinergic system.[40,41] However, we observed only limited evidence for this[42] and only negative evidence with respect to the five-choice task.[17]

Our results in both rats and monkeys imply that chronic changes in the neuromodulation of cortical, especially prefrontal, processing would also lead to alterations in higher cognitive functions. We have been pursuing this notion in several ways: First, by studying the effects of drugs that affect these systems in human volunteers, and second, by studying cognitive functioning in drug abusers themselves, particularly amphetamine abusers. One notable problem is the need to relate cognition in experimental animals to that in humans. FIGURE 6 summarizes the results of a recent study of effects of different drugs on attentional performance in normal human volunteers, illustrating how it might be possible, as in the rat, to utilize a paradigm with several different variants to discern differences in effects of agents such as the alpha-1/2 agonist clonidine, the DA receptor blocker haloperidol, the effects of depleting 5-HT (with a low tryptophan drink), and also the benzodiazepine diazepam.[43] The attentional paradigm was designed to assess different forms of attention, such as focused or divided (visual search), using a variant of Broadbent's[44] original design. Under certain conditions, clonidine acted to broaden the span of attention; haloperidol generally slowed reaction times; and low tryptophan reduced the inhibitory effects of stimulus-response compatibility. These effects are not, in fact, so very different from the types of behavioral process pos-

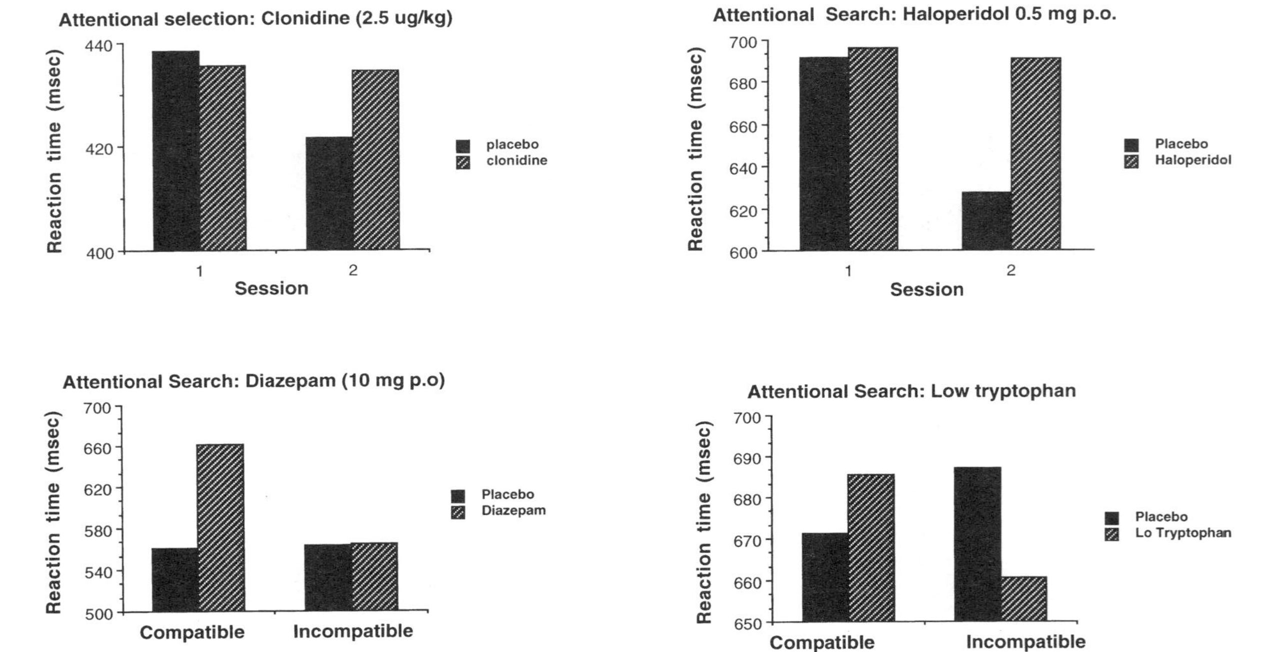

FIGURE 6. Summary of the main effects of systemic clonidine, haloperidol, diazepam, or low tryptophan on tests of selective (focused) visual attention or visual search conditions in human subjects (see ref. 43). Note the quadruple dissociation between the four manipulations, respectively, of noradrenergic, dopaminergic, GABA-ergic, or 5-HT-ergic systems, respectively. Compare with Figure 44-2 in ref. 13.

tulated to be affected by similar neurochemical manipulations in the rat. The qualitatively different effects of diazapam confirm that the effects of clonidine and haloperidol cannot be explained simply in terms of a unitary construct such as diminished arousal, or "sedation." This is consistent with the multiple arousal system model developed here from experiments using rats.

Whereas these drug effects in humans can be related to the same types of process postulated to account for differences in performance on the five-choice task, the human task was not directly based on it (and indeed employed emotive words rather than light flashes as target stimuli). In other work, it has been possible to design tasks that can be used to make more direct comparisons between animal (generally monkeys) and human subjects. One example of this is the analog of the Wisconsin Card Sorting Test just mentioned. This test has now been used to show opposite effects of prefrontal damage[36] and DA depletion[35] within the prefrontal cortex as well as a lack of effect of prefrontal cholinergic depletion in marmosets.[45] In human subjects tested with essentially the same test materials, there are expected impairments following excisions of the frontal, but not the temporal lobes[46] and also deficits in patients with basal ganglia disorders, including Parkinson's disease,[47] which suggests that the extradimensional set-shifting component might be a specific function of frontostriatal circuitry. Of possible relevance to the current topic, a group of amphetamine abusers was recently shown also to exhibit specific impairments in this phase of the test,[48] whereas a comparison group of opiate abusers with similar overall levels of intellectual deterioration are relatively unimpaired.[49] While the exact interpretation of these results in terms of causal neural mechanisms requires further elucidation, and a group of chronic amphetamine abusers might not be entirely relevant for predicting the effects of prenatal cocaine exposure, this study does illustrate the potential power of extrapolation from studies of neurochemically defined arousal systems in experimental animals to cognitive functioning in humans affected by chronic stimulant abuse.

REFERENCES

1. Scalzo, F.M. *et al.* 1990. Weanling rats exposed prenatally to cocaine exhibit an increase in D2 receptor binding associated with an increase in ligand affinity. Pharmacol. Biochem. Behav. **37:** 371–373.
2. Church, M.W. *et al.* 1991. Effects of prenatal cocaine exposure. *In* Biochemistry and Physiology of Substance Abuse. R.R. Watson, Ed.: 179–204. CRC Press. Boston, MA.
3. Minabe, Y. *et al.* 1992. The effects of prenatal cocaine exposure on spontaneously active midbrain dopamine neurons in postnatal male rats: An electrophysiological study. Brain Res. **586:** 152–156.
4. Moody, C.A. *et al.* 1992. Psychopharmacological responsiveness to the dopamine agonist quinpirole in normal weanlings and in weanling offspring exposed gestationally to cocaine. Psychopharmacology **108:** 256–262.
5. Peris, J. *et al.* 1992. Cocaine in utero enhances the behavioral responses to cocaine in adult rats. Pharmacol. Biochem. Behav. **42:** 509–515.
6. Heyser, C.J. *et al.* 1994. Responsiveness to cocaine challenge in adult rats following prenatal exposure to cocaine. Psychopharmacology **116:** 45–55.
7. Zuckerman, B. & K. Bresnahan. 1991. Developmental and behavioral consequences of prenatal drug and alcohol exposure. Pediatr. Clin. North Am. **38:** 1287–1306.
8. Pitts, D.K. & J. Marwah. 1987. Cocaine modulation of central monoaminergic neurotransmission. Pharmacol. Biochem. Behav. **26:** 453–486.
9. Steriade, H. & G. Buzsaki. 1990. Parallel activation of thalamic and cortical neurons by brainstem and basal forebrain cholinergic neurons. *In* Brain Cholinergic Systems. M. Steriade & D. Biesold, Eds.: 3–62. Oxford University Press. London.
10. Aston-Jones, G. *et al.* 1991. Discharge of noradrenergic locus coeruleus neurons in behaving rats and monkeys suggests a role in vigilance. Prog. Brain Res. **88:** 501–520.

11. JACOBS B.L. & E.C. AZMITIA. 1992. Structure and function of the brain serotonin system. Physiol. Rev. **43:** 563–578.
12. MARROCCO R. *et al.* 1994. Arousal systems. Curr. Opin. Neurobiol. **4:** 166–170.
13. ROBBINS, T.W. & B.J. EVERITT. 1995. Arousal systems and attention. *In* The Cognitive Neurosciences. M. Gazzaniga, Ed.: 703–720. MIT Press. Cambridge, MA.
14. BERLUCCHI, G. 1997. One or many arousal systems? Reflections on some of Giuseppe Moruzzi's foresights and insights about the intrinsic regulation of brain activity. Arch. Ital. Biol. **135:** 5–14.
15. BROADBENT, D.E. 1970. Decision and Stress. Academic Press. London.
16. EVERITT, B.J. & T.W. ROBBINS. 1997. Central cholinergic systems and cognition. Ann. Rev. Psychol. **48:** 649–684.
17. MUIR, J.L. *et al.* 1995. Reversal of visual attentional dysfunction following lesions of the cholinergic basal forebrain by physostigmine and nicotine but not by the 5HT-3 antagonist, ondansetron. Psychopharmacology **118:** 82–92.
18. ROBBINS, T.W. & B.J. EVERITT. 1995. Central norepinephrine neurons and behavior. *In* Psychopharmacology 4th Generation of Progress. F.E. Bloom & D. Kupfer, Eds.: 363–372. Raven Press. New York.
19. COLE, B.J. & T.W. ROBBINS. 1989. Effects of 6-hydroxydopamine lesions of the nucleus accumbens septi on performance of a 5-choice serial reaction time task in rats: Implications for theories of selective attention and arousal. Behav. Brain. Res. **33:** 165–179.
20. HARRISON, A. *et al.* 1997. Central 5-HT depletion enhances impulsive responding without affecting the accuracy of attentional performance: Interactions with dopaminergic mechanisms. Psychopharmacology **133:** 329–342.
21. HARRISON, A. *et al.* 1997. Doubly dissociated effects of median and dorsal raphé lesions on the performance of the 5-choice serial reaction time test of attention in rats. Behav. Brain Res. **89:** 135–149.
22. SOUBRIE, P. 1986. Reconciling the role of central serotonin neurons in human and animal behaviour. Behav. Brain Sci. **9:** 319–364.
23. LINNOILA, M. *et al.* 1983. Low cerebrospinal fluid 5-hydroxyindoleacetic acid concentration differentiates impulsive from non-impulsive violent behavior. Life Sci. **33:** 2609–2614.
24. ROBBINS, T.W. & B.J. EVERITT. 1992. Functions of dopamine in the dorsal and ventral striatum. Semin. Neurosci. **4:** 119–127.
25. MUIR, J.L. *et al.* 1996. The cerebral cortex of the rat and visual attentional function: Dissociable effects of mediofrontal, cingulate, anterior dorsolateral and parietal lesions on a five choice serial reaction time task in rats. Cerebral Cortex **6:** 470–481.
26. ROGERS, R.D. *et al.* 1997. Lesions of medial and lateral striatum in the rat produce dissociable deficits on attentional performance. Soc. Neurosci. Abstr. **23:** 716.8. Society for Neuroscience Annual Meeting, New Orleans, LA, USA.
27. GOEDERS, N. & J.E. SMITH. 1983. Cortical dopaminergic involvement in cocaine reinforcement. Science **221:** 773–775.
28. TASSIN, J.-P. *et al.* 1991. Relationships between mesocortical and mesolimbic dopamine neurons: Functional correlates of D1 receptor heteroregulation. *In* The Mesolimbic Dopamine System: From Motivation to Action. P. Willner & J. Scheel-Kruger, Eds.: 175–196. Wiley. Chichester, U.K.
29. CARLI, M. *et al.* 1983. Effects of lesions to ascending noradrenergic neurons on performance of a 5-choice serial reaction time task in rats: Implications for theories of dorsal noradrenergic bundle function based on selective attention and arousal. Behav. Brain. Res. **9:** 361–380.
30. COLE, B.J. & T.W. ROBBINS. 1992. Forebrain norepinephrine:role in controlled information processing in the rat. Neuropsychopharmacology. **7:** 129–141.
31. GOLDMAN-RAKIC, P.S. 1992. Dopamine-mediated mechanisms of the prefrontal cortex. Semin. Neurosci. **4:** 149–159.
32. WILLIAMS, G.V. & P.S. GOLDMAN-RAKIC. 1995. Modulation of memory fields by dopamine D1 receptors in prefrontal cortex. Nature **376:** 572–575.
33. SAHAKIAN, B.J. *et al.* 1985. Association between learning and cortical catecholamines in non-drug-treated rats. Psychopharmacology **86:** 339–343.

34. Arnsten, A. 1997. Catecholamine regulation of the prefrontal cortex. J. Psychopharmacol. **11:** 151–162.
35. Roberts, A.C. *et al.* 1994. 6-Hydroxydopamine lesions of the prefrontal cortex in monkeys enhance performance on an analog of the Wisconsin Card Sort Test: Possible interactions with subcortical dopamine. J. Neurosci. **14:** 2531–2544.
36. Dias R. *et al.* 1996. Primate analogue of the Wisconsin Card Sort Test: Effects of excitotoxic lesions of the prefrontal cortex in the marmoset. Behav. Neurosci. **110:** 870–884.
37. Taylor, J.R. & T.W. Robbins. 1986. 6-Hydroxydopamine lesions of the nucleus accumbens, but not of the caudate nucleus, attenuate enhanced responding with reward-related stimuli produced by intra-accumbens D-amphetamine. Psychopharmacology **90:** 390–397.
38. Broderick, P.A. & C.F. Phelix. 1997. I. Serotonin (5-HT) within dopamine reward circuits signals open-field behavior. II. Basis for 5-HT-DA interaction in cocaine dysfunctional behavior. Neurosci. Biobehav. Rev. **21:** 227–260.
39. Cole, B.J. & T.W. Robbins. 1987. Amphetamine impairs the discrimination performance of rats with dorsal bundle lesions on a 5-choice serial reaction time task: New evidence for central dopaminergic-noradrenergic interactions. Psychopharmacology **91:** 458–466.
40. Day, J. & H.C. Fibiger. 1993. Dopaminergic regulation of cortical acetylcholine release: Effects of dopamine receptor agonists. Neuroscience **54:** 643–648.
41. Sarter, M. 1994. Neuronal mechanisms of the attentional dysfunction in senile dementia: Two sides of the same coin? Psychopharmacology **114:** 539–550.
42. Robledo, P., R. Weissenborn, T.W. Robbins & B.J. Everitt. 1997. Effects of lesions of the nucleus basalis magnocellularis on the acquisition of cocaine self-administration in rats. Eur. J. Neurosci. In press.
43. Coull, J. *et al.* 1995. Differential effects of clonidine, haloperidol, diazepam and tryptophan depletion on focused attention and attentional search. Psychopharmacology **121:** 222–230.
44. Broadbent, D.E. 1988. Reaction time with distractors: Some possibilities for drug assessment. *In* Psychopharmacology and Reaction Time. I. Hindmarch *et al.,* Eds.: 97–102. Wiley. New York.
45. Roberts, A.C. *et al.* 1992. A specific form of cognitive rigidity following excitotoxic lesions of the basal forebrain in monkeys. Neuroscience **47:** 251–264.
46. Owen, A.M. *et al.* 1991. Extra-dimensional versus intra-dimensional set shifting performance following frontal lobe excision, temporal lobe excision or amygdalo-hippocampectomy in man. Neuropsychologia **29:** 993–1006.
47. Downes J.J. *et al.* 1989. Impaired extra-dimensional shift performance in medicated and unmedicated Parkinson's disease: Evidence for a specific attentional dysfunction. Neuropsychologia **27:** 1329–1344.
48. Iddon, J.L. *et al.* 1996. Chronic amphetamine abuse: Impact on cognition. J. Psychopharmacol. **10:** Suppl. A58, Abstr. 231. Annual Meeting of the British Association for Psychopharmacology, Cambridge, UK., July, 1996.
49. Ornstein, T. *et al.* 1997. The effects of chronic heroin abuse on cognitive function, J. Psychopharmacology **11:** Suppl.A16, Abstr. 62. Joint Meeting of the British Association for Psychopharmacology and the Canadian College of Neuropsychopharmacology, Cambridge, UK., July, 1997.
50. Muir, J.L. *et al.* 1994. AMPA-induced lesions of the basal forebrain: A significant role for the cortical cholinergic system in attentional function. J. Neurosci. **14:** 2313–2326.

Prenatal Cocaine Exposure Alters Signal Transduction in the Brain D_1 Dopamine Receptor System[a]

EITAN FRIEDMAN AND HOAU-YAN WANG

Division of Molecular Pharmacology, Department of Pharmacology, MCP ♦Hahnemann School of Medicine, Allegheny University of the Health Sciences, Philadelphia, Pennsylvania 19129, USA

ABSTRACT: Cocaine use during pregnancy may result in persistent behavioral abnormalities in the newborn. Animal studies show behavioral and neurochemical alterations in offspring that were exposed to cocaine prenatally. The monoamine neurons, including those containing dopamine, appear and become operational prenatally and mature during early postnatal life. It is therefore conceivable that exposure to cocaine during gestation may critically affect normal development and subsequently cause protracted postnatal neurochemical and behavioral changes. The data we obtained demonstrate that prenatal exposure to cocaine in the rabbit impairs signal transduction via the D_1 but not the D_2 dopamine receptor system. This is reflected in impaired dopamine-stimulated [^{35}S]GTPγS binding to Gαs without affecting binding of the nucleotide to Gαi in both cortex and striatum of rabbit offspring. This selective reduction in D_1 dopamine receptor-mediated activation of Gs protein increased in severity as the dose of cocaine administered to the pregnant dams was increased. Maximal impairment was observed after treatment with two daily injections of 3 mg/kg of cocaine HC1. The reduction in dopamine-stimulated GTP binding to Gαs did not result from a decrease in concentration of membrane Gαs protein or D_1 dopamine receptors. The data also indicate that *in utero* cocaine exposure causes persistent uncoupling of the D_1 dopamine receptors from their associated Gs protein which appears as early as gestational day 22 and persists to postnatal day 100. The reduction in D_1 dopamine receptor-mediated signal transduction may be mediated by post-translational modifications of the D_1 dopamine receptor or of Gsα such as phosphorylation, which result in altered coupling between these membrane components. The resultant attenuated D_1 dopamine receptor-mediated signaling may ultimately underlie both long-lasting behavioral dysfunction and morphologic changes which are associated with prenatal cocaine exposure in the rabbit.

INTRODUCTION

Cocaine abuse among childbearing women in the United States is a major public health issue.[1,2] Accumulated evidence suggests that use of this stimulant during pregnancy may cause long-lasting behavioral abnormalities in the newborn.[3] Similarly, animal studies show behavioral and neurochemical alterations in offspring that were exposed to cocaine prenatally.[4–7] However, few studies have addressed in detail the effect of prenatal cocaine exposure on the development of specific synaptic events that determine signal transduction in monoaminergic pathways.

The monoamine neurons, including those containing dopamine, appear and become operational prenatally and mature during early postnatal life. Cell bodies of

[a] This work was supported in part by United States Public Health Service Grant P01-DA06871 from the National Institute on Drug Abuse.

dopamine, norepinephrine, and serotonin neurons are present in rat brainstem at gestational day 14, and their axons extend rostrally thereafter.[8] These amines are also present in the human fetal brain as early as gestational week 7[9] and in the rabbit forebrain by gestational day 19.[10,11] In rat brain, postsynaptic monoaminergic receptors also develop during this early developmental period. It is therefore conceivable that exposure to cocaine during gestation may critically affect normal development and subsequently cause long-term postnatal neurochemical and behavioral changes. Neurologic and motor disorders have been observed in infants following *in utero* exposure to dopamine receptor antagonists,[12,13] and early postnatal treatment with these drugs produces motor dysfunctions in rabbits lasting well beyond the duration of treatment.[14] Furthermore, prenatal exposure of rodents to dopamine receptor inhibition affects maze learning and motor activity levels[15] as well as sensitivity to dopamine antagonists when exposed offspring were tested as adults.[16] Prenatal exposure to cocaine also produces long-lasting neurobehavioral consequences.[5,7] The ability of cocaine to bind to the dopamine transporter has been correlated with its reinforcing properties,[17] and its ability to inhibit presynaptic dopamine uptake when administered prenatally was shown as well. Enduring behavioral abnormalities involving the dopaminergic system were also reported in animals that were exposed to cocaine *in utero.*[5,18] However, these changes were not associated with persistent changes in the density or affinity of dopamine receptors,[19–21] suggesting that changes in signal transduction distal to the dopamine receptors may be responsible for the long-lasting consequences of *in utero* cocaine.[22,23]

Perturbation of the dopaminergic system *in utero* influences the development of this brain neurotransmitter system by altering both pre- and postsynaptic dopaminergic mechanisms and exerts important and far-reaching effects on the developing nervous system. In fact, stimulation of D_1 and D_2 dopamine receptors was recently shown to influence neuronal development in opposing manners.[24] In these studies, D_1 dopamine receptor stimulation suppressed axonal and neurite outgrowth in primary cortical embryonic neurons in culture, whereas D_2 dopamine receptor stimulation promoted process elongation. In cultured retinal cells, dopamine also caused neurite retraction via a D_1 dopamine receptor-mediated mechanism.[25] Recent experiments performed in our laboratory demonstrated that prenatal exposure to cocaine impairs signal transduction via the D_1 dopamine receptor system in both cortex and striatum of rabbit offspring.[22,23]

Signal transduction in the D_1 dopamine-receptor system is initiated by stimulation of guanine nucleotide regulatory protein (G protein)-coupled cell surface receptors which are characterized by seven transmembrane domains. At least two isoforms of this receptor family have been cloned to date, the D_{1A} and $D_{5/1B}$. Although these receptors are known to stimulate adenylyl cyclase, evidence suggests the existence of other D_1-like dopamine receptor-linked functional systems including phospholipase C, Ca^{+2} influx, Na^+/H^+ exchange, and Na/K ATPase activity. The third intracellular loop of the G protein-coupled receptors interacts with heterotrimeric membrane proteins which depend on GTP for activation.[26,27] The G proteins constitute a family of structurally related members each consisting of three dissimilar subunits. The α subunit binds and hydrolyzes GTP, whereas the $\beta\gamma$ dimer anchors the G protein to the membrane and terminates the action of the α subunit. The specificity of receptor-G protein and G protein-effector interactions resides with the specific combination of subunit subtypes that make up the specific trimer that couples to the receptor.

Activation of surface receptors in the presence of Mg^{2+} and GTP facilitates the exchange of GDP with GTP on the α subunit and results in the dissociation of this subunit from $\beta\gamma$. The GTP-bound α subunit or the $\beta\gamma$ complex can then interact with effector(s)—adenylyl cyclase, phospholipase C, and ion channels—to generate second messengers. In the D_1 dopamine receptor subfamily Gs stimulates adenylyl cyclase (D_1

and D_5), whereas Gq couples to phospholipase C.[28,29] We assessed dopamine receptor/G protein coupling in membranes prepared from striata or from frontal or anterior cingulate cerebrocortices of kits of Dutch-belted rabbits that were exposed to cocaine from day 8 through day 29 of gestation. The effect of prenatal cocaine exposure on the coupling of dopamine receptors to their associated G proteins was assessed by receptor-stimulated increments in [^{35}S]GTPγS binding to specific Gα proteins that were immunoprecipitated with antisera directed against select Gα proteins. In all three brain regions, the D_1 dopamine receptors were found to couple to Gs, while the D_2 dopamine receptors were associated with Gi protein. Basal and dopamine-stimulated binding of [^{35}S]GTPγS to Gαs and Gαi was assessed in brain membranes prepared from *in utero* cocaine and saline-exposed 10-, 50-, and 100-day-old rabbits. Although basal guanine nucleotide binding to these Gα proteins was not altered, dopamine-induced increases in guanine nucleotide binding to Gαs protein were reduced in the brain regions of *in utero* cocaine-exposed offspring; however, dopamine-stimulated guanine nucleotide binding to Gαi was unchanged. The apparent selective reduction in D_1 dopamine receptor-mediated activation of Gs protein increased in severity as the dose of cocaine administered to the pregnant dams was increased. Maximal impairment of D_1 dopamine receptor-stimulated GTP binding to Gαs protein was observed after treatment with 2×3 mg/kg/day cocaine HCl.[30] Furthermore, the reduction in dopamine-stimulated GTP binding to Gαs did not result from a decrease in concentration of membrane Gαs protein. An assessment of D_1 dopamine recognition sites by quantitative autoradiography using [^{3}H]SCH23390 as the ligand indicated that the density of D_1 dopamine receptors in striatum or mesocortical areas was not changed by *in utero* exposure to cocaine. The observed change in D_1 dopamine receptor-mediated response also does not appear to be associated with changes in the levels of dopamine or its metabolites.[6,31,32] These data suggest that *in utero* cocaine exposure causes persistent uncoupling of the D_1 dopamine receptors from their associated Gs protein and may be the result of an adaptive reaction to a persistent increase in synaptic dopamine which is produced by repeated cocaine exposure during the early development of the brain.

The apparent uncoupling of D_1 dopamine receptors from Gs protein in brains of *in utero* cocaine-exposed animals was further tested by directly assessing the linkage of D_1 dopamine receptors with Gαs protein. Direct coupling of receptors with G proteins was assessed by measuring the quantity of receptor protein which coimmunoprecipitated with a specific anti-Gα protein antibody. This procedure was previously used to assess receptor-G protein coupling in brain membranes.[28,29] In rat striatal membranes, the D_{1A} dopamine receptors were found to couple to Gs protein, because anti-Gαs antiserum, but not antisera which recognize Gαi, Gαo, Gαz, or Gαq, was able to coprecipitate D_{1A} dopamine receptors identified by a specific D_{1A} dopamine receptor antibody.[28] Stimulation of striatal membranes with 1 μM of dopamine increased coupling of D_{1A} dopamine receptors to Gαs. Striatal tissues obtained from rabbits at gestational days 22 and 25 as well as postnatal days 1 and 20 were tested for both basal and dopamine-stimulated coupling. Basal coupling in control tissue was observed on gestational days 22 and 25 and postnatal days 1 and 20, and dopamine elicited increases in D_{1A}/Gαs coprecipitation at these ages. Prenatal cocaine exposure did not affect coupling of D_{1A} dopamine receptor with Gαs protein. However, receptor-stimulated coupling of D_{1A} dopamine receptors with Gαs protein was markedly reduced in striatal brain membranes obtained from *in utero* cocaine-exposed rabbits at gestational day 22 to postnatal day 20. These data directly demonstrate that prenatal cocaine exposure results in reduced D_{1A} dopamine receptors/Gs coupling (FIG. 1). This impairment in transmembrane signal transduction appears as early as gestational day 22 and persists into postnatal ages.

Posttranslational alteration in D_1 dopamine receptors or Gαs protein per se may re-

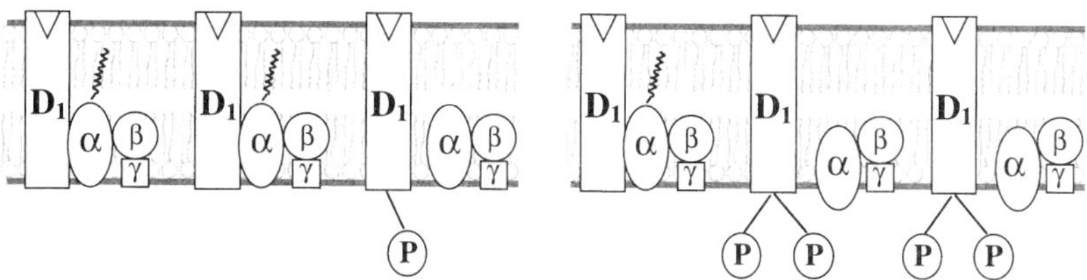

FIGURE 1. Prenatal cocaine exposure results in D_1 dopamine receptor/Gs uncoupling in rabbit brain. A schematic illustration of possible mechanisms that may contribute to the uncoupling of D_1 dopamine receptor from Gs protein. Uncoupling can result from an increase in phosphorylation of the D_1 dopamine receptors **(P)** and/or from a reduction in palmitoylation of Gα protein. **(Left)** Prenatal saline. **(Right)** Prenatal cocaine.

sult in altered signaling via D_1 receptors.[33] Previous studies have indicated that changes in plasticity of brain D_1 dopamine receptors may be mediated via alterations in G proteins or in receptor/G protein coupling[34] without affecting receptor density. It is thus possible that uncoupling of the D_1 dopamine receptors from their associated Gs protein, observed in brains of the prenatal cocaine-exposed animals, may result from changes in posttranslational modifications in D_1 dopamine receptor and/or Gs protein.

Palmitoylation is a posttranslational modification that occurs on many proteins including the heterotrimeric G proteins and neurotransmitter receptors.[33,35,36] Palmitoylation of Gαs protein is a reversibly receptor-modulated posttranslational modification that may alter the function of Gα subunits.[37,38] Interference with Gα palmitoylation has been shown to impair anchoring of the α subunit to the membrane and thus to uncouple Gs from its effector, adenylyl cyclase.[38] Dopamine and the D_1 dopamine receptor agonist SKF38393 increase [^{3}H]palmitate incorporation by membrane Gαs. This dopaminergic stimulation of Gαs palmitoylation was attenuated in striatal membranes obtained from rabbits that were exposed to cocaine at postnatal day 20 (Bhamre *et al.*, unpublished data). Changes in dopamine-stimulated palmitoylation of Gαs protein not only may reflect altered receptor/G protein coupling, but also may result from drug-induced changes in (1) D_{1A} dopamine receptors, (2) Gαs protein, or (3) enzymatic mechanisms that regulate palmitoylation and/or depalmitoylation.

In addition to lipid acylation of receptors and G proteins, phosphorylation is also an important posttranslational mechanism by which signal transduction pathways may be regulated.[39,40] Protein kinase C and protein kinase A are known to phosphorylate G proteins and surface receptors.[41–47] This ubiquitous protein modification may result in interference with signal flow and ultimately with functions associated with particular G protein-coupled receptors. In addition, receptor phosphorylation mediated by G protein-coupled receptor kinases is important in determining sensitivity of various receptors including the D_{1A} dopamine receptor.[48,49] Moreover, alterations in phosphorylation mediated by protein kinase A were reported following repeated cocaine administration in adult rats.[50,51] We found that incubation of striatal membranes with PMA or dibutyryl-cAMP inhibits D_1 dopamine receptor-mediated stimulation of [^{35}S]GTPγS binding to Gαs. Thus, it is possible that changes in membrane protein phosphorylation state contribute to the observed impairment in coupling of D_1 dopamine receptors to Gs protein in prenatal cocaine-exposed animals.

The potential role of various protein tyrosine kinases in regulating neuronal function and neurogenesis during early development was demonstrated.[52–54] Activation of neurons was shown to activate a family of mitogen-activated protein kinases such as the extracellular signal-regulated kinases (ERKs). Upon stimulation, ERKs phosphorylate other protein kinases and thus activate an array of intracellular effectors including enzymes, cytoskeletal proteins, and transcriptional factors, all of which are vital to normal neuronal development and function.[55,56] In adult rats, chronic, systemic administration of cocaine leads to a sustained increase in the ERK phosphorylation state and activity in the ventral tegmental area of the brain, which, in turn, results in drug-induced increases in tyrosine hydroxylase expression.[57] Similarly, chronic cocaine treatment also increased the levels of Janus kinase-2, a cytoplasmic protein tyrosine kinase modulated by ciliary neurotrophic factor, which is also found in the ventral tegmental area.[58] These results suggest that exposure to cocaine during early stages of neurogenesis may affect transduction of signals mediated by these protein tyrosine kinases and may critically influence neuronal development and thus mediate some of the long-lasting effects of *in utero* cocaine.

In addition to protein kinases, the phosphorylation state of proteins can also be regulated by protein phosphatases. Data emerging from diverse cell systems indicate that protein phosphatases, like kinases, are tightly regulated via intracellular second messengers and thus modulate cell function.[59] In neuronal tissue, perturbation of phosphorylation/dephosphorylation processes by various protein phosphatase inhibitors results in modification of the neuritic tree structure and reduction in synaptic number[60] as well as in inhibition of synaptic transmission.[61,62] In neostriatal neurons, D_1 dopamine receptor-regulated calcium current was found to be modulated by protein phosphatase 1.[63] Prenatal cocaine may alter protein phosphatase activity and so may not only cause changes in receptor and/or G protein phosphorylation state but also affect brain synaptic integrity and activity and have a sustained impact on brain function.

Long-term D_1 dopamine receptor/Gs uncoupling in *in utero* cocaine-exposed rabbits and its consequences are supported by the observation made by Simansky and Kachelries.[64] These authors showed in adult rabbits that prenatal exposure to cocaine diminishes amphetamine-induced D_1 dopamine receptor-associated behaviors. Furthermore, desensitization in D_1 receptor function in progeny of cocaine-treated rabbits was also observed by assessing cocaine-induced *c-fos* gene expression.[65] Similar to results obtained in rats,[66] cocaine-mediated *c-fos* mRNA expression in rabbit brain was inhibited by the selective D_1 dopamine receptor antagonist SCH23390. Furthermore, in the dopaminergically innervated anterior cingulate cortex of prenatal cocaine-exposed rabbits, excessive growth of cortical dendrites was observed.[67–69] In these studies, microtubule-associated protein 2 (MAP2) staining and dioctadecyl tetramethylindocarbocyanine (Dil)-filled neurons revealed longer dendrites which course abnormally and show reduced dendritic bundling in the anterior cingulate cortex.[67,69] The data suggest that changes in dendritic organization in the developing cortex may result from the observed uncoupling of D_1 dopamine receptors from Gs protein because stimulation of D_1 dopamine receptor was shown to cause retraction of developing neurons.[24] Thus, some of the effects of prenatal cocaine exposure on the fetus and on subsequent postnatal development of the brain may be mediated through altered dopamine receptors and/or transmembrane signaling initiated by dopamine receptors. Together, these results demonstrate a dose-related and long-lasting dissociation of D_1 dopamine receptors from Gs protein in brain of prenatal cocaine-exposed rabbits. These data, furthermore, strongly indicate that the coupling of the D_1 receptor system(s) to Gs protein is impaired as early as embryonic day 22 and that this effect may result in attenuated D_1 dopamine receptor-mediated signaling and may ultimately underlie both long-lasting behavioral dysfunctions[64,70] and morphological changes[67–69] which are associated with prenatal cocaine exposure in the rabbit.

In contrast to our finding on receptor/Gs coupling in which both cortical and striatal D_1 receptor-mediated signal transduction systems were attenuated by *in utero* cocaine administration, altered presynaptic dopaminergic function was observed only in cortex and not in striatum of *in utero* cocaine-treated offspring.[32] While the consequence of perturbation of synaptic dopamine may be critically dependent upon the precise gestational period of drug exposure,[71,72] our data indicate that pre- and postsynaptic dopamine receptors may develop at different stages during the development of the nervous system and/or that they are differentially modulated via diverse but cocaine-sensitive signaling pathways.

Exposure to cocaine during development has been shown to reduce ornithine decarboxylase activity, an enzyme that is activated during the period of neurite development, synaptogenesis, and neuronal differentiation.[73] In addition, it was also demonstrated that cocaine inhibits DNA synthesis[74] and depresses cerebral glucose utilization.[75] Although such consequences of prenatal cocaine may greatly influence the development of the central nervous system, the impact of such effects would be expected to be widely spread throughout the brain rather than limited to the D_1 dopamine receptor system. It therefore appears that fetal cocaine exposure exerts its influence on the coupling of brain D_1 dopamine receptor to Gs protein via a strikingly specific, yet unknown, mechanism(s).[22,23,30,69] The identification of the mechanism(s) by which *in utero* cocaine alters signal transduction at the D_1 dopamine receptor system will facilitate the formulation of novel specific and effective therapeutic strategies to counteract the short- and long-term neurobehavioral dysfunctions that are associated with exposure to this drug of abuse.

REFERENCES

1. KOZELL N.J. & E.H. ADAMS. 1986. Epidemiology of drug abuse: An overview. Science **234:** 970–974.
2. OSTREA, E.M., JR., M. BRADY, S. GAUSE, A.L. RAYMUNDO & M. STEVENS. 1992. Drug screening of newborns by meconium analysis: A large-scale, prospective, epidemiologic study. Pediatrics **89:** 107–113.
3. ORO A.S. & S.D. DIXON. 1987. Perinatal cocaine and methamphetamine exposure: Maternal and neonatal correlates. J. Pediatr. **111:** 571–578.
4. FOSS J.A. & E.P. RILEY. 1991. Elicitation and modification of the caustic startle reflex in animals prenatally exposed to cocaine. Neurotoxicol. Teratol. **13:** 541–546.
5. DOW-EDWARDS, D.L., L.A. FREED & T.A. FICO. 1990. Structural and functional effects of prenatal cocaine exposure in adult rat brain. Dev. Brain Res. **57:** 263–268.
6. SEIDLER, F.J. & T.A. SLOTKIN. 1992. Fetal cocaine exposure causes persistent noradrenergic hyperactivity in rat brain regions: Effects on neurotransmitter turnover and receptors. J. Pharmacol. Exp. Ther. **263:** 413–421.
7. HENDERSON, M.G. & B.A. MCMILLEN. 1993. Changes in dopamine, serotonin and their metabolites in discrete brain areas of rat offspring after *in utero* exposure to cocaine or related drugs. Teratology **48:** 421–430.
8. OLSON, L. & A. SEIGER. 1972. Early prenatal ontogeny of central monoamine neurons in the rat: Fluorescent histochemical observations. Anat. Ent.-Gesh. **137:** 301–316.
9. OLSON, L., L.O. BOREUS & A. SEIGER. 1973. Histochemical demonstration and mapping of 5-hydroxytryptamine and catecholamine containing neuron systems in the human fetal brain. Anat. Ent.-Gesh. **139:** 259–282.
10. TENNYSON, V.M., R.E. BARRETT, G. COHEN, L. COTE, R. HEIKKILA & C. MYTILINEOU. 1972. The developing neostriatum of the rabbit: Correlation of fluorescence histochemistry, electron microscopy, endogenous dopamine levels and 3H-dopamine uptake. Brain Res. **46:** 251–285.
11. TENNYSON, V.M., C. MYTILINEOU & R.E. BARRETT. 1973. Fluorescence and electron microscopic studies of the early development of the substantia nigra and area ventralis tegmenti in the fetal rabbit. J. Comp. Neurol. **149:** 233–257.

12. Hill, R.M., M.M. Desmond & J.L. Kay. 1966. Extrapyramidal dysfunction in an infant of a schizophrenic mother. J. Pediatr. **69:** 589–595.
13. Levy, W. & K. Wisniewski. 1974. Chlorpromazine causing extrapyramidal dysfunction in newborn infant of psychotic mother. N.Y. J. Med. **74:** 684–685.
14. Lundborg, P. 1972. Abnormal ontogeny in young rabbit after chronic administration of haloperidol to the nursing mothers. Brain Res. **44:** 684–687.
15. Clark, C.V., D. Gorman & A. Vernadakis. 1970. Effects of prenatal administration of psychotropic drugs on behavior of developing rats. Dev. Psychobiol. **3:** 225–235.
16. Golub, M. & C. Kornetsky. 1975. Modification of the behavioral response to drugs in rats exposed prenatally to chlorpromazine. Psychopharmacol. J. **43:** 289–291.
17. Ritz, M.C., R.J. Lamb, S.R. Goldberg & M.J. Kuhar. 1987. Cocaine receptors on dopamine transporter are related to self administration of cocaine. Science **37:** 1219–1223.
18. Hutchings, D. E., T.A. Fico & D.L. Dow-Edwards. 1989. Prenatal cocaine: Maternal toxicity, fetal effects and locomotor activity in rat offspring. Neurotoxicol. Teratol. **11:** 65–69.
19. Scalzo, F.M., S.F. Ali, N.A. Frambes & L.P. Spear. 1990. Weanling rats exposed prenatally to cocaine exhibit an increase in striatal D_2 dopamine binding associated with an increase in ligand affinity. Pharmacol. Biochem. Behav. **37:** 371–373.
20. Mayfield, R.D., G. Larson & N.R. Zahniser. 1992. Cocaine-induced behavioral sensitization and D_1 dopamine receptor function in rat nucleus accumbens and striatum. Brain Res. **573:** 331–335.
21. Leslie, C.A., M.W. Robertson, A.B. Jung, J. Libermann & J.P. Benett, Jr. 1994. Effects of prenatal cocaine exposure upon postnatal development of neostriatal dopaminergic function. Synapse **17:** 210–215.
22. Wang, H.Y., S. Runyan, E. Yadin & E. Friedman. 1995. Prenatal exposure to cocaine selectively reduces D_1 dopamine receptor-mediated activation of striatal Gs proteins. J. Pharmacol. Exp. Ther. **273:** 492–498.
23. Friedman, E., E. Yadin & H.Y. Wang. 1996. Effect of prenatal cocaine on dopamine receptor-G protein coupling in mesocortical regions of the rabbit brain. Neuroscience **70:** 739–747.
24. Reinoso, B.S., A.S. Undie & P. Levitt. 1996. Dopamine receptors mediated differential morphological effects on cerebral cortical neurons in vitro. J. Neurosci. Res. **43:** 439–453.
25. Dos Santos Rodrigues, P. & J. E. Dowling. 1990. Dopamine induces neurite retraction in retinal horizontal cells via diacylglycerol and protein kinase C. Proc. Natl. Acad. Sci. USA **87:** 9693–9697.
26. Gilman, A.G. 1987. G proteins: Transducers of receptor-generated signals. Annu. Rev. Biochem. **56:** 615–649.
27. Birnbaumer, L. 1990. G proteins in signal transduction. Annu. Rev. Pharmacol. Toxicol. **30:** 675–705.
28. Wang, H.-Y., A. Undie & E. Friedman. 1995. Evidence for the coupling of Gq protein to D_1-like dopamine sites in rat striatum: Possible role in dopamine-mediated inositol phosphates formation. Mol. Pharmacol. **48:** 998–994.
29. Friedman, E., L.-Q. Jin, G.-P. Cai, T.R. Hollon, J. Drago, D.R. Sibley & H.-Y. Wang. 1997. D_1-like dopaminergic activation of phosphoinositide hydrolysis is independent of D_{1A} dopamine receptors: Evidence from D_{1A} knockout mice. Mol. Pharmacol. **51:** 6–11.
30. Murphy, E.H., I. Fischer, E. Friedman, D. Grayson, L. Jones, P. Levitt, A. O'Brien-Jenkins, H.Y. Wang & X.H. Wang. 1997. Cocaine administration in pregnant rabbits alters cortical structure and function in their progeny in the absence of maternal seizures. Exp. Brain Res. **114:** 433–441.
31. Fung, Y. K., J.A. Reed & Y.-S. Lau. 1989. Prenatal cocaine exposure fails to modify neurobehavioral responses and the striatal dopaminergic system in newborn rats. Gen. Pharmacol. **260:** 689–693.
32. Wang, H.-Y., J.M. Yeung & E. Friedman. 1995. Prenatal cocaine exposure selectively reduces mesocortical dopamine release. J. Pharmacol. Exp. Ther. **273:** 1211–1215.
33. Ng, G.Y.K., B. Mouillac, S.R. George, M.G. Caron, M. Dennis, M. Bouvier & B.F. O'Dowd. 1994. Desensitization, phosphorylation and palmitoylation of the human dopamine D_1 receptor. Eur J. Pharmacol. **267:** 7–19.
34. Butkerait, P., H.Y. Wang & E. Friedman. 1993. Increases in guanine nucleotide binding

to striatal G proteins is associated with dopamine receptor supersensitivity. J. Pharmacol. Exp. Ther. **271:** 422–428.
35. LINDER, M.E., P. MIDDLETON, J.R. HEPLER, R. TAUSSIG, A. GILMAN & S.M. MUMBY. 1993. Lipid modifications of G proteins: α subunits are palmitoylated. Proc. Natl. Acad. Sci. USA **90:** 3675–3679.
36. PARENTI, M., M.A. VIGANO, C.M.H. NEWMAN, G. MILLIGAN & A.I. MAGEE. 1993. A novel N-terminal motif for palmitoylation of G-protein α subunits. Biochem. J. **291:** 349–353.
37. DEGTYAREV, M.Y., A.M. SPIEGEL & T.L.Z. JONES. 1993. Increased palmitoylation of the Gs protein α subunit after activation by the β-adrenergic receptor or cholera toxin. J. Biol. Chem. **268:** 23769–23772.
38. WEDEGAERTNER, P.B., D.H. CHU, P.T. WILSON, M.J. LEVIS & H.R. BOURNE. 1993. Palmitoylation is required for signaling functions and membrane attachment of Gqα and Gsα. J. Biol. Chem. **268:** 25001–25008.
39. KADATA, T., A.G. GILMAN, Y. WATANABE, S. BAUER & K.H. JACOBS. 1985. Protein kinase C phosphorylates the inhibitory guanine nucleotide-binding regulatory component and apparently suppresses its function in hormonal inhibition of adenylate cyclase. Eur. J. Biochem. **151:** 431–437.
40. CARLSON, K.E., L.F. BRASS & D.R. MANNING. 1989. Thrombin and phorbol esters cause the selective phosphorylation of a G protein other than Gi in human platelets. J. Biol. Chem. **264:** 13298–13305.
41. PYNE, N.J., M. FREISSMUTH & S. PALMER. 1992. Phosphorylation of the recombinant spliced variants of the α-sub-unit of the stimulatory guanine-nucleotide binding regulatory protein (Gs) by the catalytic sub-unit of protein kinase C. Biochem. J. **285:** 333–338.
42. PYNE, N.J., M. FREISSMUTH & S. PYNE. 1992. Phosphorylation of the recombinant spliced variants of the α-sub-unit of the stimulatory guanine-nucleotide binding regulatory protein (Gs) by the catalytic sub-unit of protein kinase A. Biochem. Biophys. Comm. **186:** 1081–1086.
43. SAUVAGE, C., J.F. RUMIGNY & M. MAITRE. 1991. Purification of g proteins from human brain: Modification of GTPase activity upon phosphorylation. Mol. Cell. Biochem. **107:** 65–77.
44. SIBLEY, D.R., J.L. BENOVIC, M.G. CARON & R.J. LEFKOWITZ. 1987. Regulation of transmembrane signaling by receptor phosphorylation. Cell **48:** 913–922.
45. BOUVIER, M., L.M.F. LEEB-LUNDBERG, J.L. BENOVIC, M.G. CARON & R.J. LEFKOWITZ. 1987. Regulation of adrenergic receptor function by phosphorylation of α_1- and β_2-adrenergic receptors by protein kinase C and the cyclic AMP-dependent protein kinase. J. Biol. Chem. **262:** 3106–3113.
46. HAGA K., T. HAGA & A. ICHIYAMA. 1990. Phosphorylation by protein kinase C of the muscarinic acetylcholine receptor. J. Neurochem. **54:** 1639–1644.
47. ZAMANILLO, D., E. CASANOVA, A. ALONSO-LLAMAZARES, S. OVALLE, M.A. CHINCHETRU & P. CALVO. 1995. Identification of a cyclic adenosine 3′, 5′-monophospate-dependent protein kinase phosphorylation site in the carboxy terminal tail of human D_1 dopamine receptor. Neurosci. Lett. **188:** 183–186.
48. HAUSDORFF, W.P., M.J. LOHSE, M. BOUVIER, S.B. LIGGETT, M.G. CARON & R.J. LEFKOWITZ. 1990. Two kinases mediate agonist-dependent phosphorylation and desensitization of the beta 2-adrenergic receptor. Symposia Soc. Exp. Biol. **44:** 225–240.
49. TIBERI, M., S.R. NASH, L. BERTRAND, R.J. LEFKOWITZ & M.G. CARON. 1996. Differential regulation of dopamine D1A receptor responsiveness by various G protein-coupled receptor kinases. J. Biol. Chem. **271:** 3771–3778.
50. TERWILLIGER, R.Z., D. BEITNER-JOHNSON, K. SEVARINO, S.M. CRAIN & E.J. NESTLER. 1991. A general role for adaptations in G-proteins and the cyclic AMP system in mediating the chronic actions of morphine and cocaine on neuronal function. Brain Res. **548:** 100–110.
51. MISERENDINO, M.J.D. & E.J. NESTLER. 1995. Behavioral sensitization to cocaine: Modulation by the cyclic AMP system in the nucleus accumbens. Brain Res. **674:** 299–306.
52. WANG, Y.T. & M.W. SALTER. 1994. Regulation of NMDA receptor by tyrosine kinases and phosphatases. Nature **369:** 233–235.
53. VOIGT, P., Y.J. MA, D. GONZALEZ, W.H. FAHRENBACH, W.C. WETSEL, K. BERG-VON DER EMDE, D.F. HILL, K.G. TAYLOR & M.E. COSTA. Neural and glial-mediated effects of

growth factors acting via tyrosine kinase receptors on luteinizing hormone-releasing hormone neurons. Endocrinology **137:** 2593–2605.

54. SERPENTE, N., M.C. BIRLING & J. PRICE. 1996. The regulation of the expression, phosphorylation, and protein associations of pp125FAK during rat brain development. Mol. Cell. Neurosci. **7:** 391–403.
55. HAYCOCK, J.W., N.G. AHN, M.H. COBB & E.G. KREBS. 1992. ERK1 and ERK2, two microtubule-associated protein 2 kinases, mediate the phosphorylation of tyrosine hydroxylase at serine-31 in situ. Proc. Natl. Acad. Sci. USA **89:** 2365–2369.
56. SEGER, R. & E.G. KREBS. 1995. The MAKP signaling cascade. FASEB J. **9:** 726–735.
57. BERSHOW, M.T., N. HIROI & E.J. NESTLER. 1996. Regulation of ERK (extracellular signal regulated kinase), part of the neurotrophin signal transduction cascade, in the rat mesolimbic dopamine system by chronic exposure to morphine or cocaine. J. Neurosci. **16:** 4707–4715.
58. BERSHOW, M.T., N. HIROI, L.A. KOBIERSKI, S.E. HYMAN & E.J. NESTLER. 1996. Influence of cocaine on the JAK-STAT pathway in the mesolimbic dopamine system. J. Neurosci. **16:** 8019–8026.
59. SIM, A.T. 1991. The regulation and function of protein phosphatases in the brain. Mol. Neurobiol. **5:** 229–246.
60. MALCHIODI-ALBEDI, F., T.C. PETRUCCI, B. PICCONI, F. IOSI & M. FALCHI. 1997. Protein phosphatase inhibitors induce modification of synapse structure and tau hyperphosphorylation in cultured rat hippocampal neurons. J. Neurosci. Res. **48:** 425–438.
61. TONG, G., D. SHEPHERD & C.E. HAHR. 1995. Synaptic desensitization of NMDA receptors by calcineurin. Science **267:** 1510–1512.
62. WANG, J.H. & P.T. KELLY. 1997. Postsynaptic calcineurin activity downregulates synaptic transmission by weakening intracellular Ca^{2+} signaling mechanisms in hippocampal CA1 neurons. J. Neurosci. **17:** 4600–4611.
63. SURMEIER, D.J., J. BARGAS, H.C. HEMMINGS, JR., A.C. NAIRN & P. GREENGARD. 1995. Modulation of calcium currents by a D_1 dopaminergic protein kinase/phosphatase cascade in rat neostriatal neurons. Neuron **14:** 385–397.
64. SIMANSKY, K.J. & W.J. KACHELRIES. 1995. Prenatal exposure to cocaine selectively disrupts motor responding to D-amphetamine in young and mature rabbits. Neuropharmacology **35:** 71–78.
65. TILAKARATNE, N., G.P. CAI & E. FRIEDMAN. 1998. Cocaine-induced activation of *c-fos* gene expression is attenuated in prenatal cocaine-exposed rabbits. Ann. N.Y. Acad. Sci. This volume.
66. GRAYBIEL, A.M., R. MORATALLA & H. ROBERTSON. 1990. Amphetamine and cocaine induce drug-specific activation of the *c-fos* gene in striosome-matrix compartments and limbic subdivisions of the striatum. Proc. Natl. Acad. Sci. USA **87:** 6912–6916.
67. JONES, L., I. FISCHER & P. LEVITT. 1997. Nonuniform alteration of dendritic development in the cerebral cortex following prenatal cocaine exposure. Cerebral Cortex **6:** 431–445.
68. WANG, X.-H., P. LEVITT, J.A. O'BRIEN & E.H. MURPHY. 1997. Normal development of tyrosine hydroxylase and serotonin immunoreactive fibers innervating anterior cingulate cortex and visual cortex in rabbits exposed prenatally to cocaine. Brain Res. **715:** 221–224.
69. LEVITT, P., J.A. HARVEY, E. FRIEDMAN, K. SIMANSKY & E.H. MURPHY. 1997. New evidence for neurotransmitter influences on brain development. Trends Neurosci. **20:** 269–274.
70. ROMANO, A.G., W.J. KACHELRIES, K.J. SIMANSKY & J.A. HARVEY. 1995. Intrauterine exposure to cocaine produces a modality-specific acceleration of classical conditioning in adult rabbits. Pharmacol. Biochem. Behav. **52:** 415–420.
71. MILLER J.C. & A.J. FRIEDHOFF. 1988. Prenatal neurotransmitter programming of postnatal receptor function. Prog. Brain Res. **73:** 509–522.
72. ROSENGARTEN, H., E. FRIEDMAN & A.J. FRIEDHOFF. 1983. Sensitive periods for the effect of haloperidol on development of striatal dopamine receptors. Birth Defects: Original Article Series **19:** 511–513.
73. KOEGLER, S.M., F.J. SEIDLER, J.R. SPENCER & T.A. SLOTKIN. 1991. Ischemia contributes to adverse effects on cocaine on brain development: Suppression of ornithine decarboxylase activity in neonatal rats. Brain Res. Bull. **27:** 829–834.

74. Anderson-Brown, T., T.A. Slotkin & F.J. Seidler. 1990. Cocaine acutely inhibits DNA synthesis in developing rat brain regions: Evidence for direct actions. Brain Res. **537:** 197–202.
75. Burchfield, D.J. & R.M. Abrams. 1993. Cocaine depresses cerebral glucose utilization in fetal sheep. Dev. Brain Res. **73:** 283–288.

A Mouse Model of Transplacental Cocaine Exposure

Clinical Implications for Exposed Infants and Children[a]

BARRY E. KOSOFSKY[b–d] AND AARON S. WILKINS[b]

[b]*Laboratory of Molecular and Developmental Neuroscience, Massachusetts General Hospital-East, Charlestown, Massachusetts 02129, USA*

[c]*Department of Neurology, Massachusetts General Hospital and Harvard Medical School, Boston, Massachusetts 02114, USA*

ABSTRACT: To characterize the effects of cocaine on developing brain we have developed a mouse model of gestational cocaine exposure. We studied pregnant dams injected twice daily with cocaine HCl at 40, 20, or 10 mg/kg/day sc from embryonic days (E)8 to E17 (COC 40, COC20, and COC10, respectively), vehicle-injected dams allowed access to food *ad libitum* (SAL) or pair-fed with the COC 40 dams (SPF 40), animals pretreated with the short-acting α-adrenergic antagonist phentolamine prior to each cocaine injection (P COC 40), and animals administered phentolamine prior to saline (PHENT). COC 40, P COC 40, and SPF 40 dams demonstrated the lowest percentage weight gain during gestation. The surrogate-fostered offspring of COC 40, P COC 40, and SPF 40 dams demonstrated transient brain and body growth retardation on postnatal days (P)1 and P9 when compared to pups born to SAL dams. We conducted behavioral tests which allowed us to dissociate the indirect effect of cocaine-induced malnutrition from a direct effect of prenatal cocaine administration in altering postnatal behavior. Pups from all groups were tested for first-order Pavlovian conditioning on P9 or P12 or for the ability to ignore redundant information in a blocking paradigm on P50. Unlike the SPF 40, PHENT, and SAL controls, COC 40 and P COC 40 mice were unable to acquire an aversion to an odor previously paired with shock on P9, a learning deficit that resolved by P12. However, on P50, COC 40 mice and, to a lesser extent, P COC 40 and SPF 40 mice demonstrated a persistent behavioral deficit in our blocking paradigm, which may reflect alterations in selective attention. We discuss how these findings in our rodent model have developmental implications for human infants exposed to cocaine *in utero.*

INTRODUCTION

Current estimates suggest that over 45,000 infants born each year in the United States have been exposed to cocaine *in utero.*[1] Numerous clinical studies have been performed, and a clear picture as to the independent role cocaine may contribute to the adverse outcomes seen in some of these infants and children is just starting to emerge (reviewed in refs. 2–11). Preliminary evidence suggests that cocaine independently contributes to impairment in brain growth which is prenatal in origin and most profound following exposure through all three trimesters, and exposure at the higher doses of drug.[12–14] Infants who sustain cocaine exposure *in utero* are at risk for alterations in

[a] This work was supported by Public Health Service Grants DA00175 and DA08648 to B.E.K.

[d] Communicating author: Barry E. Kosofsky, M.D., Ph.D., Laboratory of Molecular and Developmental Neuroscience, Massachusetts General Hospital-East, 149 13th Street, Charlestown, MA 02129. Tel, 617/724–9600; fax, 617/724–9610; e-mail, Kosofsky@helix.mgh.harvard.edu

postnatal behavior as assessed by the Brazelton NBAS[12,15,16], by more subtle measures of arousal, reactivity, and attention,[17,18] as well as the Bayley measures of cognitive function.[19–22] An underlying cocaine-induced inattention syndrome may further compromise cognitive and language skills in this cohort.[23–25] Not every child exposed to cocaine demonstrates brain growth retardation, inattention, cognitive impairments, or language delay. Even those children with a significant cocaine exposure and evidence of developmental compromise may not demonstrate all of these deficits. However, children with the greatest impairment in prenatal brain growth, which correlates with more significant cocaine exposures,[14] are more likely to demonstrate impairment in postnatal brain growth,[13] state control,[16] attention,[26] and information processing.[18] Because of the implications for medical care, psychosocial interventions, and public policy, a clearer characterization of the deficits evident in these children, and identification of the extent to which *in utero* cocaine exposure independently contributes to such outcomes, are a high priority.

We have established an animal model in mice to control the timing and dose of prenatal cocaine administration, with the goal of dissociating the growth and behavioral deficits evident in offspring exposed transplacentally to cocaine independent of other confounding (co)variables. Rodent models have been a valuable tool in leading to the characterization of a number of growth and behavioral deficits in cocaine-exposed offspring. Previous studies in rodents have demonstrated *in utero* growth retardation following prenatal cocaine exposure,[27–30] while others have described normal fetal growth.[31–33] In neonatal rodents, behavioral studies have demonstrated that prenatal cocaine exposure affects simple reflexes,[34] motor activity,[34–37] and various aspects of learning, including appetitive and aversive classical (first-order) conditioning tasks[31,38–40] (reviewed in ref. 41). Persistent behavioral deficits in adult rats exposed to cocaine *in utero* are evident in conditional discrimination,[42] the Porsolt swim test,[43] conditioned place preference,[44] and the stress response.[45]

We modified a blocking paradigm[46] for use in adult rats exposed to cocaine *in utero.* Behavioral theorists have speculated that the phenomenon of blocking is most likely explained by selective attention: training to a conditional stimulus (A) affects the extent to which an added stimulus (B) is processed ("attended to") on subsequent AB (compound conditioned) trials.[47] Successful blocking depends on the ability to attend selectively to stimuli that are informative, adaptive, and predictive of a reinforcing event (i.e., A). Disrupted performance of adult mice in a blocking paradigm (i.e., aversion to B) may reflect alterations in selective attention.[48,49]

Numerous investigators have suggested mechanisms by which gestational cocaine exposure may alter brain development following acute or chronic (recurrent) drug exposure.[2,3,5,9,28,50–63] One of the proposed mechanisms by which cocaine may alter fetal brain development is via fetal hypoxia mediated by maternal uterine artery vasoconstriction.[9,64] Alternatively, cocaine, which prevents the reuptake of norepinephrine (NE), serotonin (5-HT), and dopamine (DA), may affect the fetus by altering aminergic signal transduction in the dam and/or the fetus. According to this formulation, fetal toxicity may result from cocaine-induced alterations in the peripheral and/or central nervous system (CNS) levels of the amines NE, 5-HT, and DA,[5] neurotransmitters that may exert trophic roles during brain development,[65] and that subserve attentional mechanisms in adults.[66] In order to identify whether vasoconstriction or α-adrenergic mechanism(s) contributed to cocaine-induced alterations of fetal brain development we examined the ability of phentolamine, a short acting α-adrenergic antagonist,[67] to protect the fetus from the toxic effects of recurrent prenatal cocaine administration to pregnant mice.

In this study we examined the effects of prenatal cocaine exposure and prenatal malnutrition on food intake and weight gain in pregnant mice, and examined exposed offspring for alterations in postnatal brain and body growth, the ability of mice to first-order condition on P9 and P12, and the ability of mice to demonstrate blocking on P50. We additionally performed experiments to determine the relevance of α-adrenergic mechanisms in mediating aspects of the transplacental toxicity of gestational cocaine exposure. This publication reports a synthesis of findings from previously published work[68–70] and highlights some of the essential growth and behavioral features of our mouse model of gestational cocaine exposure.

METHODS

The methods used in the experiments described here were reported in detail[68–70] following research protocols approved by the MGH IACUC. Briefly, upon arrival, timed-pregnant Swiss Webster (SW) dams (Taconic Labs, New York) were maintained in individual cages on a 12/12-hour light/dark cycle (lights on at 7:00 AM), with food and water available *ad libitum.* Starting on E7 all animals were weighed daily and started on a liquid diet (Bio-Serv, #F1259SP). On E8 dams were assigned to one of the following treatment groups to receive twice daily injections (at 7:00 AM and 7:00 PM) from E18–E17 (inclusive):

1. SAL, administered 0.9% (physiologic) saline sc, allowed access to food *ad libitum;*
2. COC 40, administered cocaine HCl (RBI, Natick, MA) at 40 mg/kg/day sc dissolved in physiologic saline, divided twice daily (bid);
3. COC 20, administered cocaine at 20 mg/kg/day sc, divided bid;
4. COC 10, administered cocaine at 10 mg/kg/day sc, divided bid;
5. SPF 40, administered physiologic saline twice daily and pair fed with a COC 40 dam;
6. P COC 40, administered phentolamine 5 mg/kg sc 15 minutes prior to each of the two daily cocaine doses (administered at 40 mg/kg/day sc);
7. PHENT, administered phentolamine 5 mg/kg sc 15 minutes prior to each of two daily doses of physiologic saline.

Within 24 hours of delivery, between 7 and 9 pups were fostered to untreated surrogate dams that had given birth within the preceding 24–72 hours. Pup weight, sex, and biparietal diameter (measured with a micrometer placed in front of the external auditory meati) were recorded on P1 as well as behavioral testing date P9 or P50. One hundred and nine litters (dams, and a subset of exposed offspring) were used in these studies (SAL, $n = 25$; COC 40, $n = 31$; COC 20, $n = 6$; COC 10, $n = 6$; SPF 40, $n = 26$; P COC 40, $n = 8$; PHENT, $n = 7$). Behavioral testing of first-order conditioning on P9 and P12 and for blocking on P50 was conducted as previously reported.[68]

RESULTS

Maternal and Offspring Growth Data. TABLE 1 is a summary of maternal and litter data for the treatment groups studied. The percentage gestational weight gain for the period E8–E18 was decreased in COC 40 dams and in P COC 40 dams. This was likely a consequence of the cocaine-induced decrease in food intake evident in dams from these groups. Lower doses of cocaine (COC 20 and COC 10) and phentolamine pretreatment by itself (PHENT) did not significantly impair maternal weight gain. Of note, on the identical diet as COC 40 dams, SPF 40 (pair-fed) dams gained the least weight of all the dam treatment groups included in these studies. It is likely that this is a consequence of malnutrition as well as maternal stress induced by malnutrition, which has implications for the interpretation of the results from this pair-fed control group (see ref. 68). When comparing across these treatment groups, there was no difference in gestational length or litter size on P0, implying that even at the highest doses of cocaine, our drug regimen did not induce gross teratogenic effects.

TABLE 2 depicts a summary of P1, P9, and P50 weight and biparietal diameter (BPD) data for exposed offspring. Pups born to dams from the groups that demonstrated impairment in food intake and percentage gestational weight gain (TABLE 1) were the same groups in which there was a significant decrease in P1 weight of the offspring, including the COC 40, SPF 40, and P COC 40 pups. By P9 the P COC 40 pups had "caught up" to control values, and on P50 the only evidence of persistent growth retardation was in male offspring born to COC 40 and SPF 40 dams. On P1, brain growth retardation was evident in pups born to COC 40 and SPF 40 dams. This persisted through P9 in the COC 40 and SPF 40 pups and was also evident in the P COC 40 pups. Brain growth retardation was not evident in offspring from any of the treatment groups on P50.

TABLE 1. Summary of Maternal/Litter Data

Variable	SAL	COC 40	COC 20	COC 10	SPF 40	P COC 40	PHENT
Percentage gestational	37.6	25.1[a]	33.5	35.7	15.8[a]	27.9[a]	37.4
weight gain, E8–E18	(0.8)[b]	(1.2)	(1.3)	(1.4)	(1.9)	(5.0)	(1.2)
Total food intake (g),	205	157[a]	179	189		134[a]	187
E8–E16	(7.6)	(7.4)	(5.9)	(10.7)		(17.1)	(10.8)
Gestational length (d)	18.3	19.0	19.2	18.5	18.9	18.4	18.3
	(0.2)	(0.2)	(0.5)	(0.4)	(0.2)	(0.2)	(0.2)
Litter size at P0	12.6	11.4	11.5	12.3	10.9	10.9	12.6
	(0.5)	(0.5)	(1.0)	(1.2)	(0.4)	(0.7)	(0.9)

[a] $p < 0.01$ when compared with SAL controls (Dunnett t).
[b] SEMs are indicated in parentheses

TABLE 2. Summary of Offspring Data

Variable	SAL	COC 40	COC 20	COC 10	SPF 40	P COC 40	PHENT
P1 Wt (g)[a]	1.6	1.3[b]	1.7	1.7	1.2[b]	1.3[b]	1.4
	(.03)[c]	(.06)	(.07)	(.08)	(.03)	(.07)	(.03)
P9 Wt	5.0	4.4[b]	5.6	5.2	4.4[b]	5.1	5.4
	(.11)	(.13)	(.18)	(.07)	(.14)	(.17)	(.10)
P50 Wt male[e]	34.2	29.7[d]	34.9	36.0	29.5[b]	31.3	33.3
	(.98)	(1.3)	(1.5)	(.88)	(1.1)	(2.6)	(1.4)
P50 Wt female	26.4	24.3	26.5	27.7	24.2	25.5	26.3
	(.59)	(.87)	(.71)	(.66)	(1.00)	(1.2)	(.84)
P1 BPD (in)	.292	.278[b]	.303	.302	.268[b]	.279	.289
	(.002)	(.004)	(.004)	(.005)	(.003)	(.005)	(.002)
P9 BPD	.429	.405[b]	.438	.427	.403[b]	.401[b]	.416
	(.003)	(.003)	(.005)	(.003)	(.004)	(.003)	(.002)
P50 BPD male[e]	.531	.529	.538	.541	.533	.527	.533
	(.005)	(.001)	(.006)	(.004)	(.008)	(.004)	(.004)
P50 BPD female	.516	.513	.518	.525	.496	.524	.527
	(.003)	(.010)	(.013)	(.005)	(.008)	(.004)	(.002)

[a] Wt and BPD data are combined for male and female P1 and P9 pups.
[b] $p < 0.01$; treatment group smaller than SAL controls (Dunnett t).
[c] SEMs are indicated in parentheses.
[d] $p < 0.05$; treatment group smaller than SAL controls (Dunnett t).
[e] $p < 0.05$; males larger than females.

Offspring Behavioral Data. Offspring were tested on P9 for the ability to learn first-order conditioning. Pups from the COC 40 and P COC 40 groups were unable to acquire first-order conditioning (FIG. 1). However, this deficit was transient as P12 pups from the COC 40 and P COC 40 groups were able to acquire first-order conditioning (data not shown; see refs. 68 and 70).

Animals were tested in a blocking paradigm on P50. While animals from each treatment group were able to learn an aversion to the compound conditioned stimulus, animals from the COC 40 group and, to a lesser extent, animals from the SPF 40 and P COC 40 groups demonstrated a persistent deficit in blocking. Offspring from these groups were unable to ignore the redundant stimulus and spent less time over the non-novel (i.e., redundant) odor (FIG. 2).

FIGURE 3 graphically depicts a correlation analysis of the effect of prenatal exposure to cocaine on blocking performance. As the prenatal dose of cocaine increased (COC 10 vs COC 20 vs COC 40), performance in the blocking paradigm was significantly and progressively impaired. Thus, following exposure to lower doses of cocaine (e.g., COC 20), adult offspring displayed subtle yet demonstrable impairments in blocking.

DISCUSSION

Maternal Weight Gain. An inverse relationship between dose of cocaine and maternal food intake as well as maternal weight gain is evident in TABLE 1. The nutritional compromise may be one cause of altered prenatal growth in the pups, as reflected by deficits in P1 weight and BPD in the offspring of pups born to COC 40, SPF 40, and P COC 40 dams. The impairment in brain (and body) growth in these offspring persists through at least P9, suggesting that *in utero* exposure to cocaine and/or malnutrition alters mechanisms underlying brain development with consequences that are evident in the perinatal and postnatal period. One can conclude that a smaller head (i.e., decreased BPD) at birth is a marker for prenatal exposure to cocaine at increased doses (COC 40). However, the smaller head at birth is not a marker specific for the COC 40 group, as it is also seen in the SPF 40 group. Moreover, the effect of malnutrition seems to be accentuated in the SPF 40 group, as evidenced by the smallest percentage gestational weight gain in those dams despite identical food intake with the COC 40 group (and also evident by significant growth retardation in dams and their offspring following lesser degrees of malnutrition; see ref. 69).

Offspring Behavior. In support of the distinction of the high dose cocaine effect and the malnutrition effect as separable is the observation that the deficit in first-order conditioning evident on P9 was only seen in offspring exposed to the higher dose of cocaine (seen in pups from the COC 40 and P COC 40 groups) and was not seen in pups born to malnourished dams (SPF 40 pups), despite the fact that pups from all three groups demonstrated smaller heads on P9 (see TABLE 3). Thus the small head at birth may be a sensitive marker for significant *in utero* exposure to cocaine, which may have behavioral correlates, but which as already mentioned may not be a marker specific for that exposure.

Our P50 behavioral data make an additional point regarding the dissociation of growth retardation from behavioral deficits in cocaine-exposed offspring. As demonstrated by correlation analysis (FIG. 3) and additional statistical methods including path analyses and structural equation modeling (see ref. 69), exposure of developing mouse brain to cocaine at lower doses (e.g., COC 20) may result in persistent behavioral deficits in the form of impaired blocking, without any perinatal or postnatal correlates in brain or body growth retardation. This is not to say that the brains of the COC 20 (or COC 10) offspring are normal; they are just grossly normal in size. Whether there

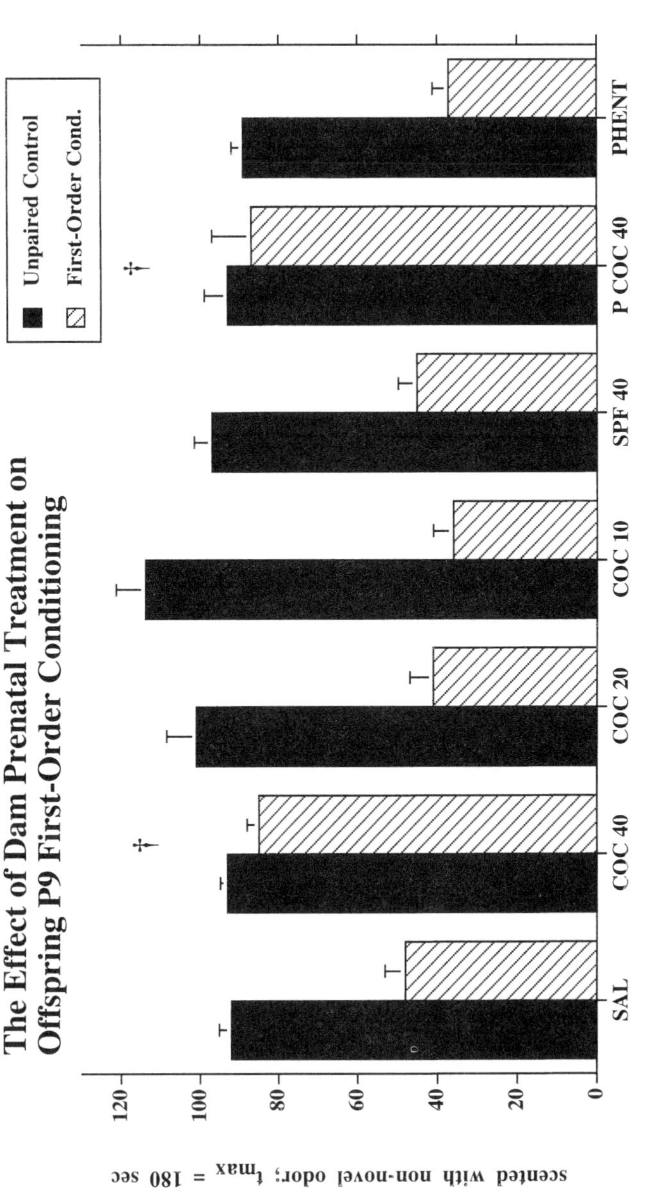

FIGURE 1. The ability of SAL, COC 40, COC 20, COC 10, SPF 40, P COC 40, and PHENT pups to demonstrate first-order conditioning on P9. Successful conditioning is reflected in animals spending less time over the non-novel scented side of the testing chamber than controls. † $p < 0.01$ between test conditions in all groups except COC 40 and P COC 40 (Dunnett t). Error bars indicate SEMs.

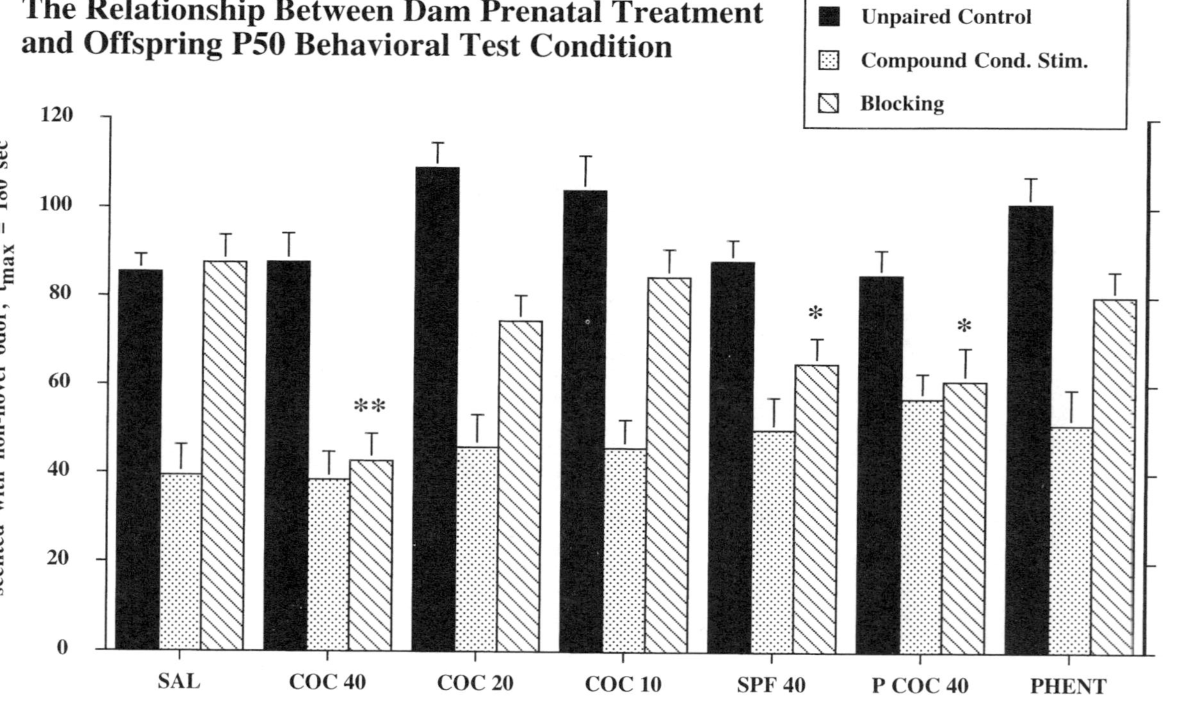

FIGURE 2. The ability of P50 SAL, COC 40, COC 20, COC 10, SPF 40, P COC 40, and PHENT adults to learn an aversion to a compcund conditional stimulus or to ignore an irrelevant stimulus in a blocking paradigm. Successful blocking is shown in animals spending no less time over the non-novel scented side of the testing chamber than animals in the unpaired control group. *$p < 0.05$, **$p < 0.01$ when compared with SAL blocking group (Dunnett t). Error bars indicate SEMs.

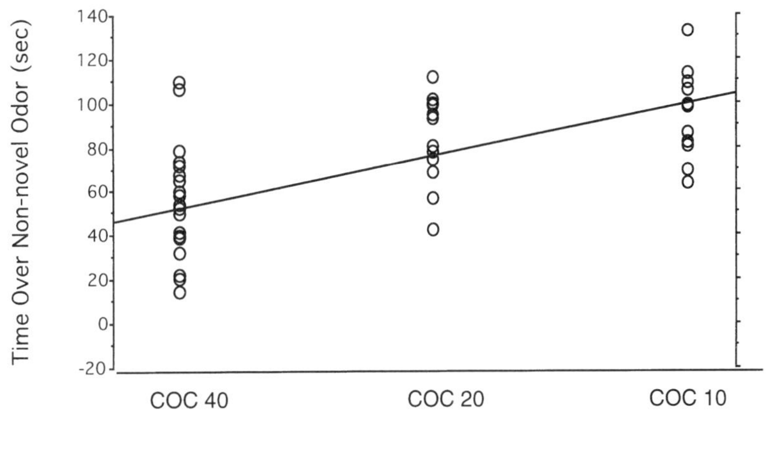

FIGURE 3. Correlation analysis depicting performance of individual P50 animals *(circles)* from COC 40, COC 20, and COC 10 treatment groups in the blocking paradigm. A significant (p <0.0001) dose-dependent correlation is evident with prenatal exposure to increasing doses of cocaine associated with progressively more impaired performance of adult mice in the blocking paradigm.

TABLE 3. Dam and Offspring Growth and Behavioral Data

Variable	SAL	COC 40	COC 20	COC 10	SPF 40	P COC 40	PHENT
Dam food intake	Normal[a] (Nl)	Less	Nl	Nl	Less	Less	Nl
Dam weight gain	Nl	Less	Nl	Nl	Least	Less	Nl
P1 Wt[b]	Nl	Small	Nl	Nl	Small	Small	Nl
P1 BPD[b]	Nl	Small	Nl	Nl	Small	Nl	Nl
P9 Wt	Nl	Small	Nl	Nl	Small	Nl	Nl
P9 BPD	Nl	Small	Nl	Nl	Small	Small	Nl
P50 Wt	Nl	Nl	Nl	Nl	Nl	Nl	Nl
P50 BPD	Nl	Nl	Nl	Nl	Nl	Nl	Nl
P9 first-order C.	Yes	No	Yes	Yes	Yes	No	Yes
P12 first-order C.	Yes	Yes	Yes	Yes	Yes	Yes	Yes
P50 blocking deficit[c]	No	Severe	Mild	±	Moderate	Moderate	No

[a] Differences reported are in comparison with SAL controls (Dunnett t), considered Normal (Nl).
[b] Wt and BPD data are combined for male and female offspring at each age.
[c] Qualitative interpretation of data from blocking experiments.

is persistent molecular dysfunction or neuropathologic abnormalities following gestational exposures to (lower doses of) cocaine, which are associated with the deficit in blocking is an area of active investigation in our laboratory. Should the molecular basis and neuropathologic correlates of the deficit in blocking be identified, the prediction is that animals exposed to lower doses of cocaine (e.g., COC 20) which demonstrate normal perinatal and postnatal BPD may demonstrate intermediate degrees of molecular and neuropathologic compromise. It is also possible that malnutrition-induced deficits in blocking may have additional and distinct molecular and neuropathologic bases and that animals exposed to high doses of cocaine *in utero* and concomitant malnutrition may bear the brunt of a compound insult with compound molecular and neuropathologic correlates.

Developmental Mechanism(s) of Cocaine Action. The phentolamine pre-treatment experiments were designed to identify mechanisms that may be relevant in mediating the growth or behavioral effects of exposure to cocaine *in utero.* The fact that PHENT animals were normal in growth and behavior implies that exposure to this agent by itself, which is likely associated with some degree of "vascular steal" and resulting fetal hypoperfusion (see ref. 70), does not alter mouse brain development as assessed by the outcomes that we measured. The fact that we detected no differences between the P COC 40 and the COC 40 animals suggests that α-adrenergic blockade prior to cocaine administration neither potentiates nor attenuates the cocaine-induced alterations in the growth or behavioral outcomes that we assessed. We conclude that in our model it is unlikely that α-adrenergic mechanisms are relevant in mediating the transplacental effects of **recurrent** cocaine administration. This would include both maternal α-adrenergic mechanisms, such as uterine artery vasoconstriction, as well as fetal α-adrenergic mechanisms, whether systemic or restricted to the developing central nervous system. This is not to say that α-adrenergic mechanisms do not in part contribute to mouse brain development. In fact, data from other laboratories (referred to by Lidow in this volume) reveal that **chronic** α_2-adrenergic antagonism results in (knockout) mice born with alterations in cortical cytoarchitecture. Equally provocative is the finding that the specific neuropathologic alterations induced in the brains of α_2-adrenergic knockout mice simulate aspects of what is seen in mice[39,71] and primates[63] consequent to gestational cocaine exposure. The most parsimonious explanation of these findings is that in our phentolamine experiments the duration of α-adrenergic blockade persisted for approximately 2 hours (see ref. 70), the window during which cocaine is circulating on the maternal and fetal side of the placenta following our subcutaneous route of administration (see ref. 68). The situation is different in the case of the knockout mice, in which there is a persistent deficit in α_2-adrenergic signal transduction.

SUMMARY

We have created a mouse model of gestational cocaine exposure which has allowed us to separate malnutrition from cocaine-induced alterations in brain growth and subsequent behavior. We have learned many lessons from our mouse model, which are coordinate with data which have emerged from other animal models (e.g., rat, rabbit, and primate). Animal models can be informative in identifying critical periods during development, dose-response relationships, and mechanisms of drug action. In addition, control over the genetic variability of subjects, environmental influences on behavior, and the specific details of drug exposure allow for elimination and/or isolation of some of the confounding variables that cloud the clinical study and interpretation of the determinants of altered behavioral outcomes in cocaine-exposed children, including:

- Genetic Predisposition
  - Novelty Seeking, Risk Taking
  - Inattention, Learning Disability, Hyperactivity
  - Personality Disorders, Psychiatric Diagnoses

- Postnatal Environment
  - Impaired Parent-Infant Interaction
  - Altered Social Supports/Chaotic Lifestyle
  - Poverty/Depression/Abuse
- *In Utero* Cocaine Exposure
  - Pattern of Cocaine Use: Quantity/Frequency/Method
  - Timing during Pregnancy of Cocaine Use
  - Concurrent Use of Other Drugs of Abuse

However, there are limitations to the interpretability and clinical relevance of data generated in preclinical models. Certain behaviors and deficits do not have relevant animal models (e.g., selective language delay). Moreover, the laboratory setting is an artificial one and may not simulate the real world challenges that tax the particular behaviors that may be compromised in cocaine-exposed offspring. Despite these "disclaimers" the second generation of preclinical and clinical research has made significant progress in identifying the independent contribution of gestational exposure to cocaine in altering brain development and subsequent behavior. As outlined below and described in the accompanying articles in this monograph, such progress has in large part resulted from:

- Better Study Design
  - Improved Controls
  - Multivariate Design and Analysis
  - Longer Study Period of Parent-Infant Interaction
  - More "Sensitive" Instruments
- Quantitating Exposure
  - Dose-Related versus Threshold Effects
  - Polypharmacy (independent effects)
  - High-Dose versus Low-Dose Effects
- Analysis of Specific Though Subtle Effects
  - Effect Size May Be Small, Requiring Study of Larger Numbers of Subjects
  - Need to Relate Exposure(s) to Outcome(s)
  - Must Analyze Cocaine-Specific Effects

CONCLUSIONS

The convergence of findings from recent preclinical and clinical studies is striking. Work in animals and humans suggests that transplacental exposure to cocaine at higher doses alters programs for brain development that may be associated with lasting alterations in brain structure and function. These effects may not be dramatic; cocaine-induced alterations are not global. Rather, there is exquisite specificity to the insult and associated behavioral deficits, presumably a consequence of molecular site(s) of cocaine action, resulting in persistent alterations in specific signal transduction pathways (e.g., aminergic). The behavioral correlates of such changes may be subtle and best demonstrated when animals and humans are placed in settings that require intact attentional, affective, reactive, and adaptive mechanisms. Deficits in such critically important systems may place exposed individuals at a significant handicap for educability and socialization. A high priority for subsequent clinical research is to identify markers of infants and children at risk for such handicaps and to design and implement appropriate and innovative interventions with the goal of normalizing behavior. A high priority for subsequent preclinical research is to identify transplacental mechanisms of cocaine action and the specific "molecular malformations" induced, as a starting point for rational (pharmaco-) therapy to prevent or attenuate the maladaptive consequences of *in utero* exposure to cocaine.

ACKNOWLEDGMENTS

We thank Cindy Tello for typing the manuscript; Andrew Mercury and Ed Tabit for expert technical assistance; Lisa Genova and Kenneth Jones for conceptual and analytic contributions to these experiments.

REFERENCES

1. National pregnancy and health survey. 1995. A National Institute on Drug Abuse report. National Institutes of Health, Department of Health and Human Services. Washington, DC. Government Printing Office.
2. Dow-Edwards, D.L. 1991. Cocaine effects on fetal development: A comparison of clinical and animal research findings. Neurotoxicol. Teratol. **13:** 347–352.
3. Gingras, J.L., D.E. Weese-Mayer, R.F. Hume, Jr. & K.J. O'Donnell. 1992. Cocaine and development: Mechanisms of fetal toxicity and neonatal consequences of prenatal cocaine exposure. Early Human Dev. **31:** 1–24.
4. Gonzalez, N.M. & M. Campbell. 1994. Cocaine babies: Does prenatal exposure to cocaine affect development? J. Am. Acad. Child Adolesc. Psychiatry **33:** 16–19.
5. Kosofsky, B.E. 1991. The effect of cocaine on developing human brain. *In* Methodologic Issues in Controlled Studies on Effects of Prenatal Exposure to Drugs of Abuse. M.M. Kilbey & K. Asghar, Eds. Washington, DC. NIDA Research Monograph #114: 128–143.
6. Lutiger, B., K. Graham, T.R. Einarson & G. Koren. 1991. Relationship between gestational cocaine use and pregnancy outcome: A meta-analysis. Teratology **44:** 405–414.
7. Mayes, L.C., R.H. Granger, M.H. Bornstein & B. Zuckerman. 1992. The problem of prenatal cocaine exposure: A rush to judgement. JAMA **267:** 406–408.
8. Robins, L.N. & J.L. Mills. 1993. Effects of *in utero* exposure to street drugs. Am. J. Public Health **83:** 3–32.
9. Volpe, J.J. 1992. Effect of cocaine use on the fetus. N. Engl. J. Med. **327:** 399–407.
10. Zuckerman, B. & K. Bresnahan. 1991. Developmental and behavioral consequences of prenatal drug and alcohol exposure. Pediatr. Clin. North Am. **38:** 1387–1406.
11. Chiriboga, C.A. 1996. Cocaine and the fetus: Methodological issues and neurological consequences. *In* Prenatal Cocaine Exposure. R.J. Konkol & G.D. Olsen, Eds. : 1–21. Boca Raton. CRC Press.
12. Chasnoff, I.J., D.R. Griffith, S. MacGregor, K. Dirkes & K.A. Burns. 1989. Temporal patterns of cocaine use in pregnancy. JAMA **261:** 1741–1744.
13. Chasnoff, I.J., D.R. Griffith, C. Freier & J. Murray. 1992. Cocaine/polydrug use in pregnancy: Two-year follow-up. Pediatrics **89:** 284–289.
14. Mirochnick, M., D.A. Frank, H. Cabral, A. Turner & B. Zuckerman. 1995. Relation between meconium concentration of the cocaine metabolite benzoylecgonine and fetal growth. J. Pediatr. **126:** 636–638.
15. Lester, B.M., L. LaGasse, K. Freier & S. Brunner. 1996. Studies of cocaine-exposed human infants. *In* Behavioral Studies of Drug-Exposed Offspring: Methodological Issues in Human and Animal Research. C.L. Wetherington, V.L. Smeriglio & L.P. Finnegan, Eds. : 164–210. U. S. Government Printing Office. Washington, DC.
16. Delaney-Black, V., C. Covington, E. Ostrea, Jr., *et al.* 1996. Prenatal cocaine and neonatal outcome: Evaluation of dose-response relationship. Pediatrics **98:** 735–740.
17. Delaney-Black, V. *et al.* Ann. N.Y. Acad. Sci., this volume.
18. Jacobson, S.W., J.L. Jacobson, R.J. Sokol, S.S. Martier & L.M. Chiodo. 1996. New evidence for neurobehavioral effects of *in utero* cocaine exposure. J. Pediatr. **129:** 581–589.
19. Azuma, S.D. & I.J. Chasnoff. 1993. Outcome of children prenatally exposed to cocaine and other drugs: A path analysis of three-year data. Pediatrics **92:** 396–402.
20. Chiriboga, C.A. 1993. Fetal effects. Neurol. Clin. North Am. **11:** 707–729.

21. CHIRIBOGA, C.A., M. VIBBERT, R. MALOUF *et al.* 1995. Neurological correlates of fetal cocaine exposure: Transient hypertonia of infancy and early childhood. Pediatrics **96:** 1070–1077.
22. MAYES, L.C., M.H. BORNSTEIN, K. CHAWARSKA & R.H. GRANGER. 1995. Information processing and developmental assessments in 3-month-old infants exposed prenatally to cocaine. Pediatrics **95:** 539–545.
23. DAVIS, E., I. FENOY & D. LARAQUE. 1992. Autism and developmental abnormalities in children with perinatal cocaine exposure. J. Nat. Med. Assoc. **84:** 315–319.
24. NULMAN, I., J. ROVET, D. ALTMANN, C. BRADLEY, T. EINARSON & G. KOREN. 1994. Neurodevelopment of adopted children exposed *in utero* to cocaine. Canad. M.A.J. **151:** 1592–1597.
25. MENTIS, M. & K. LUNDGREN. 1995. Effects of prenatal exposure to cocaine and associated risk factors on language development. J. Speech Hearing Res. **38:** 1303–1318.
26. MAYES, L. *et al.* Ann. N.Y. Acad. Sci., this volume.
27. CHURCH, M.W. & H.C. RAUCH. 1992. Prenatal cocaine exposure in the laboratory mouse: Effects on maternal water consumption and offspring outcome. Neurotoxicol. Teratol. **14:** 313–319.
28. GRESSENS, P., F. GOFFLOT, G. VAN MAELE-FABRY *et al.* 1992. Early neurogenesis and teratogenesis in whole mouse embryo cultures. Histochemical, immunocytological and ultrastructural study of the premigratory neuronal-glial units in normal mouse embryo and in mouse embryos influenced by cocaine and retinoic acid. J. Neuropathol. Exp. Neurol. **51:** 206–219.
29. HENDERSON, M.G. & B.A. MCMILLEN. 1990. Effects of prenatal exposure to cocaine or related drugs on rat developmental and neurological indices. Brain Res. Bull. **24:** 207–212.
30. AKBARI, H.M., P.M. WHITAKER-AZMITIA & E.C. AZMITIA. 1994. Prenatal cocaine decreases the trophic factor S-100*B* and induced microcephaly: Reversal by postnatal 5-HT_{1A} receptor agonist. Neurosci. Lett. **170:** 141–144.
31. HEYSER, C.J., W.-J. CHEN, J. MILLER, N.E. SPEAR & L.P. SPEAR. 1990. Prenatal cocaine exposure induces deficits in pavlovian conditioning and sensory preconditioning among infant rat pups. Behav. Neurosci. **104:** 955–963.
32. WIGGINS, R.C. & B. RUIZ. 1990. Development under the influence of cocaine. I. A comparison of the effects of daily cocaine treatment and resultant undernutrition on pregnancy and early growth in a large population of rats. Metabolic Brain Dis. **5:** 85–99.
33. KUNKO, P.M., D. MOYER & S.E. ROBINSON. 1993. Intravenous gestational cocaine in rats: Effects on offspring development and weanling behavior. Neurotoxicol. Teratol. **15:** 335–344.
34. SOBRIAN, S.K., L.E. BURTON, N.L. ROBINSON *et al.* 1989. Neurobehavioral and immunological effects of prenatal cocaine exposure in rat. Pharmacol. Biochem. Behav. **35:** 617–629.
35. HUTCHINGS, D.E., T.A. FICO & D.L. DOW-EDWARDS. 1989. Prenatal cocaine: Maternal toxicity, fetal effects and locomotor activity in rat offspring. Neurotoxicol. Teratol. **11:** 65–69.
36. SMITH, R.F., K.M. MATTRAN, M.F. KURKJIAN & S.L. KURTZ. 1989. Alterations in offspring behavior induced by chronic prenatal cocaine dosing. Neurotoxicol. Teratol. **11:** 35–
37. CHURCH, M.W., P.A. HOLMES, G.W. OVERBECK, J.P. TILAK & C.S. ZAJAC. 1991. Interactive effects of prenatal alcohol and cocaine exposures on postnatal mortality, development and behavior in the Long-Evans rat. Neurotoxicol. Teratol. **13:** 377–386.
38. GOODWIN, G.A., C.J. HEYSER, C.A. MOODY *et al.* 1992. A fostering study of the effects of prenatal cocaine exposure: II. Offspring behavioral measures. Neurotoxicol. Teratol. **14:** 423–432.
39. KOSOFSKY, B.E., A.S. WILKINS, P. GRESSENS & P. EVRARD. 1994. Transplacental cocaine exposure: A mouse model demonstrating neuroanatomic and behavioral abnormalities. J. Child Neurol. **9:** 234–241.
40. SPEAR, L.P., C.L. KIRSTEIN, J. BELL *et al.* 1989. Effects of prenatal cocaine exposure on behavior during the early postnatal period. Neurotoxicol. Teratol. **11:** 57–63.
41. SPEAR, L.P. 1995. Neurobehavioral consequences of gestational cocaine exposure: A comparative analysis. *In* Advances in Infancy Research, Vol. 9. C. Rovee-Collier & L.P. Lipsitt, Eds. : 55–105. Ablex. Norwood.

42. HEYSER, C.J., N.E. SPEAR & L.P. SPEAR. 1992. Effects of prenatal exposure to cocaine on conditional discrimination learning in adult rats. Behav. Neurosci. **106:** 837–845.
43. BILITZKE, P.J. & M.W. CHURCH. 1992. Prenatal cocaine and alcohol exposures affect rat behavior in a stress test (the Porsolt swim test). Neurotoxicol. Teratol. **14:** 359–364.
44. HEYSER, C.J., J.S. MILLER, N.E. SPEAR & L.P. SPEAR. 1992. Prenatal exposure to cocaine disrupts cocaine-induced conditioned place preference in rats. Neurotoxicol. Teratol. **14:** 57–64.
45. MOLINA, V.A., J.M. WAGNER & L.P. SPEAR. 1994. The behavioral response to stress is altered in adult rats exposed prenatally to cocaine. Physiol. Behav. **55:** 941–945.
46. KAMIN, L.J. 1969. Predictability, surprise, attention and conditioning. *In* Punishment and Aversive Behavior. B.A. Campbell & R.M. Church, Eds. Appleton-Century-Crofts. New York.
47. CRIDER, A., L. BLOCKEL & P.R. SOLOMON. 1986. A selective attention deficit in the rat following induced dopamine receptor supersensitivity. Behav. Neurosci. **100:** 315–319.
48. MACKINTOSH, N.J. 1975. A theory of attention: Variations in the associability of stimuli with reinforcement. Psychol. Rev. **82:** 276–298.
49. CRIDER, A., P.R. SOLOMON & M.A. MCMAHON. 1982. Disruption of selective attention in the rat following chronic *d*-amphetamine administration: Relationship to schizophrenic attention disorder. Biol. Psychiatry **17:** 351–361.
50. BURCHFIELD, D.J., E.M. GRAHAM, R.M. ABRAMS & K.J. GERHARDT. 1990. Cocaine alters behavioral states in fetal sheep. Dev. Brain Res. **56:** 41–45.
51. ANDERSON-BROWN, T., T.A. SLOTKIN & F.J. SEIDLER. 1990. Cocaine acutely inhibits DNA synthesis in developing rat brain regions: Evidence for direct actions. Brain Res. **537:** 197–202.
52. FANTEL, A.G., C.V. BARBER, M.B. CARDA, R.W. TUMBIC & B. MACKLER. 1992. Studies of the role of ischemia/reperfusion and superoxide anion radical production in the teratogenicity of cocaine. Teratology
53. HOYME, H.E., K.L. JONES, S.D. DIXON *et al.* 1990. Prenatal cocaine exposure and fetal vascular disruption. Pediatrics **85:** 743–747.
54. KOEGLER, S.M., F.J. SEIDLER, J.R. SPENCER & T.A. SLOTKIN. Ischemia contributes to adverse effects of cocaine on brain development: Suppression of ornithine decarboxylase activity in neonatal rat. Brain Res. Bull. **27:** 829–834.
55. KONKOL, R.J., L.J. MURPHEY, D.M. FERRIERO, D.A. DEMPSEY & G.D. OLSEN. Cocaine metabolites in the neonate: Potential for toxicity. J. Child Neurol. **9:** 242–248.
56. KOSOFSKY, B.E. & S.E. HYMAN. The ontogeny of immediate early gene response to cocaine: A molecular analysis of the effects of cocaine on developing brain. *In* Immediate Early Gene Activation by Drugs of Abuse. R.G. Grzanna & R.M. Brown, Eds. : 161–171. NIDA Research Monograph #125. Washington, DC.
57. MURPHY, E.H., J.G. HAMMER, M.D. SCHUMANN *et al.* 1995. The rabbit as a model for studies of *in utero* cocaine exposure. Lab. Anim. Sci. **45:** 163–168.
58. SEIDLER, F.J., S.W. TEMPLE, E.C. MCCOOK & T.A. SLOTKIN. 1995. Cocaine inhibits central noradrenergic and dopaminergic activity during the critical developmental period in which catacholamines influence cell development. Dev. Brain Res. **85:** 48–53.
59. THADANI, P.V. 1995. Biological mechanisms and perinatal exposure to abused drugs. Synapse **19:** 228–232.
60. SPEAR, L.P. 1993. Missing pieces of the puzzle complicate conclusions about cocaine's neurobehavioral toxicity in clinical populations: Importance of animal models. Neurotoxicol. Teratol. **15:** 307–309.
61. JONES, L., I. FISCHER & P. LEVITT. 1996. Nonuniform alteration of dendritic development in the cerebral cortex following prenatal cocaine exposure. Cerebr. Cortex **6:** 431–445.
62. RØNNEKLEIV, O.K. & B.R. NAYLOR. 1995. Chronic cocaine exposure in the fetal rhesus monkey: Consequences for early development of dopamine neurons. J. Neurosci. **15:** 7330–7343.
63. LIDOW, M.S. 1995. Prenatal cocaine exposure adversely affects development of the primate cerebral cortex. Synapse **21:** 332–341.
64. WOODS, J.R., M.A. PLESSINGER & K.E. CLARK. 1987. Effect of cocaine on uterine blood flow and fetal oxygenation. JAMA **257:** 957–961.

65. LAUDER, J.M. 1993. Neurotransmitters as growth regulatory signals: Role of receptors and second messages. Trends Neurosci. **16:** 233–240.
66. POSNER, M.I. & S.E. PETERSON. 1990. The attention system of the human brain. Annu. Rev. Neurosci. **13:** 25–42.
67. HIEBLE, J.P., A.J. NICHOLS, S.Z. LANGER & R.R. RUFFOLO, JR. 1995. Pharmacology of the sympathetic nervous system. *In* Principles of Pharmacology. P.L. Munson, R.A. Mueller, G.R. Breese, Eds. 121–144. Chapman and Hall. New York.
68. WILKINS, A.S., L.M. GENOVA, W. POSTEN & B.E. KOSOFSKY. 1998. Transplacental cocaine exposure 1: A rodent model. Neurotoxicol. Teratol. **20:** in press.
69. WILKINS, A.S., K. JONES & B.E. KOSOFSKY. 1998. Transplacental cocaine exposure 2: Effects of cocaine dose and gestational timing. Neurotoxicol. Teratol. **20:** in press.
70. WILKINS, A.S., J.A. MAROTA, E. TABIT & B.E. KOSOFSKY. 1998. Transplacental cocaine exposure 3: Mechanisms underlying altered brain development. Neurotoxicol. Teratol. **20:** in press
71. GRESSENS, P., B.E. KOSOFSKY & P. EVRARD. 1992. Cocaine-induced disturbances of corticogenesis in the developing murine brain. Neurosci. Lett. **140:** 13–116.

State Control in the Substance-Exposed Fetus

I. The Fetal Neurobehavioral Profile: An Assessment of Fetal State, Arousal, and Regulation Competency

JEANNINE L. GINGRAS[a,b,d] AND KAREN J. O'DONNELL[c,e]

[a]*Department of Pediatrics, Carolinas Medical Center, SIDS C.A.R.E. Center, P.O. Box 32861, Charlotte, North Carolina 28232.*

[b]*Department of Pediatrics, The University of North Carolina–Chapel Hill, North Carolina; and*

[c]*Department of Pediatrics, Duke University, P.O. Box 3364, Durham, North Carolina 27710.*

ABSTRACT: Behavioral states are stable structures of behaviors that become more definable and coordinated with increasing age. With ultrasound we can see the fetus move, breathe, and react to changes in its environment. Ultrasound used in conjunction with Doppler fetal heart rate recording provides behavioral and neurophysiologic data useful in state determination. The Fetal Neurobehavioral Profile (FNP) was developed by our group as an assessment of fetal behaviors reflecting CNS integrity in the drug-exposed fetus. The FNP was designed to parallel methods of examining the newborn infant, especially in state-related behaviors. The FNP measures: *fetal responsiveness and arousal* after environmental perturbation with vibroacoustic stimulation (VAS);*habituation* to VAS; *state recovery*; and *self-regulation* post-VAS. From the behavioral and physiologic recordings, the constructs of state differentiation, organization, and regulation as well as fetal arousal and regulation competency can be measured.

Previous work using the FNP showed that those fetuses with abnormal or suspect fetal state regulation demonstrated impaired performance on the NBAS (Am. J. Obstet. Gynecol. 161: 685,1989). To expand these observations, three populations are currently being studied: prenatal nicotine-exposed, prenatal cocaine-exposed, and controls. Data are from 97 women/fetus dyads and a total of 236 FNP at ages 28–30 weeks gestational age, 31–34 weeks gestational age, and > 36 weeks gestational age. Although there are no group differences in the ability to achieve state by 36 weeks, interesting trends emerge: fetuses prenatally cocaine-exposed spend less time in 1F, more time in 4F, and have fewer transitions. At FNP_1, fewer cocaine-exposed fetuses had an initial reaction to VAS, whereas fewer nicotine-exposed fetuses habituated. Although the ability to habituate to VAS did not discriminate the cocaine group from the control or nicotine groups, the number of stimuli required for habituation differed between groups: 7 for the cocaine-exposed, 3 for the nicotine, and 5 for the control groups. Thus latency, a measure of arousal, differs among these groups Preliminary data also susggest a correlation of prenatal data with postnatal outcome.

INTRODUCTION

Behavior states are distinct and mutually exclusive modes of neuronal activity reflected by specific patterns of behavior.[1,2] Behaviors that mark different states (state variables) include eye movement, body movement, heart rate, and, in the neonate, respiration. Identified patterns of state variables represent discrete sleep and wake states.

[d] E-mail, jgingras@carolinas.org; fax, 704/355-8424; phone, 704/355-1522.

[e] E-mail, kod@acpub.Duke.Edu; fax, 919/684-8559; phone 919/684-5513.

Generally, in the full-term newborn, at least three distinct states can be defined[3]: wakefulness, active sleep, and quiet sleep. Epochs of behavior that are not stable enough to classify into one of these three patterns are termed indeterminate. State organization has been shown to have a distinctive ontogeny, with states becoming more definable and coordinated with increasing age.[4] In early infancy, changes in behavioral state variables have been shown to parallel changes in EEG patterns and other measures of central nervous system (CNS) maturation.[5,6] State variables and their organization have been used to index normal versus abnormal CNS development.[5,8–14]

With the introduction of real-time ultrasound, new insights into fetal behavior have led to the knowledge that fetuses also demonstrate state variables.[15–18] With ultrasound, one can see the fetus move, breathe, and react to changes in his/her environment. From 32 weeks of gestation onward, four recognizable coordinated fetal behavior states are identified.[16,18,19] Fetuses can be observed to shift from one behavior state to another,[20,21] and the ease of these shifts are seen as reflecting the progressive maturation and integration of function in the CNS.[22,23] It follows, then, that the emergence, differentiation, and regulation of state variables could be used to assess CNS maturation in the fetus during development.

Assessment of fetal behaviors such as movement and heart rate responsivity to external stimuli have been used previously to assess fetal well-being[24] and predict perinatal outcome. The Fetal Neurobehavioral Profile (FNP) was developed by our group to provide a more sensitive assessment of fetal behavior and reactivity to be used as an index of CNS integrity in the drug-exposed fetus. We demonstrated that disrupted fetal CNS maturation is reflected by the inability of the cocaine-exposed fetus to regulate behavior state after external perturbations.[25] This work describes the theoretical basis, constructs measured, and the procedures used for the FNP. We illustrate its use with preliminary data from an on-going longitudinal study.

THEORETICAL BACKGROUND

Using ultrasound technology, the FNP assessment integrates the concept of state organization and the definitions of state variables with procedures for (1) the physiological assessment of fetal integrity and (2) the behavioral assessment of neurodevelopmental status for the preterm and full-term newborn. The content of the FNP assessment is behavioral state emergence (development), differentiation (organization), and regulation; the assessment strategy borrows from several traditions in neurological and psychological assessment of the newborn and young infant.

Current approaches to newborn and infant assessment have their roots in three historical traditions: developmental neurology, behavioral pediatrics, and developmental psychology. Each tradition contributes to the current understanding of and assessment approaches directed at fetal CNS integrity. Initially, from the early 1900s, developmental neurologists focused on the assessment of reflexes as an index of CNS integrity. The systematic neurological examinations that emerged from their work included procedures now used in the FNP. Andre-Thomas and colleagues,[26,27] for example, approached the assessment of the newborn by observing spontaneous movement then eliciting reflexes; observations extended beyond reflexes and movement to the notion that infant behavior is "governed by affect." Similarly, Saint Anne-Dargassies'[28] examination for the preterm delivered newborn included an assessment of autonomic stability (e.g., respiratory regularity and temperature control), motor status (movement and posture), and state organization. Her use of the construct of state organization referenced the infant's control over level of arousal. The Prechtl and Beintema[29] examination has as a primary assumption that state organization is an important determinant of the infant's responses. Brazelton[30,31] later integrated this notion into an examination procedure itself determined by changes in the infant's state of arousal during the examination. The actual quantitative assessment of state variables and state organization in a behavior examination was developed by Brazelton and colleagues and elaborated for the very immature neonate by Als' group.[32] The notion of changes in state variables over chronological age underpins the FNP approach.

Behavioral pediatric's approach to the assessment of child development is essentially a maturational one. Maturation is the theoretical underpinning of the Gesell schedules of developmental changes that are normative for specific ages.[33,34] The assumption of chronological age expectations for the emergence and integration of behaviors is an important aspect of the developmental neurology tradition as well and is applied in the FNP assessment of fetal neurointegrity. However, contemporary approaches to fetal and newborn development, as utilized in the FNP, are seen as more complex than the simple emergence of behaviors via maturation. Behavioral assessment also has its roots in developmental psychology with its set of assumptions about developmental processes.[32] In the past several decades, views of developmental processes and mechanisms have emphasized the importance of the developmental context and the transactional nature of developing organism and the context.[35] The following three assumptions about development[36] summarize the theoretical basis of the proposed FNP as derived from the assumptions of developmental psychology.

1. *Development is hierarchical.* Development has order, that is, predictable steps and stages. There is mutual dependence from one step or stage to the others. Each step is more complex than the preceding one and incorporates the preceding one. Als and her colleagues,[32] for example, identified a hierarchy of behavioral subsystems that represent organized and mutually dependent components of behavior. Their understanding of the state organization subsystem and its relationship with other behavioral systems, such as movement and attention, provides a theoretical framework for the use of state organization for the FNP.

2. *Development is dialectical.* Development involves complex, mutual, and ongoing negotiations between the developing fetus and his/her environment.[37] The implications of this view for assessment are very different from Gesell's maturational view, for example; Gesell saw test responses as reflecting CNS maturation or its interruption by injury.[33,34] By contrast, Als' synactive theory[38] suggests that the subsystems develop through interactions with the environment. The FNP is predicated on the assumption that fetal brain development occurs in ongoing interactions with the fetal environment, which is, in turn, affected by maternal stress and behavior.

3. *Development is teleogical.* This assumption from developmental psychology suggests that developmental changes, specifically behavior state organization, are guided by movement from diffuse undifferentiated functioning towards a complex system of differentiated and organized set of physiological and behavioral variables. The teleological assumption is not new to newborn assessment; Werner[39] suggested that development moves from globality towards increased differentiation and hierarchical integration of processes. The principle is helpful in application to fetal assessment, particularly in understanding the differentiation of identifiable patterns of state variables and their organization and integration with other behavioral subsystems.

Hence, the FNP approach has as its theoretical underpinning the assumption that fetal neurodevelopment and its behavioral manifestations of integrity and damage occur in a hierarchial sequence that is, in part, programmed by maturation. It is also assumed that fetal environmental perturbations interact with brain development in an ongoing and mutual manner and that development is organized towards complex and integrated functioning. Each level requires and leads to increased sophistication and higher CNS functioning. The FNP was developed to integrate and assess these processes (FIG. 1).

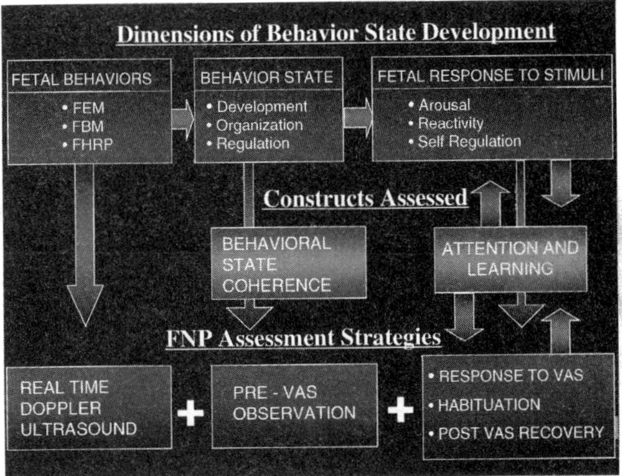

FIGURE 1.

THE FETAL NEUROBEHAVIORAL PROFILE (FNP)

Constructs Measured

The Fetal Neurobehavioral Profile (FNP) provides a comprehensive assessment of fetal neurointegrity and behavioral competence. The method involves observing the unperturbed fetus, applying an environmental perturbation, documenting the recovering fetus, and coding electrophysiologically and behaviorally the manifestations of behavior state organization.

Through FNP methodology, the examiner can observe systematically the range of fetal behaviors as well as responsiveness and regulation of the fetus with environmental perturbation. *Fetal reactivity and arousal* are measured by observing the fetus's behavioral and heart rate responses to vibroacoustic stimulation (VAS). This strategy is modeled after studies evaluating fetal heart rate and fetal movement response immediately poststimulus and is seen as an index of fetal well-being.[40–42] *Regulation and attention competence* are assessed by testing the fetus's ability to habituate, that is, to demonstrate a progressive decrease in behavioral response to repeated stimulus. The ability to habituate is seen as reflecting integrated and intact CNS functioning.[31,43] *Self-regulation competence* is assessed further by the fetus' ability to regulate behaviors postperturbation. In these ways, state differentiation and organization as well as fetal arousal, reactivity, and regulation competence are interrogated. Delay or dysfunction in state and, importantly, state regulation after perturbation is used as a marker of developmental injury.

In summary, the following dimensions of fetal behavior are measured.

Behavioral State:

Development: Coincidence of state variables in specific patterns or clusters (TABLE 1)
Organization: State variables meet state criteria
Regulation: Ability to cycle (transition) from one state to another

TABLE 1. Fetal State Assignment

	Fetal Behaviors		
State	FEM	FBM	FHRP
1F	–	–	A
2F	+	+	B
3F	+	–	C
4F	+	+	D

Abbreviations: FEM = fetal eye movement; FBM = fetal body movement; FHRP = fetal heart rate pattern.

Responsivity:

Arousal and reactivity: Initial response to external perturbation (VAS)
Habituation: Decrease in response to repeated VAS after initial response
Self-regulation competence: Progressive ability to regain state stability post-VAS

Assessment Paradigm

The FNP interrogates various features of neurobehavioral integrity by simultaneously recording physiological and behavioral observations: fetal heart rate variability, breathing patterns, body tone and flexion, quality of overall movement, and chin, mouth, and eye movements. Presumptive indicators of stress or attempts to regulate state, such as yawns, hiccups, and sucking, also are recorded. In this manner, the fetus's complete orientation and response to his/her environment is assessed. Assessment can be scored real-time or off-line, because the ultrasound studies are videorecorded. From the behavioral and physiological records, the constructs of state differentiation, organization, and regulation can be assessed.

The assessment paradigm consists of three components: an initial 21-minute observation period of fetal behaviors (pre-VAS) followed by vibroacoustic stimulation/habituation (VAS/habituation), culminating in a 21-minute post-vibroacoustic observation period (post-VAS) (FIG. 2).

Pre-VAS. The assessment conditions are standardized to control for other effects, such as diurnal variation, smoking, and metabolic conditions. At the beginning of each ultrasound, maternal glucose is measured. If the serum glucose is less than 100 mg/dl, a snack consisting of crackers and orange juice is provided. Glucose determination is repeated. Mothers are asked to restrain from smoking cigarettes and drinking caffeinated drinks for at least 1 hour prior to the FNP. Time of day is recorded.

Fetal behaviors are recorded real-time every 1 minute. A lateral-oblique transection of the fetus allows the most optimal view of the fetal face and chest for simultaneous observation of lens, mouth, and chin movement, heart motion, breathing, and flexion, trunk, and limb movement. Ultrasounds are videorecorded. Simultaneous fetal heart rate is measured by continuous wave Doppler technology (Corometrics Model 150) and recorded continuously on a strip chart recorder synchronized in time with the Doppler ultrasound (Corometrics Aloka 650 with curvilinear 3.5 MHz transducer). Maternal perceptions of fetal movement are also recorded.

VAS/Habituation. After the initial observation period and when the fetus appears in a stable state, fetal arousal and reactivity are assessed by presenting an initial VAS. Vibroacoustic stimulus is provided by the artificial larynx (Corometrics model 5c Western Electric) that emits fundamental tones of approximately 100 Hz and 85 dB for 0.5

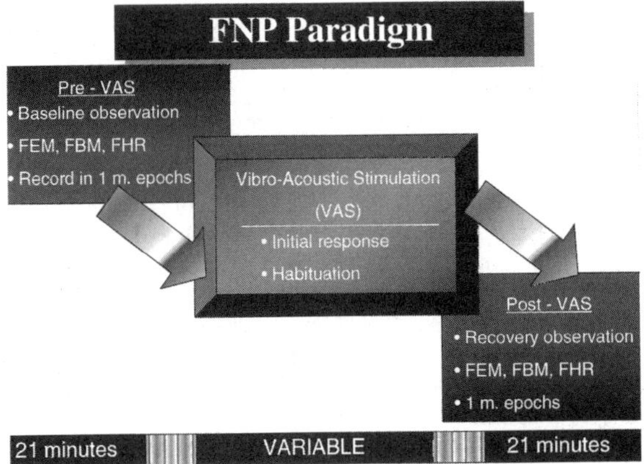

FIGURE 2.

seconds. This duration was selected because longer stimulus durations have been associated with nonphysiological state changes, excessive fetal movements, and prolonged tachycardia.[44,45] Also, a short stimulus duration is more likely to discriminate the fetus's arousal capacity.[40] No adverse effects to the fetus have been documented at this sound intensity and frequency;[45] a peak of 95 dB corresponds to the "R" wave on the maternal electrocardiogram;[47] and physiological intrauterine noise intensity is considered to be approximately 85 dB.[42]

The fetus is observed behaviorally for a blink-startle response for a duration of 10 seconds. The response components include head turning, mouth opening, tongue protrusion, cheek motion, hand-to-head movement, and eyelid blinking as well as arm movement and leg extension.[40,48,49] Most fetuses respond within 2.5–5 seconds after the first stimulus; some fetuses require up to 4 stimuli before a response is elicited.[40] Therefore, if the fetus does not respond to the initial stimulus, three additional stimuli (four total) are applied, and the response coded as suspect. If no response occurs after the fourth VAS, the response is coded as negative. After a positive response to VAS and the fetus stops reacting for 5 seconds, the stimulus is repeated to test for habituation. Behavioral habituation is defined as cessation of all components of the facial and body reaction, except eye blinking, over two sequential stimuli. Up to 12 stimuli are presented for the habituation paradigm. Fetal heart rate is simultaneously recorded so that heart rate reactivity associated with stimulation may be assessed.

Post-VAS. To assess the ability of the fetus to self-regulate after perturbation, the VAS/habituation paradigm is followed by a 21-minute poststimulation observation period; details are described in the pre-VAS portion of the paradigm.

Coding Procedures

State is coded according to the behavioral state classification previously reported.[18] Four distinct fetal behavioral states are identified: 1F, 2F, 3F, and 4F;[57,58] they correspond to postnatal behavioral states of quiet sleep, active sleep, quiet awake, and active awake, respectively.[16,17] The variables that define behavior state in the newborn include: breathing, heart rate patterns, body movement, and eye movement. Behaviors that define state for the fetus differ slightly from those for the newborn. Fetal breathing, for instance, is episodic and unsuitable for fetal state definition. If present, however, the pattern of fetal breathing is state-related. In 1F, fetal breathing is always regular, whereas in 2F, fetal breathing is irregular. Variables that do not define state but are state specific, such as fetal breathing, are termed *state concomitant.*

State variables in the fetus include: fetal eye movement (FEM), fetal body movement (FM), and heart rate (FHR) patterns (A, B, C, and D). For state to be defined, three criteria must be met: (1) coincidence of variables in specific patterns (see TABLE 1), (2) duration of stable association (minimum 3 minutes), and (3) simultaneity of change of all the variables within 3 minutes.[18] Variables present in one of the state combinations but not fulfilling state criteria are coded as *coincident.* Epochs during which state variables do not fit one of the specified combinations of state are coded as periods of *non-coincidence. Transitions* are short epochs during which one state changes into a subsequent state. State is usually achieved in the human fetus by 38 weeks of gestation, although coincidence of state-related behaviors may occur as early as 30 weeks gestational age.[19]

State Assignment

The classification of state requires three steps in the scoring of physiological and behavioral data prior to state assignment.

Assignment of Fetal Heart Rate Pattern. The first step in the determination of state is to assign heart rate patterns to each minute of the Doppler fetal heart rate tracings. Patterns are coded as A, B, C, and D based on criteria previously published.[16,18,20] The pattern determination strategy in the FNP is modified from that traditionally used, a 3-minute moving window. Heart rate pattern assignment is accomplished by viewing a 3-minute window and assigning the central minute the predominate pattern. The 3-minute window is then moved in 1-minute increments. This procedure insures that subtle transitions are not obscured and functions to smooth the "arbitrary" nature of identifying the onset of state scoring.

State Profile. Once heart rate patterns have been assigned for each minute of the recording session (A, B, C, or D), specific heart rate patterns are recorded onto the state scoring sheet. The physiological (FHRP) and behavioral (FEM, FBM) state variables are simultaneously recorded to develop a *state profile,* a graphic display of the sequence of consecutive state variables during a recording session (FIG. 3). Minute by minute assignment of state coincidence or non-coincidence is scored. From such profiles, state and state measures can be scored.

State Assignment (State Scoring). Quantitative measures of behavioral states, such as the distribution of percentages of time spent in state versus no-state (state development), the percentages of time spent in each of the four specific states (state architecture), the mean durations of state epochs, the number of state transitions (state regulation), and their direction can be derived from the state profiles. The assignment of state (state scoring) is done using a modification of the 3-minute moving window technique (FIG. 3). Each 3-minute epoch examines whether the state variables within the specific epoch fulfill state criteria. The window is then shifted to the right in 1-minute intervals. Also, because the state profile is extracted from the information recorded on the observation records from the real-time fetal ultrasounds, fetal behavior concomitants, fetal breathing, and other fetal behaviors such as hiccuping, yawning, and swallowing can be assessed.

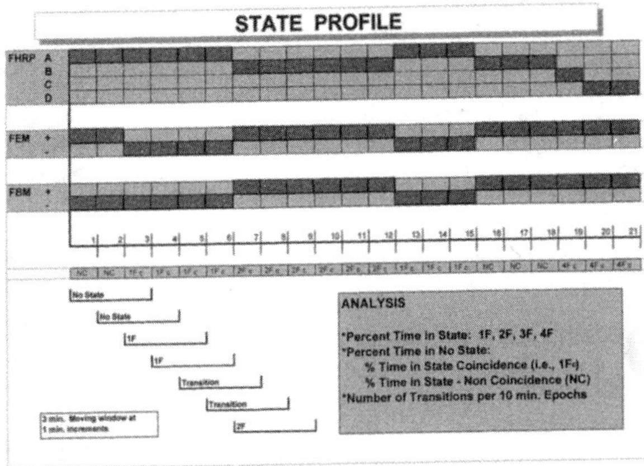

FIGURE 3.

Response to VAS

Behavioral Response. Scoring of movement responses post-VAS (blink-startle) is done in 15-second epochs or within each stimulus/response cycle if they are shorter. The fetus is offered four opportunities to initially respond to VAS with a blink/startle response.[49] The VAS at response (1, 2, 3, or 4) and the time of response (<5 seconds, 5–10 seconds) are recorded as a measure of initial response (yes, no) and of latency (time). Body movement occurring at greater than 10 seconds poststimulation is considered a spontaneous movement not synchronized to or resulting from the VAS. If no response occurs by the fourth VAS, the response is coded as negative.

Heart Rate Response. Similarly, heart rate response is scored as acceleration, deceleration, or no change. The percentage change from baseline is calculated as is the duration of the heart rate response.

Habituation

Behavioral. Habituation is defined as complete cessation of all body movement in response to VAS for two consecutive stimuli. The number of stimuli to habituation is also recorded. Additionally, the quality of the fetal behavioral response is coded by a scoring system developed by our group. The Behavioral Reactivity Score measures fetal reactivity in response to stimulation and is based on a scale of 0–5. A score of 5 represents complete habituation. A score of 3–4 reflects a fetus that can attenuate his/her behavioral response post-stimulus but does not meet the habituation criteria of cessation of body movement over two consecutive stimuli. A score of 1 or 2 represents behavioral "activation" or increased arousal poststimuli with the highest reactivity scored as 1. A score of 5 represents the optimal response of habituation and a score of zero, non-habituation. Scores between 1 and 4 represent decreasing behavioral and physiological reactivity in response to the vibroacoustic stimuli.

Physiological. Heart rate acceleration in response to stimuli is measured as the delta change from baseline. Heart rate habituation or attenuation is scored by observing cessation or diminution in the delta change in response from baseline after repeated VAS.

PRELIMINARY DATA: APPLICATION OF THE FNP

The SIDS Risk Study (SRS) is a prospective longitudinal study testing the hypotheses that (1) arousal deficits underpin altered neurodevelopment and SIDS risk; (2) deficits are present prenatally; and (3) prenatal deficits predict postnatal outcome. Although called the SIDS Risk Study, the SRS goes beyond SIDS risk and is a study of neurodevelopment, of CNS injury, and of efforts to identify biological markers of developmental risk.

Enrollment into the SRS occurs at or before 28 weeks of gestational age. Three groups are recruited: a gestational cocaine use group, a gestational nicotine use group, and a comparison group with no known cocaine or nicotine use. The mother/fetus, mother/infant dyad is studied during seven encounters (FIG. 4). Three encounters are prenatal at which times prenatal assessment of state, arousal, reactivity, and regulation is performed by the FNP. The four postnatal assessments of state (sleep), heart rate reactivity, behavior, and respiratory control are performed at 6 days, 6, 12, and 24 months.

Enrollment into the SRS is currently ongoing. The data presented below are preliminary; they are used as examples of applications for the FNP. Preliminary data are derived from over 200 observations across three gestational ages (GA): 29–31 weeks GA = FNP_1; 32–35 weeks GA = FNP_2; > 36 weeks GA = FNP_3. Statistical methods include: Chi-square (Fisher's Exact Test), Kruskal-Wallis, ANOVA, MANOVA, or Cochran's Q test, when appropriate. Significance level is defined as $p < 0.05$.

Findings

State Development/Ontogeny and State Architecture. The percentage time in state increases with increasing gestational age: 39%, 61%, and 79%, respectively, at 29–31 weeks, 32–35 weeks, and >36 weeks gestational age. No group differences (prenatal cocaine exposure, prenatal nicotine exposure, and comparisons) were found. However, the *quality* of state differs between groups at the third ultrasound (FNP_3, ie, the most mature US): those fetuses prenatally exposed to cocaine alone with or without other substances showed a tendency to demonstrate more state 4F (active awake, 2.5% and 2%,

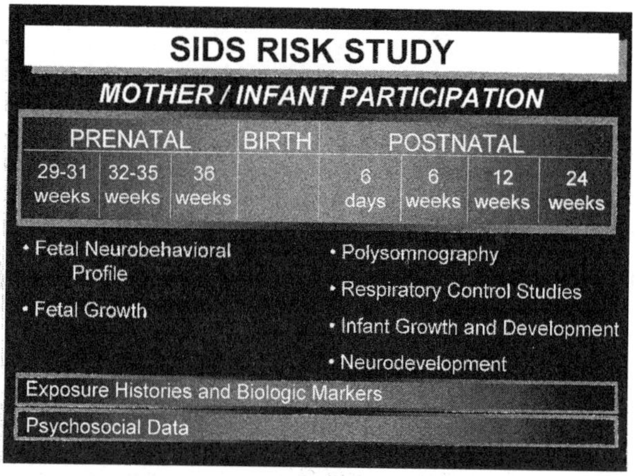

FIGURE 4.

respectively, for the comparisons and nicotine group, 5.5% for the cocaine-exposed group) than 1F (quiet sleep; 11% for both the comparison and nicotine groups, 0% for the cocaine-exposed group).

Response to VAS/Habituation. Significant differences among groups were seen at the first FNP evaluation. Those infants prenatally cocaine exposed had less initial reaction to VAS (75% = 9 of 12) than did the nicotine-exposed (100% = 22 of 22) and comparison fetuses (94% = 32 of 34);($X^2 = p < 0.05$).

Although not statistically significant at this interim data analysis, nicotine-exposed fetuses appear to have a decreased ability to habituate after initially responding to VAS (59% = 13 of 22) than did the cocaine-exposed (78% = 7 of 9) and comparison groups (78% = 25 of 32). It is of interest that although the ability to habituate did not discriminate the cocaine group from the comparison group, the latency to habituation, that is, the number of stimuli required to habituate, differed between groups with cocaine-exposed fetuses requiring seven stimuli compared to three for the nicotine group and five for the comparison group. It seems that latency, a measure of arousal, may differ among these groups.

Another measure of reactivity or arousal is obtained from an analysis of the quality of behavioral response. A Behavioral Reactivity Score of 0–5 was developed and based on the quality of the behavioral response. A score of 5 represents complete habituation. A score of 3–4 reflects a fetus that can attenuate his/her behavioral response poststimulus but does not meet habituation criteria of cessation of body movement over two consecutive stimuli. A score of 0–2 represents behavioral "activation" or increased arousal poststimuli. Interestingly, of those infants who did not habituate, those in the cocaine-exposed group demonstrated greater reactivity (or less optimal responses) in response to VAS, as reflected by lower Behavioral Reactivity Scores, than did the nicotine and comparison groups: 70% of the cocaine fetuses demonstrated a behavioral reactivity score of 0–2 in response to VAS compared to 51% and 52% of the comparison and nicotine groups, respectively. That is, instead of demonstrating an attenuation of their behavioral and heart rate responses, the fetuses gestationally cocaine exposed demonstrated increased behavioral activity and increased heart rate. Some fetuses were so "aroused" that termination of the paradigm was necessary secondary to fetal tachycardia in excess of 200 beats/minute.

These data suggest that initial arousal, reactivity, and ability to habituate are altered by prenatal exposure to cocaine and/or nicotine.

Prenatal Measures Predict Postnatal Behaviors. The ability to initially respond to VAS and the ability to habituate did correlate with performance on the Neonatal Behavioral Assessment Scale (TABLE 2), particularly in the domains of newborn habituation, autonomic stability (at the early FNP), and state regulation. Although these data are not statistically significant at this time, the trends support the finding that the fetal assessments might provide predictive power. Interestingly, those infants who, at the third and most mature FNP, did not respond to the initial VAS or who did not habituate if demonstrating an initial response, demonstrated lower scores on autonomic stability and orientation domains than did those fetuses who responded to VAS and who habituated. Perhaps these fetuses are less able to demonstrate the range of newborn behavioral repertoire. Fetal responses were also associated with increased motor scores on the newborn INFANIB scale ($p > 0.05$).

DISCUSSION

Behavior state in the human fetus is defined in terms of the clustering of specific behaviors, including fetal eye movement, fetal body movement, and fetal heart rate pat-

TABLE 2. Prenatal Response and Postnatal Outcome

	NBAS Subscale					
Fetal Response	Habituation	Autonomic Stability[a]	State Regulation	Orientation	Range of State[b]	Autonomic Stability[b]
VAS						
Yes	6.8	5.3	4.2	5.2	No Trend	4.8
No	4.3	4.0	3.3	6.2		5.7
Habituation						
Yes	7.2	5.3	No trend	5.8	3.8	4.6
No	4.4	5.0		4.2	4.4	6.3

[a]Data from FNP # 1 and 2.
[b]Data from FNP # 3.

terns and parallels postnatal infant state. A large body of evidence exists that suggests an association between behavioral state organization in the fetus and newborn and maturation, integrity, and functional status of the CNS.[5,11,17] Fetal behavioral state analysis has been useful in the differentiation of normal and obviously at-risk fetuses, including the fetuses of diabetic women,[8] the fetuses of alcoholic women,[9,12] and those with evidence of growth retardation[10,21] and hydrocephaly.[7] However, the large but normal variability in state measures and state control that exists between subjects[51] makes state assessment, in itself, a poor predictor of more subtle developmental risk.

Not all individuals within a high risk group will ultimately demonstrate risk. This is particularly true for infants prenatally cocaine exposed; a spectrum of infant outcomes was reported.[52] The FNP examination, described in this report, was developed as a fetal assessment tool that would offer increased sensitivity and discriminative power; that is, the goal is that the FNP examination will discriminate who, within a high risk group, is at greatest risk. Preliminary data from the SRS suggest that the FNP provides greater discriminatory potential derived from the strategies of habituation, latency, and regulation; the paradigm allows enhanced discrimination above the more traditional measures of state. Hence, the FNP shows potential to be used as a predictive tool.

The strengths of the FNP are as follows: (1) The FNP integrates validated neurophysiological and behavioral concepts and assessments from established scientific traditions. The conceptualizations of state and state regulation and habituation have been studied extensively, and the fetal and preterm delivered infant responses appear consistent. (2) The FNP allows for scoring of both physiological and behavioral data. This is especially important for research purposes. The FNP examination can look at a number of items in the repertory of fetal behaviors and fetal responsivity: state and state transitions, ability to respond to an external stimulus, habituation, a measure of learning, and heart rate variability. Simultaneous recording of physiological and behavioral data allows for the interrogation of possible linkages in behavior and physiology as well as possible "dissociations." Recent data suggest that the dissociation of two or more variables that normally occurs together will provide a more sensitive index of pathological conditions and, therefore, provide a more sensitive marker of CNS integrity.[23,53] (3) Real-time and off-line analyses can be used effectively for research as both behavioral and physiological data are simultaneously recorded. Off-line assessment can be used to investigate subtleties not able to be interrogated during real-time recording. Also, videorecording and off-line analysis are useful in training and reliability assessment. (4) The FNP paradigm, lasting 45–60 minutes, interrogates a number of variables and could easily be adapted for clinical settings. (5) The FNP can easily be computerized and techniques such as artificial intelligence applied. (6) Multiple analyses strategies can be performed; between/within group, cross-sectional, and longitudinal analyses are all possible. (7) The FNP can be used to engage women in prenatal care by enhancing their knowledge of and relationship with their fetus.

A few limitations must be considered. (1) There is potential interference from the dual Dopplers used for real-time ultrasound and fetal heart rate recording. This interference can be corrected by positioning and by utilizing a curvilinear ultrasound transducer. (2) The ability to visualize the fetal lens and, therefore, to determine fetal eye movement is dependent on fetal position. If the fetal lens cannot be seen and therefore scoring of fetal eye movement impossible, an alternative scoring system must be employed. Alternately, this time can be coded as "indeterminate." In our own scoring system, two approaches are used. The first is interpolation of the data obtained in the minute before and the minute after the interference. For instance, if the pre- and postinterference minute show eye movement, the minute of interference is coded as positive for fetal eye movement. If the pre- and postinterference minutes differ, then interpolation is not possible. For these occasions, scoring is based on the fetal heart rate pattern and the presence or absence of fetal movement.[54] (3) The FNP is personnel and labor intensive. However, artificial intelligence and voice activation may ultimately decrease the labor- and personnel-intensive nature of the assessment.

SUMMARY

1. The Fetal Neurobehavioral Profile (FNP) is reproducible and well tolerated by the mother and the fetus. Most women were comfortable during the procedure and tolerated the procedure without incident. A few experienced nausea or discomfort; most of these women were near term. Simple interventions such as a pillow behind their back or shifting to their side resolved the symptoms of discomfort.

2. Preliminary data suggest that the FNP can differentiate groups. More importantly, the FNP can discriminate within group differences to address the important question of "Who within a group is at greatest developmental risk?"

3. The FNP shows promise in the detection of early regulation and attention/arousal disorders.

REFERENCES

1. PRECHTL, H.F.R. 1974. The behavioral states of the newborn infant: A review. Brain Res. **76:** 185–212.
2. THEORELL, K., H.F.R. PRECHTL, A.W. BLAIR & J. LIND. 1973. Behavioral state cycles of normal newborn infants. Dev. Med. Child Neurol. **15:** 597–605.
3. ANDERS, T., R. EMDE & A. PARMELEE. 1971. A Manual of Standardized Terminology, Techniques and Criteria for Scoring of State of Sleep and Wakefulness in Newborn Infants. UCLA Brain Information Service. Los Angeles, CA.
4. SWARTJES, J.M., H.P. VAN GEINJN, R. MANTEL, E.E. VAN WOERDEN & H.C. SCHOEMAKER. 1990. Coincidence of behavioral state parameters in the human fetus at three gestational ages. Early Human Dev. **23:** 75–83.
5. NIJHUIS, J.G. 1986. Behavioral states: Concomitants, clinical implications and the assessment of the condition of the nervous system. Eur. J. Obstet. Gynecol. Reprod. Biol. **21:** 301–308.

6. Watanabe, K., S. Miyazaki, K. Hara & S. Hakamada. 1980. Behavioral state cycles, background EEGs and prognosis of newborns with perinatal hypoxia. Electroencephal. Clin. Neurophysiol. **49:** 618–625.
7. Arduini, D., G. Rizzo, L. Caforio & S. Mancuso. 1987. Development of behavioral states in hydrocephalic fetuses. Fetal Ther. **2:** 135–143.
8. Mulder, E.J.H., G.H.A. Visser, D.J. Bekedam & H.F.R. Prechtl. 1987. Emergence of behavioral states in fetuses of type-1 diabetic women. Early Human Dev. **15:** 231–251.
9. Mulder, E.J.H., A. Kamstra, M.J. O'Brien, G.H.A. Visser & H.F.R. Prechtl. 1986. Abnormal fetal behavioral state regulation in a case of high maternal alcohol intake during pregnancy. Early Human Dev. **14:** 321–326.
10. van Vliet, M.A.T., C.B. Martin, Jr., J.G. Nijhuis & H.F.R. Prechtl. 1985. Behavioral states in growth-retarded human fetuses. Early Human Dev. **12:** 183–197.
11. Prechtl, H.F.R. 1992. The organization of behavioral states and their dysfunction. Sem. Preinatol. **16:** 258–263.
12. Rurak, D.W. 1992. Fetal behavioral states: Pathological alterations with drug/alcohol abuse. Sem. Perinatol. **16:** 239–251.
13. Bocking, A.D. 1992. Fetal behavioral states: Pathological alteration with hypoxia. Sem. Perinatol. **16:** 252–257.
14. Groome, L.J., M.J. Swiber, L.S. Bentz, S.B. Holland & J.L. Atterbury. 1995. Maternal anxiety during pregnancy: Effect on fetal behavior at 38 to 40 weeks of gestation. Dev. Behav. Pediatr. **16:** 391–396.
15. Nijhuis, J.G., C.B. Martin, Jr. & H.F.R. Prechtl. 1984. Behavioural states of the human fetus. *In* Continuity of Neural Functions from Prenatal to Postnatal life. Clin. Dev. Med. **94:** 65–79.
16. Pillai, M. & D. James. 1990. Are the behavioral states of the newborn comparable to those of the fetus? Early Human Dev. **22:** 39–49.
17. Prechtl, H.F.R. 1988. Assessment of fetal neurological function and development. *In* Fetal and Neonatal Neurology and Neurosurgery. M. Levene, M. Bennett & J. Punt, Eds.: 33–40. Churchill Livingstone. New York, NY.
18. Nijhuis, J.G., H.F.R. Prechtl, C.B. Martin, Jr. & R.S.G.M. Bots. 1982. Are there behavioral states in the human fetus? Early Human Dev. **6:** 177–195.
19. Visser, G.H.A., G. Poelman-Wessjes, T.M.N. Cohen & D.J. Bekedam. 1987. Fetal behavior at 30 to 32 weeks of gestation. Pediatric Res. **22:** 655–658.
20. Arduini, D., G. Rizzo, M. Massacesi, C. Romanini & S. Mancuso. 1991. Longitudinal assessment of behavioral transitions in healthy human fetuses during the third trimester of pregnancy. J. Perinatol. Med. **19:** 1967–1972.
21. Arduini, D., G. Rizzo, L. Caforio, M.R. Boccolini, C. Romanini & S. Mancuso. 1989. Behavioural state transitions in healthy and growth retarded fetuses. Early Human Dev. **19:** 155–165.
22. Groome, L.J., L.S. Bentz & K.P. Singh. 1994. Behavioral state organization in human term fetuses: Evidence of relatively tight control of state cycling. J. Matern. Fetal Med. **3:** 49–55.
23. Groome, L.J., L.S. Bentz & K.P. Singh. 1995. Behavioral state organization in human term fetuses: The relationship between periods of undefined state and other characteristics of state control. Sleep **18:** 77–81.
24. Bocking, A.D. & R. Gagnon. 1991. Behavioural assessment of fetal health. J. Dev. Physiol. **15:** 113–120.
25. Hume, R.F., K.J. O'Donnell, C.L. Stanger, A.P. Killam & J.L. Gingras. 1989. In utero cocaine exposure: Observation of fetal behavioral states may predict neonatal outcome. Am. J. Obstet. Gynecol. **161:** 685–690.
26. André-Thomas, J., & S. Saint Anne Dargassies. 1952. Etudes Neurologiques sur le Nouveau-né et le Jeune Nourrission. Paris. Masson.
27. André-Thomas, J., Y. Chesni & S. Saint Anne-Dargassies. 1960. The neurological examination of the infant. Medical Advisory Committee of the National Spastics Society. London, England.
28. Saint Anne-Dargassies, S. 1965. Neurologic examination of the neonate. Proc. Roy. Soc. Med. **58:** 5.

29. Prechtl, H.F.R. & D. Beintema. 1964. The Neurological Examination of the Full Term Newborn Infant. Heinemann/Spastics International Publications. London.
30. Brazelton, T.B. 1973. Neonatal Behavioral Assessment Scale. Clinics in Developmental Medicine 50. J.B. Lippincott Co. Philadelphia, PA.
31. Brazelton, T.B. 1984. Neonatal Behavioral Assessment Scale, 2nd Ed. Clinics in Developmental Medicine 88. J.B. Lippincott Co. Philadelphia, PA.
32. Als, H., B.M. Lester, E.Z. Tronick & T.B. Brazelton. 1982. Toward a research instrument for the assessment of preterm infants' behavior (APIB). *In* Theory and Research in Behavioral Pediatrics. Vol. **1:** H. Fitzgerald, B.M. Lester & M.W. Yogman, Eds.: 35–132. Plenum. New York, NY.
33. Gesell, A. 1940. The first five years of life: A guide to the study of the preschool child. Harper & Brothers. New York.
34. Gessell, A. & C. Amatruda. 1941. Developmental Diagnosis. Hoeber. New York.
35. Sameroff, A. & M. Chandler. 1975. Reproductive risk and the continuum of caretaking casualty. *In* Review of Child Development Research. Vol. 4. F. Horowitz, M. Hetherington, S. Scarr-Salapatek & G. Siegel, Eds. :187–244. University of Chicago Press. Chigaco, IL.
36. O'Donnell, K.J. 1996. Neurobehavioral assessment of newborn infants. *In* Assessing Infants and Preschoolers with Special Needs. M. McLean, D.B. Bailey & M. Wolery, Eds. 2nd Ed. Merrill/Prentice Hall. Englewood Cliffs, NJ.
37. Sameroff, A.J. 1983. Developmental systems: Contexts and evolution. *In* Handbook of Child Psychology. Vol. 1. History, Theory, and Methods. P. Mussen, Ed. John Wiley & Sons. New York, NY.
38. Als, H., G. Lawhon, E. Brown, R. Gibes, F. Duffy, G. McAnulty & J. Blickman. 1986. Individualized behavioral and environmental care for the very low birth weight preterm infant at high risk for bronchopulmonary dysplasia. Neonatal intensive care unit and developmental outcome. Pediatrics **78:** 1123–1132.
39. Werner, H. 1957. The concept of development from a comparative and organismic point of view. *In* The Concept of Development. D.B. Harris, Ed. 125–148. University of Minnesota Press. Minneapolis, MN.
40. Kuhlman, K.A & R. Depp. 1988. Acoustic stimulation testing. Obstet. Gynecol. Clin. North Am. **15:** 303–319.
41. Devoe, L.D., C. Murray, D. Faircloth & E. Ramos. 1990. Vibroacoustic stimulation and fetal behavioral state in normal term human pregnancy. Am. J. Obstet. Gynecol. **163:** 1156–1161.
42. Romero, R., M. Mazor & J.C. Hobbins. 1988. A critical appraisal of fetal acoustic stimulation as an antenatal test for fetal well-being. Obstet. Gynecol. **71:** 781–786.
43. Leader, L.R., P. Baillie, B. Martin & E. Vermeulen. 1982. The assessment and significance of habituation to a repeated stimulus by the human fetus. Early Human Dev. **7:** 211–219.
44. Lecanuet, J.P., C. Grainier-Deferre & M.C. Busnel 1989. Differential fetal auditory reactiveness as a function of stimulus characteristics and state. Sem. Perinatol. **13:** 421–429.
45. Visser, G.H.A. & E.J.H. Mulder. 1993. The effect of vibro-acoustic stimulation on fetal behavioral state organization. Am. J. Indust. Med. **23:** 531–539.
46. Shaw, J.K. & R.H. Paul. 1990. Fetal responses to external stimuli. Obstet. Gynecol. Clin. North Am. **17:** 235–248.
47. Visser, G.H.A., H.H. Mulder, H.P. Wit, E.J.H. Mulder & H.F.R. Prechtl. 1989. Vibroacoustic stimulation of the human fetus: Effect on behavioural state organization. Early Human Dev. **19:** 285–296.
48. Westgren, M., H. Almstrom, M. Nymon & U. Ulmsten. 1987. Maternal perception of sound-provoked fetal movements as a measure of fetal well-being. Br. J. Obstet. Gynecol. **94:** 523–527.
49. Kuhlman, K.A., K.A. Burns, R. Depp & R.E. Sabbagha. 1988. Ultrasonic imaging of normal fetal response to external vibratory acoustic stimulation. Am. J. Obstet. Gynecol. **158:** 47–51.
50. Groome, L.J. & J.E. Watson. 1992. Assessment of in utero neurobehavioral development. I. Fetal behavioral states. J. Matern. Fetal Invest. **2:** 183–194.

51. Groome, L.J., L.S. Bentz, S.B. Holland, M.J. Swiber, K. P. Singh & R. F. Trimm, III. 1995. Individual consistency in behavioral state profiles in human fetuses between 38 and 40 weeks gestation. J. Matern. Fetal Med. **4:** 247–251.
52. Gingras, J.L., D.E. Weese-Mayer, R.F. Hume, Jr. & K.J. O'Donnell. 1992. Cocaine and development: Mechanisms of fetal toxicity and neonatal consequences of prenatal cocaine exposure. Early Human Dev. **31:** 1–24.
53. Groome, L.J., D.M. Mooney & R.A. Dykman. 1994. Motor and cardiac response during habituation testing: Demonstration of exaggerated cardiac reactivity in a subgroup of normal human fetuses. Am. J. Perinatol. **11:** 73–79.
54. DiPietro, J.A., D.M. Hodgson & K.A. Costigan. 1996. Fetal antecedents of infant temperament. Child Dev. **67:** 2568–2583.

Prenatal Coke: What's Behind the Smoke?

Prenatal Cocaine/Alcohol Exposure and School-Age Outcomes: The SCHOO-BE Experience[a]

VIRGINIA DELANEY-BLACK,[b,f] CHANDICE COVINGTON,[d] TOM TEMPLIN,[d] JOEL AGER,[c,e] SUE MARTIER,[c] SCOTT COMPTON,[b] AND ROBERT SOKOL[c]

Departments of Pediatrics[b] and Obstetrics,[c] School of Medicine; College of Nursing;[d] Department of Psychology,[e] College of Science; Wayne State University, Detroit, Michigan 48201, USA

ABSTRACT: Despite media reports and educators' concerns, little substantive data have been published to document or refute the emerging reports that children prenatally exposed to cocaine have serious behavioral problems in school. Recent pilot data from this institution have indeed demonstrated teacher-reported problem behaviors following prenatal cocaine exposure after controlling for the effects of prenatal alcohol use and cigarette exposure. Imperative in the study of prenatal exposure and child outcome is an acknowledgment of the influence of other control factors such as postnatal environment, secondary exposures, and parenting issues. We report preliminary evaluation from a large ongoing historical prospective study of prenatal cocaine exposure on school-age outcomes. The primary aim of this NIDA-funded study is to determine if a relationship exists between prenatal cocaine/alcohol exposures and school behavior and, if so, to determine if the relationship is characterized by a dose-response relationship. A secondary aim evaluates the relationship between prenatal cocaine/alcohol exposures and school achievement. Both relationships will be assessed in a black, urban sample of first grade students using multivariate statistical techniques for confounding as well as mediating and moderating prenatal and postnatal variables. A third aim is to evaluate the relationship between a general standardized classroom behavioral measure and a tool designed to tap the effects thought to be specific to prenatal cocaine exposure. This interdisciplinary research team can address these aims because of the existence of a unique, prospectively collected Perinatal Database, funded in part by NIAAA and NICHD. The database includes repeated measures of cocaine, alcohol, and other substances for over 3,500 births since 1986. Information from this database is combined with information from the database of one of the largest public school systems in the nation. The final sample will be composed of over 600 first grade students for whom the independent variables, prenatal cocaine/alcohol exposures, were prospectively assessed and quantified at the university maternity center. After informed consent, the primary dependent variable, school behavior, is assessed, using the PROBS-14 (a teacher consensus developed instrument), the Child Behavior Check List, and the Conners' Teacher Rating Scale. The secondary dependent measure, school achievement, is measured by the Metropolitan Achievement Text and the Test of Early Reading Ability. Control variables, such as the environment and parenting, are measured by several instruments aimed at capturing the child and family ecology since birth. All analyses will be adjusted as appropriate for prospectively gathered control variables such as perinatal risk, neonatal risk, and other prenatal drug and cigarette exposures. Further adjustment will be made for postnatal social risk factors which may influ-

[a] This study was supported by grants from the National Institute on Drug Abuse.

[f] Address for correspondence: Virginia Delaney-Black, M.D., Children's Hospital of Michigan, 3901 Beaubien, Detroit, MI 48201. Phone, 313/745-5638; fax, 313/745-5867; e-mail, vdelaney@med.wayne.edu

ence outcome. Of particular concern are characteristics of the home (adaptation of HOME), parent (depression, stress), and neighborhood (violence exposure). Finally, postnatal exposure to lead and other drugs is being considered.

INTRODUCTION

Despite the escalating use of cocaine, especially among pregnant women,[1] and warnings of a public health emergency,[2] no systematic studies were available to evaluate the outcome of children at early school age when we submitted a grant to the National Institute on Drug Abuse in 1993. Although substance abuse was not a new problem, within our urban, low socioeconomic maternity population, cocaine had emerged as the predominant illicit drug of abuse in the mid-1980s. At its height the cocaine epidemic affected as many as 31% of the maternity clients at our center.[3] Although other illicit drugs of abuse have reappeared, cocaine continues to have a significant impact on our NICU admissions. At its peak, national media provided chilling statistics and predictions suggesting that children prenatally exposed to cocaine would have permanent and irreversible effects.[4] Early school educators also reported that the cocaine-exposed child displayed characteristics such as poor concentration, labile stimulatory overload, and delayed speech.[5] Of concern were the reports of unique behaviors thought to be related to prenatal cocaine exposure.[6] Evidence to support the teachers' claims came from substantial increases in special education referrals from communities across the country thought to be largely related to the epidemic of prenatal cocaine abuse.[6–10] Although new curricula were designed and teaching strategies for these children were discussed, little substantive data were available to indicate that these behaviors were in fact more prevalent among children with prenatal exposures. Furthermore, the information that was available came from case reports and referral centers for childhood problems. Bias was a likely problem, as no blinded studies were available to approach the hypothesis that children prenatally exposed to cocaine did indeed have more behavioral problems. Following their landmark paper, "A Rush to Judgment," Mayes and her colleagues were challenged to provide scientific inquiry with longitudinal, prospective design that could control for covariates and provide adequate power to answer the urgent research questions.[11]

SPECIFIC AIMS

Within this framework, we sought to develop a research protocol that would address the relationship between prenatal cocaine/alcohol exposure and school-age outcomes, taking advantage of the prospectively collected data from Wayne State University's Fetal Alcohol Research Center. The specific aims of the research protocol were: (1) to determine if a relationship exists among prenatal exposure to cocaine/alcohol and school behavior; (2) to determine if a dose-response relationship exists between prenatal exposure to cocaine/alcohol and school behavior; and (3) to evaluate the relationship between prenatal cocaine/alcohol exposures and school achievement.

The study sought to direct inquiry towards an area of significant interest and controversy: child behavior. Neonatal studies at that time had focused significant effort on the behavioral effects of prenatal cocaine exposure.[12–15] Additionally, other authors had provided interesting research evidence of behavioral differences later in infancy.[16,17] No prospective, long-term, controlled studies in humans were available, however. Subsequent evidence of behavioral problems following prenatal exposure now exists. Griffith *et al.*[18] reported more aggressive and destructive behavior and higher externalizing scores on the Child Behavior Checklist in children prenatally exposed to cocaine. Additionally, Richardson *et al.*[19] have suggested that the exposed child may have attention problems.

SAMPLE IDENTIFICATION

At the time of our grant submission, Wayne State University's Fetal Alcohol Research Center (FARC) had prospectively screened over 17,000 consecutive pregnancies at the University's maternity center for alcohol, drug, and cigarette exposure. A stratified statistical sample of 3,500 pregnancies had been repeatedly screened at each pregnancy visit for exposure status using both dichotomous (yes/no) and quantitative reporting. All data were obtained by trained research staff members using the structured interview previously reported.[20] The sample chosen for this study consisted of the singleton offspring of the FARC-participating women born between September 1, 1989 and August 31, 1991. The dates for inclusion took into account the estimated sample size required for a medium-size effect,[21] the age of the subjects, and the Detroit Public School calendar. The Detroit Public School limits first grade entry to children who attain 6 years of age on or before December 1 of the year of school entry. Additionally, as the overwhelming majority of women receiving prenatal care at the University Health Center are African-American, the sample was limited to this racial group as there would be inadequate representation of other ethnic groups. The limited economic, geographic, and housing variability of the sample at study entry was thought to add to the relative homogeneity of the sample. Women receiving care at the University's maternity center were Medicaid recipients and with few exceptions lived in the central Detroit area. Unlike some other urban centers, Detroit has little high-rise public housing. Housing stock in Detroit is primarily pre-1960 single family units, duplexes, or small apartment buildings. Furthermore there is limited diversity in the origin of Detroit's African-American population with few Hispanic African-Americans.

OUTCOME MEASURES

Behavior

Child behavior was defined in three settings: the school, the home, and the research laboratory. To define behavior in these three sites standardized measures were sought that would include both parent and teacher versions for assessing child behavior. Additionally, the research staff, who were blinded to the exposure status of the child, was also asked to provide descriptive information using questions from the parent version of the behavior measures. Two standardized and one-investigator developed behavior measures were identified for study use. The standardized measures were the Conners Parent and Teacher Rating Scales[22,23] and the Achenbach Child Behavior Checklist and Teacher Report Form. Each of these measures takes into account the age and gender of the child in computing a final score. The 39-item version of the Conners Teacher Rating Scale (CTRS) and the 48-item version of the Conners Parent Rating Scale were used. Behaviors are scored on a 4-point Likert scale from 0 (not at all like) to 3 (very much like). In general, the Conners scale utilizes negative phraseology such as "sassy to grown-ups," "steals," and "bullies others." The 48-item parent version is made up of five subscales and a hyperactivity index. It can be completed in less than 15 minutes. Both parent and teacher versions consist of a single page. The Conners scales were selected because of their widespread use in the educational literature as well as their ease of completion. Whereas there was wide experience with the use of the CTRS, the Detroit Public School staff expressed concern with the negative wording of many of the available measures, but particularly the Achenbach.

Within the research literature, the Achenbach report forms have been a standard measure. For this reason, teacher ratings using both the Conners and Achenbach scales were trialed for a 3-month period at the beginning of the grant. No reduction in teacher compliance was observed over that experienced in a pilot study when the Achenbach was omitted. Hence both measures were included in the final study design.

The Child Behavior Checklist (1991 profile for ages 4–18) consists of 113 items scored as 0 (not true), 1 (somewhat or sometimes true), or 2 (very true or very often). In addition, the parent is asked to provide information on the child's activities (sports, hobbies, organizations, and chores) as well relationships and school work. Two open-ended sections permit the parent to identify things about the child that concern them and qualities that they like best. The authors report an average time for completion of the form to be 15–17 minutes. The parent version is scored into eight problem scales with five scales collapsed into internalizing (withdrawn, somatic complaints, and anxious/depressed) and externalizing (delinquent, aggressive) behaviors. Higher scores reflect more problems. As with the parent version, the Teacher Report Form consists of 113 items in addition to descriptive information on the child's school performance. Open-ended comments are also solicited for the teacher's primary concerns as well as the child's best characteristics. As with the parent version, five of the eight scales are used to create internalizing and externalizing behaviors.

The third teacher rating form utilized was the Problem Behavior Scale. As children prenatally exposed to cocaine entered the school system, media reports of unique behaviors were attributed to the epidemic.[4] Three competing hypotheses were available.[26] Children prenatally exposed to cocaine could (1) demonstrate the same types of behavior problems as could unexposed children; (2) share some problem behaviors as could unexposed children but also demonstrate some unique behaviors; or (3) have unique behaviors that were unlike those of the unexposed child.

If either of the later two scenarios was true, then available measures might be inadequate to assess the variability in the cocaine-exposed sample. Consideration of these three hypotheses led to the formation of research questions that guided instrument development of a tool specific to the behaviors described by elementary school teachers. A consensus group process was used to derive descriptive information from teachers regarding their real-life experiences of problem behaviors demonstrated by cocaine-exposed children within their own classroom. The consensus group was composed of teachers outside the Detroit Public School to avoid biasing the sample to be tested in the grant. However, the moderate-sized communities from which the 19 first grade, 2 resource room, and 3 special education teachers were recruited had significant substance abuse indicators. A more extensive description of the consensus process utilized has been published.[26] From an initial list of 25 problem behaviors identified by the teachers, a final list of 14 were selected using T-scores. A visual analog scale with four verbal anchors (not at all like, just a little like, pretty much like, and very much like) was devised (FIG. 1). For each item a score of 0–10 may be identified by placing an "x" at the selected level. Analysis of the measure demonstrated interitem correlations from 0.35–0.65 with a Cronbach's alpha of 0.96.

Achievement

The Detroit Public Schools provide achievement testing with the Metropolitan Achievement Test in the spring of each school year. Although parents provided us with consent for accessing school records, changes in Detroit Public School enrollment oc-

CHILD CODE: — — — —
TEACHER'S ID: — — — —

CHILD'S AGE: ——— YEARS ——— MONTHS
CHILD'S GENDER: — M — F

PROBS - 14

Instructions: Rate the student's behaviors. Where does this child's behavior fall? Mark clearly with an "X."

Example:
0 | | | | 2.5 | | | | 5.0 **X** | | | 7.5 | | | | 10

Not at all like	Just a little like	Pretty much like	Very much like

Scale	Item
0 | | | | 2.5 | | | | 5.0 | | | | 7.5 | | | | 10	1. High Distractibility
0 | | | | 2.5 | | | | 5.0 | | | | 7.5 | | | | 10	2. Inappropriate Social Skills
0 | | | | 2.5 | | | | 5.0 | | | | 7.5 | | | | 10	3. Severe and/or inconsistent inability to retain academic material
0 | | | | 2.5 | | | | 5.0 | | | | 7.5 | | | | 10	4. Unpredictable and inconsistent behavioral responses
0 | | | | 2.5 | | | | 5.0 | | | | 7.5 | | | | 10	5. Hyperactivity
0 | | | | 2.5 | | | | 5.0 | | | | 7.5 | | | | 10	6. Extremely disorganized on task
0 | | | | 2.5 | | | | 5.0 | | | | 7.5 | | | | 10	7. Difficulty internalizing a personal code of behavior and abilities

Not at all like	Just a little like	Pretty much like	Very much like

Scale	Item
0 | | | | 2.5 | | | | 5.0 | | | | 7.5 | | | | 10	8. Inability to respond to concrete abstract thought stimulus
0 | | | | 2.5 | | | | 5.0 | | | | 7.5 | | | | 10	9. Passive to animate/inanimate environment
0 | | | | 2.5 | | | | 5.0 | | | | 7.5 | | | | 10	10. Delayed speech and language development
0 | | | | 2.5 | | | | 5.0 | | | | 7.5 | | | | 10	11. Frequently demand attention inappropriately
0 | | | | 2.5 | | | | 5.0 | | | | 7.5 | | | | 10	12. Inability to handle transitions or change, need for constant redirection
0 | | | | 2.5 | | | | 5.0 | | | | 7.5 | | | | 10	13. Overall motor skill problems
0 | | | | 2.5 | | | | 5.0 | | | | 7.5 | | | | 10	14. Inability to handle sensory overload at school assemblies, lunch, gym, playground, bus rides

Not at all like	Just a little like	Pretty much like	Very much like

FIGURE 1. Visual analog scale.

curred between the pilot study (when more than 80% of our subjects attended Detroit Public Schools) and the funding of this grant. State funding became available for "charter schools." These charter schools exist separate from the Detroit Public Schools but are supported by public funds. Each makes its own regulations and testing decisions. As a result, the number of children for whom MAT scores were available fell. Several areas of concern were considered in choosing a replacement for the MAT. Although a variety of achievement measures have been used in previous research, the Wide Range Achievement Test is perhaps most commonly used for elementary school children. However, because of the early educational level of the 6-year-old subjects in this study, concern was expressed that subjects might be clustered at the basal level. A reliable test with ease of administration and with inclusion of pre-primary items was sought. Ethnic sensitivity was also a concern. The Test of Early Reading Ability (second edition) met these selection criteria.[27] It can be administered in 15–30 minutes and uses familiar logos for pre-primary items, hence providing a measure of reading readiness as well as reading achievement. The mean score is 100 with standard deviation of 15.

INDEPENDENT VARIABLE

Drug use during pregnancy was determined by history as well as maternal and infant urine. During the later stages of subject recruitment, infant meconium was also available. A woman was considered cocaine exposed if any of the three identification sources, history or maternal or infant laboratory test, were positive. Detailed drug histories including the frequency of drug use were obtained at the initial and each subsequent prenatal visit. In addition to their use of cocaine, women were queried regarding use of marijuana, heroin, and a variety of other prescription drugs. Hence, a dichotomous cocaine as well as an ordinal quantified exposure variable could be derived for each drug of interest.

CONTROL VARIABLES

Prenatal/Perinatal

Alcohol. Prenatal alcohol exposure is one of the most important control variables for any study evaluating the effects of illicit substance exposure during pregnancy. In addition to the observation that women who use cocaine are more likely to abuse alcohol, prenatal alcohol exposure has important and serious consequences that may obscure the effects of prenatal cocaine exposure. Since the classic papers describing fetal alcohol syndrome (FAS),[28,29] substantial data have been published linking maternal alcohol use with short- (neonatal)[30–32] and long-term (childhood) effects.[33–35] A direct, dose-response effect[36–38] as well as individual variability in the fetus' susceptibility[39] has been described. Not all alcohol-exposed pregnancies result in the birth of a child with FAS. More subtle findings of the effects of fetal alcohol exposure have been reported including alterations of growth,[40] intelligence,[41,42] achievement,[41,43,44] and behavior.[45,46] Even after exclusion of children with FAS, verbal IQ was negatively related to maternal alcohol consumption.[38] In a large, well-controlled study of 7-year-old, their IQ was significantly lower when mothers had used more than an ounce of alcohol per day during pregnancy.[43] In addition, achievement scores were negatively affected by maternal alcohol intake.[41,43,47] Thus, careful consideration must be taken of the child's prenatal exposure to alcohol. Specific information was obtained for periconceptual and later pregnancy alcohol consumption using previously described structured interview format.[20]

Cigarettes. Prenatal exposure of our clients to cocaine is also associated with a greater likelihood of cigarette smoking. Substantial evidence exists to suggest that prenatal and perhaps postnatal smoking may have serious consequences. Prenatal smoking has been associated with alterations in fetal growth[48,49] and child cognitive outcome,[49–51] achievement,[48,49] and behavior.[52,53] Hence, control for maternal smoking is essential in attempting to identify causality for any of the outcomes affected by both prenatal cocaine and cigarette exposure.

Prenatal/Perinatal Risk. Evaluation of other prenatal and perinatal risk factors was considered in the study design. In our sample as well as that of Eyler and colleagues,[54] women with cocaine exposure were older and had more children. Other perinatal risk factors may be mediators of the effects of cocaine exposure rather than true control variables. Included in this list might be abruptio placenta,[48] prematurity,[55] meconium,[3] and low Apgar scores.[54] Control for these variables may inappropriately reduce the variance associated with maternal cocaine exposure. Other factors such as maternal hypertension, lack of prenatal care, and nutritional deficits may be associated with but not caused by maternal drug use.

Neonatal Risk. Neonatal abnormalities associated with prenatal drug exposure include early gestational age and reduction in intrauterine growth.[54] Prematurity, fetal distress, and its subsequent neonatal complications may also be associated with an increased risk of admission to the neonatal intensive care unit as well as other neonatal complications. Some of the effects of prenatal cocaine exposure may be mediated by the reduction in the length of gestation and fetal growth. Controlling for these factors may inappropriately reduce the risk attributed to prenatal cocaine exposure.

Postnatal

A variety of postnatal factors may affect child outcome including maternal characteristics (depression, support) and family characteristics (family functioning). Children prenatally exposed to alcohol and drugs may also be affected by continuing family use as well as personal exposure. A list of the primary postnatal control variables selected for inclusion in the SCHOO-BE study are provided in TABLE 1.

METHODS

Data from the FARC study were utilized to identify a sample of children with known prenatal exposure to alcohol, drugs, and cigarettes. As described earlier, women receiving care at the University Maternity Center were queried at their initial prenatal visit using a structured research interview. Women with moderate and heavy alcohol use as well as those with drug exposure were oversampled. Alcohol, drug, and cigarette exposure was queried at each subsequent visit using both dichotomous and frequency data for each exposure. Maternal and infant urine specimens and, in the later stages of the study, infant meconium were ordered when clinically indicated. Drug use was identified by any positive (history or laboratory) report. Pregnancy, intrapartum, and neonatal complications were recorded. Six years later families were contacted by phone, mail, and, when needed, by home visit to evaluate childhood outcome. Once contacted, the study was explained by a research nurse and consent was requested for further follow-up. Families who declined to be interviewed in the laboratory setting were asked for permission to obtain the teacher's reports and/or parent interviews were conducted by phone. In the laboratory the biologic mother, father, or primary caretaker was tested and interviewed, while the child was tested by a second trained research assistant. Research assistants were blinded to perinatal information until the mother's testing was complete. As the interview contained questions about the child's exposures to drugs and alcohol, it was not possible to maintain blinding for the remainder of the session. When both mother and primary caretaker were available, both were tested and inter-

TABLE 1. Primary Variables of Interest for SCHOO-BE Study

	Operational Measure
Independent variable	
Prenatal Cocaine Exposure (dichotomous/quantitative)	% Days of exposure
Dependent variables	
School Behavior	
Achenbach (CBC, TRF)	Total score
Conners' Rating Scales	Scale scores
PROBS-14 (teacher/only)	Total score
Secondary Outcome	
Achievement	
MAT	Total score
Grade Retention	No, yes
Special Education Referrals	No, yes
Control Variables	
Perinatal factors	Perinatal risk score
Prenatal alcohol exposure	Absolute alcohol, ounces/day
Prenatal smoking	Cigarettes/day
Prenatal drug exposure	Interview % days of exposure
Perinatal/neonatal risk	Neonatal risk score
Other drug exposures	Yes on any drug exposure variable
Prenatal smoking	Maternal cigarettes/day
Postnatal exposures	
Postnatal drug exposure	Interview % days of exposure
Postnatal alcohol exposure	Absolute alcohol, ounces/day
Postnatal smoking exposure	Cigarettes/day
Maternal characteristics/home environment	
Maternal IQ	WAIS-R/PPVT-R
Demographic at birth	Hollingshead
	Maternal age
	Insurance status
Demographic at follow-up	Hollingshead
	Insurance status
	Child guardianship
Child health status	Chronic illness
	Chronic medication
Family functioning	FACES-II
Attitudes toward parenting/parenting stress	Parenting-stress index
Home environment	HOME—lab adaptation
Maternal social support	Norbeck Social Support Questionnaire
Daily stress	Daily Hassles-Index
Neighborhood/environment	Neighborhood survey, violence exposure
Child measures	
Cognitive-Child IQ	WPPSI FS IQ
	KABC
Hearing	Audiogram
	Tympanogram
Weight	Weight (kg)
Height	Height (cm)
Head circumference	Head circumference (cm)
Self-concept	Pictoral Scales of Perceived Competence

viewed. The primary testing measures are provided in TABLE 1. A standard format for testing was utilized with breaks and snacks provided for both adult and child. To avoid transportation difficulties biasing the research results, all families were offered cab transportation to the testing site. Testing was provided 6 days a week with morning and afternoon appointments Monday through Friday. Each family was provided with gift certificates as a stipend for their participation.

Teachers were identified by the parent or guardian during the laboratory portion of testing. A single research assistant called each school prior to sending the teacher report forms. This enabled us to verify the name and address of the school as well as alert the principal and first grade teacher to the mailing. All materials sent to the school were placed on letterhead from the Children's Hospital. As pediatric forms are frequently sent by this institution for teacher completion, we hoped to avoid inappropriately identifying a child as problematic. The teacher was questioned about medical conditions of the child including but not limited to allergies, asthma, attention deficit hyperactivity disorder, absences, and lead, alcohol, and drug exposure. The questions pertaining to family exposure to drugs were embedded in the list of medical problems to obtain evidence of potential teacher bias. Forms not returned within the month were followed up by a phone call and when needed a visit was scheduled with the teacher. During the 20-minute visit the teacher filled out the forms while the research assistant waited. Questions regarding the nature of the study were answered honestly; the study is developing a new, shortened version of a behavior measure. No information was provided about the child's testing; no information was available to the research assistant at the time of her visit. Teachers were paid a small stipend for form completion.

SAMPLE CHARACTERISTICS

The sample consisted of 1,076 singleton children born to the women participating in the FARC and born between September 1, 1989 and August 31, 1991. Of these, 378 were considered cocaine exposed and 688 controls. Women using cocaine during the pregnancy were older (28 ± 5 *vs* 24 ± 6, $p < 0.001$), had a lower pre-pregnancy weight (135 ± 30 *vs* 145 ± 38, $p < 0.001$), smoked more cigarettes (13 ± 10 *vs* 6 ± 9, $p < 0.001$), and drank more ounces of absolute alcohol per day (1.0 ± 1.6 *vs* 0.6 ± 1.4, $p < 0.001$). As in previous studies, their offspring were smaller (2,759 ± 658 *vs* 3,090 ± 616, $p < 0.001$), shorter (47.2 ± 3.8 *vs* 48.8 ± 3.2, $p < 0.01$), and had smaller head circumferences (32.8 ± 2.4 *vs* 33.7 ± 2.0, $p < 0.001$) and shorter gestational ages (38 ± 3 *vs* 39 ± 2, $p < 0.001$).

RESULTS

At the time of this writing only the first year of subject testing was complete (date of birth September 1, 1989 to December 1, 1989). Year two testing was drawing to an end; however, not all data had been entered and verified. The first 279 subjects studied by the project are described below; however, extreme care must be taken in evaluating the results, as this represents less than half the final projected study sample. For that reason, outcome variables were not analyzed.

The sample included 107 children with prenatal exposure to cocaine and 172 without. In the following description the cocaine-exposed group is presented first. At discharge from the hospital nursery, 96% of both groups were released to their biologic mother. At follow-up 6 years later few caretakers were married (25% and 29%, NS), although more acknowledged living with a partner (34% and 40%, NS). Fewer cocaine-exposed children were accompanied to the testing by a biologic parent (79% *vs* 93%, p <0.03), but subsequent testing of the biologic parent was often possible. The primary caretaker also was less likely to be a biologic parent in the cocaine group (76% *vs* 94%, p <0.001). In most cases the child remained with a relative, particularly a grandparent. Three percent of the cocaine sample and less than 1% of controls had been adopted. In addition, caretaker status was more likely to have changed since hospital discharge for the child with prenatal cocaine exposure (44% *vs* 15%, p <0.001). Only 53% of the cocaine-exposed children had always been in the custody of their biologic mother compared to 81% of the controls (p <0.001).

The test results of the primary caretaker were evaluated with ANOVA. No relationship was found between cocaine exposure, child custody, or the interaction of custody and exposure and the primary caretaker's verbal (PPVT) or performance IQ (-WAIS-R), education in years, or income per year. However, subscales of the adapted HOME measure were related to either cocaine exposure (one subscale approached significance, p =0.059) or custody (three subscales were significantly related (p <0.02).

CONCLUSION

The SCHOO-BE experience is a work in progress. As a result, our summary statements must of necessity be very general. Understanding the school-age outcomes of children prenatally exposed to cocaine is a much more complicated undertaking than is evaluating neonatal complications. Postnatal exposure of the child to the effects of ongoing substance abuse in the family (alcohol, drugs, and cigarettes) is essential. So too is the child's exposure to violence in both the home and the neighborhood. The child self-concept may also mediate the prenatal effects and must be considered in understanding child outcome. Of paramount importance is the concern regarding the effects of changes in custody status, particularly when multiple changes occur. Separating the effects of changes in custody from prenatal exposure will perhaps be the greatest challenge as it is likely that change in custody is also a surrogate which correlates with increasing prenatal drug exposures. Even after careful control and adequate sample size, questions are likely to remain. If behavioral effects are identified, will they persist? Is there a relation between the parent's drug exposure and underlying behavioral problems? As often happens even at this study's conclusions, more questions are likely to be raised than answered. Do underlying behavior problems of the parent lead to drug abuse? And, if so, how does this affect child behavior?

REFERENCES

1. CHASNOFF, I. 1987. Perinatal effects of cocaine. Contemporary OB/GYN 163–179.
2. HOROWITZ, R. 1990. Prenatal substance abuse. Children Today **4:** 9–12.
3. OSTREA, E.M., M. BRADY, S. GAUSE *et al.* 1992. Drug screening of newborns by meconium analysis: A large-scale, prospective, epidemiologic study. Pediatrics **89:** 107–113.
4. TOUFEXIS, A. 1991. Innocent victims. Time Magazine May 13: 56–60.
5. RIST, M. 1990. The shadow children. American School Board J. **177:** 19–24.
6. 102ND CONGRESS: COMMITTEE ON THE JUDICIARY, U.S. SENATE. MAY 16, 1991. COCAINE KINDERGARTNERS: PREPARING FOR THE FIRST WAVE (SERIAL NO. J-102-16). U.S. GOVERNMENT PRINTING OFFICE. WASHINGTON, DC.
7. 102ND CONGRESS. SELECT COMMITTEE ON NARCOTICS ABUSE AND CONTROL. JULY 30, 1991. DRUG EXPOSED CHILDREN IN THE SCHOOLS: PROBLEMS AND POLICY (SCNAC-102-1-9). U.S. GOVERNMENT PRINTING OFFICE. WASHINGTON, DC.

8. GREGORCHIK, L. 1992. The cocaine-exposed children are here. Phi Delta Kappa **18:** 60–64.
9. ELLIOT, K. & D. COKER. 1991. Crack babies: Here they come, ready or not. J. Inst. Psychol. **18:** 60–64.
10. BARTH, R. 1991. Educational implications of prenatally drug-exposed children. Soc. Work Ed. **13:** 130–136.
11. MAYES, L.C., R.H. GRANGER, M.H. BORNSTEIN *et al.* 1991. The problem of prenatal cocaine exposure: A rush to judgement. JAMA **267:** 406–408.
12. MAYES, L.C., R.H. GRANGER, M.A. FRANK *et al.* 1993. Neurobehavioral profiles of neonates exposed to cocaine prenatally. Pediatrics **91:** 778–783.
13. COLES, C.D., K.A. PLATZMAN, I. SMITH *et al.* 1992. Effects of cocaine and alcohol use in pregnancy on neonatal growth and neurobehavioral status. Neurotoxicol. Teratol. **14:** 23–33.
14. NEUSPIEL, D.R., S.C. HAMEL, E. HOCHBERG *et al.* 1991. Neurotoxicol. Teratol. **13:** 229–233.
15. EISEN, L., T.M. FIELD, E.S. BANDSTRA *et al.* 1991. Perinatal cocaine effects on neonatal stress behavior and performance on the Brazelton Scale. Pediatrics **88:** 477–480.
16. HANSEN, R.L., J.M. STRUTHERS & S.M. GOSPE. 1993. Visual evoked potentials and visual processing stimulant drug exposed infants. Dev. Med. Child Neurol. **35:** 798–805.
17. ALLESANDRI, S.M., M.W. SULLIVAN, S. IMAIZUMI *et al.* 1993. Learning and emotional responsivity in cocaine-exposed infants. Dev. Psychol. **29:** 989–997.
18. GRIFFITH, D.R., S.D. AZUMA & I.J. CHASNOFF. 1994. Three-year outcome of children exposed prenatally to drugs. J. Am. Acad. Child Adolesc. Psychiatry **33:** 20–27.
19. RICHARDSON, G.A., M.L. CONROY & N.L. DAY. 1996. Prenatal cocaine-exposure: Effects on the development of school-age children. Neurotoxicol. Teratol. **18:** 627–634.
20. SOKOL, R.J., S. MARTIER & C. ERNHART. 1985. Identification of alcohol abuse in the prenatal clinic. *In* Research Monograph No 17: Early identification of alcohol abuse. N. Chang & N. Chao, Eds. I.S. Department of Health and Human Services Publication No. (ADM) 85-1258. Washington, D.C.
21. COHEN, J. 1988. Statistical Power Analysis for the Behavioral Sciences. Lawrence Erlbaum Associates. Hillsdale, NJ.
22. TRITES, R.L., A.G. BLOUIN & K. LAPRADE. 1982. Factor analysis of the Conners' Teacher Rating Scale based on a large normative sample. J. Consult. Clin. Psychol. **50:** 615–623.
23. CONNERS, C.K. 1990. Rating scales. Multi-Health Systems.
24. ACHENBACH, T.M. 1991. Manual for the Child Behavior Checklist/4–18 and 1991 Profile. University of Vermont Department of Psychiatry. Burlington, VT.
25. ACHENBACH, T.M. 1991. Manual for the Teacher's Report Form and 1991 Profile. University of Vermont Department of Psychiatry. Burlington, VT.
26. COVINGTON, C., V. DELANEY-BLACK, R.J. SOKOL, *et al.* 1996. Development of an instrument to assess problem behavior in first-grade students prenatally exposed to cocaine: Part I. Substance Abuse **17:** 87–99.
27. REID, D.K., W.P. HRESKO & D.D. HAMMILL. 1989. Test of Early Reading Ability, 2nd Ed. Pro-ED. Austin, Texas.
28. JONES, K.L. & D. SMITH. 1973. Recognition of the fetal alcohol syndrome in early infancy. Lancet **2:** 999–1001.
29. JONES, K.L., D.W. SMITH, C.N. ULLELAND, *et al.* 1973. Patterns of malformation in offspring of chronic alcoholic mothers. Lancet **1:** 1267–1271.
30. PIEROG, S., O. CHANDAVASU & I. WEXLER. 1977. Withdrawal symptoms in infants with the fetal alcohol syndrome. J. Pediatr. **90:** 630–633.
31. STREISSGUTH, A.P., D.C. MARTIN & H.M. BARR. 1983. Maternal alcohol use and neonatal habitation assessed with Brazelton Scales. Child Dev. **54:** 1109–1118.
32. OUELLETTE, E.M., H.L. ROSETT, N.P. ROSMAN *et al.* 1977. Adverse effects on offspring of maternal alcohol abuse during pregnancy. N. Engl. J. Med. **297:** 528–530.
33. ARONSON, M., M. KYLLERMAN, K.G. SABEL, *et al.* 1985. Children of alcoholic mothers: Developmental, perceptual, and behavioral characteristics as compared to matched controls. Acta Paediatr. Scand. **75:** 27–35.
34. STREISSGUTH, A.P., H.M. BARR, D.C. MARTIN *et al.* 1980. Effects of maternal alcohol, nicotine, and caffeine use during pregnancy on infant mental and motor development at eight months. Alcoholism **4:** 152–154.

35. ABEL, E.I. & R.J. SOKOL. 1990. Is occasional light drinking during pregnancy harmful? Controversy in the addition field. R.C. Engs, Ed. Kendall-Hunt Publishing Co. Dubuque.
36. STREISSGUTH, A.P., P.D. SAMPSON & H.M. BARR. 1989. Neurobehavioral dose-response effects of prenatal alcohol exposure in humans from infancy to adulthood. Ann. N.Y. Acad. Sci. **562:** 145–158.
37. AUTTI-RAMO, I. & M.L. GRANSTROM. 1991. The psychomotor development during the first year of life of infants exposed to intrauterine alcohol of various duration. Fetal alcohol exposure and development. Neuropediatrics **22:** 59–64.
38. AUTTI-RAMO, I. & M.L. GRANSTROM. 1991. The effect of intrauterine alcohol exposition in various durations of early cognitive development. Neuropediatrics **22:** 203–210.
39. CHERNOFF, G.F. 1980. The Fetal Alcohol Syndrome in mice: Maternal variables. Teratology **22:** 71–75.
40. NATIONAL HEALTH/EDUCATION CONSORTIUM. 1991. Health brain development: Precursor to learning. National Commission to Prevent Infant Mortality and Institute for Educational Leadership. Washington, DC.
41. SCOTT, K. *et al.* 1991. Long-term psychoeducational outcome of prenatal substance exposure. Semin Perinatol. **15:** 317–323.
42. LAPKE, J., T.B. GOLEMAN, J.C. ALDAG & A.M. MORGAN. 1992. Developmental follow-up of cocaine exposed infants in foster care. Pediatr. Res. **31:** 95A.
43. HUTCHINGS, D.E. 1993. The puzzle of cocaine's effects following maternal use during pregnancy: Are there reconcilable differences? Neurotoxical. Teratol. **15:** 281–286.
44. ANDERSON, G.D., I.N. BLINGER, M.A. MCCLEMONT *et al.* 1998. Determinants of size at birth in a Canadian population. Am. J. Obstet. Gynecol.
45. RONA, R.J., S. CHINA & C. DU VE FLOREY. 1985. Exposure to cigarette smoking and children's growth. Int. J. Epidemiol. **14:** 402–409.
46. TAYLOR, B. & J. WASSWORTH. 1987. Maternal smoking during pregnancy and lower respiratory tract illness in early life. Arch. Dis. Child. **62:** 786–791.
47. ROBINSON, S. 1992. Grant #R01 DA04746-03.
48. RANTAKILLO, P. 1983. A follow-up study up to the age of 14 of children whose mothers smoked during pregnancy. Acta Paediatr. Scand. **72:** 747–753.
49. FOX, N.L., M. SEXTON & J.R. HEBEL. 1990. Prenatal exposure to tobacco. I. Effects on physical growth at age three. Int. J. Epidemiol. **19:** 66–71.
50. BUTLER, N.R. & H. GOLDSTEIN. 1973. Smoking in pregnancy and subsequent child development. Br. Med. J. **4:** 573–575.
51. DUNN, H.G., A.K. MCBURNEY, S. INGRAM *et al.* 1977. Maternal cigarette smoking during pregnancy and the child's subsequent development. II. Neurological and intellectual maturation to the age of 6 1/2 years. Can. J. Public Health **68:** 43–50.
52. FERGUSSON, D.M. & M. LLOYD. 1991. Smoking during pregnancy and its effect on child cognitive ability from the ages of 8 to 12 years. Paediatr. Perinatol. Epidemiol. **5:** 189–200.
53. WEITZMAN, M., S. GORTMAKER & A. SOBEL. 1992. Maternal smoking and behavior problems of children. Pediatrics **90:** 342–349.
54. EYLER, F.D., M. BEHNKE, M. CONLON *et al.* 1994. Prenatal cocaine use: A comparison of neonates matched on maternal risk factors. Neurotoxicol. Teratol. **16:** 81–87.
55. FERGUSSON, D.M., L.J. HORWOOD & M.T. LYNSKEY. 1993. Maternal smoking before and after pregnancy: Effects on behavioral outcomes in middle childhood. Pediatrics **92:** 815–822.

Round Table 4. Levels of Vulnerability in Functional Deficits: Specificity of Dysfunctional Brain Systems

Moderator: E. HAZEL MURPHY
Panelists: TREVOR W. ROBBINS, EITAN FRIEDMAN, BARRY E. KOSOFSKY, JEANNINE L. GINGRAS, VIRGINIA DELANEY-BLACK
Discussants: DONNA FERRIERO *(UCSF)*, CLAUDIA CHIRIBOGA *(Columbia)*, IRA CHASNOFF *(Chicago)*, CHANDICE COVINGTON *(Detroit)*, RACHELLE TYLER *(LA)*, GIDEON KOREN *(Toronto)*, PENNY MAZA *(Children's Bureau)*, LINDA WRIGHT *(NIDA)*, BERNARD KARMEL *(Staten Island)*

E. HAZEL MURPHY: It seems to me from the range of things that have been described that when comparing molecular studies in animal models to behavioral studies in children, there are two directions that need to be addressed: (1) We don't have enough knowledge of the basic effects of exposure to drugs on the developing system. As one of our speakers stated earlier, we know typical responses such as hypersensitivity to perturbations in the mature system, but we don't know those effects in the developing system. We're just beginning to understand the effects of monoamines on growth, and I think there's a lot of very basic work that needs to be done to help us understand these mechanisms. (2) Regardless of what is damaged or whatever the mechanisms, we know from long-term studies on early lesions that the developing brain has an extraordinary capacity for change and there are compensatory mechanisms. What sort of compensatory mechanisms are possible and given that there are compensatory mechanisms, what treatments can we use and how can we make use of the systems that are functional to compensate for those that are not?

BARRY KOSOFSKY: We go back and forth; is it nature, is it nurture, is it the womb? It's all three. There is clear evidence that there are genetic determinants, postnatal determinants, and *in utero* determinants that interact and influence behavior. The swing of the pendulum is in some ways artificial; we must recognize the importance of all of these factors. I think Hazel is getting to what is the bottom line: in what ways can we selectively intervene to improve outcomes? First, we need to know what kinds of outcomes are cocaine-exposed children at risk for, so we can demonstrate which selective interventions are most appropriate. We don't want to just study this problem; we want to fix this problem. Last night Floyd Bloom gave us our marching orders; it is important for those of us working in the field to increase our collective knowledge base and get a better mechanistic understanding of cocaine-induced alterations in brain development. However, we must proceed in parallel to educate clinicians, educators, parents, legislators, and the lay public that many cocaine-exposed children are handicapped. These children may be at risk for compromise of specific behaviors for many reasons, and we must try to develop and disseminate appropriate and effective intervention strategies. I was intrigued by the data Linda Spear presented which suggested that the response of cocaine-exposed animals to handling and early stimulation was greater than that seen in control animals, suggesting that you may get more therapeutic "bang for your buck" when you tailor the right intervention to the right groups.

Additionally we need to identify "markers" in the early perinatal period of the infant at risk and to define "at risk for what" Then we may be in a better position to provide resources and interventions in selective ways for populations that are at risk for particular outcomes. Delivering those resources may well be a very complex task. However, if Claudia Chiriboga is correct, and the "stiff baby" at birth and during the first year of life is the marker of the child who was cocaine exposed, albeit at higher doses, that's an important point for child neurologists and developmental pediatricians to know. Then a clinician who sees a stiff baby can consider if that stiffness is a consequence of *in utero* exposure to significant quantities of opiates and/or cocaine, but not alcohol. Perhaps clinical researchers will find more of these perinatal and postnatal markers and identify the extent to which they are specific. That will help us sort out some predictors of the adverse outcomes these children are at risk for and which interventions might be most appropriate. We want to fix the problem, and living in an environment of greatly constrained financial and personal resources as we do, we need to allocate resources such as occupational therapy, physical therapy, and speech therapy or whatever else we can do in a more cost-effective, user-friendly, outcome-improving fashion. In short, how can we better identify those infants and children at risk, target appropriate resources and interventions, and improve outcomes?

DONNA FERREIRO: I agree with you 100–1,000% on your overall aims and goals. As a child neurologist, I was geared to proving Claudia Chiriboga's point about cocaine-induced hypertonicity and was shocked and amazed in our prospective study that the hypertonicity evident at 6 weeks of age was not due to cocaine, but rather to the presence of cigarette smoking. We measured cotinine as the marker for smoking, not history, and we don't know if it's nicotine or some other component of cigarettes, but in our study sample we know that the stiff babies didn't just have cocaine on board. What is unfortunate is that we've been parading around in our Child Neurology best telling everybody that this hypertonicity is probably due to cocaine, which excludes or at least separates out those infants exposed to significant amounts of alcohol. Now we've got to step back from that. It still allows us to use the information that other people are finding in the animal models. Maybe this hypertonicity that is having an impact on systems is a marker of some of the cognitive stuff that we see later on. I would love to know in Dr. Chasnoff's study and everybody else's who are heavily into neurobehavior who the hypertonic infants turn out to be in terms of their specific behavioral deficits.

SPEAKER: The question of whether hypertonicity is a marker for kids who need help is a different question from whether it is a marker for kids who have been prenatally exposed. We have data in our cohort that the kids who do terrible on their MAIs do terrible on the Bayley's motor assessment of infants at 4 months, and do terrible in their mental development index (MDI) at 2, regardless of drug exposure. The issue is not whether or not you are drug exposed but whether or not you have this behavioral constellation. You have to be very careful about doing retrospective stigmatization to go back to find this point of a baby on the basis of their neurologic finding, but that's very different from saying whatever got this baby here, we need to do something for this baby now for the future.

DONNA FERREIRO: You have to get away from the idea that it's a stigmatizing label. Calling hypertonicity an abnormality is not stigmatizing, but rather identifying.

SPEAKER: I agree. I don't think calling a baby hypertonic is stigmatizing; that's descriptive. But saying hypertonic must be cocaine, that's stigmatizing.

CLAUDIA CHIRIBOGA: Could I talk about some opposite results? We also look at tone and jitteriness in newborns and 4–6 weeks after birth. If we separate our infants with serious injuries and our preemies and look at our "healthy" term cohort, look at babies who have been cocaine exposed, and also look at our healthy term kinds, women without tobacco use, women without prenatal care, women without proper nutrition, and women with a lot of high-risk factors, what we find is, yes, increased tone at birth. However, by the 6-week point, the only kids who are really showing elevated levels of stiffness are not the cigarette-exposed kids, but mostly the cocaine-exposed kids. Now that excludes our SGA infants and our postmature infants, who, as all the child neurologists know, also show increased tone at birth. So in essence what we're saying is that we're getting opposite results because what we're left with between 1 and 2 months are the cocaine-exposed kids. Yes, their moms also smoked cigarettes, but when we look at the infants born to moms who smoked cigarettes, but did not use cocaine, they didn't show the increased tone at 1–2 months of age. Methadone babies were in the middle; alcohol babies tend to look much more like RCF-injured infants and not like the cocaine-exposed or the cigarette-exposed infants.

SPEAKER: We've been looking at children with hypertonicity for a long time, and I think it should be considered a marker of some nonspecific event rather than a specific marker for cocaine or prematurity or whatever. As such, we don't have to label it as a good or a bad, but as Deborah Frank pointed out, something that obviously is different. We did a study many years ago of neurologic findings in cocaine-exposed infants and found hypertonicity, but most of my hypertonic babies are in the low-birth weight follow-up clinic rather than the cocaine clinic.

JEANNINE GINGRAS: I would like to add to that work which I did not present that substantiates the fact that it's a marker irrespective of group. In babies that we studied as fetuses, who have difficulty in regulation, who do not habituate, and who do not arouse initially, we looked at the data for 6-day and 6-week-old infants and found no group differences, but there was clearly an association on the fourth subscale of increased tone and the fifth subscale which is increased leg tone, with the inability to habituate, which we think reflects CNS injury independent of exposure group. So I do agree that it's a marker of CNS injury, but is not specific for cocaine. However, there are data to suggest that children who have the transient hypertonicity of prematurity have cognitive deficits later in development.

IRA CHASNOFF: We published some data on 4-month olds in our population, and using the MAI, saw muscle tone changes in cocaine-exposed children. Now at 6 years of age, those children who had abnormalities on the MAI are not the ones in whom we're seeing any kind of difficulties in that arena now. In fact, our NBAS data is not predictive of anything. One problem with our study is that if we did find a child who had muscle tone problems at 4 months of age, then that child was put into early intervention. Clinically one of the most interesting groups we are seeing is not the cocaine-exposed or the alcohol-exposed, but the children who have been exposed to cocaine and alcohol together. Based on my clinical experience, those are the children I have the greatest concern about.

BARRY KOSOFSKY: Could we then avoid the problem of stigmatization by saying that a stiff infant is at risk; although it's not a marker specific for *in utero* cocaine exposure, it is a marker sensitive to a child at risk. Likewise, a smaller head circumference, at birth or with impaired postnatal growth, identifies an infant at risk, a sensitive, but not a specific marker of *in utero* cocaine exposure. The lack of specificity implies that such clinical "labels" are not stigmatizing, but the sensitivity for detecting an infant at risk allows appropriate referral of infants to occupational and physical therapy services who are in need of such interventions. The child who is stiff during the first year of life or who has a head circumference 2 standard deviations below the mean needs interventions. Are we on safer ground there?

IRA CHASNOFF: I think so, because when we looked at head circumference we found that small head circumference over the first 6 months of life was predictive of development compromise at 3 years of age, but it was not predictive of overall global cognitive developmental compromise at 6 years of age. We keep talking about global cognitive functioning when, in fact, everyone knows that there are a lot more aspects to child development than global cognitive functioning. I'm glad to see that Virginia Delaney-Black was showing results of questioning teachers about students' behavior and school performance.

SPEAKER: In our state of Alabama, custody and family reunification is a very politicized issue. In Michigan does the connection between exposure and custody have to do with the home situation or does it have more to do with scrutiny by social services? Is it a "social marker" that we should be watching more closely because these are more troubled homes or homes where there is ongoing (passive) drug exposure?

VIRGINIA DELANEY-BLACK: The policy in the State of Michigan is to maintain families together. Whether that's good or bad I don't think anyone has been able to demonstrate. It's hard even to know if it's cheaper, because we don't know what the effects are on the children. Clearly I don't think anyone has the data to indicate that one is better than the other. That's the problem with the political issue of changing these laws from state to state. No one has data to suggest which is better.

As to scrutiny, more scrutiny was applied to children who were cocaine exposed. In another study that we did, there's about a 15% change in custody status during the first year of life. Many of the children who are removed initially return, and about 15% of the children who weren't removed initially were removed between birth and the first year. I don't know if it's because there's a lot of scrutiny.

CHANDICE COVINGTON: There's more monitoring because these infants are identified as drug exposed and a case is filed, but there may not be much scrutiny.

RACHELLE TYLER: Going back to the hypertonicity, I'm curious whether anyone has looked at African-American children who have not had prenatal cocaine exposure versus African-American children who have had prenatal drug exposure, because classically African-American children are hypertonic at birth.

DONNA FERREIRO: In our population in San Francisco, most of our cocaine-exposed babies are African-American. As a child neurologist, I know that African-American babies have more tone. We actually looked at how tone segregated with race, and you are 100% correct that African-American babies have more tone. But if you do the appropriate statistical analyses, matching your data, the tone abnormalities seem to be related to maternal cocaine use and to maternal cigarette smoking. When we looked for interactions, there were none, and when we conducted a logistic regression model, cocaine fell out as not being the cause of the increased tone. You're 100% correct that racial differences are evident in muscle tone, and all clinicians must take that into consideration when they do their motor exams.

SPEAKER: My question pertains to whether there is bias due to cocaine on custody.

VIRGINIA DELANEY-BLACK: All the children in the State of Michigan who are known to be cocaine exposed at birth have what's called a CD3200 filed. It means that the state has to investigate the case and deem that the child can go home to that family. However, how much scrutiny occurs after the child is discharged is related to the case load of the assigned staff, and much of the custody decisions that are reported are not state-directed custody changes, but family-directed custody changes. So we are not talking about someone having to go to the state to get a court ruling; we're talking about whether the mother passed the child on to another family member.

IRA CHASNOFF: Yes, this reflects on our population more or less the same. Because of the numbers we are talking about, most jurisdictions will take the approach of maintaining the wholeness of the family. Of course, the question of cost is much more complex, and how do you measure cost? It may ultimately be more costly for the system to have the child maintained in the home; if there are synergistic effects of intrauterine drug exposure and environmental risks, the cost of not "rescuing" a child may be in the millions.

VIRGINIA DELANEY-BLACK: I don't think there are any data to really look at child outcome or cost outcome. Very few of our children were actually in out-of-home placements. In both the exposed and the non-exposed groups, most children were with some family member whether it was a cousin or an aunt or, in the cocaine-exposed group, grandparents primarily.

GIDEON KOREN: Margaret Johnson, a social worker with the Children's Aid Society in Toronto, published a prospective study of 25 children given back to high cocaine-using mothers. In terms of optimal conditions for the child, 24 of the 25 were judged by a prospective, objective analysis not to be appropriately placed. I'll talk about our adoption study in the next session which will be the mirror image in a way for this question.

PENNY MAZA: I'm with the U.S. Children's Bureau which is the Federal agency that runs the Federal foster care program. I'm particularly interested in the custody question and whether or not you included in your data collection just formal custody arrangements or whether you looked at informal, relative care, for example, which is used very extensively in Michigan.

VIRGINIA DELANEY-BLACK: Yes, we looked at informal custody, any change in the custody, because the child really doesn't care whether it's the court or the family that required it. From our perspective we thought that it was the number of homes that the child was in rather than who requested it.

CHANDICE COVINGTON: I just wanted to clarify why so many of our children who may be born to substance-abusing women go home with their mothers. We have a rich history and tradition in Detroit and in Michigan in family reunification as well as family preservation. But I agree with a previous comment that what might initially be cheaper for the state may not be cheaper later on. One of the issues that came up about 8 years ago was the need for unification for substance-abuse models with child-abuse models. There was a statewide effort, especially centered in Detroit, to train caseworkers with Federal money, to combine those two models aimed at keeping families together. That was well tolerated because the majority of our caseworkers in the Detroit area are from Detroit, they are African-American, and they believe strongly in their African-American heritage and in keeping families together. So we have a rich tradition that may not always be seen in other places of the country; it may seem a little different at first, but you can see from our numbers that families then make decisions within themselves about who should take care of the child. In the long run it may be an excellent model.

Also in our state, the past director of our DSS program, which is now called the Family Independence Agency, is in Texas setting up an independent, private management company for DSS sort of functions. The popularity and success of his program, I think, herald for all the states the issue that this is very popular with voters; by empowering extended families you cut down costs and you may improve outcomes. That's what is happening in Michigan.

SPEAKER: I wanted to comment that the Maternal Lifestyles Study to be discussed in the next session will be looking at the impact of different policies in the different sites in terms of what the placement and movement situation is for each of the children and will eventually relate those factors to outcomes, so that some of the questions that have been raised here are being studied.

SPEAKER: As a clinician the most fascinating part of this conference for me is to learn something about the underlying basic science mechanisms. I am really interested in how much compensation and recovery can occur given the plasticity of the young brain. That brings me to consider the postnatal environment, which relates to custody issues. We have to look at the care-giving environment. Rather than hearing about the effect of multiple changes in care-giving environments, I'm interested in knowing what qualities in the care-giving environment are important and how they can help a baby develop in an optimal way, despite a biologic insult. I am worried that when we start to talk about custody issues, and what is better for the child, there is no acknowledgment of the very inadequate maternal substance abuse treatment programs that address the barriers for women. Currently in Connecticut many of the babies that test positive for drugs, though not most, are removed from the nursery. I direct a well-newborn nursery in a hospital that has 5–10 deliveries a day, and I also run an intervention program for substance-exposed children. I am concerned that Medicaid/Managed Care Plans now make a woman eligible for 20 visits, which if she is in an ambulatory day treatment program covers her for 4 weeks. However, some long-term treatment programs are showing some benefits if women stay in those programs for several months. That is an important thing whenever we talk about custody issues.

TREVOR ROBBINS: When we talk about brain plasticity issues, we have to consider both the extent to which the damaged system is able to recover under perhaps optimal postnatal conditions, but also the extent to which other systems can take over the function of a permanently damaged system. Those are two separate issues that really need to be investigated.

BARRY KOSOFSKY: Trevor, have you ever looked at developmental insults in your experiments?

TREVOR ROBBINS: Yes, we've looked at effects of early maternal separation in the rat and that may be another variable that experimentally needs to be considered, because it does produce profound changes in behavior when the animals have grown up. This is correlated with changes in some of the monoamine systems.

If I could address the general point about compensation. You need a conceptual classification of the types of compensative mechanisms involved. For example, one kind of compensation occurs when a completely different system takes over the function. You can see this in maybe the lateral hypothalamic lesioned rats where the cortex takes over the functions of feeding, which it doesn't normally have much to do with. Another type of compensation is when another related system that is changed, maybe the serotonergic system, compensates for the dopaminergic system, and is changed in opposition to the perturbation; you can manipulate that. The third type of compensation is when there is recovery intrinsic in the system. This is like the supersensitivity phenomenon with receptor proliferation. You can also sometimes capitalize on that. So, you need to consider these three somewhat separate mechanisms.

BERNARD KARMEL: Dr. Robbins, most of the tests that we currently use to evaluate outcome in humans are based on lesion studies and evolved mainly for the study of hypoxic injuries or things of this nature. They certainly weren't written or developed at the time when we had drug effects that were very specific to CNS mechanisms, as you described. How would you propose to modify our current methods to evaluate such things as competence, performance, cognitive organization, and perhaps intelligence quotients?

TREVOR ROBBINS: That's quite a big agenda. Unfortunately, because I didn't have enough time I wasn't able to describe how we're trying to tackle that problem in Cambridge. One approach is to try to take existing tests that are sensitive clinically. For example, take frontal lobe dysfunction, which is a major problem and is not assayed properly by intelligence tests, and break these tests down into their constituents in a way that can be given to experimental animals, but also to children, for example. We first got into this problem because of the need to assess demented patients, where you've got the opposite end of the developmental spectrum. When you've worked with animals, you know how they can fail cognitive tests. It can be so simple, you just can't believe that they could fail. With demented patients, you can readily understand that. Our philosophy has been to design tests that are so easy you can actually define what people can do as well as what they can't do. Because defining what they are capable of helps to define the specificity of the deficit. So, our basic approach has been neuropsychological; we have actually modified human tests for animals and then fed them back to humans. It's actually just as easy, I think, to study these in a pharmacologic sense. For example, in the case of Parkinson's disease, there are a number of tests that are very sensitive to cognitive deficits in Parkinson's disease, which by the way correlate to some degree with clinical motor disability. And there are tests that are sensitive to frontal lobe lesions such as planning, working memory, and attentional set shifting like the Wisconsin Card Sorting Test. We found that L-dopa seems to remediate functions that are produced by frontal lobe lesions, but not other deficits in Parkinson's disease which are associated with other neural changes, such as deficits in recognition memory. It's interesting to think of how the (brainstem) neurochemical systems do interface quite nicely with their neural targets in the forebrain. There are many other examples of this such as 5-HT which interfaces very nicely with tests of orbitofrontal dysfunction and affects decision making and reversal learning. I think the neurotransmitters will fit nicely into the way the forebrain as a whole organizes behavioral functions.

MODERATOR: I'd like to thank all of the speakers for a wonderful session.

The Maternal Lifestyles Study[a]

BARRY M. LESTER[b]

Infant Development Center, Women & Infants' Hospital, 101 Dudley Street, Providence, Rhode Island 02905–2499, USA

INTRODUCTION

Despite early reports suggesting that prenatal cocaine exposure had devastating effects on the developing child, findings from the literature continue to show an inconsistent pattern of results. Concerns about this literature led us to develop a computerized database for the Robert Wood Johnson Foundation of the published literature of studies of prenatal cocaine exposure and child development outcome to provide a systematic analysis and description of the characteristics and findings from these studies. The database can be used to summarize and compare the literature, resulting in a more objective understanding of the findings, as well as to identify methodologic problems in order to shape the direction of future studies. In this article, we summarize findings from the database and then describe the ongoing National Institutes of Health Maternal Lifestyles Study that addresses many of the shortcomings in the literature.

DATABASE OF PUBLISHED STUDIES

The first report from this database was published in 1996 as part of a National Institute on Drug Abuse monograph[1] and was based on 50 studies that met the inclusion

[a] Conducted under the auspices of the NICHD Neonatal Research Network. Supported by NIH National Institute of Child Health and Human Development through cooperative agreements: U10HD2704,[1] U10HD21397,[2] U10HD21385,[3] U10HD27856,[4] and U01HD19897,[5] interagency agreement with the National Institute on Drug Abuse (NIDA), Administration on Children, Youth and Families (ACYF), Center for Substance Abuse Treatment (CSAT), NICHD contract #N01-HD-2-3159,[1] and a grant from the Robert Wood Johnson Foundation.[1] The Maternal Lifestyles Study Investigators include Principal Investigators at the study sites; Charles R. Bauer, MD,[2] Seetha Shankaran, MD,[3] and Henrietta S. Bada, MD,[4] a biostatistics coordinating center, Joel Verter, PhD,[5] NICHD project officer Linda L. Wright, MD,[6] and the following collaborators: Loretta P. Finnegan, MD,[7] Linda LaGasse, PhD,[1] Penelope L. Maza, PhD,[8] Ronald Seifer, PhD,[1] Vincent L. Smeriglio, PhD,[9] and Edward Z. Tronick, PhD[10]

[1] *Brown University School of Medicine, Providence, Rhode Island*
[2] *University of Miami, Miami, Florida*
[3] *Wayne State University, Detroit, Michigan*
[4] *The University of Tennessee, Memphis, Memphis, Tennessee*
[5] *George Washington University, Washington, DC*
[6] *National Institute of Child Health and Human Development*
[7] *Center for Substance Abuse Treatment*
[8] *Administration of Children, Youth and Families*
[9] *National Institute on Drug Abuse*
[10] *Harvard University, Cambridge, Massachusetts*

[b] Phone, 401/453–7640; fax, 401/453–7646; e-mail, Barry_Lester@Brown.edu

criteria. In our second report[2] the database was expanded to 76 studies that met the inclusion criteria. Our most recent review includes 118 studies in the database published from 1985 through August 1997. An additional 52 studies were excluded for methodologic reasons.

The method includes a literature search from Medline and Psyclit. Each article is reviewed to determine eligibility for inclusion in the final database contingent on the inclusion criteria to be described. Information from the articles is then abstracted, coded, and entered into the database. Variables are defined that represent any characteristics of the study such as sample size, method of drug detection, or behavioral outcomes such as an IQ score. Summary statistics are then generated across studies.

Criteria for Inclusion

Seven criteria are used to identify studies to be included in the final database: (1) cocaine use during pregnancy, (2) human subjects, (3) neurobehavioral measures, (4) original research, (5) inclusion of control or comparison group, (6) statistical analysis of data, and (7) publication in a peer-reviewed or refereed journal.

Arguably, the most important question about prenatal drug-exposed infants is their long-term developmental outcome. Yet most of the published literature has not followed children beyond infancy. Of the 118 studies in the database only 8 (7%) followed the children beyond 4 years of age.

Confounding Factors

Cocaine use is often associated with three classes of potential confounding variables: other drugs, medical factors, and sociodemographic factors. These factors could provide alternative explanations for effects attributed to cocaine and therefore need to be controlled if cocaine effects are to be isolated. The initial problem of prenatal cocaine exposure has been redefined as a problem of polydrug exposure. Of the 118 studies, cocaine was reported as the only drug used in only 10 studies (8%). Alcohol (61%), marijuana (55%), and tobacco (58%) are the drugs most commonly used along with cocaine. Opiate use was reported in 19% of the studies.

History (including self-report) and/or toxicology analysis of urine, meconium, or hair are the methods used to detect maternal use of cocaine during pregnancy. Most studies do not rely on a single index; 90 (76%) used some combination of these methods. The most common was urine and self-report which was used in 77 studies (65% of the studies using multiple indices). The meconium assay provides a record of drug use from approximately 20 weeks' gestational age in contrast to the urine assay which only provides a 72-hour record of drug use. However, most of these studies were conducted before the meconium assay was in widespread use. Meconium was used in eight studies, seven of which also used self-report. Similarly, most studies have not controlled for obstetrical and perinatal factors including prenatal care, parity, and gravida. Factors such as birth weight, gestational age, and medical complications are mediator variables because they can be a consequence of prenatal drug exposure. Sociodemographic factors have not been well controlled and may provide yet another set of explanations for effects attributed to cocaine. Finally, given the high risk nature of this population it would be reasonable to expect that many of the infants and mothers in these studies are receiving intervention services. Although intervention may affect the outcome of the child, information about intervention provided to the child or the mother was only mentioned in 28 (37%) of the studies.

Neurobehavioral Outcome

TABLE 1 shows the neurobehavioral measures used in the studies including the number of times each measure was used and if statistically significant cocaine effects were found. It is apparent from this table that a wide range of measures has been used with few measures used across studies. The most frequently used measures, Neonatal Behavioral Assessment Scale (NBAS) and Neonatal Intensive Care Unit Network Neurobehavioral Scale (NNNS) and stress abstinence measures, as expected pertain to early infancy. The NBAS/NNNS does show cocaine effects in 17 of 19 studies. Abstinence or withdrawal effects were reported in 12 of 21 studies and may be related to the additional effects of opiates as a confounding variable. It is also interesting that 6 of 12 studies using measures of developmental level such as the Bayley Scales did not find cocaine effects. By contrast, measures of more subtle function such as temperament showed cocaine effects in 8 of 13 studies and attention in 7 of 8 studies. With older children, 4 of 9 language studies and 3 of 7 IQ studies showed cocaine effects.

Database Summary

To summarize, the initial outcry about the devastating effects of prenatal cocaine exposure on child development have now started to shift to proclamations about the benign effects of cocaine. However, we have seen from this review that our knowledge base is virtually confined to early infancy with a striking absence of long-term follow-up studies. Findings are limited and compromised by methodologic problems that mitigate any conclusions about whether or not or how prenatal cocaine exposure affects child outcome.

The neurobehavioral findings are scattered across a wide array of measures, most of which have been used in only a few studies. There is a clear need for measures to be used across studies to determine if there is a consistent pattern of findings. There is also a question as to how measures are selected; few appear to have been theoretically or hypothetically driven, and some measures may be too gross to detect the more subtle effects that have been attributed to cocaine. Factors such as high attrition rates in longi-

TABLE 1. Neurobehavioral Measures ($n = 118$)

	Significant (*n*)	Not Significant (*n*)	Total (*n*) (%)
• Stress/Abstinence/ Withdrawal	12	9	21 (18)
• NBAS/NNNS	17	2	19 (16)
• Cry	2	2	4 (3)
• Feeding/Sucking	2	2	4 (3)
• Sleep	4	1	5 (4)
• Temperament	8	5	13 (11)
• Attention/Info Processing	7	1	8 (7)
• Mother/Child Interaction	1	1	2 (2)
• Developmental Level	6	6	12 (10)
• Motor Assessment	1	2	3 (3)
• Attachment	3	0	3 (3)
• Play	3	1	4 (3)
• Language	4	5	9 (8)
• IQ	3	4	7 (6)
• Caregiving Environment	3	2	5 (4)

tudinal studies, failure to control for examiner blindness, and intervention effects further cloud interpretation of the findings.

THE MATERNAL LIFESTYLES STUDY

The Maternal Lifestyles Study (MLS) was designed to address many of these methodologic issues. MLS is a prospective, multisite, longitudinal study of the effects of drug use during pregnancy on acute neonatal events and long-term neurodevelopmental outcome. The MLS is being conducted under the auspices of the Neonatal Research Network involving a scientific and fiscal collaboration among four Federal agencies (National Institute of Child Health and Human Development, National Institute on Drug Abuse, Administration on Children Youth and Families, and Council on Substance Abuse Treatment). The four study sites and their principal investigators include Brown University (Barry Lester), University of Miami (Charles Bauer), University of Tennessee, Memphis (Henrietta Bada), and Wayne State University (Seetha Shankaran). George Washington University (Joel Verter) provides biostatistical support, and the National Institute of Child Health and Human Development project officer is Linda Wright. MLS co-investigators include Loretta Finnegan, Linda LaGasse, Penelope Maza, Ronald Seifer, Vincent Smeriglio, and Edward Tronick. Special features of the MLS include drug use based on self-report and meconium with gas chromatography/mass spectroscopy (GC/MS); the inclusion of preterm as well as term infants; and the measurement of potentially confounding variables including drugs other than cocaine (opiates, marijuana, alcohol, and tobacco), sociodemographic factors (such as social class, race, and ethnicity), and the effects of interventions provided for the mother and the child.

Another strength of the MLS is the development of a neurodevelopmental battery specifically designed for drug-exposed and high risk infants. The neurodevelopmental battery is based on the model[3] shown in FIGURE 1 and views cocaine as a marker variable for a lifestyle that includes polydrug use and as a marker variable for a lifestyle that includes environmental factors that have been shown to affect child development without drug exposure. In this model, the hypothesis is that cocaine affects neuroregulatory

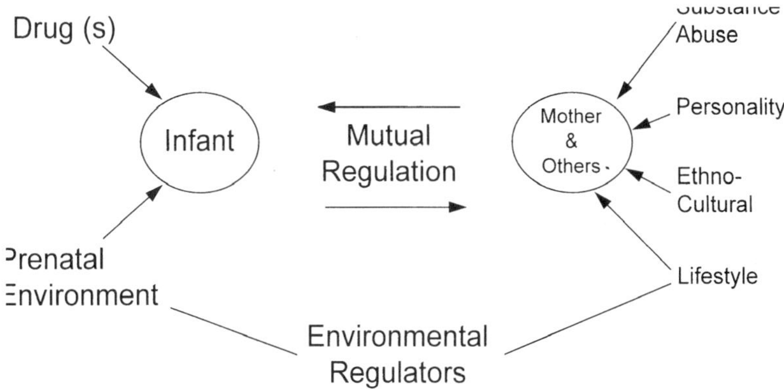

FIGURE 1. Systems approach to the effects of prenatal cocaine exposure.

mechanisms which in turn result in disorders of behavioral regulation. These disorders of behavioral regulation are manifest as the "Four A's of Infancy": Attention, Arousal, Affect, and Action. These four areas seem to be most affected by prenatal drug exposure. As explained later in this chapter, the ability of the drug-exposed infant to recover from disorders in behavioral regulation will require regulatory input from the caregiving environment.

Attention refers to visual and auditory abilities that relate to the intake and processing of information from the environment.

Arousal includes control and modulation of behavioral states from sleep to waking to crying and the ability to display the entire range of states from excitation to inhibition to incoming stimuli.

Affect relates to the development of sociability and emotion, the mutual regulatory processes of social interaction and social relationships.

Action indicates perceptual-motor function, the development of fine and gross motor skills, and the acquisition of knowledge and social exchange through motor patterns.

The MLS study design includes an acute outcome phase in which 11,811 subjects consented to participate and, initially, a 36-month follow-up phase involving 1,400 of these subjects. The follow-up has now been extended to age 7. Exclusion criteria for the acute outcome phase were teenage mothers (<18 years old) and mothers who were institutionalized for retardation or emotional disturbance or who showed evidence of psychosis. Infants were excluded if they were unlikely to survive, multiple gestation, or born at an outlying hospital. For the follow-up phase, subjects were excluded if there were plans to move out of the catchment area or if the infant was born at greater than 43 weeks' gestational age, had a major life-threatening congenital anomaly, a chromosomal abnormality associated with mental, neurologic, clinical deficiency, or overt TORCH infection. For the acute outcome phase, the mother was approached in the hospital after delivery and consent was obtained. A hospital interview was conducted by trained examiners to collect demographic information and maternal history of drug use during this pregnancy. Meconium was collected from the infant's diaper and sent to a central laboratory for toxicology analysis. Meconium was collected from 8,803 of the 11,811 subjects. Maternal and infant medical charts were reviewed and approximately 400 items (60% infant, 40% maternal) were abstracted. Drug exposure for this study was defined as cocaine and/or opiate use in the current pregnancy based on self-report during the maternal hospital interview or the presence of cocaine or opiate metabolites in the infant's meconium based on a positive toxicology screen confirmed by GC/MS. Alcohol, nicotine, and marijuana exposure occurred as background exposure in both the exposed and the comparison groups because these drugs are known to covary with cocaine/opiate exposure and we wanted to determine the effects of cocaine/opiate exposure given the presence of these background drugs.

For the long-term follow-up phase, exposed subjects were matched to comparison subjects for gestational age, race, and sex. Comparison subjects had to have denied cocaine and opiate use during the current pregnancy and their infant had to have had a negative meconium. Enrollment in this phase was defined by virtue of participation in the 1-month clinic visit. At the 1-month visit, the infant was examined with the NNNS, acoustical cry analysis, and the auditory brain response (ABR). The infant's medical history was taken and a physical examination was conducted. The mother was interviewed for demographic information, history of drug use, and involvement with social services. Additional follow-up visits were conducted at 4, 8, 10, 12, 18, 24, 30, and 36 months. Three domains of function were measured at the follow-up visits. These include measures of the child, mother (or caregiver), and context shown in TABLE 2.

TABLE 2. Domains of the MLS Study

Child	Maternal	Context
Physiology	Psychological Distress	Social Class
Attention	Depression	Neighborhood
Temperament	Self-Esteem	Social Support
Social Interaction	Interaction with Child	Household
Attachment	Attachment	Home
Motivation	Parenting Stress	Social Services
Cognition	Parenting Values	Acculturation
Language	IQ	Violence
Motor Development	Drug History/Use	
Neurologic Status	Treatment	
Medical Status		

SUMMARY OF RESULTS

Acute Outcome Phase

Demographics. The mothers were 50% Black, 37% White, and 13% Hispanic, 48% were 18–25 years of age, 62% were single, 63% were on Medicaid, and 33% had less than 12 years' education. The infants included term and preterm infants with 7% born at less than 33 weeks' gestational age.

Drug Exposure. Of the infants for whom sufficient quantity meconium was available for toxicologic analysis, 1,185 (7.4%) were in the exposed group. There were 642 mothers who reported that they used cocaine. However, only 16 mothers (2%) reported that cocaine was the only drug that they used. One hundred twenty mothers (19%) reported the use of cocaine and one other drug; 272 mothers (42%) used cocaine and two other drugs, 72% of which were alcohol and tobacco; 221 mothers (35%) used cocaine and three other drugs, 86% of which were marijuana, alcohol, and tobacco.

Maternal and Infant Findings. Bauer *et al.*[4] found that the exposed group had more medical conditions such as gonorrhea, chronic psychotic/nervous disorders, and abruptio placenta; however, the overall prevalence of complications was low. Bauer *et al.*[5] reported similar findings for acute infant outcome. The prevalence of adverse medical outcomes, such as gastrointestinal, genitourinary, and cardiac, that have been associated with prenatal cocaine exposure previously reported were low. Prevalence rates were low for newborn physical abnormalities and were not elevated in the exposed infants. However, there was an increase in subtle physical findings such as hypertonicity and tremors in the exposed group. Exposed infants were also born, on the average, 1 week earlier than the comparison infants, birth weight was 449 gm less, length 2.3 cm less, and head circumference 1.3 cm less. The prevalence of CNS/ANS signs, such as hypertonia and jitteriness, in these infants was studied by Bada *et al.*[6] Although the prevalence of these signs was increased in the exposed group, the rates were less than 5% for most of the signs.

One-Month Follow-Up

The sample at 1 month included 636 in the exposed group and 721 in the comparison group. Frequency of cocaine use by trimester was reported by 394 mothers. One hundred thirty-four mothers (34%) reported that they used cocaine 3 or more days per week during the first trimester, 94 mothers (24%) reported this heavy usage pattern during the second trimester, and 62 mothers (16%) reported this pattern during the third trimester.

Environmental risk factors, including less education and public assistance, were higher in the exposed than in the comparison group. There were slight differences in global ratings of health status and motor development. However, neither these nor the environmental risk factors were related to physical growth at 1 month as shown by Wright *et al.*,[7] and Maza *et al.*[8] found that the living arrangements of the exposed infants were more unstable at 1 month, that they were more often in foster care or in other alternative living arrangements.

Neurobehavioral outcome was analyzed by comparing scores of infants in the exposed group versus the comparison group with the following factors covaried: site, birth weight, alcohol, tobacco, and marijuana. On the NNNS there were subtle (less than 1 point) but statistically significant differences between exposed and comparison infants on summary scores of handling, state regulation, and self-regulation controlling for the effects of the covariates. Similarly, small magnitude but statistically significant differences were found between infants in the exposed and comparison groups on the acoustical cry analysis. Exposed infants required fewer cry stimuli (more reactive) and had fewer short utterances, longer period of breath holding following the cry stimulus, less vocal control, and higher frequencies in the cry sound controlling for the effects of the covariates. On the auditory brainstem response, there were no statistically significant effects between exposed and comparison groups. However, there were statistically significant effects for two of the drug covariates. At both 70 and 50 dB, interpeak latencies (I–III and I–V) were longer related to alcohol exposure. Tobacco exposure had the opposite effect, resulting in a shorter I–III interpeak latency at 70 and 50 dB.

To summarize, preliminary results of the MLS study suggest that cocaine/opiate use during pregnancy is associated with other maternal high risk conditions, behaviors, and diagnoses; however, the prevalence rates of these conditions are low. Prevalence rates are also low for newborn physical abnormalities; however, subtle physical findings such as hypertonia may be increased. Cocaine/opiate-exposed infants are more likely to live in nontraditional households. Neurobehavioral effects are statistically significant, but the effect size is small. It is possible that environmental conditions in cocaine/opiate-exposed infants may exacerbate these subtle physical and neurobehavioral effects. The MLS provides the opportunity to study this problem in a way not previously possible.

THE MEANING OF SUBTLE EFFECTS

The results of the MLS are beginning to suggest that the effects of cocaine/opiate exposure may be subtle. We can estimate how these subtle effects impact on society by using meta-analysis techniques on studies of cocaine-exposed school age children. To date, there are eight studies with school age children; IQ was measured in five studies, receptive language in four studies, and expressive language in five studies. As shown in TABLE 3, the difference in IQ between cocaine-exposed and control groups across available studies is 3.26 IQ points. This difference, although small, is statistically significant and can have a substantial impact on society.

Early intervention and special education services are typically provided for children who score less than 2 standard deviations (SD) (or in some cases less than 1.5 SD) on standardized tests. This would correspond to IQ scores of <70 or <78, respectively. In a normal distribution (a good model for IQ scores), 2.28% of children will score <70

TABLE 3. Increase in Number of Children Affected by Prenatal Cocaine Exposure

		Percent <2 SD		Number	Percent <1.5 SD		Number
	Effect	(Normal 2.28%)	Increase	of Children	(Normal 6.68%)	Increase	of Children
Measure							
IQ Difference ($n = 5$)	3.26	3.75	1.6×	3,750–14,062	10.03	1.5×	10,030–37,612
Effect Size							
IQ	.33	4.75	2.0×	4,750–17,812	12.10	1.8×	12,100–45,375
Receptive Language ($n = 4$)	.71	9.85	4.3×	9,850–36,938	21.48	3.2×	21,480–80,550
Expressive Language ($n = 5$)	.60	8.08	3.5×	8,080–30,300	18.14	2.7×	18,140–68,025

(2 SD) and 6.68% of children will score <78 (1.5 SD). When the IQ distribution is shifted downward by 3.26 IQ points, the number of children at the low end of the distribution will increase (TABLE 3) to 3.75%. This results in a 1.6-fold increase in the number of children with IQs <70 and to 10.03% or a 1.5-fold increase in the number of children with IQs <78. Using the U.S. Government Accounting Office[9] estimate that between 100,000 and 375,000 cocaine-exposed children are born each year, the number of children affected by this 3.26 IQ point difference is estimated to be 3,750–14,062 at <2 SD and 10,030–37,612 for children <1.5 SD.

Another way to think about these IQ differences is as an effect size. An effect size may be expressed in terms of standard deviation units.[10] For example, the standardized IQ score has a mean of 100 and an SD of 15. A difference of 7.5 IQ points would represent an effect size of .50. Effect size is a useful construct because all measures are expressed in the same units (SD units); therefore, effects across different measures can be compared even if they use different scales of measurement. Effect sizes are divided into small (<.5 SD), medium (.5–.75 SD), and large (>.75 SD). TABLE 3 also shows the mean effect sizes weighted for the number of children in the exposed groups, for the IQ studies as well as the studies of receptive and expressive language. The table also shows the follow-up calculations for the percentage of children affected at <2 SD and <1.5 SD and the number of children affected.

The language studies showed a medium effect size compared with the small effect size for the IQ studies, with the effect size for receptive language more than twice that of the effect size for IQ; expressive language showed a 1.8 times greater effect size than did IQ. These moderate effect sizes in language result in a 2.7–4.3-fold increase in children who will be affected at clinically significant levels. Between 8,080 and 68,025 will need special education services.

In summary, the published follow-up studies of cocaine-exposed children show reliable differences that are subtle in two ways. First, subtlety can mean "small magnitude" as shown by the IQ findings. This small magnitude variant of subtlety is in sharp contrast to the more sensationalistic reports in popular media on the effects of prenatal cocaine exposure.[11] Second, subtlety can mean "more subtle function" suggested by the larger effect sizes for specific language domains relative to global IQ. The public health consequences of both of these kinds of subtle effects are substantial, indicating that we should not equate small magnitude with unimportant. Prenatal cocaine exposure may not cause irreversible brain damage, but it will significantly increase the number of children who will fail in school and need special education services.

Although it seems as if the cocaine problem has been with us for a long time, it has been less than 10 years since most of the literature was published. In that time we have become acutely aware of the magnitude of this problem that affects a substantial number of children in our society, mostly children in poverty, and concern for the welfare of these children has led to increased research. We may not have definitive findings about the effects of cocaine exposure on child development, but our knowledge has advanced considerably. We have learned that the cocaine problem is more complicated than first envisioned. It is a multifactorial problem including the use of other drugs and parenting and environmental lifestyle issues. The long-term developmental outcome of these children is likely to be a function of how the caregiving environment responds to the behavioral constellation of the infant with the understanding that both the behavior of the infant and the caregiving environment are making dynamic adjustments to each other as well as being influenced by other forces. We have also learned that the effects of prenatal cocaine exposure are probably more subtle than first anticipated. Understanding these issues will enable us to design better, more theoretically driven studies and gain a clear understanding of the processes by which prenatal cocaine exposure affects child outcome.

REFERENCES

1. LESTER, B.M., L. LAGASSE, C. FREIER & S. BRUNNER. 1996. Studies of cocaine- exposed human infants. *In* Behavioral Studies of Drug Exposed Offspring: Methodological Issues in Human and Animal Research: 175–210. NIDA Research Monograph 164. Washington, DC.
2. LESTER, B.M., L. LAGASSE & S. BRUNNER. 1997. Data base of studies on prenatal cocaine exposure and child outcome. J. Drug Issues **27:** 487–499.
3. LESTER, B.M. & E.Z. TRONICK. 1994. The Effects of Prenatal Cocaine Exposure and Child Outcome: Lessons from the Past. Infant Mental Health J., **15:** 107–120.
4. BAUER, C. *et al.* 1997. Maternal Lifestyles Study (MLS): The Effects of Substance Exposure during Pregnancy on Acute Infant Outcomes. Collected Abstract of the New York Academy of Sciences Conference, Washington, DC: no. P2. Allegheny University of the Health Sciences.
5. BAUER, C. *et al.* 1997. Maternal Lifestyles Study (MLS): Effects of Substance Exposure during Pregnancy on Acute Maternal Outcomes. Collected abstract of the New York Academy of Sciences Conference, Washington, DC: no. P3. Allegheny University of the Health Sciences.
6. BADA, H. *et al.* 1997. Maternal Lifestyles Study: Central/Autonomic Nervous Systems (CNS/ANS) Signs Associated with Antenatal Cocaine/Opiates (C/O) Exposure. Collected abstract of the New York Academy of Sciences Conference, Washington, DC: no. P34. Allegheny University of the Health Sciences.
7. WRIGHT, L. *et al.* 1997. Maternal Lifestyles Study (MLS): Health status of substance exposed infants at one-month corrected age. Collected abstract of the New York Academy of Sciences Conference, Washington, DC: no. P5. Allegheny University of the Health Sciences.
8. MAZA, P. *et al.* 1997. Maternal Lifestyles Study (MLS): Caretaking environment and stability of substance-exposed infants at one-month corrected age. Collected abstract of the New York Academy of Sciences Conference, Washington, DC: no. P4. Allegheny University of the Health Sciences.
9. U. S. GENERAL ACCOUNTING OFFICE. 1990.
10. COHEN, J. 1988. Statistical Power Analysis for the Social Sciences, 2nd Ed. Lawrence Erlbaum. Hillsdale, NJ.
11. New York Times, May 19, 1990: **1**; May 25, 1990: **1**; August 19, 1990.

Long-Term Neurodevelopmental Risks in Children Exposed *in Utero* to Cocaine

The Toronto Adoption Study[a]

GIDEON KOREN,[b] IRENA NULMAN,[b] JOANNE ROVET,[c] RACHEL GREENBAUM, MICHAL LOEBSTEIN, AND TOM EINARSON[d]

[b]Motherisk Program, [b]Divisions of Clinical Pharmacology, and [d]Psychology Research, [b,d]The Research Institute; The Hospital for Sick Children, and [b,c,d]Department of Pediatrics, [b]Pharmacology and [c]Psychology, University of Toronto; and [d]Faculty of Pharmacy, University of Toronto, Toronto, Ontario, Canada

ABSTRACT: Children exposed *in utero* to cocaine are at risk for long-term neurobehavioral damage not just because of the drug itself, but also because of clustering of other health determinants, including low socioeconomic status, low maternal education, and maternal addiction, to mention a few. One methodologic approach to separate the direct neurotoxic effects of cocaine from these synergistic insults is to follow up a cohort of children exposed *in utero* to cocaine and given up for adoption to middle-upper class families.

The Toronto Adoption Study, supported by Health Canada, has proven the direct neurotoxic effects of cocaine on IQ and language. These effects are mild to moderate as compared to those measured in children exposed *in utero* to cocaine and reared by their natural mothers.

THE COCAINE EPIDEMIC

Cocaine is an alkaloid prepared from the leaves of the *Erythroxylon coca* plant. The most common modes of administration are the intranasal and inhalation routes; peak concentrations are achieved almost immediately with a mean elimination half-life of 1 hour. Cocaine is a powerful central nervous system stimulant and has the ability to increase heart rate, blood pressure, and body temperature. Subjects using cocaine experience euphoria, reduced fatigue, sexual stimulation, increased mental ability, and increased sociability. These characteristics account for the very wide recreational use of the drug and its addictive potential.[3]

The last two decades have seen a dramatic increase in the recreational use of cocaine. It is estimated that more than 10 million Americans currently use cocaine. As a rapid increase in use has occurred in women of child-bearing age, much concern has been expressed about the potential effects of the drug in pregnancy.[4-8] Addiction Research Foundation reports revealed that during the last decade cocaine use in women of Ontario increased significantly[9]; in young females aged 18–29, 11.5% reported use in 1987 compared to 3.5% in 1984 ($p < 0.05$). Among all adults in Ontario, highest use is reported in Metropolitan Toronto (11%), whereas outside Toronto it is 5% or less.[9]

[a] This work was supported by a grant from Health Canada.

[b] Address for correspondence: Gideon Koren, MD, ABMT, FRCPC, Division of Clinical Pharmacology/Toxicology, The Hospital for Sick Children, 555 University Avenue, Toronto, Ontario, M5G 1X8. Phone, 416/813–5781; fax, 416/813-7562.

EFFECTS OF COCAINE IN PREGNANCY

Animal studies show that cocaine affects fetal growth and brain development. A study in pregnant mice showed increased eye and skeletal defects, whereas a study by Fantal and Marphail[10] using both rats and mice showed no increase in congenital abnormalities but only a reduction in fetal weight and increased resorption frequencies. Cocaine injections to the pregnant ewe,[11] which decreased uterine blood flow and increased uterine vascular resistance, resulted in marked fetal hypoxemia, hypertension, and tachycardia. Because these effects on fetal heart rate and blood pressure were greater than those from direct cocaine administration to the fetus, it appears that adverse outcome is associated to a greater degree with changes in maternal uterine blood flow than with direct pharmacologic effects on the fetus. Behavioral studies of animals exposed to cocaine *in utero* indicate increased motor activity and impaired learning.[12]

In most human reports published to date, subjects were typically poor, black, inner-city addicted women. The first study linking maternal cocaine use with adverse neonatal outcome was reported from Chicago.[8] These researchers found that cocaine exposure *in utero* was associated with significant depression of interactive behavior and a less effective organizational response to environmental stimuli, suggestive of effects on neurologic integrity. In a more recent study on a different population by the same authors, growth parameters at birth were significantly altered by cocaine exposure, but catch-up occurs by 1 year of age.[13]

In a recent study conducted by us in Toronto, comparing 37 infants exposed to cocaine *in utero* to 563 unexposed infants, we found that the cocaine-exposed group had significantly lower birth weights. However, this difference was nullified after correction for maternal smoking, with babies exposed to cocaine, but not cigarette smoke, being similar to the unexposed controls. Of clinical importance, we also found that mothers using cocaine were significantly more likely to test positive for hepatitis B and the cocaine-exposed infants needed resuscitative measures significantly more often.[14]

An early study of infants of mothers with a history and positive screen for cocaine showed no signs of teratogenicity.[15] In a recent prospective study,[16] the incidence of stillbirth was significantly higher in the group abusing cocaine near term, and all stillbirths were related to abruptio placentae. Birth weight, length, and head circumference were also significantly decreased in infants exposed to cocaine or cocaine plus other drugs, whereas the rate of congenital malformations was significantly higher in users of cocaine only than in the drug-free group. Several groups describe increased lethargy, irritability, tremulousness, hypertonicity, poorer social responsivity, and disorganized patterns of feeding and sleeping among cocaine-exposed infants.[17,18] A recent study observed long-term neurologic sequelae including rigidity and visual dysfunction.[19] Respiratory pattern abnormalities have also been described,[20] potentially explaining cocaine association with sudden infant death syndrome.[21]

Eisen *et al.*[22] showed that habituation was impaired in cocaine-exposed infants during the first week of life. However, a study of infants at 1 day and 1 month of age[23] failed to differentiate between cocaine-exposed and unexposed infants. Deficits in motor function and abnormal reflexes[24] have also been observed during the first month. Although studies of older children show that intrauterine cocaine exposure increases the risk of behavioral and social problems as well as intellectual impairment, they have not accounted for differences in parenting and other background variables. For example, a recent study[25] compared the environments of mothers who were drug users with that of mothers who were poor. Children of the former were more likely to be victims of emotional and physical neglect. Drug-abusing mothers were more depressed, had fewer resources, spent less time with their children, and moved more. The home environments were more chaotic; there were fewer toys, less adequate housing, poorer care, and less contact with fathers.

In older children, mother-child interactions are atypical in cocaine-exposed children, reflecting an increased incidence of disorganized and insecure attachments[26,27] and the children show more immature and deviant play,[28] more difficult temperaments,[23] and more behavior problems.[29] Cognitively, poorer outcome has also been described, although the findings are not consistent across studies. Most studies employing the Bayley Scales of Infant Development have failed to detect differences between infants exposed to cocaine versus control groups.[17] Report of a 2-year follow-up[13] concluded that whereas cocaine-exposed infants differed from controls on the Bayley at 6 and 24 months, no differences were observed at 3, 12, or 18 months of age, the reason for which was not clear. Overall however, cocaine exposure was associated with increased risk of subnormal intelligence in about 15% of the children.

The lack of consistent results on cognitive testing with young children does not necessarily signify that cocaine has had no effect on the developing brain. It is possible that deleterious effects on limbic, hypothalamic, and extrapyramidal systems will address themselves in domains other than global cognitive and perceptual-motor functions, as assessed by the Bayley. Although areas such as attention, emotional control, learning, memory, and language may be affected, infant tests may not be sufficiently sensitive to detect these subtle effects. On the other hand, assessment during infancy may precede the emergence of more advanced skills.[25,29,30]

INTERACTION BETWEEN *IN UTERO* COCAINE EXPOSURE AND CRITICAL HEALTH DETERMINANTS

The main problem in identifying the effects of *in utero* cocaine exposure on child neurodevelopment is the clustering of many other unfavorable health determinants in the same population. These include other reproductive risks taking place during pregnancy as well as a variety of determinants affecting the environment of the child postnatally. These health determinants are summarized in TABLE 1.

Any attempt to address the role of cocaine on child neurodevelopment must therefore take into account the relationship and potential interaction among these determinants and cocaine itself.

For example, many cocaine users also smoke cigarettes which increases by themselves the risk of prematurity and intrauterine growth retardation. We recently showed that the birth weight of children of cocaine users who do not smoke in pregnancy is only marginally different from the general population mean of 3,400 g; those who were exposed to cigarettes alone were at a mean birth weight of 3,200 g, yet when the mother consumed both cocaine and cigarettes, the average birth weight was 2800 g, implying a synergistic adverse relationship between cocaine and cigarettes.[14]

In a similar way, Singer and colleagues showed that maternal use of cocaine and alcohol in combination was the best predictor of fetal linear growth after controlling for prematurity.[48]

Numerous studies have shown that postnatally, low socioeconomic status and especially poverty strongly predict children's achievements in standard neurodevelopmental tests. When Hurt and colleagues recently compared early language development at 2 1/2 years of age among a cohort of children of low socioeconomic status exposed or unexposed to cocaine *in utero,* no differences were noted between the subgroups in expressive or receptive language scores,[32] suggesting that the effects of poverty are by far stronger than those of cocaine itself. Similar conclusion were reached by Fetters and Tronick[33] in a longitudinal study.

Poor children have a higher likelihood of prenatal exposure to cocaine as compared to their non-poor peers; however, with or without cocaine exposure, children of poverty

TABLE 1. Health Determinants Clustered in Cocaine-Using Women

Determinant	Recent Reference
Maternal addiction	Hofkosh *et al.*[31]
Socioeconomic status	Fetters *et al.*[32,33]
Poverty	Hurt *et al.*[32]
Maternal education	Richardson *et al.*[34]
Maternal compliance/participation in intervention program	Hofkosh *et al.*[31]
Maternal infection	Bunkhead *et al.*[35]
Maternal STD	Ball *et al.*[36]
Maternal race (minority status)	Hurt *et al.*[37]
Maternal age	Bendersky *et al.*[38]
Prenatal care	Chazotte *et al.*[39]
Cigarette use	Kistin *et al.*[40]
Parity	Bendersky[4]
Psychiatric comorbidity	Killeen *et al.*[41]
Employment	Bendersky *et al.*[38]
Time of exposure during pregnancy	Barton *et al.*[42]
Dose of exposure	Sallee *et al.*[43]
Single motherhood	Ingersoll *et al.*[44]
Disruptive parenting (caretaking)	Ingersoll *et al.*[44]
Home environment	Howard *et al.*[45]
Postnatal maternal bonding	Scafidi *et al.*[46]
Prematurity	Jacobson *et al.*[47]
Alcohol use	Singer *et al.*[48]

are more likely than their more advantaged peers to exhibit low birth weight, prematurity, malnutrition, anemia, and congenital infections.[49]

Maternal addiction leads to increased rates of poverty, disruptive home environment,[45] and reduced parenting or caretaking skills,[44] and is often associated with psychiatric comorbidity.[45]

Another aspect that must be addressed in establishing cocaine effects is the drug's direct (primary) versus indirect (secondary) effects on neurodevelopment.[19] Primary effects are those that are direct on brain development. Examples of secondary effects of cocaine are the strong association between drug exposure and either prematurity or increased risk of abruptio placentae, both of which may impair child development. Therefore, any attempt to address direct cocaine neurotoxicity must control for these adverse effects.[47]

An example of the complex interaction between health determinants in cocaine-exposed children has been documented in a study by Chazotte *et al.*,[39] showing that among cocaine-using pregnant women, those attending prenatal care had a significantly fewer low birth weight infants than did those who failed to attend prenatal care. In a similar manner, in substance-exposed infants whose mothers were receiving support services, developmental skills were not different from those of the general population.

Based on all of the foregoing, it is generally accepted that the effects of cocaine on the fetus will not be related in a simple linear fashion to cocaine exposure per se, but rather will reflect interactions of the drug with a variety of health determinants, both perinatally and postnatally. It is biologically plausible that the primary or secondary effects of cocaine itself on neurodevelopment may be overcome by the fetus/child because of tremendous brain plasticity and by providing that optimal environmental health determinants surround the child.[49] Conversely, suboptimal or poor caretaking, socioeconomic status, etc. may render children susceptible to long-term developmental dysfunction.

THE TORONTO ADOPTION STUDY

Because many of the health determinants placing children exposed *in utero* to cocaine at risk exert their effect postnatally, our ability to follow-up children after adoption into a typically middle-upper class environment should nullify these risks. These include the risks of poverty, broken family, disruptive parenting, low maternal education, addiction, and a variety of other determinants listed in TABLE 1. Similar research approaches are often used to separate genetic from environmental effects in addressing questions such as the etiology of alcoholism or schizophrenia.

In trying to separate intrauterine cocaine insults from suboptimal postnatal home conditions, we carried out a study in children exposed *in utero* to cocaine who were given up for adoption soon after birth and were being raised by middle-to-upper class families.[2] The aim of this approach was to answer directly the question of whether intrauterine exposure to cocaine by itself results in measurable effects on neurodevelopment.

We studied all families referred to the Motherisk Program at The Hospital for Sick Children, Toronto, for counseling and follow-up after adopting children whose biologic mothers had used cocaine during pregnancy. At the initial visit none of the parents reported having perceived any physical or developmental abnormalities in their children, and in no case were such problems the reason prompting the consultation.

Each adoptive mother was paired with the first woman in the Motherisk Program database who matched the index mother on socioeconomic class, IQ, and age of the child, to allow use of the same cognitive tests. Both IQ and socioeconomic class of the mothers strongly predict the home environment of the child. The matched control women attended the Motherisk Clinic during pregnancy for counseling regarding nonteratogenic exposures (e.g., penicillins, acetaminophen), and their children were tested with the same tests as those of the study children.

The control women were identical to the adoptive mothers in IQ and socioeconomic class (as these were the matching variables); however, the former were significantly younger than the latter ($p < 0.0001$). None of the biologic mothers or control women reported heavy alcohol use during the pregnancy; however, three of the biologic mothers reported moderate alcohol use (up to 0.5 g/kg of ethanol per day).

Eighteen of the biologic mothers reported having smoked cigarettes during pregnancy, whereas only one of the control women smoked ($p = 0.0001$). All the biologic mothers were reported to have used cocaine throughout pregnancy. None of the control women reported using alcohol or any recreational drug during pregnancy.

The children exposed to cocaine had a significantly lower mean birth weight ($p = 0.005$) and gestational age ($p = 0.002$) than the control subjects (TABLE 2).

At the time of testing, cocaine-exposed children were not different from control children in body weight or stature (both nominal and percentile for age). However, the former had a significantly smaller fronto-occipital head circumference than did the latter in both nominal values ($p = 0.002$) and percentile for age ($p = 0.001$) (TABLE 2). Nine of the cocaine-exposed children, compared with only two of the control children ($p < 0.01$), had a head circumference under the 11th percentile for age and sex. Eight of the children exposed to cocaine were considered microcephalic. Cocaine-exposed children were eight times as likely as control children to be microcephalic (95% confidence interval 1.5–42.3).

TABLE 2. Anthropometric Characteristics of Cocaine-Exposed and Control Children

Characteristic	Group; Mean (and SEM) Cocaine-Exposed ($n = 23$)	Control ($n = 23$)	p Value
At birth			
Weight (g)	2,597 (200)	3,415 (106)	0.005
Gestational age (wk)	37.3 (0.8)	40.1 (0.37)	0.002
At testing			
Age (mo)	34.0 (3.3)	33.3 (2.5)	NS
Weight (kg)	13.8 (0.72)	15.4 (0.84)	NS
Percentile	56.7 (7.6)	69.5 (6.6)	NS
Height (cm)	89.8 (2.0)	92.6 (2.2)	NS
Percentile	39.2 (6.2)	52.3 (7.1)	NS
Head circumference (cm)	47.7 (0.5)	49.8 (0.4)	0.002
Percentile	30.7 (7.0)	63.4 (6.6)	0.001

No differences were noted between the study and control groups in global IQ (TABLE 3). However, among the children tested with the McCarthy scales there was a trend towards lower IQ in the cocaine-exposed group (107 [SEM 4.8] vs. 117 [SEM 2.0]) ($p = 0.1$). No differences were found between the study and control groups in mean scores on the Bayley scales. Cocaine-exposed children had significantly lower scores than did the control children on both the verbal comprehension scale ($p = 0.003$) and the expressive language scale ($p = 0.001$) of the Reynell language test (TABLE 3).

No correlation was noted between gestational age, birth weight, or moderate alcohol use and achievement on the cognitive or language tests or in percentile of head circumference at testing. ANCOVA failed to show effects of prematurity on head circumference or of prematurity and number of siblings in the home on IQ or achievement on the language tests.

Our study, after controlling for the postnatal environment of children exposed *in utero* to cocaine, detected clinically significant language delay and a trend towards decreased IQ as measured in preschool children. These effects were not due to prematurity, which may be caused by cocaine. Because mothers using cocaine also smoke heavily and consume ethanol, it is impossible to separate the effects of cocaine from those

TABLE 3. Results of Cognitive and Language Testing in Cocaine-Exposed and Control Children

Variable	Group; Mean (and SEM) Cocaine-Exposed		Control		p Value
Global IQ* (Bayley	$n = 23$		$n = 23$		
and McCarthy scales)	109	(3.0)	112	(2.2)	NS
McCarthy global IQ*	$n = 11$		$n = 11$		
	107	(4.8)	117	(2.0)	0.1
Score on Reynell					
language test	$n = 23$		$n = 23$		
Verbal comprehension	0.4	(0.19)	1.2	(0.18)	0.003
Expressive language	−0.58	(0.14)	0.4	(0.17)	0.001

of other chemicals. However, it is noteworthy that neither cigarette smoking nor moderate alcohol consumption has been associated with cognitive and language delay.

It is possible, however, that a synergistic effect exists between cocaine and cigarettes or alcohol. For example, esterification of cocaine and ethanol results in the production of cocaethylene which is more neurotoxic than is either cocaine or ethanol.

Further and longer studies of larger cohorts of adopted children exposed *in utero* to cocaine will help to better identify the risks on various domains of child neurodevelopment.

REFERENCES

1. Graham, K., A. Feigenbaum, A. Pastuszak *et al.* 1992. Pregnancy outcome and infant development following gestational cocaine use by social cocaine users in Toronto. Clin. Invest. Med. **15:** 384–394.
2. Nulman, I. 1994. Can. Med. Assoc. J. **151:** 1591–1597.
3. Haddad, L.M. 1983. Cocaine. *In* Clinical Management of Poisoning and Drug Overdose. L.M. Haddad & J.F. Winchester, Eds.: 445. W.B. Saunders Co., Philadelphia, PA.
4. Wallis, C. 1986. Time Magazine. Jan. 20: 44.
5. Szabo, P. 1987. Cocaine babies differ significantly. The Journal. April 1: 4.
6. McConnell, H. 1986. Women's cocaine use is probably underestimated. The Journal. Feb. 1: 3.
7. Neuspiel, D.R. 1994. Behavior in cocaine-exposed infants and children: Association versus causality. **36:** 101–107.
8. Chasnoff, I.J., W.J. Burns, S.H. Schnoll *et al.* 1985. Cocaine use in pregnancy. N. Engl. J. Med. **313:** 666–669.
9. Smart, R.G. *et al.* 1987. Alcohol and other drug use among Ontario adults 1977–1987. Alcoholism and Drug Addiction Research Foundation. Toronto.
10. Fantel, A.G. & B.J. Macphail. 1982. The teratogenicity of cocaine. Teratology **26:** 17–19.
11. Woods, J.R., M.A. Plessingey & K.E. Clark. 1987. Effect of cocaine on uterine blood flow and fetal oxygenation. JAMA **257:** 957–961.
12. Neuspiel, D., S.C. Hamel, E. Hochberg *et al.* 1991. Maternal cocaine use and infant behavior. Neurotoxicol. Teratol. 1991.
13. Chasnoff, I.J., M.E. Bassey, R. Savicho *et al.* 1986. Perinatal cerebral infarction and maternal cocaine use. J. Pediatr. **108:** 456–459.
14. Forman, R., J. Klein, D. Meta *et al.* 1993. Maternal and neonatal characteristics following exposure to cocaine in Toronto. Reprod. Toxicol. **7:** 619–622.
15. Chasnoff, I.J., D.R. Griffith, C. Freier *et al.* 1992. Cocaine/polydrug use in pregnancy. 1991. Two year follow-up. Pediatrics **89:** 284–289.
16. Bingol, N., M. Fuchs & V. Diaz. 1987. J. Pediatr. **110:** 93–96.
17. Dixon, S.D., R. Bejar *et al.* 1989. Echoencephalographic findings in neonates associated with maternal cocaine and methamphetamine use: Incidence and clinical correlates. **115:** 770–778.18. Singer, L.T., R. Garber & R. Kliegman. 1991. Neurobehavioral sequelae of fetal cocaine exposure. J. Pediatr. **119:** 667–6.
19. Volpe, J.Y. 1992. Effect of cocaine on the fetus. N. Engl. J. Med. **327:** 399–407.
20. Chasnoff, I.J., C.E. Hunt, R. Kletter, *et al.* 1989. Prenatal cocaine exposure is associated with respiratory pattern abnormalities. AJDC **143:** 583–587.
21. Doberczak, T.M., S. Shanzer, R.T. Senile & S.R. Kandall. 1988. Neonatal neurologic and electroencephalopeptic effects of intrauterine cocaine exposure. J. Pediatr. **113:** 354–358.
22. Eisen, L.N., T.F. Field, S.E. Bandstra *et al.* 1989. Prenatal cocaine effects on neonatal stress behavior and performance on the Brazelton Scale. Pediatrics **13:** 229–233.
23. Woods, N.S., F.D. Eyler, M. Behnke *et al.* 1993. Cocaine use in pregnancy: Maternal depressive symptoms and infant neurobehavior over the first month. Infant Behav. Dev. **16:** 83–98.
24. Coles, C., K.A. Platzman, I. Smith *et al.* 1992. Effects of cocaine and alcohol use in pregnancy on neonatal growth and neurobehavioral status. Neurotoxicol. Teratol. **14:** 23–33.

25. FAWLEY, H.T.L. 1993. Children of the crack epidemic: The cognitive, language, and emotional development of preschool children of addicted mothers. Presented at the meeting of the Society for Research in Child Development. New Orleans, March, 1993.
26. RODNING, C., L. BECKWITH & J. HOWARD. 1989. Characteristics of attachment organization and play organization in prenatally drug exposed toddlers. Dev. Psychopathol. **1:** 277–289.
27. RODNING, C., L. BECKWITH & J. HOWARD. 1989. Prenatal exposure to drugs: Behavioral distortions reflecting CNS impairment. Neurotoxicity **10:** 629–634.
28. BECKWITH, L. 1990. Spontaneous play in two-year-olds born to substance-abusing mothers. Presented at the meeting of the Society for Research in Child Development, New Orleans. March 1993. Centers for Disease Control. MMWR **39:** 225–227.
29. CRAWFORD, S.D. 1993. Developmental characteristics of prenatally drug exposed young children. Presented at the meeting of the Society for Research in Child Development, New Orleans. March 1993.
30. AHL, V. 1993. Classification by infants prenatally exposed to cocaine. Presented at the Meeting of the Society for Research in Child Development, New Orleans. March 1993.
31. HOFKOSH, P., J.L. PRINGLE, H.P. WALD *et al.* 1995. Early interaction between drug-involved mothers and infants. Arch. Pediatr. Adolesc. Med. **149:** 665–672.
32. HURT, H., N.L. BRODSKY, L. BETANCOURT *et al.* 1997. Cocaine-exposed children; Follow-up through 30 months. Pediatrics **130:** 310–312.
33. FETTERS, L. & E.Z. TRONICK. 1996. Neuromotor development of cocaine-exposed and control infants from birth to 15 months. Pediatrics **98:** 938–943.
34. RICHARDSON, G.A., S.C. HAMEL, L. GOLDSCHMIDT, N.L. DAY *et al.* 1996. The effects of prenatal cocaine use on neurobehavioral status. Neurotoxicol. Teratol. **18:** 627–34.
35. BURKHEAD, J., J.L. ERICKSEN & J.D. BLANCO. 1995. Cocaine use in pregnancy and the risk of intraamniotic infection. Reprod. Med. **40:** 198–200.
36. BALL, S.A., R.S. SCHOTTENFELD *et al.* 1997. A fine factor model of personality of addiction, psychiatric and AIDS risk severity in pregnant and postpartum cocaine misusers. Subst. Use Misuse **31:** 25–41.
37. HUNT, H. *et al.* 1995. J. Dev. Behav. Pediatr. **16:** 29–35.
38. BENDERSKY, M., S. ALESSANDRI, P. GILBERT, M. LEWIS *et al.* 1996. Characteristics of pregnant substance abusers in two cities in the northeast. Am. J. Drug Alc. Abuse **22:** 349–362.
39. CHAZOTTE, C., J. YOUCHAH & M.C. FREDA. 1995. Cocaine use during pregnancy and low birthweight: The impact of prenatal care treatment. Semin. Perinatal. **19:** 293–300.
40. KISTIN, N., A. HANDLER, F. DAVIS & C. FERRES. 1996. Cocaine and cigarettes; A comparison of risks. Paediatr. Perinat. Epidemiol. **10:** 269–278.
41. KILLEEN, J., K.T. BRADY & A. THEVOS. 1995. Addiction severity, psychopathy and treatment compliance in cocaine-dependent mothers. Addict. Dis. **14:** 75–84.
42. BARTON, S.J., R. HARRIGAN & A.M. TSE. 1995. Prenatal cocaine exposure: Implication for practice, policy development and needs for future research. J. Perinatol. **15:** 10–22.
43. SALLEE, F.R., L.P. KATINKANENI, P.D. MCARTHUR *et al.* 1995. Head growth in cocaine-exposed infants: Relationship to neonate hair level. J. Dev. Behav. Pediatr. **16:** 77–81.
44. INGERSOLL, K., K. DAWSON & D. HALLER. 1996. Family functioning of perinatal substance abusers in treatment. J. Psychoact. Drugs **28:** 61–71.
45. HOWARD, J., L. BECKWITH, M. ESPINOSA & R. TYLER. 1995. Development of infants born to cocaine abusing women: Biologic/maternal influences. Neurotoxicol. Teratol. **17:** 403–411.
46. SCAFIDI, F.A., T.U. FIELD, A. WHEEDER *et al.* 1996. Cocaine-exposed preterm neonates show behavioral and hormonal differences. Pediatrics **97:** 851–855.
47. JACOBSON, S.W., J.L. JACOBSON, R.J. SOKAL *et al.* 1996. New evidence for neurobehavioral effects on *in utero* cocaine exposure. J. Pediatr. **129:** 581–590.
48. SINGER, L., R. ARENDT, L.Y. SONG *et al.* 1994. Direct and indirect interactions of cocaine with childbirth outcomes. Arch. Pediatr. Adolesc. Med. **148:** 959–964.
49. FRANK, D., K. BRESNAHAN & B.S. ZUCKERMAN. 1993. Maternal cocaine use: Impact on child health and development. Adv. Pediatr. **40:** 65–99.

Prenatal Exposure to Cocaine and Other Drugs

Outcome at Four to Six Years[a]

IRA J. CHASNOFF,[b] AMY ANSON, ROGER HATCHER, HERB STENSON, KAI IAUKEA, AND LINDA A. RANDOLPH

National Association for Families and Addiction Research and Education, 122 South Michigan Avenue, Suite 1100, Chicago, Illinois 60603, USA

ABSTRACT: In a longitudinal, prospective study, 95 children born to mothers who used cocaine and other drugs during pregnancy and 75 matched, nonexposed children born to mothers who had no evidence of alcohol or illicit substance use during pregnancy were evaluated for cognitive and behavioral outcome at 6 years of age. Prenatal exposure to cocaine and other drugs had no direct effect on the child's cognitive outcome (measured as IQ), but it had an indirect effect as mediated through the home environment. However, prenatal exposure to cocaine and other drugs *did* have a direct effect on the child's behavioral characteristics at 4–6 years of age, with the home environment having little impact. This study helps us to understand the fragile interaction of biological and environmental factors affecting the cognitive and behavioral development of children prenatally exposed to cocaine and other drugs.

INTRODUCTION

Children prenatally exposed to maternal substances of abuse make up an important subset of the United States' population of children. The most recent data from the National Institute on Drug Abuse suggest that up to 221,000 children per year are exposed to illicit substances during gestation, 45,000 of them to cocaine.[1] The impact of prenatal cocaine exposure on pregnancy and the neonate has been described in a variety of studies,[2–5] and the long-term implications of prenatal cocaine exposure for the child are just beginning to be explored.[6–9] Woven throughout this research is the realization that multiple factors mediate the impact of cocaine on the exposed child's neurologic and behavioral development. However, no comprehensive evaluation of the multiple factors that affect developmental outcome for children beyond 3 years of age who were prenatally exposed to cocaine has been published.

This study identifies the potency and direction of biological and environmental factors on cognitive and behavioral development in children aged 4–6 years who were born to mothers who used cocaine and other drugs during gestation. The hypothesis is that prenatal exposure to cocaine and other drugs has both a direct and an indirect effect on the child's intellectual and behavioral functioning and that these effects are mediated by the home environment as defined by the level of developmental support in the home, the mother's psychological status, and the mother's ongoing use of alcohol or illicit substances.

[a]This work was supported by Grant S184U30001 from the U.S. Department of Education, Safe and Drug Free Schools.

[b]Address for correspondence: Ira J. Chasnoff, M.D., 122 South Michigan Avenue, Suite 1100, Chicago, IL 60603. Phone, 312/431–0013; fax, 312/431–8697; e-mail, irajc@smtp.bmai.com

SUBJECTS

The children enrolled in this longitudinal study were described in previous publications.[2,3,6,7] In brief, the initial subjects were born to women who were referred to the project during pregnancy before 15 weeks' gestation from a general obstetric clinic. Referral to this group was based on the patient's self-report or a physician's diagnosis of cocaine use. Informed consent as approved by the Institutional Review Board (IRB) of the Illinois Department of Alcoholism and Substance Abuse was obtained from all women upon enrollment in the project and renewed when the child reached 4 years of age. IRB approval, including review of human subjects' protection, has been renewed on an annual basis since inception of the project.

Following enrollment, all women received intensive obstetric and psychotherapeutic interventions through the remainder of the pregnancy. The goal of the interventions was to have the women cease all use of alcohol and illicit substances. Complete drug and alcohol use evaluations were performed at the time of enrollment and at subsequent intervals throughout the pregnancy. Toxicologic analyses for nicotine, barbiturates, cocaine and its metabolites, opiates, benzodiazepines, propoxyphene, phencyclidine, amphetamines, and marijuana were performed at enrollment for all women and repeated on a random basis throughout pregnancy. Current substance use history was reviewed at each prenatal visit.

A population of pregnant women matched to the study population on race and socioeconomic status but with no history or evidence of alcohol or illicit drug use were enrolled to serve as a comparison group. Urine toxicologic analyses were performed as part of the clinical care of the drug-free women in the prenatal period, and extensive substance use evaluations were performed throughout gestation by trained interviewers to insure that none of the women in the comparison group had in fact used alcohol or illicit drugs.

The study cohort (Group 1) and comparison group (Group 2) are predominantly from a low socioeconomic class, with approximately 70% in both groups receiving public aid. The study subjects and the controls all live in the central inner city of Chicago and share the same neighborhoods, schools, and general community environment.

At 4, 5, and 6 years of age, the growth and cognitive and behavioral developmental outcomes of 170 children were evaluated. Ninety-five of these children had been born to women who used cocaine, but no opiates, during pregnancy (Group 1). Most of these women also had used additional nonopiate substances, including marijuana, alcohol, and/or tobacco, in various combinations with the cocaine. Thus, we refer to this group as cocaine/polydrug (C/P) exposed because few of the children were exposed only to cocaine. The remaining 75 children had been born to women with no evidence of alcohol or illicit substance use, although 10 smoked tobacco during gestation (Group 2).

The children included in this present analysis represent 60% of the original cohort recruited in the prenatal period and a slight increase over the number of cocaine-exposed children included in analysis at 3 years of age.[7] The maternal drug use patterns, marital status, and socioeconomic status and the mean neonatal gestation age, birth weight, and head circumference of the subjects who were evaluated at 4, 5, and 6 years of age did not differ from those of the subjects who had been lost to follow-up.

PROCEDURES

All children were evaluated at the research clinic of the National Association for Families and Addiction Research and Education (NAFARE), a comprehensive program of health care and developmental follow-up for substance-abusing women and their children. All growth, developmental, behavioral, and environmental data were collected prospectively according to the established protocol (TABLE 1) and entered into a computerized database. Those staff responsible for child evaluation were blind to the past and current drug histories and urine toxicologic results of all women and children.

To aid in retention of the subjects and controls in the project, families were contacted by telephone and mail before all appointments. Bus tokens and cab fares for families who required transportation support were provided, and all families were paid $20 per visit for their participation. In addition, all attempts were made to accommodate the time frame of the family in terms of scheduling evaluations. Routine immunizations and general pediatric care were provided to all children in conjunction with collection of research data, an incentive for the families to continue in the project.

At the 4- and 5-year visits, measurements of the child's weight, standing height, and frontooccipital head circumferences were collected by the pediatrician. Psychologists administered the Wechsler Primary and Preschool Scales of Intelligence-Revised[10] which provides a global index of a child's level of cognitive ability (Full Scale IQ) and subscale scores on performance (Performance IQ) and verbal (Verbal IQ) capabilities.

A research assistant administered the Structured Maternal Interview, an instrument created by the research team to evaluate maternal health, psychosocial status, and ongoing drug use patterns. To evaluate the current level of maternal psychopathology, seven questions from the Structured Maternal Interview were chosen *a priori* and summed, the total score based on one point given for each positive answer and zero for each negative answer with a possible range of scores from 0–7:

Not counting the effects from drug or alcohol use, have you ever experienced:

Serious depression?
Serious anxiety or tension?
Hallucinations—hearing or seeing things that others thought were your imagination?
Trouble understanding, concentrating, or remembering?
Trouble controlling violent behavior?

TABLE 1. Evaluation Protocol

4 Years
Medical evaluation with standing height, weight, and occipitofrontal head circumference
Home Screening Questionnaire
Structured Maternal Interview
Wechsler Primary and Preschool Scales of Intelligence-Revised (WPPSI-R)
Achenbach Child Behavior Checklist
5 Years
Medical evaluation with standing height, weight, and occipitofrontal head circumference
Home Screening Questionnaire
Structured Maternal Interview
WPPSI-R
Achenbach Child Behavior Checklist
6 Years
Medical evaluation with standing height, weight, and occipitofrontal head circumference
Structured Maternal Interview
Wechsler Intelligence Scales for Children-III (WISC-III)
Achenbach Child Behavior Checklist

Serious thoughts of suicide?
Attempts at suicide?

Degree of postnatal alcohol or illicit drug use was evaluated using a five-point Likert-type scale developed for the SMI and based on the response of the mother to the question:

Which of the following best describes your drug use pattern since ____ was born?

1. never used drugs again
2. occasional but not consistent use over the years
3. consistent, occasional use over the years
4. stopped altogether for periods, then began to use again
5. continued to use drugs on a consistent basis.

The Child Behavior Checklist (CBCL)[11] was completed by the mother or primary caretaker at each visit for each child at 4, 5, and 6 years. The CBCL contains 112 specific problem items and two open-ended problem items scored on a three-step response scale (0,1,2). It was designed to record, in a standardized fashion, children's problems in behavioral terms as reported by their parents or other caretakers. With empirical techniques, this instrument derived "syndromes," or groups of items that covary together at high levels, and designated them with appropriate labels. Eight such "syndromes" were identified with this instrument, in addition to two larger groupings of the syndromes, into "internalizing" and "externalizing" domains. Full validity and reliability studies have been conducted on this instrument, with excellent results.[11]

The mother or primary caretaker also completed the Home Screening Questionnaire (HSQ) at the 4- and 5-year visits.[12] The HSQ is a screening instrument completed by the caretaker that identifies factors within a young child's home environment related to the child's growth and development. It was designed to identify children at risk for developmental delay secondary to negative environmental influences. Total HSQ scores less than 41 are considered an indication of environmental risk.

At 6 years of age, each child again underwent full physical evaluation, and standing height, weight, and occipitofrontal head circumference were recorded. Cognitive functioning was evaluated using the Wechsler Intelligence Scales for Children-III (-WISC-III),[13] with Full Scale, Performance, and Verbal IQs calculated. The mother or primary caretaker completed the CBCL and responded to the Structured Maternal Interview.

STATISTICAL METHODS

Two groups of subjects were formed based on the subjects' prenatal exposure to cocaine and other drugs (Group 1) versus no prenatal exposure (Group 2). Group differences were analyzed by a variety of statistical techniques including *t* tests, Chi-square tests, analyses of variance, Pearson correlations, factor analysis, and path analyses, depending on the nature of the dependent variables and the goals of the analyses. In all cases the SYSTAT statistical package was used.

A major focus of this paper is a series of path analyses that were performed to better understand the data. It should be noted that such "causal" analyses are fraught with both philosophical and statistical problems. The models that we present are not the only possible models, and we do not believe that we can prove causality in any final sense. However, the models do provide plausible structures with which to understand the effects of prenatal substance exposure on the offspring of the substance-abusing women.

In each path model the group variable (prenatal cocaine/polydrug exposure *vs* nonexposed) provides the first node in a path. We combine this starting point with nodes representing environmental variables and behavioral variables in various combinations in order to predict a specific outcome such as IQ or behavioral problems. In all cases the path coefficients shown are standardized coefficients, so that comparison of the sizes of the various coefficients are scale-free. We also show the statistical significance of these coefficients as well as relevant multiple regression coefficients that are involved in the path structure.

In a longitudinal study such as this, the loss of subjects along the way is inevitable as is the problem of missing data of one kind or another for some subjects. In order not to lose statistical power we performed analyses on all of the data that were available for the particular variables involved in an analysis. This procedure resulted in some analyses being based on a slightly different subset of subjects than other analyses. However, there is no reason to suspect that the missing data for a particular subject on a few variables is the result of systematic causes. Thus, we reason that the omission of a subject from one analysis and the inclusion of the same subject in another creates no bias in the interpretation of data. In all cases we show sample sizes for the analyses performed.

RESULTS

Maternal Descriptors and Home Environment

Mean maternal age at delivery (Group 1: mean = 26.7, SD = 4.7 years, $n = 95$ *vs* Group 2: mean = 25.9, SD = 4.8 years, $n = 75$), racial distribution (approximately 75% African-American in each group), mean income (below poverty level for both groups), marital status, and mean education level (approximately 11.5 years for each group) were similar for the two groups. The two groups of children had a similar distribution of male and female.

Among the cocaine/polydrug-using women in Group 1, all had used cocaine plus other drugs during pregnancy, the most common substances being marijuana, alcohol, and tobacco. Women who had used opiates or who had used alcohol or illicit substances but no cocaine are not included in this study cohort. Overall the women were heavy cocaine users with an average estimated frequency of cocaine use in the first trimester of pregnancy of 2.5 times per week with a range of .25 g to 1 g with each use. Forty percent of the women ceased all alcohol and illicit drug use by the beginning of the third trimester. However, from the time of delivery to follow-up at 6 years postdelivery, all women in Group 1 had relapsed to cocaine use at least once. At the 6-year assessment, 40% of Group 1 women were currently drug and alcohol free an average of 2 years. The remaining 60% continued to use cocaine, alcohol, or some other substance on an occasional to a weekly basis. Among Group 2 women, although none used alcohol or illicit drugs during pregnancy, five had begun to use cocaine during the 6 years of follow-up. The mean postnatal drug use score was significantly higher ($F = 2.1$, $p < 0.05$) for Group 1 women (mean = 3.1, SD = 1.2, $n = 92$) than that for the five Group 2 women (mean = 2, SD = 1) who had used drugs.

The level of current maternal psychopathology was similar for the two groups of women as documented via mean scores on the *a priori* summed scores from the Structured Maternal Interview (mean = 1.9, SD = 1.8, $n = 92$ *vs* mean = 1.2, SD = 1.2, $n = 70$, Groups 1 and 2, respectively). Mean Home Screening Questionnaire (HSQ) scores for the two groups also were similar, with both groups scoring in the at-risk range (mean = 34.1, SD = 5.3, $n = 90$ *vs* mean = 36.1, SD = 7.3, $n = 72$, Groups 1 and 2, respectively).

There was a high inverse correlation between HSQ score and the degree of maternal drug use over the 6 years of follow-up ($r = 0.60$, $n = 160$, $p < 0.01$).

Child Growth Data

Mean weight and standing height for the two groups at 4, 5, and 6 years were similar, both groups' mean weight and height falling well within the normal range on standardized growth charts. At 4 years of age, Group children children had a mean head circumference (mean = 49.8, SD = 1.6 cm) that was significantly smaller than that for Group 2 (mean = 50.9, SD = 2.7 cm) children ($F = 3.3$, $p < 0.01$). Through univariate and multivariate repeated measures analysis, no difference was found between the two groups of children in the rate of growth of weight, height, or head circumference over the 3 years, and by 6 years of age, children in Group 1 had a head circumference that continued to be marginally smaller ($F = 3.9$, $p = 0.05$).

Cognitive Development

The mean IQ scores on the WPPSI-R at 4 and 5 years of age and on the WISC-III at 6 years of age for both groups were at the lower end of the normal range, and no significant differences were noted between the two groups at any age. However, the mean Full Scale IQ, Performance IQ, and Verbal IQ scores for both groups showed a steady decline over the 3-year period. To summarize findings for children's cognitive development, Full Scale IQ, Performance IQ, and Verbal IQ data for each child were averaged over ages 4, 5, and 6 years (TABLE 2). Each child's score is the average of those scores available for the three ages. This averaged score was utilized for further analyses.

Behavioral Data

On behavioral assessment utilizing the CBCL completed by the mother or primary caretaker, children in both groups demonstrated consistent patterns of behavior across the 3 years of evaluation (multivariate repeated measures analysis). To summarize the findings for the children's behavioral ratings for the home, data for each of the CBCL scales for each child were averaged over ages 4, 5, and 6 years. The average scores for behavioral variables for which significant differences existed for the two groups are shown in TABLE 3. Children prenatally exposed to cocaine and other drugs (Group 1) had significantly higher scores on the internalizing and externalizing domains, several individual items, and total CBCL score. In addition, the proportion of children scoring above a clinical cutoff of the 98th percentile was significantly greater in Group 1 than in Group 2 (Chi square = .292, $p < 0.03$).

TABLE 2. Average IQ Scores for Ages 4, 5, and 6 Years

	Group 1: Cocaine/Polydrug Exposed ($n = 64$)	Group 2: Nonexposed ($n = 54$)
Full Scale IQ	88.1 ± 12.3 (SD)	90.4 ± 15 (SD)
Performance IQ	89.1 ± 13.6 (SD)	91.4 ± 14.6 (SD)
Verbal IQ	88.6 ± 11.8 (SD)	91.3 ± 14.8 (SD)

TABLE 3. Average Behavioral Scores for Ages 4, 5, and 6 Years

	Group 1: Cocaine/Polydrug Exposed ($n = 66$)		Group 2: Nonexposed ($n = 56$)	
	Mean	± SD	Mean	± SD
Anxious/Depressed***	3.70	2.89	2.03	2.79
Social problems**	2.53	1.70	1.79	1.57
Thought problems***	1.18	1.27	0.46	0.98
Attention problems***	4.17	2.78	2.54	2.89
Delinquent behavior***	2.65	1.89	1.47	1.31
Aggressive behavior***	11.67	6.63	7.25	5.53
Internalizing composite*	6.71	4.47	4.74	6.41
Externalizing composite***	14.32	8.00	8.72	6.62
Total problems***	34.34	16.08	21.72	17.36

* t test, $p < 0.05$; ** t test, $p < 0.01$; *** t test, $p < 0.001$.

Correlations

The zero-order correlation matrix for maternal and environmental variables and IQ and behavior (averaged over 3 years) regardless of group classification is presented in TABLE 4. The Pearson correlations represent the relationship between the variables. Examination of the correlations indicates a moderate but consistent correlation between continued postpartum drug use by the mother and child behavioral problems; between maternal postpartum drug use and lower Full Scale IQ, Performance IQ, and Verbal IQ scores; and between maternal psychopathology and child behavioral problems.

Factor Analysis of Child Behavior Checklist

Factor analysis of all CBCL scores for each child over the 3-year period revealed that four of the eight scales (aggressive behavior, delinquent behavior, attention problems, and social problems) formed a cohesive cluster (TABLE 5). This cluster includes the two scales that are considered to measure “externalizing behaviors” by Achenbach, but also includes the attention problems and social problems scales. This pattern suggests an array of behaviors indicative of a child with problems in *self-regulation,* or the ability to manage their behaviors and impulses in ways that are considered adaptive for their age. The inability to regulate or inhibit responses leads to the range of behaviors tapped by these four scales. Somatic complaints and withdrawal, two of the three scales making up Achenbach’s internalizing behaviors composite, also formed a distinct cluster, suggesting a child with a tendency to *internalize* problems, or direct them inwardly. The anxious/depressed scale and the thought problems scale both appeared to be related to each of the two distinct clusters just described. For model analysis, all behavioral data were collapsed and analyzed via this pattern of behavioral clusters: self-regulation problems, internalizing style, anxious/depressed, and thought problems.

TABLE 4. Correlation Matrix for Maternal and Environmental Factors and Behavioral Assessment and IQ Scores

		Behavior			Cognitive Development			Environmental Factors		
		Internal	External	Total Problems	Performance IQ	Verbal IQ	Full Scale IQ	Postpartum Drug Use	Psychopathology	HSQ
Behavior	Internal	1								
	External	.429	1							
	Total Problems	.741	.866	1						
	Performance IQ	–.107	–.096	–.103	1					
Cognitive Development	Verb IQ	–.147	–.097	–.137	.704	1				
	Full Scale IQ	–.110–	.038	–.098	.893	.878	1			
	Postpartum Drug Use	.299	.294	.394	–.315	–.269	–.330	1		
Environmental Facts	Maternal Psychopathology	.115	.295	.320	–.022	–.104	–.062	.206	1	
	HSQ	–.104	–.227	–.214	.279	.214	.280	–.125	.038	1

TABLE 5. Factor Analysis of Behavioral Scores Averaged Over 4, 5, and 6 Years of Age

		Factor 1	Factor 2
Self-regulation problems	Aggressive behavior	0.870	0.104
	Delinquent behavior	0.836	0.052
	Attention problems	0.757	0.370
	Social problems	0.712	0.290
	Anxious/Depressed	0.561	0.653
	Thought problems	0.519	0.595
Internalizing style	Somatic complaints	–0.028	0.771
	Withdrawn	0.226	0.695

Model Assessment

To understand some of the more interesting relationships in our data we constructed a number of path diagrams. We present here those diagrams that seemed to elaborate in a sensible way the statistical relationships in the data. In each, the coefficients shown on the path arrows are standardized regression coefficients. Thus, their relative sizes can be meaningfully compared. Multiple regression coefficients are shown for the prediction of a variable from more than one prior variable in the path.

FIGURE 1 shows the relationship of group membership (GROUP) and the Home Screening Questionnaire scores (HSQ) to each of three measures of intelligence: Full Scale IQ (FSIQ), Verbal IQ (VERB), and Performance IQ (PERFORM). The group variable was coded so that 0 represented each child in the control group and 1 repre-

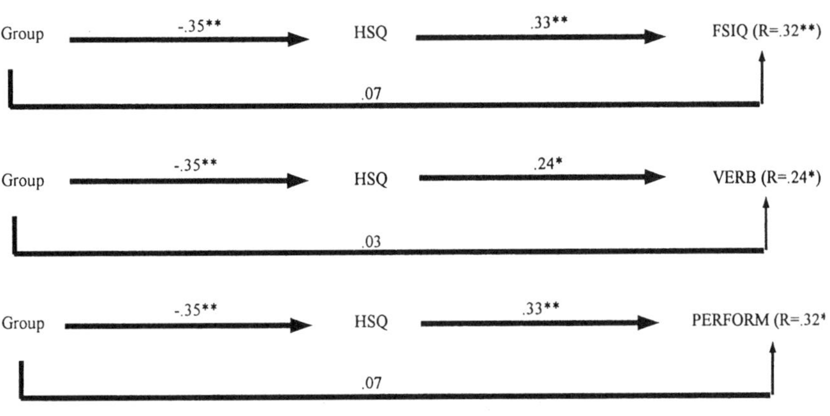

FIGURE 1. Path diagrams showing the relationship of intelligence to prenatal drug exposure and quality of home environment.

sented a child prenatally exposed to cocaine and other drugs. High scores on the HSQ indicate a positive, supportive home environment. Each diagram in FIGURE 1 is based on the same 110 cases (59 drug-exposed and 51 control children) for which there were complete data on all the relevant variables.

FIGURE 1 shows that prenatal exposure to cocaine and other drugs is not directly related to later IQ scores, but that an indirect effect is mediated through the quality of the home environment. Children from homes in which there is prenatal drug use have a lower quality home environment and this in turn is related to lower performance on all three IQ measures. Whether this is treated as a true causal relationship or not, the multiple regression coefficients show that each of the three measures of I are significantly predictable from the two independent variables.

We next examined GROUP and HSQ as predictors of behavioral indices. These diagrams are shown in FIGURE 2. We used four different measures of behavior: self-regulation, internalizing style, anxious/depressed, and thought. These are all based on the factor analysis performed previously. Self-regulation, based on the scale constructed through factor analysis, is the sum of a child's scores on the Aggressive Behavior, Delinquent Behavior, Attention Problems, and Social Problems scales of the CBCL, which all relate to a child's ability to control his/her behavior and impulses and the resulting difficulty in peer relationships. Internalizing style, also derived from factor analysis, is the sum of the Withdrawn and Somatic Complaints scales of the CBCL, an index of the degree to which a child turns his or her problems or feelings inward. It is not a measure of introversion in the usual sense of that word, but rather the tendency to turn feelings, especially anger, inwardly, which is often also reflected in insecurity and/or difficulty engaging in relationships. The Anxious/Depressed variables are the Achenbach checklists for behaviors often associated with anxiety and/or depression, although as

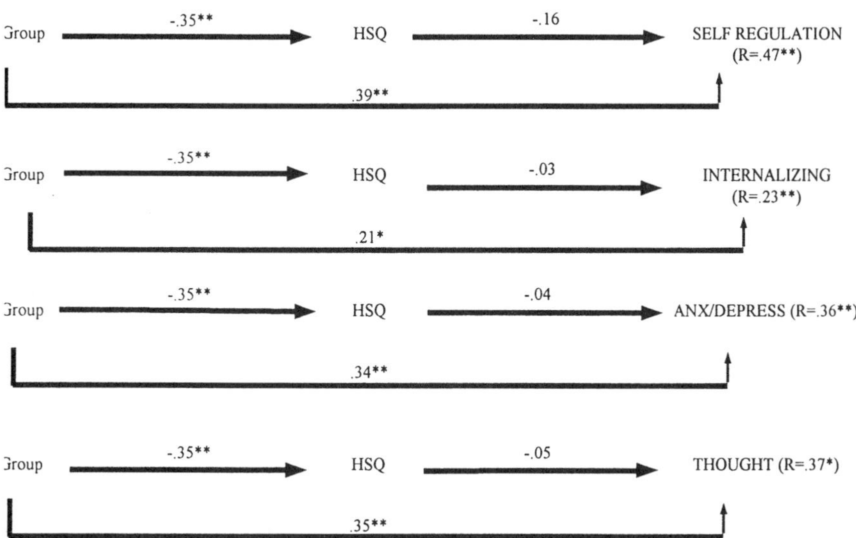

FIGURE 2. Path diagrams showing the relationship of four sets of behavioral problems to prenatal drug exposure and quality of home environment.

with all scales in this measure, some levels of behavior are expected and considered normal and not indicative of "problems" or psychopathology. The Thought Problems scale identifies behaviors or ideas that are considered strange by the caretaker as well as staring and hallucinations. Each of the diagrams presented in FIGURE 2 is based on the same 114 cases (61 drug-exposed and 53 control children) for which there were complete data on all the relevant variables.

FIGURE 2 shows a markedly different pattern from that in FIGURE 1 in that the quality of the home environment is not related to behavioral problems, but that prenatal drug exposure, or the lack of it, *is* related to such problems. In fact, the diagrams show that even though HSQ is related to GROUP, it may as well not be in the equation for predicting behavior because the coefficients on the direct path from GROUP to the behavioral variables are almost as large as the whole multiple R in three of the four diagrams. It is interesting to note that the one exception to this is the mediating role of the home environment on self-regulatory capacities. The better the home environment, the more self-control capacity is reported in the child.

DISCUSSION

Although the modern description of the Fetal Alcohol Syndrome was published initially in 1973[14] and newborn heroin withdrawal was first described in the mid-1970s,[15] until relatively recently little attention has been paid to the long-term implications of prenatal substance exposure. Fried and Watkinson[16] examined the effects of prenatal exposure to marijuana, tobacco, and alcohol on developmental outcome at 3 and 4 years of age. In their sample, these authors found cigarette smoking to be related to poor language development and cognitive functioning at both 3 and 4 years. Alcohol exposure was related to decreased cognitive abilities at 3 years, and marijuana exposure was associated at 4 years with lower scores in the verbal and memory domains.

Streissguth *et al.*[17] examined the effects of prenatal exposure to alcohol and/or tobacco on IQ scores of 4-year-old children. They found a significant negative relationship between alcohol consumption during pregnancy by white, middle class women and the IQ scores of their offspring at 4 years of age. This relationship held after controlling for various prenatal and postnatal confounding variables.

In the last decade, cocaine has become a primary substance of abuse among relatively large numbers of women of childbearing age. A variety of problems in neonates born to cocaine-using women has been described, including increased rates of preterm delivery, low birth weight, and small head circumference.[2–5,18,19] The present study confirmed findings of smaller head circumference at 4–6 years of follow-up, although we note less statistically significant results, suggesting a trend toward catch-up growth.

Infants born to cocaine-using women also demonstrate impaired neurobehavioral functioning in the newborn period, with poor state regulation, orientation, and habituation capabilities.[2,3,20–22] Subsequently, over the last 5 years, more information on the developmental outcomes of cocaine-exposed infants and children has begun to emerge. A study of 3-month-old infants who had been prenatally exposed to cocaine found that prenatal cocaine exposure had effects on arousal and attention regulation rather than on early cognitive processes.[8]

Early data from the University of California at Los Angeles[23] indicate that a group of 18-month-old children who had been exposed prenatally to cocaine had significantly lower developmental scores than those of a group of non-drug–exposed infants from similar family and socioeconomic backgrounds. However, these children still fell within the low-average range on standardized developmental scores. The drug-exposed children also showed deficits in the context of free play. They were reported to have less representational play than did the control group, and most drug-exposed children demonstrated a high rate of scattering, batting, and picking up and putting down of toys rather than sustained combining of toys, fantasy play, or curious exploration.

As in earlier studies, a recent study by Hurt *et al.*[9] of 30-month-old children prenatally exposed to cocaine demonstrated statistically lower mean weights and smaller mean head circumferences than those of control children throughout the follow-up period. Mean developmental scores achieved on the motor and mental scales of the Bayley Scales of Infant Development (BSID)[24] showed no differences between the two groups. It was noted, however, that mean scores on the Mental Developmental Index for both cocaine-exposed and control infants were lower than the standardized norms, a finding the authors attributed to low socioeconomic status and related deprivation rather than prenatal exposure.

A group of adopted, cocaine-exposed children studied by Nulman *et al.*[25] were compared to an unexposed matched control of mother-child pairs. The researchers found that intrauterine exposure to cocaine resulted in a significantly smaller mean head circumference in the exposed children and an increased rate of microcephaly. Children prenatally exposed to cocaine also showed significant delays on both expressive and verbal comprehension tasks.

Through a longitudinal, prospective research study, our research group has followed a prenatal group of children whose mothers used cocaine and other drugs during pregnancy. Although significant growth impairment and neurobehavioral deficiencies were documented in the neonatal period,[2,3] long-term follow up consistently showed normal global cognitive development.[6,7] However, utilizing path analytic procedures to analyze the 3-year outcome of the children in the research cohort, the study showed that prenatal cocaine exposure had minimal direct influence on cognitive development as measured with the Stanford Binet,[26] but that home environment, as measured on the Home Screening Questionnaire, was the single most important predictor of cognitive development.[7] The study highlighted the multivariate nature of the effect of prenatal drug exposure and documented the relationships of the home environment to intellectual development of the child at 3 years of age.

Data from all these investigations raise two critical issues. First, currently published studies on cocaine/polydrug-exposed children generally concern cognitive outcome and lack comprehensive assessment of behavioral functioning. Second, current investigations do not include clear definitions of factors that potentially affect behavioral outcome, especially the family environment. Longitudinal research with other populations has shown that family functioning is a critical independent variable in the prediction of childhood behavioral outcome.[27] These studies have shown that family variables such as socioeconomic status, history of psychological problems, and number of adults in the household are significantly related to behavioral characteristics and school success in early and middle childhood.

The data presented in the current study demonstrate the multiple difficulties faced by children born into impoverished homes. Scores on the HSQ for both groups of families were well below accepted range indicating developmental support in the home, and both groups of women demonstrated similar levels of maternal psychopathology. The fact that 60% of the women who had used cocaine during pregnancy continued their substance use 6 years after delivery adds one more risk factor with the potential to impede the children's development.

Within the home environment, a correlation was found between the mother's continuing drug use and the child's IQ and behavioral problems at 6 years of age. In addition, maternal psychopathology correlated with behavior problems. On further analysis through path analytic techniques, prenatal cocaine/polydrug exposure did not have a direct effect on global cognitive functioning but a strong indirect effect as mediated through the home environment. This interaction of the biological factor, prenatal drug exposure, with environmental factors is an important point to make, documenting the need for early intervention programs to include intervention strategies for the mothers of high risk children as well as for the children themselves.

In contrast to the indirect influence of prenatal drug exposure on cognitive functioning, prenatal cocaine/polydrug exposure had a significant *direct* effect on the children's behavior at 4, 5, and 6 years of age. A significant number of the exposed children demonstrated clinically significant levels of behavior on one or more scales on the CBCL. This means that their caretaker reported a frequency of behavior at or above the 98th percentile when comparing their scores to others in their same age group. It is interesting that one of the neurobehavioral difficulties consistently documented in this and other populations of prenatally cocaine-exposed children at birth was a deficiency in state regulation capabilities.[2,3,21,22] Now, 6 years later, the children continue to demonstrate behaviors associated with regulatory difficulties, including difficulty managing impulses and frustration, as well as difficulty with tension regulation and arousal.

The findings in the present study are supported by our understanding of the pathophysiology of cocaine. Cocaine blocks the reuptake of the biogenic amines serotonin, dopamine, and norepinephrine,[28–30] in this way increasing the availability of these transmitters at the receptor sites and producing the cocaine "high" by increasing neuronal excitability. Over a period of chronic exposure, a dampening effect may be produced by downregulation of the postsynaptic dopaminergic receptors in the brain.[31] In studies of pregnant rat dams and fetuses, it was found that cocaine levels in the fetal brain are 109% to 151% those in the maternal blood.[32] The impact of exposure to such levels of cocaine during critical periods of early development could place the fetal central nervous system at risk for abnormal differentiation of key neurotransmitter systems, abnormal glial cell function, altered migrational events, and abnormal neuronal growth.[33–36] Recent studies in adult rats who were exposed to cocaine at the period of gestation comparable to the third trimester in human pregnancy demonstrated altered brain metabolism in the motor, limbic, and sensory systems, suggesting the possibility of long-term effects on central nervous system function in children exposed *in utero* to cocaine.[37]

The results of this study cannot be generalized to the overall population of children prenatally exposed to cocaine and other drugs. The pregnant women who voluntarily enrolled in our study were all heavy cocaine users and most used alcohol, tobacco, and marijuana in various combinations in addition to cocaine. Because we cannot isolate any of the findings to cocaine in particular but rather to the use of cocaine in conjunction with other substances, we utilized the term cocaine/polydrug to indicate polydrug exposure. However, this is the most frequent pattern of use in most substance-abusing populations, making the information applicable to a broad array of clinical situations.

The women in our study all were enrolled in an intensive treatment program and received comprehensive prenatal care. From the outset of the study, any of the children who demonstrated significant motor or language difficulties were referred for early intervention. If anything, their outcomes represent a "best case" scenario for prenatally exposed children living with their biological families.

In working with substance-abusing populations, the chaotic lifestyle interferes with long-term follow-up. The children who we retained in the study over the 6 years, however, are representative of the entire cohort, because their early neonatal and infant medical and developmental outcomes were similar to those of the children who we subsequently lost to follow-up.

This study helps us to understand the fragile interaction of biological and environmental factors affecting the cognitive and behavioral development of children prenatally exposed to cocaine and other drugs. In the early years of our research we hypothesized that mechanical insults via intrauterine hypoxia served as the basis for the difficulties exhibited by the cocaine-exposed infants. That hypothesis clearly does not address the larger picture, however, for it appears that the impact of prenatal cocaine exposure is more subtle an insult, occurring at the level of the neurotransmitters and perhaps affecting the organization of neuronal transmission from subcortical regions to higher cortical control areas. Home environment can positively influence overall cognitive development, but only through ongoing longitudinal studies will it be determined to what extent the cognitive and behavioral findings at 4–6 years of age are affected by ongoing environmental influences, especially the home and school settings.

REFERENCES

1. National Institute on Drug Abuse. 1994. National Pregnancy and Health Survey. Rockville, Maryland. U.S. Department of Health and Human Services.
2. Chasnoff, I.J., W.J. Burns, S.H. Schnoll & K.A. Burns. 1985. Cocaine use in pregnancy. N. Engl. J. Med. **313:** 666–669.
3. Chasnoff, I.J., D.R. Griffith, S. MacGregor *et al.* 1989. Temporal patterns of cocaine use in pregnancy. JAMA **161:** 1741–1744.
4. Chavez, G.F., J. Mulinare & J. Cordero. 1989. Maternal cocaine use during early pregnancy as a risk factor for congenital urogenital anomalies. JAMA **262:** 795–798.
5. Frank, D.A., H. Bauchner, S. Parker, A.M. Huber *et al.* 1990. Neonatal body proportionality and body composition after in-utero exposure to cocaine and marijuana. Pediatrics **117:** 622–626.
6. Chasnoff, I.J., D.R. Griffith, C. Freier & J. Murray. 1992. Cocaine/polydrug use in pregnancy: Two year follow-up. Pediatrics **89:** 284–289.
7. Azuma, S.D. & I.J. Chasnoff. 1993. Outcome of children prenatally exposed to cocaine and other drugs: A path analysis of three-year data. Pediatrics **92:** 396–402.
8. L.C. Mayes, M.H. Bornstein, K. Chawarska & R.H. Granger. 1995. Information processing and developmental assessments in 3-month-old infants exposed prenatally to cocaine. Pediatrics **95:** 539–545.
9. Hurt, H., N.L. Brodsky, L. Betancourt, L.E. Braitman *et al.* 1995. Cocaine-exposed children: Follow-up through 30 months. J. Sub. Abuse. **7:** 267–280.
10. Wechsler, D. 1989. WPPSI-R Manual. Western Psychological Services. Chicago, IL.
11. Achenbach, T.M. 1991. Manual for the Child Behavior Checklist and 1991 Profile. University of Vermont, Department of Psychiatry. Burlington, VT.
12. Coons, C.E., E.C. Gay, A.W. Fandal *et al.* 1981. The Home Screening Questionnaire Reference Manual. John F. Kennedy Child Development Center. Denver, CO.
13. Wechsler, D. 1991. WISC-III Manual. Western Psychological Services. Chicago, IL.
14. Jones, K.L., D.W. Smith, C.N. Ulleland & A.P. Streissguth. 1973. Pattern of malformation in offspring of chronic alcoholic mothers. Lancet **1:** 1267–1271.
15. Finnegan, L.P., J.F. Connaughton, R.E. Kron *et al.* 1975. Neonatal abstinence syndrome: Assessment and management. *In* Perinatal Addiction. R.D. Harbison, Ed.: 141–158. Spectrum Publications. New York, NY.
16. Fried, P.A. & B. Watkinson. 1990. 36- and 48-month neurobehavioral follow-up of children prenatally exposed to marijuana, cigarettes, and alcohol. Dev. Behav. Pediatr. **11:** 49–58.
17. Streissguth, A., P. Sampson & H. Barr. 1989. Neurobehavioral dose-response effects of prenatal alcohol exposure in humans from infancy to adulthood. Ann. N.Y. Acad. Sci. **562:** 145–158.
18. Zuckerman, B., D.A. Frank, R. Hingson *et al.* 1989. Effects of maternal marijuana and cocaine use on fetal growth. N. Engl. J. Med. **320:** 762–768.
19. Bingol, N., M. Fuchs, V. Diaz *et al.* 1987. Teratogenicity of cocaine in humans. J. Pediatr. **110:** 93–96.
20. Eisen, L.N., T.M. Field, E.S. Bandstra, J.P. Roberts *et al.* 1991. Perinatal cocaine effects

on neonatal stress behavior and performance on the Brazelton Scale. Pediatrics **88:** 477–480.

21. LESTER, B.M., M.J. CORWIN, C. SEPKOSKI *et al.* 1991. Neurobehavioral syndromes in cocaine-exposed newborn infants. Child Dev. **62:** 694–705.
22. SINGER, L.T., R. GARBER & R. KLIEGMAN. 1991. Neurobehavioral sequelae of fetal cocaine exposure. J. Pediatr. **119:** 667–672.
23. HOWARD, J., L. BECKWITH, C. RODNING *et al.* 1989. The development of young children of substance-abusing parents: Insights from seven years of intervention and research. Zero to Three **9:** 8–12.
24. BAYLEY, N. 1993. Bayley Scales of Infant Development. Second Edition. Psychological Corporation. New York, NY
25. NULMAN, I., J. D. ROVET, D. ALTMANN *et al.* 1995. Neurodevelopment of adopted children exposed in utero to cocaine. J. Dev. Behav. Pediatr. **16:** 418–424.
26. THORNDIKE, R.L., E.P. HAGEN & J.M. SATTLER. 1986. Stanford-Binet Intelligence Scale. 4th Edition. Riverside Publishing Co. Chicago, IL.
27. STANGER, C., S. MCCONAUGHYM & T. ACHENBACH. 1992. Three year course of behavioral/emotional problems in a national sample of 4- to 16-year olds. II. Predictors of syndromes. J. Am. Acad. Child Adolesc. Psychiatry **31:** 941–950.
28. FRIEDMAN, E., S. GERSHON & J. ROTROSEN. 1975. Effects of acute cocaine treatment on the turnover of 5-hydroxytryptamine in the rat brain. Br. J Pharmacol. **54:** 61–64.
29. KOMISKEY, H.L., D.D. MILLER, J. B. LAPIDUS *et al.* 1977. The isomers of cocaine and tropacocaine: Effect on 3H catecholamine uptake by rat brain synaptosomes. Life Sci. **21:** 1117–1122.
30. PITTS, D.K. & J. MARWAH. 1987. Cocaine modulation of central monoaminenergic neurotransmission. Pharmacol. Biochem. Behav. **26:** 453–461.
31. SPEAR, L.P., C.L. KIRSTEIN & N.A. FRAMBES. 1989. Cocaine effects on the developing central nervous system: Behavioral psychopharmacological and neurochemical studies. Ann. N.Y. Acad. Sci. **56:** 290–307.
32. WIGGINS, R.C., C. ROLSTEN, B.V. RUIZ *et al.* 1989. Pharmacokinetics of cocaine: Basic studies of route, dosage, pregnancy and lactation. Neurotoxicology **10:** 367–382.
33. COYLE, J.T. & D. HENRY. 1973. Catecholamines in fetal and newborn rat brain. J. Neurol. **21:** 61–67.
34. LAUDER, J.M. & F.E. BLOOM. 1974. Ontogeny of monoamine neurons in the locus coeruleus, raphe nuclei and substantia nigra of the rat. I. Cell differentiation. J. Comp. Neurol. **155:** 469–482.
35. LANIER, L.P., A.J. DUNN & C. VANHARTESVELDT. 1976. Development of neurotransmitters and their function in brain. Rev. Neurosci. **2:** 195–256.
36. JOHNSTON, M.V. & F.S. SILVERSTEIN. 1986. New insights into mechanisms of neuronal damage in the developing brain. Pediatr. Neurosci. **12:** 87–89.
37. DOW-EDWARDS, D.L. 1989. Long-term neurochemical and neurobehavioral consequences of cocaine use during pregnancy. Ann. N.Y. Acad. Sci. **562:** 280–289.

Prevention and Treatment Issues for Pregnant Cocaine-Dependent Women and Their Infants

KAROL KALTENBACH[a,c] AND LORETTA FINNEGAN[b]

[a]*Maternal Addiction Treatment Education and Research, Department of Pediatrics, 1201 Chestnut St. 9th Fl., Philadelphia, Pennsylvania 19107, USA*

[b]*Women's Health Initiative, National Institutes of Health, Federal Building, Room 6A09, 7550 Wisconsin Avenue, Bethesda, Maryland 20892, USA*

ABSTRACT: The increase in cocaine use among pregnant women has created significant challenges for treatment providers. Drug-dependent women tend to neglect general health and prenatal care. Perinatal management is often difficult due to medical, obstetrical, and psychiatric complications. Research has demonstrated that comprehensive care, including high risk obstetrical care, psychosocial services, and addiction treatment can reduce complications associated with perinatal substance abuse. Research investigating the effectiveness of residential and outpatient treatment for pregnant cocaine-dependent women also suggests that many biopsychosocial characteristics and issues influence treatment outcomes. Homelessness and psychiatric illness require a more intensive level of care, and abstinence is difficult to maintain for many women in outpatient treatment as they continue to live in drug-using environments. To optimize the benefit of comprehensive services, services should be provided within a multilevel model of substance abuse treatment including long- and short-term residential, intensive outpatient, and outpatient settings.

INTRODUCTION

The prevalence of cocaine abuse among pregnant and parenting women presents a major health care problem in general and a tremendous challenge to substance abuse treatment providers in particular. In recent years the number of cocaine-abusing clients admitted to publicly funded drug treatment programs has risen dramatically.[1] The 1992 National Pregnancy and Health Survey[2] on drug use during pregnancy found that 1.1% of pregnant women used cocaine during their pregnancy. Of the 5.5% of pregnant women who used an illicit drug during pregnancy, cocaine use was second only to marijuana.

TREATMENT ISSUES

Meeting the needs of pregnant substance-abusing women is especially challenging as drug-dependent women tend to neglect their general health and are often noncompliant with prenatal care. The threat of involvement with legal and child protection authorities, often with punitive outcomes, keeps many drug-dependent women from seeking prenatal care. Perinatal management is difficult due to medical, obstetric, and psychiatric complications, and failure of substance-abusing women to receive comprehensive health care during pregnancy is a known cause of increased morbidity and mortality in both mother and infant.[3] Many medical complications, including anemia, bac-

[c] Phone, 215/955–4068; fax, 215/568–6414; e-mail, kaltenb1@jeflin.tju.edu

teremia/septicemia, cardiac disease, cellulitis, depression, diabetes, edema, hepatitis B and C, TB, hypertension, phlebitis, STDs, urinary tract infections, and vitamin deficiency compromise many drug-involved pregnancies.[3] Obstetrical complications associated with substance abuse, such as abruptio placentae, placenta previa, intrauterine death, spontaneous abortion, premature labor and delivery, premature rupture of membranes, and intrauterine growth retardation, are also a threat to both mother and fetus. In addition, the lives of many substance-abusing women are chaotic and involve multiple factors that may adversely affect their health and well-being as well as the health and well-being of their infants. These include poverty, homelessness or inadequate housing, lack of education, domestic violence, and social and emotional problems. A large percentage are single heads of households, have less than a high school education, and are progeny of substance-abusing parents.[4,5] Drug-dependent women have experienced a high incidence of physical abuse, childhood rape, and sexual molestation[4,6–8] and a majority also have moderate to severe depression.[4,5,8,9]

The recognition that substance-abusing women have special needs has led to the development of gender-specific treatment models.[10–12] One model developed at Jefferson Medical College of Thomas Jefferson University reflects a multisystems approach designed to provide medical and psychosocial outpatient services to drug-dependent pregnant women.[13]

In this model, treatment is organized into four service components (FIG. 1). Comprehensive medical services include a prenatal clinic staffed by physicians specifically trained in the field of maternal addiction and high risk pregnancy. In addition, a perinatal nurse facilitates the provision of general health care guidance and the prevention of STDs and coordinates educational programs that address health concerns during pregnancy as well as nutritional counseling and family planning. An HIV counselor provides HIV counseling and testing. Methadone maintenance is provided to opioid-dependent women. A psychiatrist evaluates all patients and provides services to those women with dual diagnoses.

Intensive psychosocial counseling services are provided by master level professionals trained in social work, psychology, or addictions counseling. Treatment aims are directed at reducing/eliminating substance abuse, developing resources, improving family and interpersonal relationships, and reducing/eliminating socially destructive behavior.

A clothing bank and a small food bank are available to patients. Tokens are provided for transportation if needed, and patients are linked with agencies that assist in providing shelter living space and vouchers for more permanent housing. Treatment approaches are modified and the staff are culturally and racially diverse in order to respond to gender-, race-, and culture-specific issues.

Parent/child services are provided to reduce the intergenerational transmission of substance abuse and the incidence of child abuse and neglect to children of drug-dependent women. A Parent Child Center, staffed by early childhood specialists, provides developmental classes for infant, toddlers, and preschoolers to promote the children's development and to demonstrate appropriate nurturing and play strategies with children. Consultation is available to parents concerning child behavior and management techniques. Parent/child play group sessions are organized to stimulate positive interaction and mutual enjoyment of play between mother and child. Parent education groups which focus on the basic tenets of growth and development are conducted. The Center also provides childcare during group and individual counseling sessions as needed.

This outpatient model has been most successful in reducing both maternal and infant morbidity associated with pregnancies complicated by opioid dependence.[14,15] However, given the lack of an effective pharmacological agent in the treatment of co-

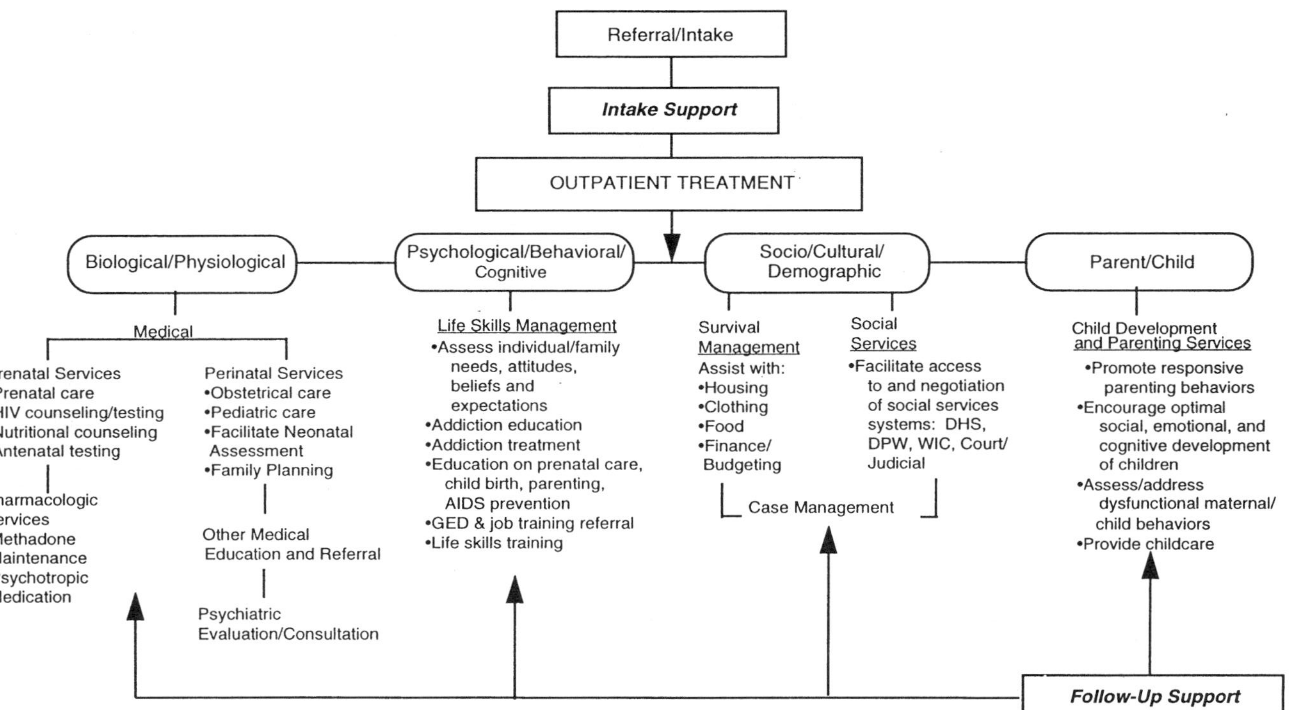

FIGURE 1. Family center treatment model for drug-dependent pregnant and parenting women and their children. Reprinted with permission from Kaltenbach & Comfort.[23]

caine dependence, many women require more intensive treatment to begin and sustain recovery than can be offered in an outpatient setting. The difficulty in engaging pregnant and parenting cocaine-dependent women in treatment, poor compliance and retention among those who seek treatment, and a dearth of residential treatment facilities for women and their children led to federal initiatives under the National Institute on Drug Abuse (NIDA), Center for Substance Abuse Prevention (CSAP), and the Center for Substance Abuse Treatment (CSAT) to support the development of residential treatment services for pregnant and parenting substance-abusing women and their children.

Although research investigating the effectiveness of residential and outpatient treatment for pregnant cocaine-dependent women is limited, the available evidence suggests that a number of biopsychosocial characteristics and issues influence treatment utilization and outcomes. An important mediating factor in the utilization of residential treatment is the need for immediate housing. In one study, only 38% of phone referrals appeared in person to enroll in treatment. Telephone inquiries focused on availability of housing as much as, if not more than, treatment needs. Of the 38% assessed for intake (99 women), 69% requested residential services. Twenty-four of 35 women who did not complete the intake process requested residential placement.[16] Within the sample of women enrolled in treatment ($n = 64$), more women in residential treatment were homeless in the last 3 years and/or dissatisfied with their housing accommodations.[17] A study by Haller *et al.*[18] indicated that the provision of transition housing was a critical factor in retention in a day treatment program among a sample of poly-substance-abusing women, the majority for whom cocaine was the primary drug of abuse. Women who lived in the community were 6.125 times more likely ($p < 0.0001$) to drop out of treatment than were those who lived in the program's shelter. Similarly, Chavkin *et al.*[19] found that safe shelter was identified as a top priority for women's treatment services in a sample of inner city pregnant and parenting cocaine-dependent women.

Psychiatric comorbidity has also been identified as an important factor in treating cocaine-dependent women. Women utilizing residential treatment have more total psychiatric symptoms and suffer more from depression than do women enrolled in outpatient treatment.[17] Women who engage in intensive outpatient treatment also have a higher incidence of psychopathology than do women who reject such treatment.[20] However, among women who were in treatment, Killeen *et al.*[8] found lower rates of Axis II psychopathology among pregnant cocaine-dependent women who were treatment compliers than treatment noncompliers.

Since length of time in treatment has consistently been related to positive outcomes,[21,22] it is important to identify patterns of treatment retention that may be specific for pregnant drug-dependent women. Although Comfort and Kaltenbach[17] found no difference in the total number of months that residential and outpatient women participated in treatment, two critical periods were identified. First, approximately 30% of both outpatient and residential patients left treatment before delivery. These statistics represent not only a "treatment dropout" but also a high risk pregnant woman who very likely will not continue to receive the prenatal care and other medical and/or psychiatric services she may need. Therefore, pregnant cocaine-dependent women may require targeted assistance during the first few months of treatment to ensure engagement in treatment and participation in medical/obstetric care critical to the healthy outcome of both mother and infant. Second, differences were found between groups in the rates of dropout during the early postpartum period. Twice as many outpatients (31%) as residential patients (16%) left treatment within 2 months postpartum. The reasons for this difference are unclear. It is possible the women in residential treatment were in greater need of treatment, had greater motivation to remain in treatment, and/or were more engaged in treatment. It is also possible that the birth of a healthy infant represented a "treatment success" for women attending outpatient treatment. For some women, a successful infant outcome may negate other reasons for treatment participation. Clearly, these findings have important implications if treatment programs are to be successful in matching patients to the most appropriate level of care and in retaining patients for whatever time is necessary to be effective.

Few data are available to help determine whether residential treatment is more effective than outpatient treatment in improving the health of pregnant cocaine-dependent women and their children. In a study that compared outcomes of pregnant cocaine-dependent women enrolled in residential and outpatient treatment,[17] less than half the women receiving outpatient treatment (47%) were successful in remaining abstinent during the entire course of treatment as compared to 94% of the women receiving residential treatment. Although the two programs differed in their drug use policy (i.e., drug use was a reason for discharge in the residential program; drug use was not a reason for discharge in the outpatient program if a women showed signs of commitment to and progress in treatment), no women enrolled in the residential program were discharged for drug use. Residential treatment may be a necessary option to assist some women living in adverse environments to accomplish and maintain abstinence during pregnancy.

Unfortunately, studies pertaining to neonatal outcomes of cocaine-exposed infants provide relatively no information on treatment effects (i.e., infants born to cocaine-dependent women who received comprehensive treatment services during their pregnancy). In a review of 359 articles published between 1993 and September 1997 reporting on the effects of cocaine use during pregnancy, less than .01% evaluated the outcome of infants in relation to their mother's participation in treatment services. Comfort and Kaltenbach[17] found no differences in birth outcomes among infants born to mothers participating in residential or outpatient treatment. Eighty-five percent of the infants were full term. Means for birthweight, gestational age, head circumference, and body length were similar between groups with the birthweights for both groups >3,000 g. The incidences of preterm birth and low birth weight for the infants in this study compare favorably to the 1994 national norms in the general population. The most meaningful difference in birth outcomes related to treatment modality was in discharge custody. All infants born to women in residential treatment were discharged to their mothers, whereas only 81% of infants born to women in outpatient treatment were discharged to their mothers.

SUMMARY

Data suggest that comprehensive treatment services for cocaine-dependent pregnant women can reduce the perinatal morbidity associated with prenatal cocaine abuse. Moreover, shorter length of hospital stays for newborns and less need for neonatal intensive care, foster care, and child protective services elucidate the critical role treatment services play in effective prevention efforts. Variable patterns of retention suggest that (1) further research is needed to clarify how maternal characteristics influence treatment outcome and (2) a model of comprehensive services is necessary but not sufficient. Services must be provided within a multilevel of substance abuse treatment including long- and short-term residential, intensive outpatient, and outpatient settings. It is also critical that longitudinal studies be conducted on the outcome of infants born to cocaine-dependent women who receive comprehensive treatment services in order to identify effective child intervention strategies within treatment services.

REFERENCES

1. Substance Abuse and Mental Health Services Administration. 1995. Substance Abuse and Mental Health Statistics Sourcebook. DHHS Pub. No. (SMA) 95-3064. Department of Health and Human Services. Rockville, MD.
2. NIDA. 1996. National Pregnancy & Health Survey: Drug Use Among Women Delivering Livebirths: 1992. NIH Pub. No. 96-3819. Department of Health and Human Services. Rockville, MD.
3. Finnegan, L.P. & S.R. Kandall. 1992. Maternal and neonatal effects of alcohol and drugs. *In* Substance Abuse, A Comprehensive Textbook. J.H. Lowinson, P. Ruiz & R.B. Millman, Eds.: 628–656. Williams & Wilkins. Baltimore, MD.
4. Comfort, M.L. & K. Kaltenbach. 1996. Longitudinal outcomes for pregnant and parenting women in substance abuse treatment. Presented at the American Psychological Association Women's Health Conference. Washington DC, Sept 19–21, 1996.
5. Haller, D.L., J.S. Knisely, M.S. Dawson & S. Schnoll. 1993. Perinatal substance abusers: Psychological and social characteristics. J. Nerv. Ment. Dis. **81:** 509–513.
6. DePetrillo, P.B. & J.M. Rice. 1995. Methadone dosing during pregnancy: Impact on program compliance. Int. J. Addict. **30:** 207–217.
7. Hagan, T. 1988. A retrospective search for the etiology of drug abuse: A background comparison of a drug-addicted population of women and a control group of non-addicted women. NIDA Res. Monogr. **81:** 254–261.
8. Killeen, T.K., K.T. Brady & A. Thevos. 1995. Addiction severity, psychopathology and treatment compliance in cocaine-dependent mothers. J. Addict. Dis. **14:** 75–84.
9. Hoegerman, G. & S. Schnoll. 1991. Narcotic use in pregnancy. Clin. Perinatol. **18:** 51–76.
10. Beschner, G.M., B.G. Reed & J. Mondanaro Eds. 1981; 1982. Treatment Services for Drug Dependent Women. Vols. 1–2. US Department of Health and Human Services. Rockville, MD.
11. Nelson-Zlupko, L., E. Kauffman & M.M. Dore. 1995. Gender differences in drug addiction and treatment: Implications for social work intervention with substance abusing women. Social Work. **40:** 45–54.
12. Zankowski, G.L. 1987. Responsive programming: Meeting the needs of chemically dependent women. Alcohol Treatment Q. **4:** 53–65.
13. Finnegan, L.P., T. Hagan & K. Kaltenbach. 1991. Scientific foundation of clinical opiate use in pregnant women. Bull. N.Y. Acad. Med. **67:** 223–239.
14. Connaughton, J.F., D.S. Reeser, J. Schut & L.P. Finnegan. 1997. Perinatal addiction: Outcome and management. Am. J. Obstet. Gynecol. **129:** 679–685.
15. Kaltenbach, K. & L.P. Finnegan. 1989. Prenatal narcotic exposure: Perinatal and developmental effects. Neurotoxicology **10:** 597–604.
16. Kaltenbach, K., M.L. Comfort & S. Balis. 1994. Cocaine, Pregnancy and Progeny Project: Treatment and Evaluation. Final Report. #5R18 DA06363, NIDA. Rockville, MD.
17. Comfort, M. & K. Kaltenbach. 1997. Biopsychosocial characteristics and treatment outcomes of pregnant cocaine dependent women in residential and outpatient substance treatment. In press.
18. Haller, D.L., J.S. Knisely, R.K. Elswick, K.S. Dawson & S. Schnoll. 1997. Perinatal substance abusers: Factors influencing treatment retention. J. Subst. Abuse Treat. In press.
19. Chavkin, W., D. Paone, P. Friedman & I. Wilets. 1993. Reframing the debate: Toward effective treatment for inner city drug-abusing mothers. Bull. N.Y. Acad. Med. **70:** 50–68.
20. Ingersoll K., D. Haller & K. Dawson. 1996. Psychological differences between perinatal substance abuse treatment acceptors and rejectors. NIDA Res. Monogr. **162:** 257.
21. Hubbard, R.L., M.E. Marsden, J.V. Rachel, H.J. Harwood, E.R. Cavanaugh & H.M. Ginzburg. 1989. Drug Abuse Treatment: A National Study of Effectiveness. University of North Carolina Press. Chapel Hill, NC.
22. Simpson, D.D. 1981. Treatment for drug abuse: Follow-up outcomes and length of time spent. Arch. Gen. Psychiatry **38:** 875–880.
23. Kaltenbach, K & M.L. Comfort. 1996. Comprehensive treatment for pregnant substance-abusing women: An enhanced model to address multiple health and human service needs. Final Report, Center for Substance Abuse Treatment.

Policies towards Pregnancy and Addiction

Sticks without Carrots

WENDY CHAVKIN,[a,c] PAUL H. WISE,[b] AND DEBORAH ELMAN[a]

[a]*Columbia University, Center for Population and Family Health, New York, New York 10032, USA*

[b] *Department of Pediatrics, Boston University School of Medicine, Boston, Massachusetts, USA*

ABSTRACT: Throughout this century in the United States, tension has existed between those who believe drug abuse is best combatted through the criminal justice system and those who emphasize a medical/public health model of prevention and treatment. In the last decade this debate has centered around the person of the pregnant addict. The former have construed her addiction as willful harm to the fetus punishable on criminal and child abuse grounds. The latter have countered that pregnancy is a moment of increased motivation for treatment and focused on expansion and improvement of treatment options. Both managed care and welfare reform have exacerbated conditions between these opposing policy approaches. The addicted woman is increasingly caught between policies that punish her drug use without options for overcoming addiction.

INTRODUCTION

Policy, by definition, is dependent on social context. In the dozen years that *in utero* cocaine exposure has had star billing, the context has changed in several dramatic ways. The crack epidemic of the mid-1980s differed from preceding drug waves in the high level of involvement of young women, many of whom were mothers.[1,2] Social consternation about this development centered on the consequences for young children and then shifted to the fetus. The construction of the fetus as the central protagonist marks a significant shift in social perception. Some have attributed this phenomenon to the development of perinatal medicine, heroic neonatal interventions, and technologies such as ultrasound and *in utero* surgery associated with constructs such as the "fetus as patient."[3] Others have emphasized the role of the antiabortion movement. In efforts to legally constrain the availability of abortion and affect its public acceptability, this movement has both stressed fetal personhood and concurrently characterized pregnant women as so selfish that their indifference to fetal welfare must be constrained by outside intervention.[4]

POLICY EVOLUTION

The 1980s then witnessed two parallel policy responses towards crack use by women. One reiterated the points made a decade earlier by treatment pioneers such as Loretta Finnegan, Richard Brotman, and Beth Reed who had both described the inadequacies of prevailing drug treatment programs for women and established models that re-

[c]Address for correspondence: Wendy Chavkin, MD, MPH, Professor of Clinical Public Health, Columbia University, Center for Population and Family Health, 60 Haven Ave., B-3, New York, NY 10032. Phone, 212/304-5220; fax, 212/304-5609.

dressed these gaps by incorporating reproductive health care, therapy for past abuse, and concern for relationships with children.[5–7] The other approach involved sanctions—within both the criminal justice and child protective systems—for the new construct of harming a fetus by using drugs when pregnant. Many of those advocating penalties claimed that these sanctions served as sticks to propel drug users into the carrot of treatment.[8] Opponents of sanctions argued that such an approach had grave implications for the social status of women and that it was likely to be ineffective, as treatment programs not only were sparse and inadequate, but also indeed often categorically excluded pregnant women.[9] We confirmed this in 1987 by showing that most New York City treatment programs refused to admit pregnant women.[10] It is important to underscore that although the two sides differed on critical issues such as the nature of addiction, autonomy of the pregnant woman, status of the fetus, and utility of punitive measures, they concurred that treatment was an essential component of the social response.

On the federal level, this consensus translated into funding for treatment and treatment-oriented research. In 1988, Congress mandated that states (1) increase from 5% to 10% the portion of the block grant budget "set-aside" for the treatment of pregnant women and women with children, (2) give pregnant women priority enrollment in treatment as well as specific services such as prenatal care and child care, and (3) establish demonstration treatment programs for drug-using women.[11]

DEVOLUTION TO THE STATES

We conducted surveys of Directors of Substance Abuse (SAS) and Child Protective Services (CPS) from all 50 states in 1992 and again in 1995.[12,13] The Congressional elections in 1994, ensuing budget cuts, and devolution of budgetary and regulatory authority to the states led to a marked shift regarding drug users and treatment. State Directors of both services indicated that there had initially been a move to increase services for pregnant women and women with children. Most SAS Directors reported that their states had begun or expanded treatment for pregnant women and mothers. CPS Directors described renewed emphasis on family preservation and heightened standards of care. These State Directors attributed both trends to increased Federal funding and Federally imposed standards of care.

At the same time as services available to substance-using pregnant and parenting women expanded, a dramatic shift occurred towards Medicaid-managed care in the provision of these services. This, in turn, had consequences for women's choices regarding drug treatment. By 1995, state-by-state, the majority were in the process of converting to Medicaid-managed care. Twenty-five states had implemented waivers, and waivers were pending in another 22 states. These waivers from previously universal Federal regulations permitted states to bypass freedom-of-choice provisions that had been intended to safeguard Medicaid enrollees' choice of providers or permitted states to mandate enrollment in managed care plans while altering the benefit package they offered.[14] Four SAS Directors reported that the waivers would reduce funding and eligibility for programs for women.

Many of the Medicaid waivers were linked with eligibility for other services. Some states mandated that recipients of Aid to Families with Dependent Children participate in managed care; others required women to remain in drug treatment in order to receive social security and Medicaid. Yet, 33 CPS Directors were completely unfamiliar with Medicaid waivers, and many could not explain how the waivers were related to changing welfare policies. Some explained that even when drug treatment was court ordered, managed care may not have covered the mandated treatment.

Furthermore, Directors reported conflicting trends in funding and oversight. As previously mentioned, federal funding for substance abuse services had initially increased in 18 states. Ten SAS Directors described heightened federally imposed standards of care in conjunction with increased funding. More than half the CPS Directors reported increases in funding or more rigorous standards of care. Conversely, these state Directors reported that most recently, states had assumed control of services with reduced local funding. About one third of SAS Directors reported recently increased local control coupled with reductions in local funding. Similarly, six CPS Directors reported decreased funding, and 15 reported increased local control of child protective services.

Concurrently, state intervention against pregnant drug users had increased dramatically from our previous survey in 1992. Respondents from 34 states reported that cases of criminal prosecution for using drugs when pregnant had transpired in their states, an increase of 12 states since 1992. Reporting positive toxicology results had increased significantly and was widespread. In 1995, eight states required mandatory reporting of positive maternal toxicology results to Child Protection authorities (cf., one in 1992), and almost two thirds of states described this to be actual practice. Ten states mandated that positive newborn toxicology results be reported to the criminal justice system (significantly more than the three that did so in 1992), and almost two thirds of states reported positive newborn toxicology results to the Child Protective Service or Department of Health. Approximately a quarter of the states reported that pregnant drug users and mothers were mandated to treatment.

WELFARE REFORM AND DRUG-USING MOTHERS

The Personal Responsibility and Work Reconciliation Act of 1996 (PRWRA) ended standard entitlement and most regulatory oversight of traditional welfare mechanisms in the United States. Paralleling what I have just described in the treatment context, federal regulations had been both the major conduit for societal resources and the major protection for the reproductive autonomy of childbearing women. The devolution of responsibility to the states means that they will develop their own welfare programs with state-specific eligibility and benefit mechanisms.

The PRWRA subjects families formerly eligible for welfare to 5-year lifetime limits on benefits, strict work requirements, and a host of potential sanctions. Certain groups, such as immigrants and those with drug-related felony convictions, are not eligible; however, states can opt out of these exclusions. Thirty-five states will deny Temporary Assistance to Needy Families (TANF) to drug felons; 18 plan to opt out of this provision. The new law will also allow states to test TANF applicants for drug use; seven states plan to test under specified circumstances.[15] Medicaid eligibility has been decoupled from eligibility for TANF. States will have great latitude in designing their own programs with block grant monies. Each state will receive a capped amount based on 1994 funding levels.[16]

The profound changes occurring in the structure of welfare and health care strike directly at the relationship between women's and children's interests. The "end of welfare as we know it" and the rapid implementation of managed care in both public and private health insurance systems together represent a historic shift in how human services are to be delivered in the United States. The public debate and the structure of the revised programs will both reflect the way in which women's and children's interests are framed. These new state programs will be vulnerable to impulses to functionally separate the interests of children from those of their mothers by compelling women to act in accordance with specific reproductive and parenting behaviors and then providing a "safety net" of benefits that is confined to children alone.

This "irresponsible mother," be she drug addicted, a teen, a welfare recipient, unmarried, or HIV infected, has become a familiar icon in American political discourse and a common target of newly adopted welfare regulations. Eligibility criteria exclude teen mothers who do not live at home and women who do not use prenatal care or obtain the recommended battery of immunizations for their children. Benefit caps prohibit benefits to any child born to a woman already receiving welfare. The work requirement and time limits pertain even during the third trimester of pregnancy and the newborn period.

Certain provisions of these new rules will particularly affect drug-using mothers. Research by the Urban Institute and others has documented that a significant proportion of the TANF population, an estimated 15–20%, have drug problems severe enough to impair their ability to work.[17,18] The Substance Abuse and Mental Health Services Administration has also reported that drug treatment improves employability.[19] As previously described, drug treatment for this population, even when universally endorsed, has been inadequate in quantity and quality. Many treatment programs rely on money from the drug and alcohol treatment block grants and Medicaid reimbursement, and residential programs depend on the public assistance benefits and food stamps to pay for room and board of those in their care. Reductions in these block grants as well as ineligibility for benefits resulting from sanctions will cut the funds available for treatment programs and this may further shrink the treatment system.

How do state health and welfare programs shape eligibility and benefit mechanisms to separate or integrate children's and women's concerns? Specifically, is maternal eligibility conditioned upon compliance with specified maternal behaviors (prenatal carefare, shotfare, learnfare, family cap, etc)? Do children remain eligible if the mother is not or if she has been sanctioned for noncompliance? Are TANF, Medicaid, and CPS authorities aware of the implications of their own agency's policies for the other agencies; for example, does involvement with CPS render women ineligible for TANF and thus Medicaid? If women are under CPS supervision because of positive drug toxicology at delivery, will Medicaid managed care cover drug treatment? Will this render her ineligible for TANF and thus unable to demonstrate to CPS that she has sufficient resources to care for her baby?

An important step is for those responsible for TANF and those responsible for drug treatment to plan jointly. The service gaps and policy contradictions need to be addressed. For example, TANF regulations exclude all those with felony convictions, and they sanction parole and probation violators.[15] How might a drug-addicted woman ineligible for TANF because of a prior drug felony or sanctioned because of a dirty urine specimen while in treatment proceed down the road to self-sufficiency without benefits and without treatment? Even if she is covered by a Medicaid managed care plan that covers drug treatment, what happens if she lives in a state where the block grant-funded treatment has no openings.

CONCLUSION

The welfare debate has been characterized by a striking disjuncture between a symbolic focus on women and a programmatic absence of interest in them. Even those advocating for the poor or evaluating the impact of the repeal of entitlements have not confronted this contradiction. Yet, welfare policies punish the sexual and reproductive activities of poor women and then construe the resulting poverty of children to be their mothers' fault. Welfare policies and practices attempt to dramatically alter the reproductive, parenting, and economic behaviors of poor women while simultaneously asserting concern for the "innocent children" who will now face poverty without public assistance. This has led to programmatic contradictions and to tensions between advocates for women and for children. These policies will have consequences for children's health, for women's health, and for the public health of the community.

Changes in the social role of women over the last several decades have sparked advocacy for reproductive autonomy, economic opportunity, and recognition of women's health needs. Reformist groups in the United States have long been concerned with the health and well-being of children and have increasingly focused on children alone such as income and nutritional support for young children, child protection, education, and early health and developmental services.[20] This divergence serves neither women nor children well. Constructive revision of welfare policy in the United States requires an alliance between those concerned with the health and rights of women and those concerned with the health and well-being of children.

REFERENCES

1. Chasnoff, I.J., W.J. Burns, S.H. Schnoll & K.A. Burns. 1985. Cocaine use in pregnancy. N. Engl. J. Med. **313:** 666–669.
2. United States General Accounting Office. Drug exposed infants: A generation at risk: Report to the chairman. Washington, DC. Committee on Finance, US Senate, June 1990.
3. Callahan, D. 1986. How technology is reframing the abortion debate. Hastings Center Report. February: 33–43.
4. King, P.A. 1991. Helping women helping children: Drug policy and future generations. Milbank Q. **69:** 595–621.
5. Finnegan, L.P. (Ed). 1978. Drug dependence in pregnancy: Clinical management of mother and child. National Institute on Drug Abuse, Service Research Branch, Rockville, MD. Government Printing Office. Washington, DC.
6. Reed, B. & R. Moise. 1980. Implications for treatment and future research in addicted women. *In* Family Dynamics, Self-Perception, and Support System. National Institute on Drug Abuse, DHEW Pub No. (ADM) 80-762:114–130. Government Printing Office. Washington, DC.
7. Suffet, F. & R. Brotman. 1984. A comprehensive care program for pregnant addicts: Obstetrical, neonatal, and child development outcomes. Int. J. Addict. **19:** 199–219.
8. Horger, E., S. Brown & C. Condon. 1990. Cocaine in pregnancy: Confronting the problem. J. South Carolina Med. Assoc. **86:** 527–531.
9. Chavkin, W. 1990. Drug addiction and pregnancy: Policy crossroads. Am. J. Pub. Health **45:** 55–57.
10. Breitbart, V., W. Chavkin & P. Wise. 1994. The accessibility of drug treatment for pregnant women: A survey in five cities. Am. J. Pub. Health **84:** 1658–1661.
11. United States General Accounting Office. ADMS Block Grant: Drug Treatment Services Could Be Improved by New Accountability Program. Report to Chairman, Select Committee on Narcotics Abuse and Control, House of Representatives, 1991.
12. Chavkin, W., V. Breitbart & P. Wise. 1995. Efforts to reduce perinatal mortality, HIV, and drug addiction: Survey of the states. JAMWA **50:** 164–166.
13. Chavkin, W., V. Breitbart, D. Elman & P. Wise. 1998. National survey of the states: Policies and practices regarding drug-using pregnant women. Am. J. Pub. Health. **88:** 117–119.
14. Gold, R.B. & C.L. Richards. 1996. Improving the fit: Reproductive health services in managed care settings. Alan Guttmacher Institute. Washington, DC.
15. 1997. National Governors' Association Center for Best Practices: Summary of Selected Elements of State Plans for Temporary Assistance for Needy Families. National Governors' Association. Washington, DC.
16. P.L. 104–193 Personal Responsibility and Work Opportunity Reconciliation Act of 1996.
17. Pavetti, L., K. Olson, N. Pindus & M. Pernas. 1996. Designing welfare-to-work programs for families facing personal or family challenges: Lessons from the field. The Urban Institute. Washington, DC.

18. U.S. Department of Health and Human Services. 1994. Patterns of substance abuse and substance-related impairment among participants in the Aid to Families with Dependent Children Program. U.S. Department of Health and Human Services. Washington, DC.
19. YOUNG, N.K. 1996. Alcohol and other drug treatment: Policy choices in welfare reform. Substance Abuse and Mental Health Services Administration, Center for Substance Abuse Treatment. Rockville, MD.
20. D'EMILIO, J. & E.B. FREEDMAN. 1989. Intimate matters: A history of sexuality in America. Harper and Row. New York.

Round Table 5. Nature-Nurture Issues

Moderator: JOSEPH COYLE
Panelists: BARRY M. LESTER, GIDEON KOREN, IRA J. CHASNOFF, KAROL KALTENBACH
Discussants: BERNARD KARMEL (*Staten Island*), NAIMAH WEINBERG (NIDA), ABIGAIL SNYDER-KELLER (*Albany*), LINDA WRIGHT (NICHD), DEBBIE LUBIN (UNC), VINCE SMERIGLIO (NIDA), DEBORAH FRANK (*Boston*)

JOSEPH COYLE: To start this round table discussion, I might try to stir the pot a little bit. What has been extremely powerful about this conference is the melding of basic scientists with clinical researchers. My background is more in the basic sciences, and I think we know a great deal now about the molecular mechanisms of action of a number of these substances of abuse in the developing brain. It's quite clear that they interact with receptors that in the adult brain are involved in the euphoric effect and reinforcing effects of the drugs. But in the developing brain they may play a very important role in modulating neuronal differentiation. At the same time, when you walk out of the laboratory into the urban environment, it is extremely difficult to carry out the type of controlled studies you can in the laboratory. There is increasing resonance between what is being found in the experimental animal and what is being observed in the very complicated real world situation.

It seems to me that an extremely important outcome of science is not just knowledge, but knowledge that can be used to shape policy. In recent years, there has been increasing concern about the impact of knowledge and how that knowledge could be used both positively and negatively against individuals who may be at risk. The negative consequences, of course, could be stigma. On the other hand, in the absence of knowledge or denial of knowledge, there can be a significant negative impact in terms of not informing people about behaviors that put them at risk, undermining the ability to carry out preventive interventions, and finally, justifying state and national government support for postnatal treatment programs for those at risk if the perception is that there is no risk.

If the product of this conference is to be informative, I was a little bit concerned about the recent article in the *Washington Post,* one of the newspapers of record in the United States, which reported on this conference stating that, "Crack Baby Fears May Have Been Overstated: Children of Cocaine-Abusing Mothers Are No Worse Off Than Others in Urban Poverty." With that I'd like to open the discussion.

BERNARD KARMEL: Can the panel address the following issue, which you just raised? Should we be using a deviant approach as opposed to a discriminant approach in assessing the effect of cocaine on the outcome of a child? The particular tests that we tend to use, such as global IQ, are essentially tests that have been normed. Essentially, they've gone out and determined that this is what the average population does. Deviation from that is defined as abnormal. This contrasts with an approach in which one takes the particular things that may go abnormal and does a discriminative analysis against a criterion population, a normal versus a criterion group (i.e., you use two groups rather than one to define a difference as opposed to a deviant from one group to define a difference). If you just use a deviant from normal, for instance, you may find you're measuring the wrong things. For instance, the IQ may be measuring the effects of poverty but not the specific effects of cocaine. So, having answered that question partially myself, I would like the panel to answer it.

GIDEON KOREN: Well, first and foremost, any attempt at new testing methods has to validate them and follow many other procedures that we do for new tests. From what we have heard here, we cannot even verify dose and, needless to say, which drugs are involved or the 300 confounders; so I agree with you, but we are not there yet. For us now to decide is whether we would rather use the well verified developmental tests available or create new benchmark tests. How can you do testing before you know even what Mom took? Coming back to integrity of biology, if any of these fundamental scientists went to their laboratory and found out that the previous night instead of cocaine, nicotine was given and the next day alcohol was given with both, they would throw out the whole experiment and would restart it.

We have to incorporate all that, and pharmacologically it's a nightmare. It's clear that all we try to do is to get the best estimate, and all of this group and many other groups around the country try their best. We are in a statistical nightmare, and it is not going to get any better because we have populations that are just not necessarily telling us everything, and there are reasons not to tell us.

The fundamental biology is so crucial to allow us to see where we should aim. The one thing that comes to mind, as someone who does both animal and human work, is some neuropathology of kids who are exposed to cocaine *in utero* and who die for other reasons. Namely, we need a brain bank. It should be national and well coordinated, to obtain data, as done for other diseases and afflicted populations. Otherwise, we have a huge gap between the animal biology and the behavioral outcomes we are measuring. We are still missing the human neuroscience, and I'm sure there are cases. If 10% to 15% of kids are exposed to these drugs, hundreds of them die every year all over the country for other reasons, such as road accidents or just anything that happens in the normal cycle of life. I haven't seen any attempt to collect that data and bring it into the laboratory.

The point you make about new benchmarks to measure the role of drugs should be the case, no question. But how are you going to validate such benchmarks before you even know what drugs to measure? That's my main issue.

JOSEPH COYLE: Gideon, I just wanted to respond to your last point on postmortem studies. Although they can be useful, they are awfully complicated to do. Having been interested in autism, I think in the entire United States there are about 10 autistic brains that have been acquired over the last 15 years. But the beauty is that we now have technologies that can address these very issues, not in dead people but in live people, and that includes functional brain imaging with MRI (fMRI), which does not involve any radiation at all, MR spectroscopy, and quantitative morphometry. There are real opportunities to start looking at substantial populations from a developmental perspective.

BARRY LESTER: Just to comment on the newspaper quote and in partial response to Bernie's question, we went through a period when the effects of cocaine were overexaggerated. To some extent we may be witnessing a backlash of all of that. It's just as dangerous and as premature to watch the pendulum swing to the other side, and now everybody's going to say okay, there are no effects and it's all environment. That's probably the nature of the media and the press and how things get interpreted. We have to be aware of these cycles and we need to understand that one position is probably as inaccurate and dangerous as the exaggeration on the other end.

One of the things that concerns me is the extent to which we take advantage of what we know from other areas in other fields, other studies about risk populations. Some of you may remember an article written years ago by Anastasy around the debate of

IQ. The question was heredity and environment, and she wrote that instead of asking which one, let's start asking how.

Maybe that's what we should start thinking about with the issues around cocaine, that what we're really interested in asking is, how does cocaine affect development, and get away from this either/or kind of mentality. Bernie's question depends on your hypothesis and what you're trying to get at. There certainly are people who want to know how "cocaine kids" stack up against a standard IQ measure, and so we may want to answer that question, but then we may also want to answer the question with reference to other kinds of descriptive information and other kinds of sampling procedures and norms.

In the Maternal Lifestyles Study we deliberately have our comparison group with background drug variables, because we knew that if we compared our sample with white, middle class, pure, non-drug–exposed infants and children, they would look different. But that's not the issue. We want to see if there are cocaine drug effects in the context of these other variables, because that's the environment in which these kids grow up.

IRA CHASNOFF: Yes, I read the newspaper article and Barry referred to it. If we look at the history of this whole issue, unfortunately it's been a very interesting ride. We published our first article in 1985, and it was a very simple comparison of three groups of children, and we saw emerge from that all of these articles about crack babies. And this study says this, and these babies are doomed forever. There was something in the *Washington Post* that described these children as the biologic underclass. Clearly if you look at all that historically, much of the media hysteria over this was racist and racially based. This became very clear when we published our Pinellas County study which showed the bias of physicians in selecting out who are the drug users. Editorials were written about how this wasn't at all possible and that our data were flawed because everyone knows that African-Americans use drugs and whites don't. Then we published our 2-year study, and I reviewed not only our articles, but also a few others, and compared them to newspaper accounts of those articles. It was very clear that the writers of the newspapers had read nothing more than the abstract; they had never read the paper and never tried to understand it. All of us get telephone calls, and they do an interview over the telephone. The data that you publish in a peer-reviewed journal becomes a political issue: now read it and let's talk about it. The political issue that is emerging is that there are many states that are looking at early intervention services for children and don't want to pay for them. Managed care companies do not want to pay for early intervention services for children. They are identifying specific children as the ones who are using up all the money and we know who they are: it's the African-American kids. That is the agenda. So there is a real purpose out there in writing something like this. They may be no worse than any other kid growing up in poverty, and poverty is a crime.

I don't know exactly how we can communicate with the media and take the kind of information that is here and translate it for public consumption as something that everybody can understand. I'm afraid it's an issue that we are all going to struggle with, but I hope that coming out of this meeting might be some idea of how we approach these issues, because these issues have to be understood in the context of what's happening in this country with poverty, with racial issues, with managed care, and with the almighty dollar, that nobody wants to spend on children.

GIDEON KOREN: Just to be fair to the discussion, many of our colleagues rushed to publish partially positive results. I call it teratophyllia, because in the area of teratology, negative results are not publishable and are not fundable. You're not going to sustain your research program if you find negative results. And so we publish . . . The bias against the null hypothesis is not just the media; it's physicians, it's editorial boards of journals, and granting agencies. So we have to do our share. Actually this is one of the most responsible meetings I have ever attended, but there is a trend towards positive results, and unfortunately our scientific community is part of it and we have to do a better job, too.

NAIMAH WEINBERG: I have a couple of questions on a somewhat different topic. As I listened to the presentations I was wondering about the possible biologic contributions of the father. I did hear references to genetics, a genetic role in the susceptibility of the fetus to whatever they're exposed to *in utero,* and that genetic predispositions could come from either parent. In the area of alcohol abuse, we have documentation of associative mating so that women who use alcohol heavily tend to marry or associate with men who use alcohol heavily, although the reverse is not as strong. Have any patterns of assortative mating been looked at? Also, what other contributions may be made by the father—(temperament and impulsivity have been mentioned in terms of the mother)? What about the father who's likely a drug abuser; perhaps his impulsivity is being passed on. Other factors involved may be resilience as well as social supports.

DEBORAH FRANK: We have data on associative mating in our sample as well as for cocaine and alcohol use as well as for anything else. You're right; dads tend to get ignored in the literature because it's so hard to get a hold of and measure them. Our work was turned down once for publication because they asked why we hadn't obtained urine samples and so on, on the dads? Again, obviously those people don't work in a community where it's hard to find dads, and mothers are afraid to identify them for fear they'll get beat up. So there's a lot of uncertainty, but in fact in terms of mother's report of dad's use, we got it.

SPEAKER: I also mentioned that 70% of our women reported that their partners were users.

SPEAKER: I'm left wondering about the fathers' exposure to drugs.

SPEAKER: Long ago Ruth Little in Seattle did some work with alcoholic fathers and showed about a 200-g decrease in birth weight of the infants. I don't know of any other human studies.

SPEAKER: The cocaine data are that it binds to the sperm and is a relative cause of male infertility, but as far as I know, no one has looked at outcomes in children.

SPEAKER: Let's get real: men don't want to give up their specimens. Even if you found the fathers (Barry just made a comment to me that in their study they know 100% of their babies have fathers), they are the putative fathers. In both our residential and outpatient programs we have had programs for the fathers, but they're the person the mother names as the father. When it comes down to it, I'm working with the women. In our population, in reality they're not sure who is the father and that makes it very difficult for us.

SPEAKER: In fairness, in the psychology literature, there is good concordance between maternal and paternal IQ and many other things, such as cigarettes and alcohol. Therefore, there is predictive value in one set of data. Indeed we cannot find the other, so it's quite theoretical to find people who don't want to come to any of these tests.

ABIGAIL SNYDER-KELLER: The issue of what kind of barrier the placenta poses was just raised again. Because of studies in the rat which show that with repeated administration of cocaine, there is an increase in the delivery of cocaine to the brain. This is work done by Nancy Zahniser and Jay Justis. In experiments in adult rats, my husband Rick Keller at Albany Medical has shown that with prenatal cocaine exposure, when these animals are challenged with cocaine within the first month after birth, the amount of cocaine that gets into the brain is about doubled. So I'm wondering if, with repeated use of cocaine during pregnancy, the placental barrier might also change. There would be a change in the passage of cocaine through the placenta, and it could go in either direction. That is something we have to consider.

SPEAKER: Most placental perfusion studies in humans are done with term placenta because of difficulties in procuring samples. However, now with fetal sampling (choriocentesis), we and other people are embarking on getting human data earlier, when you can look at the maternal-fetal unit. By and large we have little knowledge on the ontogeny of placenta. The unit is there and is functioning, but the placenta develops throughout pregnancy and actually rejuvenates itself. So these are very crucial studies. Clearly there is a dose response. No one has tried to say that 5 mg/kg does not make more than 20, but the variability can be so huge, as my simple example showed, that in some cases maybe huge amounts would not make it. In the animal situation, when you breed and you know where it's coming from, you can probably control much more of that variability than in the much more difficult state with humans.

SPEAKER: I'd like to extend Dr. Chasnoff's excellent point about the sociopolitical and media agendas in terms of findings that have been reported. Clearly, one effect of the early studies, not to mention some of the later ones, was to demonize drug-abusing women, and clearly that has not worked in anybody's interests. What I have seen in the literature is almost a backlash to that in terms of trying to portray these women as victims, and I am concerned about whether a unilateral focus on the victimization issue is necessarily productive. Yes, these women incur an incredible amount of victimization. Clearly, that must be a target of any interventions geared towards these women giving them services. But where do we find a suitable stance that encourages women and trains, teaches, and empowers women to assume increasingly responsible collaboration in the raising of their children and the managing of their own lives without, on the one hand, demonizing them and, on the other, what I feel might be infantilizing them by casting them so completely as victims that we don't expect them to take the responsibility for their own lives?

SPEAKER: One of the issues that emerges is the tendency to characterize these women, whether it's as victims or as horrible mothers. We really run the same risk when we say that the environments are all terrible, the mothers are all terrible, they are all inadequate parents, they are all victims, they are all this or that. This mentality is just as erroneous as thinking that all these kids are damaged because they had cocaine *in utero.*

Drug-using mothers are very variable in how they parent, in what they're like as people, and in what their personalities are like. You find a lot of variability in their home environment; some are stressed, some are not. We really have to appreciate the variability in parenting and in environmental factors that are going to interact with whatever predisposition cocaine may or may not have.

SPEAKER: I don't think we should minimize the fact that drugs do produce very specific kinds of effects, not just neurological, as we have been talking about, but also psychiatric. There are patterns of behavior associated with drug use, so that anyone using drugs, and it depends on the kind of drugs they're using, has an entire ecology and associated with that is an entirely new kind of behavior and way of adjusting to the environment. I don't think that that is inconsequential. There is another dimension with a very different kind of way of looking at life, of adjusting to the social situation.

JOSEPH COYLE: If I could just amplify that, we actually know a lot about where these drugs act in the developing brain and how they act. What's very interesting is that they can actually have very opposite effects. For example, ethanol acts at a glutamate receptor and activation of that glutamate receptor has trophic effects on nerves. Ethanol blocks those trophic effects. You can show it in a dish and you can show it in the experimental animal. We have compelling evidence in humans that can account for the failure to develop certain structures. Ironically, nicotine acts as an acetylcholine receptor. If you activate acetylcholine receptors in the developing brain, they have trophic effects. That doesn't mean that nicotine is good because it has a trophic effect that is occurring out of the normal developmental symphony, so to speak. I found it very interesting that in fact you saw different effects of ethanol and nicotine, which said to me that the basic science actually may be telling us something that is meaningful.

My second point regards stigmatization. Virtually all of these women and their mates are poly-substance abusers. I'm curious about why cocaine is used as a demonizing drug when we already have out there in advertising for smoking and ethanol "do not use this if you're pregnant," and there are signs in bars. It seems to me that the issue is linkage and not isolation. The bottom line of this conference is that these drugs act at receptors in the developing brain. That's bad for the developing brain, and you shouldn't use any of them if you're pregnant.

SPEAKER: I want to go back to the point that Ira Chasnoff was making that got a round of applause, and present an alternative possibility. It's always dangerous to consider what's happening at a particular time and view it within a political context without considering the longer historical perspective. The bottom line is that the same dire consequences, flash back to no consequences, working back towards the middle, have happened with every single drug of abuse. With alcohol the same thing happened; with lead, the same thing happened. Lead's bad; no it's not bad; well it's somewhere in between.

Hazel Murphy has talked about this as a matter of philosophy, so it's important for us to consider the science history, that this happens with all drugs, and that this happens with many different kinds of scientific issues. Although I have issues with the health care system too, it may not just be a political thing that's causing this particular reaction in the *Washington Post.*

SPEAKER: I agree with you to a point, but what happened as cocaine was emerging in the early 1980s was that it was also the time of the War on Drugs. By definition, at a policy level the War on Drugs defined the good drugs and the bad drugs. The good drugs were alcohol and tobacco. They were not included in the War on Drugs. The bad drugs were cocaine and opiates, and marijuana literally just kind of floated in between, depending on whether you inhaled or not. As the War on Drugs was further defined, it became very clear that the terminology in and of itself was defining the issue. No one was going to touch alcohol and tobacco because they were the white man's drugs, and no one was going to interfere with those profits because those profits fed into the political system. So I agree with you to a point, but I think cocaine appeared when our political system was looking for a demon and they found it with cocaine. And we had kids that literally suffered because of that.

LINDA WRIGHT: I thought it encouraging yesterday when our basic science colleagues got to the microphone and tried to make some translation into clinical science. I heard one of them ask, please clinicians tell us what to look for, tell us what to ask. I hope that we do not leave this meeting without some attention to that laundry list of questions. We must acknowledge their constraints. They use very high doses because they want to get funded. Basically, however, we should try to devote some attention to the questions that we would like our basic science colleagues to explore and spend some time on models, translation, and that kind of thing.

JOHN HARVEY: I would like to take exception; I can't let that go by. We don't use very high doses. In fact, I calculated that our dose is 42 mg/kg a week, the same number I heard as a dose of one addict. We are very sensitive to that issue. I really think it's a bad thing to say.

SPEAKER: Also, it's not the delivered dose that's critical; the critical thing is the plasma level, and many of these animal models that have been reported deal with plasma levels that are in the range of human use.

LINDA WRIGHT: Precisely. I mean that wasn't meant in any way to be criticism, and there's been a lot of diversity in the doses presented. But this is particularly the kind of thing we need to talk about—quantitating intake and polydrug exposure. It is only becoming clear to some of our basic science colleagues that the challenge that this represents is to establish cross-talk here.

SPEAKER: I found Ira Chasnoff's study where he disassociated effects of IQ from issues of aggression, impulsivity, and overactivity very intriguing because it points to systems that use dopamine. Cocaine may interact with those systems that regulate affect, impulsivity, and aggressivity.

DEBBIE LUBIN: I'm a student in Dr. Joey John's lab at the University of North Carolina at Chapel Hill. I have learned quite a bit at this conference over the last 3 days and I want to raise one point relative to a comment that Dr. Chasnoff made. He said that it might be important to look at maternal attachment as a factor in the outcome in children. We are looking at some of those aspects at the basic science level. We're looking at using a rat model and those animals that have been exposed not only to acute cocaine but also to chronic cocaine. We are finding that there are some significant disruptions in the onset of maternal behavior as well as some disruptions in the maintenance, but mostly in the onset. Also, we look at aggressive behavior in the postpartum period which we find to be elevated at around 6–12 days postpartum. I just wanted to mention those aspects, that research is going on at the basic science level, and that we are getting at some of those issues.

SPEAKER: If you could cause attachment problems in the little baby female mice before they become pregnant and exposed to cocaine, that would help address the problem. Actually, I was trying to take it a generation back and look at the mother's experiences as a child and her attachment experiences and see how they affect all that we're trying to understand.

VINCE SMERIGLIO: Just a brief comment and what I hope is a clarification. I've heard a couple of times this question of whether NIDA would fund a polydrug model in the animal. Obviously, we can ask Alan Leshner directly. I don't know where the question comes from, maybe your experience with previous applications, I don't know. Somebody raised the question with skepticism that a combined alcohol/cocaine model would be funded. I've checked with people in basic research and I briefly mentioned it to Alan. We would fund a polydrug model if a peer review group judged it to be sound science and good work. The one caveat from an administrative point of view is that, if it's an alcohol study with a little bit of other drug, NIDA probably wouldn't get it, so NIDA probably wouldn't fund it. If it's a true polydrug study with emphasis on illicit substances, NIDA would get it and be very interested in it.

JOSEPH COYLE: I'd like to thank the speakers. It's been truly an extraordinary set of presentations.

Round Table 6. Where Do We Go from Here and How Do We Get There?

Moderator: ALAN I. LESHNER
Panelists: LORETTA P. FINNEGAN, WENDY CHAVKIN
Discussants: JOHN HARVEY *(Allegheny)*, DONNA FERRIERO *(UCSF)*, GIDEON KOREN *(Toronto)*, BERNARD KARMEL *(Staten Island)*, DEBORAH FRANK *(BMC)*, J.T. JABBOUR *(Memphis)*

LORETTA FINNEGAN: When considering how to improve services for pregnant substance abusers and their infants, we can learn from the whole business of heart disease. You can study congestive heart failure, myocardial infarctions, however much you want, but the real change that took place to improve (cardiac) health was a change in the diet and activity of the population and the education of the population to prevent heart disease. There are two different issues here; we can do all the longitudinal studies that we want, and we can document what's wrong with these kids, but our real concern is not to have any more kids come down the pipeline. The first thing is to educate the public, starting with our fellow colleagues, about the lack of treatment programs and resources for pregnant women or for women with children. A very separate problem is to understand what cocaine does to the developing brain and what it does to children, and to identify what kinds of help they're going to need later on in school. Maybe we can just start with our pediatricians and obstetricians, so that they know in their own communities how few programs really are concretely available. A lot of them are unaware of that and don't advocate because they assume that programs exist that don't actually exist. It's only going to get worse with changes in funding.

JOHN HARVEY: I would like to say something more from a drug abuse perspective, sitting here in a room with no smoking. The hardest thing is not to give up heroin, but to give up smoking. We need that kind of public campaign. We give warnings but it doesn't have the kind of social pressure that changes habits.

The other point is that in a sense we don't really need any more data. We know from the animal experiments that there's a dose effect curve; even with low doses of cocaine, you are at least potentiating all the other kinds of problems these children are facing. You have impoverished environments, domestic violence, malnutrition, smoking, alcohol, and cocaine. It's clear that exposure to cocaine and alcohol would potentiate what is already a bad situation. If we are to make progress with basic science, we should be looking not only at pre- but also postnatal exposure, and we should be looking at it in terms of multidrug abuse and to see how these factors such as cocaine exposure and malnutrition may be synergistic. Nobody wants to include malnutrition in animal studies, because that would complicate looking at just the effects of cocaine. But as Barry Kosofsky has demonstrated in his mouse model, a subthreshold dose of cocaine plus malnutrition is going to cause long-term trouble. So if we think of it not simply as a cocaine effect, which at high doses exists, but that even at low doses, the potentiating effect it has on all of these other kinds of environmental problems must be studied.

LORETTA FINNEGAN: You and I are thinking along the same lines in many areas. I wanted to comment on how one gets this kind of information out? You said let's teach the pediatricians. Well how do you do that? I was on a group at Jefferson that wanted to get something about substance abuse into the medical school curriculum, and we were considered rebels. The fact is that there is so much for physicians to learn in their early years, as well as during their later education, that you're always in competition. So, unless you're dealing with these problems on a day-to-day basis, you are not well informed. We must think of ways to be very innovative, trying to be sure that we get into medical societies, not just the American Society on Addiction Medicine. Several hundred physicians who are interested and are the ones who really know the problem come to that meeting. What about internal medicine meetings and what about cardiology meetings where they're talking about the heart? There are cardiomyopathies in people who are using drugs. We must try to think long and hard and to have meetings where we can discuss translational research not only between animal and clinical researchers, but also between all of us as researchers and clinicians and all of us as clinicians and scientists to the general public.

DONNA FERREIRO: I wanted to get back to the concrete question: Where does science go from here and what can we do and what can you guys do? We still need animal models, translational research from the neuron all the way through the MR image, and we have lots of data on the human experience that we can use to develop models, polydrug models. But in order to do that, we have to get back to descriptive research, not mechanistic, because we have to develop models. That means you have to take a risk; you have to bet on us that we might be able to develop a good model. You have to give us a chance to explore an area without having lots of preliminary data, and I would say that something concrete would be to put out a proposal to develop models for polydrug exposure using the foundations that have been developed by the people here, in the mouse, rat, rabbit, Rhesus monkey.

SPEAKER: It behooves us to pay attention to the common theme of findings from the animal work. Yes, I agree that there should be more polydrug work, and, yes, we have to deal with malnutrition and all the other social issues. I don't know if I could cope with anything that broad at the moment. But as a baby researcher, I can try to learn from the themes that seem to be present in the animal work, where the deficits are being found, either in alcohol abuse or in cocaine abuse or in the combinations of cocaine and all the other polydrugs that the moms are using; they seem to be in areas that deal with arousal, attention, impulsivity, and behavior. Ira Chasnoff showed great data; in the 6-year olds it wasn't the cognitive deficits as much as the impulsiveness and the aggressiveness. Rather than using our standard tools so to speak, we can design studies that will probe these areas; there have to be precursors in the infants; these behavioral deficits may not just emerge when you reach school age. If we're smart enough, if we do it well enough, by probing these areas we can figure out the appropriate interventions for dealing with it. Yes, we need the interventions for the moms, and the moms are not isolated, and it has to be in the family context because no matter how good the program, the moms are going to go back to the environment, they are going to be re-exposed, and everything is going to fall apart. But you also have to deal with the kids and their parents, and their parents are just as impulsive and just as aggressive. Only by devising and showing that those lines of research have really identified where the deficits are, and by demonstrating where we have to work can we then get the programs and the interventions going that target those kinds of things.

GIDEON KOREN: I would like to make a couple of methodologic suggestions and then a remark on the public domain. Methodologically, the animal results are fascinating, and on the other end of the spectrum we have the longitudinal human studies with all the confounders. But if 10%–20% of kids in this country and in Canada are really exposed to polydrugs and cocaine, every year many of them will die from unrelated causes, and we have to see these brains. These brains, I believe, will give a lot of clues to the insult. As Joe Coyle mentioned, there are 10 autistic brains going around, and everyone looks at them, but autism occurs in 1 in 20,000 and drug exposure occurs in 10%–20% and none of us have seen these brains. This is something we have to do.

With respect to longitudinal studies, all of us know that it's a cumulative effect. The question is the relative contribution to the cumulative effect. At least 20 or 30 longitudinal studies have been conducted, many funded by NIDA, and others in Canada and other countries. This group of people have to sit together because there are a lot of commonalities. We have done it here, but not in a methodologic manner. I wouldn't suggest a meta-analysis because the data are not necessarily combinable, but we have to be more microscopic in comparing our results. We may find out much more if we scrutinize the data that is looked at just in the context of such a symposium as this.

As to the public domain, Loretta Finnegan mentioned the main issue, citing the cardiac example. In Toronto, I was summoned by our foundation at the Hospital for Sick Children to talk to a group of philanthropic donors who had just given $500,000 to provide safety helmets for children. Of course I went with my best slides and three-piece suit. After three sentences, it was clear from how they were looking at me that they were thinking, "this doesn't happen to people we know . . . we don't know anyone that has these issues with cocaine." The bottom line is that mainstream America/Canada does not identify with this issue; the problem is that if the middle class does not identify with an issue, as they did with smoking and with heart disease, then you will have a hard time mobilizing public attention and action.

The fact is that we as both scientists and socially aware people don't understand that most people think this problem is far, far on the left side of the arena. If we are to bring this problem to the public's attention, we must identify the ways in which it is their problem. These kids will cost our society billions of dollars. Ira Chasnoff was probably correct when he stated that it's easier for the journalists to take an approach that prenatal exposure to drugs is not having an effect because it means that we as a society don't have to invest so much. In Toronto we are counseling about 140 women a day. Most of these professional people do not think that these things happen to them or to their fellow man. They are much more interested in the rain forest in Brazil than in what happened to the kids in the neighborhood nearby.

Alan Leshner: One of the points made today that might have an interesting hook as a way to bring this to greater public attention is that prenatal cocaine or other drug exposure doesn't occur in a vacuum; it occurs as part of a variety of negative occurrences that are going on simultaneously. And people appear to be a bit more able to identify with one or more of those individual occurrences. The point made by John Harvey earlier that what normally might be a subthreshold cocaine effect, in combination with some other bad stuff that society has already decided is okay to worry about (like poor prenatal nutrition, that's acceptable), may provide one way to slide this issue in the side door by seeing it in a broader context.

Prof. Nichols: You started to get to the point I was going to raise about the we-versus-they mentality, and I was even guilty of it myself. When I went to my hotel last night, there were two prostitutes standing on the sidewalk, and I realized that I didn't think that I was the same, but I think we need to get past thinking that people are not us. One thing that has come out of this conference is emphasizing the similarities between attention deficit disorders (ADD) and some of the effects of cocaine; that I think middle class parents can relate to. Whether their child has been properly diagnosed or not, at least they think their kid has ADD, and they might start to pay attention to a few of those similarities. Another analogy is tobacco addiction; all of a sudden tobacco is addictive. Well, it killed my grandfather 20 years ago, but now the concept of addiction as a biologic process is a little more out in the open. Maybe people who are addicted to tobacco can better understand how someone can get addicted to crack. Finally, we see a little bit different view of poverty. Despite your depressing facts, at least for right now, until everyone forgets about Mother Theresa, we might be able to remember that there are other ways to look at poverty besides a "blame" mentality.

SPEAKER: Often times because substance abuse or substance dependence is so ingrained in our society and politics, it's often difficult to get down to some of the real issues. Just as public policy changed in the medical field with regard to HIV, requiring us to take courses in HIV and risk management to be accredited for relicensure, we should be able to promote certain avenues for ongoing CMEs (Continuing Medical Education) in the field of substance abuse, proposing that a certain amount of physician training be required within a given period of time. We could work through the American Academy of Pediatrics and the AMA to make that mandatory education. We have too much competition within the medical school curriculum, though I think a lot more of the medical schools are getting to the point where they are trying to integrate substance abuse into the curriculum.

Just as advancement in our feelings about drunk driving was promoted by MADD (Mothers Against Drunk Driving), this is a public policy issue, and if we are very clever and sophisticated and have a good spokesperson that people in general can identify with, it helps to forward the cause. In the current climate of back-to-work welfare reform, or whatever you want to call it, working in Baltimore where you have 67,000 people who are in need of alcohol and drug treatment and only 1,500 beds, it's extremely frustrating. You have beautiful models, but if there's no money to support expansion and access to healthcare and to rehabilitation, then it's almost a losing battle. We did have model programs and then the funding left, and there was no one to pick up that slack.

LORETTA FINNEGAN: You're absolutely right; we were able to get HIV-Aids into curricula. That movement had spokespersons, the gay community, the ACT-UP community; there was someone to speak on behalf of these individuals. With the women that we speak of today, we have few advocates, we have few individuals that will speak on their behalf. Money talks, and in Washington it talks loud. The point is that we should calculate the dollar savings that we could have; maybe you can't hit them immediately with the human side of this, but maybe you can hit them in their pockets. It's costing all of us in this room, and everybody else in this country, a great deal of money to care at the back end, and for life, for these children. So we really need to think about the preventive part. By investing our dollar there, not only will we reduce the human cost but we will also reduce the financial cost.

WENDY CHAVKIN: People have made various suggestions that folks other than addiction specialists have to become educated about this matter, and I agree with that. I'm talking particularly about care givers and physicians, and talking about the fact that internists, cardiologists, and gynecologists all need to learn something about addiction.

I would also suggest though that people who have technical imperatives that they care about, like all of you here, do have to care about public policy, too. In the same way that this context is determining your ability to do your own work, and just as the last discusser talked about how frustrating it was to be in a city that had some tiny proportion of the needed slots for drug treatment, you have to take this on in some fashion; you have to be aware of the fact that these broad public policy issues are determining what you can do in your clinical or laboratory settings.

SPEAKER: I'd like to follow up on a point that Dr. Koren and Dr. Nichols were addressing in terms of the us-versus-them kind of dichotomy. Who are the pregnant women who are doing cocaine and who are the cocaine-exposed babies? Dr. Chasnoff published an eloquent paper some years ago where he showed that positive toxicology screens for cocaine among pregnant women cut across ethnic lines and across social class lines. He's not the only one who has demonstrated that. The point is that it does happen to middle class, white, private, obstetric patients, even ones who have planned their pregnancies. And yes, the consequences may be less; it may be less likely to be identified as a function of bias on the part of clinicians as to who they suspect, but it does happen. So it really isn't an us-versus-them at all, it's us and us. We have to find some way, and I'm not sure what that way is, of conveying that and making people, not just scientists, not just policy makers, not just fundraisers, but the general population, whatever that means, aware of that fact.

BERNARD KARMEL: Dr. Finnegan, you question why we do this research when everything is going to be cut out from under us. When you talk about comprehensive services for women and children with drug abuse, my immediate thought is that what we should be dealing with is comprehensive services. Period. When I look at a baby on a neonatal intensive care unit, I look at a baby who has been drug exposed, a baby who may have an intraventricular hemorrhage, and I look at all of the various possible things that could happen to this infant and then I try to think about how we might treat this infant. So, when we talk about comprehensive characteristics, we have to begin to talk about the comprehensive nature of the problems in infants and children that are related to drug exposure.

My second point regards the differentiation of perhaps something like a syndrome. To call it a "cocaine syndrome" is not very good, but serves to differentiate it from the other kinds of effects that we might have, which might be very useful. Early on we differentiated (poor) kids who had problems of genetic origin from others with genetic problems. So in terms of treatment facilities, we cut out things related to genetic and metabolic problems, Down's and so forth. Then we found that we were getting more and more premature babies and babies who had hemorrhages or bad birth problems, and this also crossed strata. Each time before we found out that it crossed strata, we always blamed the problem on the poor people. They were the ones who weren't so smart; they were the ones who had the premature babies. Then we found out that wasn't quite true; it crossed strata. In Dr. Leshner's remarks, you have a very comprehensive summary of many of the issues in terms of assessment, intervention, and so forth. What we are struggling with is how to get this across to others, and what I would argue is that you have to take out this poverty problem. Poverty is itself a problem, but it's not the problem that we are trying to deal with—the effect of this syndrome. Once you eliminate the poverty component, this thing left over, call it a frontal syndrome, a dopaminergic syndrome, etc., perhaps not a cocaine syndrome, but it is something we know that affects certain parts of the nervous system due to perturbations at certain points in development. Then we begin to say, okay, now how do we deal with that problem comprehensively in the context of all the other problems we see when these babies are born?

DEBORAH FRANK: The first thing to do is to reframe the Pollyanna that there's no problem; okay? As I have been known to say on a lot of measures, although not all, the good news is that the cocaine-exposed kids in our cohort don't look a lot worse than the unexposed kids, but the bad news is that they all look awful and they get progressively awfuller as poverty corrodes them. Listening to all of this and reflecting on some data which suggest that if you can get people to stick with prenatal care, even if you can't give them drug treatment, their babies come out better, even if they are still using. So the research question is comprehensive, nonspecific, nontargeted vs targeted services, and the results may be different for mothers and children. I don't think any of us would argue that drug-using, alcohol-using women need interventions targeted towards their addiction. But one of the things you could test is whether generic kinds of interventions for children at biological/social risk or ones specifically targeted to the theory about dopaminergic neurons make a difference in the outcome of the kids. First, you've got to reframe the Pollyanna and then you have to say, okay, that's testable.

J.T. JABBOUR: It seems that you've touched on many points that are pertinent to this problem. But, as a neurologist, most of the patients that come to me don't necessarily come from the pediatrician. You've overlooked one group of people who are more involved in this than anyone and those are the educators, the teachers. I've always had the idea that if you looked at these children, as Dr. Leshner mentioned, not as drug children, but just as a whole population of children, you have to conclude that they have some syndrome. These children present to me at very early ages, before school age, at 2, 3, and 4. I previously mentioned that I see alterations in sleep patterns in many of these children. Several people have mentioned impulsivity and something akin to Attention Deficit Disorder. It is truly a temperament problem; nobody defined temperament for me, but I know what temperament is, and at the extreme there is significant aggressivity. So you've got the problem with attention, with temperament, and with those who are sleeping in school. You have to get children early by educating teachers in what to look for. Saying no to drugs isn't what we're talking about; we're talking about devastation of the brain. You can't fix it with medicines alone; you can't fix it with the facilities that we have, the mental health centers. Pediatricians don't have enough time and are being pressured to take less time seeing each child and family. You have to have interest and you have to have time. So the point is to get educators involved very early as they have a great ability to communicate.

The second group of people, one that Dr. Bada works with, are the nurses. The public health nurses have a better feel for this than anybody and refer more people to us early than anyone. They know the families, the educators know the families, and the pediatricians know certain families. I recommend strongly that early on we get the nurses, the educators, and the pediatricians involved. And more importantly, Dr. Leshner, give some of those grants to the chief resident in pediatrics and in family medicine, and let him/her get interested in this because that's where the beginning will have to be. If you go to a hospital and look at the developmental records and the histories, they're going to have information on where the patients live and how they live, but they're not going to get into all of these problems and know what's happened unless you give them the time and the interest to do it.

WENDY CHAVKIN: I'm actually a little disturbed that several people have talked about how depressing my talk was. The reason I'm disturbed is that I didn't intend to leave people depressed, because depressed to my mind means hopeless and overwhelmed and feeling as if there is nothing available to do, and that is very much not what I intended. I don't mind, however, leaving you alarmed. I'm perfectly happy if I leave you alarmed and yet with the feeling that there is something you can do.

I've described some of the negative tendencies with the devolution of authority to the state. The hope in all this, however, is that you might have an impact at your state level. These shifts that I have described are so momentous, they are going to be fluid for a good while. Everything that I talked about is not written in stone. A lot of it is not going to work, and it's not going to work really fast. So there will be an opportunity, I suspect, in every state to reshape it. So rather than depress you, I would leave you with some sense that you might better do your work if you take some of this on in your home states.

LORETTA FINNEGAN: I agree with Wendy, that it is all of our responsibility as concerned scientists and clinicians and as citizens of the United States. But the New York Academy of Sciences has spent a great deal of effort in putting together with the cochairs an excellent forum. We hope that this would not stop at this point; perhaps some of these suggestions would be picked up, particularly with regard to the education of the various professional groups.

I also wanted to pick up on something that John Harvey said and direct it to Alan Leshner, that perhaps we ought to look at the portfolio of the past NIDA studies to see what we have already determined, not redo some of the same work, but to build on the work that has been done and what has been presented here, and move forward in that way.

Finally, I only know one person here from Los Angeles, Rachelle, and there may be one other. As Gypsy Rose Lee said, we need a gimmick, and ones we could really use are people who could be spokespersons. There is Elizabeth Taylor for HIV. There is Mary Tyler Moore for Diabetes. Kim Bassinger who doesn't want us to do any experiments on animals. There must be one out there in California who cares and who may even have a child exposed to cocaine. There might be one who would be very good at this.

SPEAKER: It's really important that we incorporate in our future research endeavors at changing social systems. Welfare reform really concerns me in terms of where are the children going to be? They are going to be out of their mother's care a lot sooner because of the compelling nature of drug addiction. We need to address this in terms of drug treatment or family treatment. We need to bring other people into that whole model—foster parents, relative caregivers. I deal with a lot of relative caregivers, and there are some really significant issues with respect to relative caregivers and outcomes in these children.

Prenatal Cocaine Exposure Produces Long-Term Impairments in Brain Serotonin Function in Rat Offspring[a]

GEORGE BATTAGLIA,[b] THERESA M. CABRERA-VERA, LOUIS D. VAN DE KAR, FRANCISCA GARCIA, ALEKSANDRA VICENTIC, AND WILFRED PINTO

Department of Pharmacology, Stritch School of Medicine, Loyola University Chicago, Maywood, Illinois 60153, USA

Because of cocaine's prominent actions on catecholamine systems, these systems have been the focus of attention in most studies investigating the consequences of prenatal exposure to cocaine. However, cocaine also exerts profound effects on brain serotonin (5-HT) neurons[1] primarily via blockade of 5-HT uptake. Indeed, cocaine is a more potent blocker of serotonin uptake than of catecholamine uptake.[2] Prior to assuming its role as a neurotransmitter, 5-HT in fetal brain influences the development of both serotonergic neurons and the target tissues with which these neurons make synaptic connections.[3] Indeed, perturbation of fetal 5-HT systems by administration of serotonergic drugs during pregnancy alters the development of 5-HT systems in offspring.[3] Cocaine can readily cross the fetoplacental barrier, thereby entering fetal brain and blocking 5-HT uptake sites. Therefore, prenatal cocaine-induced perturbations of fetal 5-HT levels would likely result in marked alterations in the development of serotonin pathways. We hypothesized that exposure to cocaine during pregnancy would produce long-term neurochemical and functional impairments in brain serotonergic systems in offspring. As dysfunction of brain serotonin systems has been implicated in psychiatric disorders (e.g., depression, anxiety, aggression, eating disorders, and premenstrual syndrome), prenatal cocaine-induced changes in serotonin function in offspring may have significant clinical consequences.

Pregnant Sprague-Dawley rats were administered saline solution or 15 mg/kg (–) cocaine (sc, bid) from gestational day 13 through 20, and offspring were fostered to non-drug–treated dams to preclude any confounding effects of cocaine-induced differences in nurturing. Offspring were tested at prepubescent (postnatal day 28) and adult (postnatal day 70) ages. Functional impairments in pre- and postsynaptic components of serotonin pathways were assessed by neuroendocrine challenge tests. Offspring exposed prenatally to saline solution or cocaine were compared for differences in the magnitude of elevation of the plasma hormones adrenocorticotropin (ACTH), corticosterone, renin, and prolactin following challenge with the 5-HT releaser *p*-chloramphetamine (PCA) or the 5-HT_{1A} agonist 8-hydroxydipropylaminotetralin (8-OH-DPAT). Biochemical measurements of neurotransmitter levels as well as 5-HT receptors and uptake sites were also determined.

[a] This research was supported by National Institute on Drug Abuse Grant DA 07741.

[b] Address for correspondence: Dr. George Battaglia, Department of Pharmacology, Stritch School of Medicine, Loyola University Chicago, 2160 South First Avenue, Maywood, IL 60153. Phone, 708/216 5680; fax, 708/216-6596; e-mail, gbattag@luc.edu

Marked reductions in the ability of the 5-HT releaser PCA to elevate plasma levels of ACTH (–43%) and renin (–50%) were observed in adult male offspring exposed to cocaine prenatally. This impaired functional response of 5-HT terminals to the challenge drug occurred in the absence of alterations in basal levels of hormones.[4] Deficits in hormone responses to a 5-HT releaser were also observed in immature female offspring exposed prenatally to cocaine,[5] indicating that 5-HT terminal impairments occur in both males and females. In contrast to the presynaptic deficit, neuroendocrine responses to a directly acting postsynaptic 5-HT_{1A} receptor agonist, 8-OH-DPAT, were potentiated (+28 to 53%) in offspring exposed to cocaine prenatally.[6] This potentiated response of plasma hormones to a 5-HT_{1A} agonist exhibited gender specificity as it was observed in male but not female offspring at an immature developmental time. These data are consistent with the hypothesis that the postsynaptic hyperresponsiveness may be compensatory to the presynaptic impairment. Taken together, the implication of these data is that the degree of reduction observed after challenge with the 5-HT releaser may represent an underestimate of the magnitude of the presynaptic deficit. Indeed, the neuroendocrine responsiveness of postsynaptic receptors appeared to normalize to control values following maturation. These functional alterations occurred independent of changes in 5-HT uptake sites, 5-HT receptors, or 5-HT levels in the hypothalamus. However, a reduction in 5-HT_{1A} receptors and 5-HT content was observed in other brain regions after *in utero* exposure to cocaine.

Taken together, our data indicate that prenatal exposure to cocaine produces long-term functional impairment in brain serotonin systems in offspring, as evidenced by the blunted hormone responses to a 5-HT releaser and the potentiated hormone responses to a 5-HT receptor agonist. Furthermore, the effects of prenatal cocaine exposure on 5-HT systems appear to differ in male and female offspring and as a consequence of developmental age. An additional point that emerges from our studies is that some of the impairments in serotonin systems produced by prenatal exposure to cocaine may only be revealed when the system must respond to a challenge imposed on it. Despite the marked alterations in hormone responses to pharmacologic challenges, prenatal cocaine exposure produced few if any changes in basal hormone levels or regional densities of 5-HT uptake sites or 5-HT receptor subtypes. Presumably, the ability of 5-HT systems to maintain or regulate densities of uptake sites or receptors may also be compromised in response to chronic drug treatments, physiologic adaptations, or environmental situations in cocaine-exposed offspring.

These findings suggest that prenatal exposure to cocaine can produce impairments in the serotonin system of offspring that may compromise the ability of individuals to respond to subsequent biologic or situational challenges. Comparable deficits in human offspring may render these individuals vulnerable to psychiatric or other clinical disorders associated with impaired serotonin function. Our data suggest that such vulnerability may differ between genders and at different stages of the life cycle. These findings indicate the need to investigate the effectiveness of currently prescribed antidepressant drugs, such as fluoxetine (Prozac®) or paroxetine (Paxil®), to restore normal function to serotonin systems impaired by prenatal exposure to cocaine.

REFERENCES

1. Cunningham, K.A. & J.M. Lakoski. 1988. Electrophysiological effects of cocaine and procaine on dorsal raphe serotonin neurons. Eur. J. Pharmacol. **148:** 457–462.
2. Ritz, M.C., E.J. Cone & M.J. Kuhar. 1990. Cocaine inhibition of ligand binding at dopamine, norepinephrine and serotonin transporters: A structure-activity study. Life Sci. **46:** 635–645.

3. Whitaker-Azmitia, P.M., M. Druse, P. Walker & J.M. Lauder. 1996. Serotonin as a developmental signal. Behav. Brain Res. **73:** 19–29.
4. Cabrera, T.M., J.M. Yracheta, Q. Li, A.D. Levy, L.D. Van de Kar & G. Battaglia. 1993. Prenatal cocaine produces deficits in serotonin mediated neuroendocrine responses in adult rat progeny: Evidence for long-term functional alterations in brain serotonin pathways. Synapse **15:** 158–168.
5. Cabrera, T.M., A.D. Levy, Q. Li, L.D. Van de Kar & G. Battaglia. 1994. Cocaine-induced deficits in ACTH and corticosterone responses in female rat progeny. Brain Res. Bull. **34:** 93–97.
6. Battaglia, G. & T.M. Cabrera. 1994. Potentiation of 5-HT_{1A} receptor-mediated neuroendocrine responses in male but not female progeny after prenatal cocaine: Evidence for gender differences. J. Pharmacol. Exp. Ther. **271:** 1453–1461.

Maternal Lifestyles Study (MLS)

Caretaking Environment and Stability of Substance-Exposed Infants at One Month Corrected Age[a]

PENELOPE L. MAZA,[b] LINDA L. WRIGHT,[c] CHARLES R. BAUER,[d] SEETHA SHANKARAN,[e] HENRIETTA S. BADA,[f] BARRY LESTER,[g] HEIDI KRAUSE-STEINRAUF,[h] VINCENT L. SMERIGLIO,[i] ANN BOWLER,[j] AND VASILIS KATSIKIOTIS[k]

[b]*Administration on Children, Youth and Families (ACYF), Box 1182—Children's Bureau, Washington, DC 20013. Phone, 202/205-8172; fax, 202/401-5917; e-mail, PMAZA@ACF.DHHS.GOV*

[c]*National Institute on Child Health and Human Development (NICHD), 6100 Executive Blvd., Room 4B03G, Rockville, MD 20852. Phone, 301/496-5575; fax, 301/496-3790; e-mail, LWRIGHT@hd01.nichd.nih.gov*

[d]*University of Miami School of Medicine, Jackson Memorial Hospital, Department of Pediatrics, Maternal Lifestyles Study, Dominion Towers, Room 813, 1400 NW 10th Avenue, Miami, FL. 33136. Phone, 303/243-4841; fax, 305/243-6032; e-mail, CBAUER@peds.med.miami.edu*

[e]*Wayne State University School of Medicine, Children's Hospital of Michigan, Division of Neonatal and Perinatal Medicine, 3901 Beaubian Boulevard, Room 401, Detroit, MI 48201. Phone, 313/745-1436; fax, 313/745-5867; e-mail, SSHANKA@cms.cc.wayne.edu*

[f]*University of Tennessee School of Medicine, E.H. Crump Hospital, New Born Center 853 Jefferson Avenue, Room 201, Memphis, TN 38163. Phone, 901/448-5950; fax, 901/448-1691; e-mail, HBADA@utmem1.utmem.edu*

[g]*Brown University, Women's and Infants Hospital, Department of Pediatrics, 101 Dudley Street, Providence, RI 02905. Phone, 401/453-7640/41; fax, 401/453-7646; e-mail, BARRY__LESTER@brown.edu*

[h]*George Washington University Biostatistics Center, 6110 Executive Blvd., Suite 750, Rockville, MD 20852. Phone, 301/881-9260; fax, 301/ 816-0385*

[i]*National Institute on Drug Abuse (NIDA), Clinical Medicine Branch, 5600 Fishers Lane, Room 10A-08, Rockville, MD 20857. Phone, 301/443-1801 9; fax, 301/594-6566; e-mail, VS240@nih.gov*

[j]*George Washington University Biostatistics Center, 6110 Executive Blvd., Suite 750, Rockville, MD 20852. Phone, 301/881-9260; fax, 301/816-0385; e-mail, BowlerA@hd01.nichd.gov*

[k]*George Washington University Biostatistics Center, 6110 Executive Blvd., Suite 750, Rockville, MD 20852. Phone, 301/881-9260; fax, 301/816-0385; e-mail, KATSIKIO@biostat.bsc.gwu.edu*

This report identifies the differential impact of and interactions between *in utero* drug exposure, particularly cocaine/polydrug exposure, and social environment on child de-

[a] This study was supported by the National Institute on Child Health and Human Development through cooperative agreements as well as intra-agency agreements with the National Institute on Drug Abuse (NIDA), Administration on Children, Youth and Families, and The Center for Substance Abuse Treatment (CSAT).

velopment. Although some studies found minimal or equivocal environmental effects,[1–7] others suggested that the environment may have a stronger effect on child development than drug exposure status. This hypothesis is based on a combination of theoretical discussions[8–12] and empirical studies.[13–21] This body of empirical and theoretical literature is directly related to general research findings on the effect of social environment on at risk children.[9,22,23]

The Maternal Lifestyles Study is studying 1,400 children almost evenly divided between cocaine/opiate exposed (EXP) infants and a group-matched comparison (COMP) cohort at 1 month corrected age (CA). Major features of the method include the following: cocaine/opiate exposure was defined by maternal hospital interview or GCMS positive meconium; the caretaker was considered to be the biologic mother if living in the household with the infant, otherwise the caretaker is the household member with primary responsibility for the infant; caretaker and social service involvement is ascertained at discharge from the hospital and at 1 month CA; certified interviewers administered the Addiction Severity Index (adapted) and social/environmental instruments developed for the study.

The study found that 42% of the EXP infants were reported to child protective services, but that sites had different reporting rates related to state reporting policy. Most of both the EXP and COMP infants were living with their biologic mothers at discharge, and almost all were still living with their mothers at 1 month CA. However, 113 EXP infants were not discharged to their mothers and 41% of these infants were in nonrelative foster care (TABLE 1).

Although the mothers of the EXP and COMP infants came from roughly the same communities, the mothers of EXP infants experienced greater economic insecurity than did the mothers of COMP infants. They were less likely to have worked during the 3 years before the infant's birth. When they worked, they earned less money and were less likely to return to work before the infant reached 1 month CA than were mothers of comparison infants (TABLE 2).

The caretakers of EXP infants were older, more likely to be Medicaid recipients, more likely to be African-American, and less likely to be high school graduates than were caretakers of COMP infants. Although caretakers of EXP and COMP infants received about the same number of services, caretakers of EXP infants were more likely to be referred for Medicaid, food stamps, and Aid to Families with Dependent Children than were caretakers of COMP children.

The environments of EXP infants differ in important ways from the environments

TABLE 1. Disposition of Infants at Discharge and at One Month

Disposition of Infants	Exposure	Comparison
Living with biologic mother:	$n = 632$	$n = 731$
At discharge	82%	100%
At 1 month	80%	99%
If discharged to mother, at 1 mo with:	$n = 519$	$n = 728$
Mother	95%	99%
Other relatives	2%	<1%
Congregate care/no stable home	2%	<1%
If *not* discharged to mother, at 1 mo with:	$n = 113$	$n = 3$
Mother	13%	33%
Other relatives	32%	0%
Nonrelative foster care	41%	67%
Other	14%	0%

TABLE 2. Mother's Employment/Income at One Month

	Exposure (n=537)	Comparison (n=719)
Usual employment status		
Unemployed	30%	15%
Employed		
Full time	26%	39%
Part time	18%	22%
Student	2%	7%
Monthly *pre-pregnancy* income (mean[a])	$745	$812
No pre-pregnancy income	25%	15%
Source of *current* income (mean %[a])		
Employment	4%	12%
Unemployment compensation	2%	2%
Welfare	70%	56%
Social Security	8%	6%
Family/friends	17%	24%
No current income	3%	8%
Biologic mother returned to work	5%	11%

[a]Of those reporting income.

of COMP infants. Future analyses of Maternal Lifestyles Study data will assess the impact of the differences identified here and others to determine their impact on child development. The analyses will also examine the role of child welfare policies regarding reporting of drug-exposed infants in the long-term safety and development of drug-exposed and comparison children.

REFERENCES

1. Hack, M.B., N. Breslau, D. Aram, B. Weissman, N. Klein & E. Borawski-Clark. 1992. The effect of very low birth weight and social risk on neurocognitive abilities at school age. J. Dev. Behav. Pediatr. **13:** 412–420.
2. Howard, J., L. Beckwith, C. Rodning & V. Kropenske. 1989. The development of young children of substance abusing parents: Insights from seven years of intervention and research. Zero to Three **9:** 8–12.
3. Kolar, A.F., B.S. Brown, C.A. Haertzen & B.S. Michaelson. 1994. Children of substance abusers: The life experiences of children of opiate addicts in methadone maintenance. Am. J. Drug & Alcohol Abuse **20:** 159–171.
4. Kronstadt, D. 1989. Pregnancy and cocaine addiction: An overview of impact and treatment. Far West Lab. Ed. Res. & Dev. San Francisco, CA.
5. Myers, B.J., H.C. Olsen & K. Kaltenbach. 1992. Cocaine-exposed infants: Myths and misunderstandings. Zero to Three **13:** 1–15.
6. Nulman, I., J. Rovet, D. Altmann, C. Bradly, T. Einarson & G. Koren. 1994. Neurodevelopment of adopted children exposed in utero to cocaine. Can. Med. Assoc. J. **151:** 1591–1597.
7. Zuckerman, B. 1991. Drug exposed infants: Understanding the medical risk. Future of Children **1:** 26–35.
8. Griffith, D.R. 1992. Prenatal exposure to cocaine and other drugs: Developmental and educational prognoses. Phi Delta Kappan Sept 1992: 30–34.
9. Kaplan-Sanoff, M., S. Parker & B. Zuckerman. 1991. Poverty and early childhood development: What do we know, and what should we do? Infants & Young Child. **4:** 68–76.

10. KALTENBACH, K.A. & L. FINNEGAN. 1989. Prenatal narcotic exposure: Perinatal and developmental effects. Neurotoxicology **10:** 597–604.
11. MATHIAS, R. 1992. Developmental effects of prenatal drug exposure may be overcome by postnatal environment. NIDA Notes January/February: 14–16.
12. ZUCKERMAN, B. & D. FRANK. 1992. "Crack kids": Not broken. Pediatrics **89:** 337–339.
13. AZUMA, S.D. & I.J. CHASNOFF. 1993. Outcome of children prenatally exposed to cocaine and other drugs: A path analysis of three year data. Pediatrics **92:** 396–402.
14. BARTH, R.P. 1991. Adoption of drug-exposed children. Children & Youth Serv. Rev. **13:** 323–342.
15. BILLING, L., M. ERIKSSON, B. JONSSON, G. STENEROTH & R. ZETTERSTROM. 1994. The influence of environmental factors on behavioural problems in 8-year-old children exposed to amphetamine during fetal life. Child Abuse & Neglect **18:** 3–9.
16. FRANCK, E. 1996. Pre-natally drug-exposed children in out-of-home care: Are we looking at the whole picture? Child Welfare **75:** 19–34.
17. GIUSTI, L.M. 1996. Development of children in foster care: Comparison of Battelle screening test performance of children prenatally exposed to cocaine and non-exposed children. L.S. Chandler & S.J. Lane, Eds.: 155–171. Haworth Press, Inc. New York, New York.
18. GRIFFITH, D.R., S.D. AZUMA & I.J. CHASNOFF. 1994. Three year outcome of children exposed prenatally to drugs. J. Am. Acad. Child. & Adolesc. Psychol. **33:** 20–27.
19. HAWLEY, T.L., T.G. HALLE, R.E. DRASIN & N.G. THOMAS. 1995. Children of addicted mothers: Effects of the "crack epidemic on the caregiving environment and the development of preschoolers. Am. J. Orthopsychiatry **65:** 364–379.
20. HURT, H., N.L. BRODSKY, L. BETANCOURT, L.E. BRAITMAN, E MALMUD & J. GIANNETTA. 1995. Cocaine-exposed children: Follow-up through 30 months. J. Dev. Behav. Pediatr. **16:** 29–35.
21. ORNOY, A., V. MICHAILEVSKAYA, I. LUKASHOV, R. BAR-HAMBURGER & S. HAREL. 1996. The developmental outcome of children born to heroin-dependent mothers, raised at home or adopted. Child Abuse & Neglect **20:** 385–396.
22. AYLWARD, G.P. 1990. Environmental influences on the developmental outcome of children at risk. Infants & Young Child. **2:** 1–9.
23. LIAW, F & J. BROOKS-GUNN. 1994. Cumulative familial risks and low-birthweight children's cognitive and behavioral development. J. Clin. & Child Psychol. **23:** 360–372.

Sequential Neuromotor Examination of Children with Intrauterine Drug Exposure[a]

HAROLYN M.E. BELCHER,[b,c,i] BRUCE K. SHAPIRO,[b,c] MARY LEPPERT,[b,c] ARLENE M. BUTZ,[c] SHERRY SELLERS,[b,c] ELLEN ARCH,[b,c] KEN KOLODNER,[d] MARGARET PULSIFER,[e] KATE LEARS,[f] AND WALTER E. KAUFMANN[c,e,g,h]

[b]The Kennedy Krieger Institute, [c]Department of Pediatrics, [d]School of Hygiene and Public Health, [e]Department of Psychiatry, [f]School of Nursing, [g]Department of Pathology, and [h]Department of Neurology, The Johns Hopkins University School of Medicine, Baltimore, Maryland 21205 USA

Polydrug use is a frequent occurrence among women using illicit drugs. Illicit drug use patterns in Baltimore include a substantial number of persons who use opiates as well as cocaine. The distribution of illicit drug use in women admitted to drug rehabilitation programs in Baltimore between 1993 and 1995 ranged from 18.6% to 29.4% for heroin, 18.9% to 30.5% for crack cocaine, 11.1% to 30.5% for other forms of cocaine, and 0.2% for marijuana.[1] A variety of neuromotor outcomes have been documented in cocaine/polydrug-exposed children including: transient hypertonia, poorer functioning on the motor subtest of the Brazelton Neonatal Assessment Scale, and less than optimal function on the Alberta Infant Motor Scale and the Movement Assessment of Infants Test.[2-4] No studies to date have reported the sequential differences in neurologic status of children with cocaine/non-opiate exposure versus cocaine and opiate exposure.

METHODS

The objectives of this study were to: (1) describe the longitudinal neuromotor development of a cohort of children with intrauterine polydrug exposure, and (2) determine whether neuromotor outcome is associated with drug exposure patterns.

A prospective cohort design with examiners blind to drug of exposure and status of neonatal drug screen was used. Subjects were admitted to The Johns Hopkins Hospital and Bayview Hospital Center from 1994 to 1996. Total population enrolled in the study was 188. Data are presented on 157 newborns followed sequentially in a randomized home-based nursing interventional trial for drug-exposed infants with subsequent 3- ($n = 118$), 6- ($n = 124$), and 12-month ($n = 77$) examinations (TABLE 1).

Serial neuromotor examinations were performed during the newborn period and at 3, 6, and 12 months. Infants were grouped on the basis of maternal drug use pattern and the presence of drug metabolites in the neonatal drug screen. The Sequential Neu-

[a] This research was supported by a National Institute of Nursing Research Grant (NR03442-01A1) "Home Nursing Intervention for Infants with Intrauterine Drug Exposure."

[i] Address for correspondence: Harolyn M.E. Belcher, M.D., The Kennedy Krieger Institute, 707 North Broadway, Baltimore, MD 21205. Phone, 410/502-8012; fax, 410/502-9884; e-mail, BELCHER@KENNEDYKRIEGER.ORG

TABLE 1. Infant and Maternal Demographics ($n = 188$)

	Percentage of Population	Mean	SD	Z-Score
Infant				
Birth weight (g)		2,817	427	–0.96
Head circumference (cm)		33	1.4	–1.47
Length (cm)		48.3	2.4	–0.86
Gestational age (wk)		38.4	1.5	
Mean length of stay (days)		9	6.5	
Gender (female)	51			
Apgar 1 minute <7	18			
Apgar 5 minute <7	3			
Maternal				
Age (yr)		28	4	
Education (≤HS grad)	47.8			
Unemployed	94.5			
Never married/single	85			
Tobacco use	84.2			
Race (African-American)	97			

romotor Exam (SNE) was used at each age to evaluate the neuromotor status of six domains: (1) axial tone; (2) peripheral tone; (3) tremors/abnormal movement patterns; (4) state; (5) feeding/swallowing; and (6) deep tendon reflexes and define categorical classifications of normal, suspect, and abnormal. The SNE is a comprehensive pediatric neurologic examination based largely on the work of Dubowitz and Dubowitz,[5] Prechtl,[6] Amiel-Tison and Grenier,[7] Capute,[8] and Allen and Capute.[9] Interrater reliability (Kappa) was .82. The dataset was reduced and analyzed using descriptive and χ^2 statistics.

RESULTS

Multiple patterns of neuromotor abnormalities were present during the neonatal period. Most of these patterns resolved over time. Axial hypotonia (31%) was a prominent finding in the neonatal period; however, it is found in only 10% of examinations at 12 months. Increased lower extremity tone (5%) was a less frequent finding during the neonatal period. Three-month-old children with positive urine drug screens were more likely to have peripheral hypertonia than were children with negative drug screens ($p < 0.05$). Persistence of increased leg extensor tone was found in 67% of the abnormal examinations at 12 months. Children who had a urine drug screen that was positive for cocaine and heroin were more likely to have an abnormal SNE score at 6 months of age compared to children with negative, cocaine-positive only, or heroin-positive only urine drug screens ($p < 0.05$). Rolling prone to supine and supine to prone as well as walking were significantly delayed in the polydrug-exposed cohort than in a similar non-drug-exposed peer group (TABLE 2).

CONCLUSION

Children with intrauterine polydrug exposure have numerous early suspect and abnormal patterns of neuromotor development. Most tone and movement abnormalities

TABLE 2. Gross Motor Milestones ($n = 73$)

Motor Milestone	Infants with Polydrug Exposure (SD)	Normative Population (SD)
Roll (prone to supine)[a]	4.57 (1.95) ($n = 61$)	3.8 (1.3) ($n = 90$)
Roll (supine to prone)[a]	5.2 (1.88) ($n = 58$)	4.4 (1.3) ($n = 90$)
Sit independently	6.05 (1.66) ($n = 68$)	5.9 (1.3) ($n = 95$)
Crawl	7.15 (1.59) ($n = 66$)	7.4 (1.8) ($n = 93$)
Cruise	8.78 (1.52) ($n = 67$)	8.7 (1.4) ($n = 96$)
Walk[b]	11.38 (2.01) ($n = 73$)	10.9 (1.7) ($n = 96$)

[a] $p < 0.001$, by two-tailed t test.
[b] $p < 0.05$, by two-tailed t test.

resolve over time. Children who had an abnormal score on the SNE are more likely to have a positive urine drug screen for cocaine and heroin at 6 months. Increased lower extremity extensor tone at 12 months was a prominent finding in children with an abnormal SNE. Mild, but significant delays are noted in the acquisition of motor milestones in the drug-exposed cohort.

REFERENCES

1. Trends and Patterns in Maryland Alcohol and Drug Abuse Treatment, Fiscal Year 1995. 1996. Maryland Department of Health and Mental Hygiene. Baltimore, MD.
2. Chiriboga, C.A., M. Vibbert, R. Malou *et al.* 1995. Neurological correlates of fetal cocaine exposure: Transient hypertonia of infancy and early childhood. Pediatrics **96:** 1070–1077.
3. Delany-Black, V., C. Covington, E. Ostrea *et al.* 1996. Prenatal cocaine and neonatal outcome: Evaluation of dose-response relationship. Pediatrics **98:** 735–740.
4. Fetters, L. & E.Z. Tronick. 1996. Neuromotor development of cocaine-exposed and control infants from birth through 15 months: Poor and poorer performance. Pediatrics **98:** 938–943.
5. Dubowitz, L. & V. Dubowitz. 1981. The neurological assessment of the preterm and full-term newborn infant. Clinics in Developmental Medicine No. 79. Spastics International. J.B. Lippincott. Philadelphia.
6. Prechtl, H.F.R. 1977. The neurological examination of the full term newborn infant (second edition). Clinics in Developmental Medicine 63. Spastics International Medical Publications. J.B. Lippincott. Philadelphia.
7. Amiel-Tison, C. & A. Grenier. 1986. Neurological Assessment during the First Year of Life. Oxford University Press. New York, NY.
8. Capute, A.J. 1986. Early neuromotor reflexes in infancy. Pediatr. Ann. **15:** 3, 217–226.
9. Allen, M.C. & A.J. Capute. 1989. Neonatal neurodevelopmental examination as a predictor of neuromotor outcome in premature infants. Pediatrics **83:** 489–506.

Prenatal Cocaine Exposure and Impulse Control at Two Years

MARGARET BENDERSKY AND MICHAEL LEWIS[a]

Institute for the Study of Child Development, UMDNJ-Robert Wood Johnson Medical School, New Brunswick, New Jersey 08903–0019, USA

Impulse control is a mediator of interpersonal relationships, motivation, and learning ability. Prenatal exposure to cocaine disrupts development of the fetal central nervous system, in particular monoaminergically innervated regions such as the mesolimic, which may underly this capacity.[1,2] However, impulse control may be affected by many factors, both biologic and environmental, that are more prevalent in cocaine-exposed children. This study examined whether prenatal exposure to cocaine, independent of other potential explanatory variables, resulted in poorer impulse control at 2 years of age.

METHOD

Subjects

Seventy-seven subjects, 51 of whom were prenatally exposed and 26 unexposed to cocaine, were studied. Of the exposed subjects, 27 were heavily exposed (≥ twice a week) and 24 were lightly exposed (< twice a week on average throughout gestation). Subjects were recruited from inner-city, predominantly African-American populations. They were full-term and healthy, with no congenital anomalies. Cocaine exposure was determined by neonatal meconium screens and maternal interviews.

TABLE 1 presents the sample characteristics. Subjects whose mothers used cocaine during pregnancy had more neonatal medical complications, were exposed to more alcohol and cigarettes, and had significantly higher general environmental risk in the second year of life. Lightly and heavily exposed subjects did not differ on these variables.

Procedure

At 24 months of age subjects were seated at a table upon which the examiner placed a cookie and were told not to take the cookie until the examiner returned. The subjects were given a toy and the examiner left. Caregivers remained in the room. The examiner returned after 2 minutes. The procedure was videotaped from behind a one-way mirror. Videotapes were coded to quantify the subjects' responses and the amount of time the caregiver spent distracting the subject.

[a] Address for correspondence: 97 Paterson Street, New Brunswick, NJ 08903-0019. Phone, 732/235-7700; fax, 732/235-6189; e-mail, LEWIS@UMDNJ.EDU

TABLE 1. Sample Characteristics, Frequencies, or Means (SD)

	Unexposed ($n = 26$)	Cocaine-Exposed ($n = 51$)
Males/females	13/13	22/29
Gestational age (wk)*	39.2 (2.4)	38.1 (2.1)
Birth weight (g)*	3,059 (552)	2,741 (533)
Neonatal Medical Risk*[a]	0.7 (1.5)	1.4 (2.1)
Average no. Drinks/Day–Pregnancy**	0.02 (0.07)	1.1 (1.8)
Average no. Cigs/Day–Pregnancy**	2.3 (3.7)	9.4 (10.3)
Average no. Joints/Day–Pregnancy	0.01 (0.04)	0.32 (1.65)
Environment Risk*[,b]	47.5 (10.5)	51.8 (7.1)

*p <.05; **p <.001.

[a]Neonatal Medical Risk Score is the weighted sum of 31 neonatal medical complications. Log transformed scores are used in statistical analyses.

[b]Environmental Risk Score is the sum of 11 proximal and distal environmental risk variables, including race, parental education, occupation, social support, life stress, and continued drug use, as well as the stability and regularity of the child's daily environment based on caregiver report at 18 months.

RESULTS

Impulse control was operationalized as the latencies to reach, take, and eat the cookie (seconds). The amount of time caregivers interacted with their children affected the latencies to reach ($r = 0.24$, $p < 0.05$), to take ($r = 0.30$, $p < 0.01$), and to eat the cookie ($r = 0.23$, $p = 0.05$), so that the greater the time the caregivers spent interacting with their children, the longer the children delayed reaching for, taking, or eating the cookie. The exposure groups did not differ in the amount of time the caregivers spent interacting with their children. However, to account for the effect the caregiver's presence during the procedure may have had on the subject's behaviors, the amount of time the caregiver actively distracted the child was included as a covariate in subsequent analyses.

TABLE 2 presents the means and standard deviations of the dependent variables for the unexposed and exposed groups. Because the cocaine-exposed groups differed in the amount of exposure to alcohol and cigarettes, neonatal medical risk, and environmental risk, the mean latencies also are adjusted for these variables in analyses of covariance. As TABLE 2 indicates, cocaine-exposed subjects were quicker to reach for ($F(1,70)=17.2$, $p < 0.001$), take ($F(1,70) = 7.1$, $p = 0.01$), and eat the cookie ($F(1,70) = 4.9$, $p < 0.04$).

The amount of exposure to other substances, neonatal medical risk, and environ-

TABLE 2. Latencies (seconds) and Adjusted Means[a] (SD)

	Unexposed	Cocaine-Exposed
To reach***	81.2 (45.9)	30.4 (43.2)
To take**	87.6 (47.0)	51.4 (50.0)
To eat*	90.2 (49.1)	57.6 (53.6)

*p <0.05; **p = 0.01; ***p <0.001.

[a]Means are adjusted for amount of exposure to alcohol and cigarettes, neonatal medical risk, environmental risk, and amount of time the caregiver actively distracted the child.

mental factors may provide additional explanations of impulse control differences. Regression analyses indicated that the amount of prenatal alcohol exposure was independently related to latency to reach ($\beta = 8.9$, $p < 0.02$), so that increased alcohol exposure was associated with longer latencies. Increased caregiver distraction was associated with longer latency to reach for the cookie ($\beta = 0.36$, $p < 0.07$), take the cookie ($\beta = 0.57$, $p < 0.02$), and eat the cookie ($\beta = 0.47$, $p = 0.05$).

CONCLUSIONS

The findings suggest that impulse control is a function of both brain biology and how children are trained by their parents. Prenatal cocaine exposure resulted in poorer impulse control at 24 months of age, when medical factors, other substance exposures, as well as the caregiver's concurrent behavior were controlled. The amount of time the caregiver spent engaging her child in distracting interactions also had an independent effect on the impulse control measures. Thus, caregivers may be able to help children develop some measure of impulse control whether or not there is a biologic tendency for poor behavioral regulation.

REFERENCES

1. Dow-Edwards, D. 1991. Cocaine effects on fetal development: A comparison of clinical and animal findings. Neurotoxicol. Teratol. **13:** 347–352.
2. Mayes, L.C. & M.H. Bornstein. 1995. Developmental dilemma for cocaine-abusing parents and their children. *In* Mothers, Babies and Cocaine: The Role of Toxins in Development. M. Lewis & M. Bendersky, Eds.: 251–272. Erlbaum. Hillsdale, NJ.
3. Hobel, C., M. Hyvarinen, D. Okada & W. Oh. 1973. Prenatal and intrapartum high-risk screening. Am. J. Obstet. Gynecol. **117:** 1–9.

Cocaine-Induced Activation of *c-fos* Gene Expression Is Attenuated in Prenatal Cocaine-Exposed Rabbits[a]

NANDA TILAKARATNE, GUOPING CAI, AND EITAN FRIEDMAN[b]

Division of Molecular Pharmacology, Department of Pharmacology, MCP ◆ Hahnemann School of Medicine, Allegheny University of the Health Sciences, Philadelphia, Pennsylvania 19129, USA

Developmental and neurobehavioral abnormalities have been shown in newborns exposed to cocaine *in utero.*[1,2] These deficits could be caused by indirect effects of cocaine, which elicit uterine vasoconstriction either directly on smooth muscle cells or via maternal vasoactive factors that reduce blood flow to the fetus, or by direct cocaine-mediated modulation of fetal brain synaptic neurotransmitters. Cocaine blocks presynaptic uptake of neurotransmitters such as dopamine, norepinephrine, and serotonin, resulting in synaptic accumulation of these amines and stimulation of synaptic receptors. Systemic administration of cocaine in adult rodents elicited rapid induction in expression of immediate-early genes, such as *c-fos* and *zif*-268.[3,4] Immediate-early gene products function as transcription factors and regulate subsequent target gene expression. This mechanism has been suggested to mediate the short- and long-term effects of central stimulants.[3] Therefore, changes in cocaine-induced genomic responses may reflect on developmental and neurobehavioral alterations attributable to prenatal cocaine exposure. In this study, cocaine-induced *c-fos* gene expression was examined in 20-day-old prenatal saline-exposed as well as prenatal cocaine-exposed rabbits.

Female Dutch Belted rabbits were bred and randomly distributed into two treatment groups. One group was given two daily iv injections of 4 mg/kg cocaine HCl and the other received two daily iv saline injections from day 8 through day 29 of gestation. Kits were nursed by their respective dams and removed from their cages on postnatal day 20. Kits were sacrificed 60 minutes after a single intraperitoneal (ip) injection of 40 mg/kg cocaine HCl or saline solution. In testing receptor antagonists, rabbit offsprings received an ip injection of a specific antagonist 30 minutes before the injection of cocaine. Brain frontal cortex and striatum were dissected out for extraction of total RNA. Ten micrograms of RNA were size fractionated by electrophoresis on 1% agarose–6% formaldehyde gel and transferred onto a Nytran membrane. *c-fos* mRNA was detected by hybridization with a ^{32}P-labeled DNA probe which was a 500-bp fragment of the *c-fos* cDNA. The membrane was exposed to X-ray film, and the relevant autoradiographic signals were quantitated by soft laser densitometry. The mean ± SEM optical density, in arbitrary units, was calculated and data were analyzed by ANOVA followed by the Newman-Keuls test.

Acute cocaine administration (40 mg/kg, ip) induced *c-fos* gene expression in brain frontal cortex and striatum of both prenatal saline-exposed and prenatal cocaine-

[a] This work was supported in part by United States Public Health Service Grant P01-DA06871 from the National Institute on Drug Abuse.

[b] To whom correspondence should be addressed. Phone, 215/842–4203; fax, 215/843–1515; e-mail: FRIEDMANE@AUHS.EDU

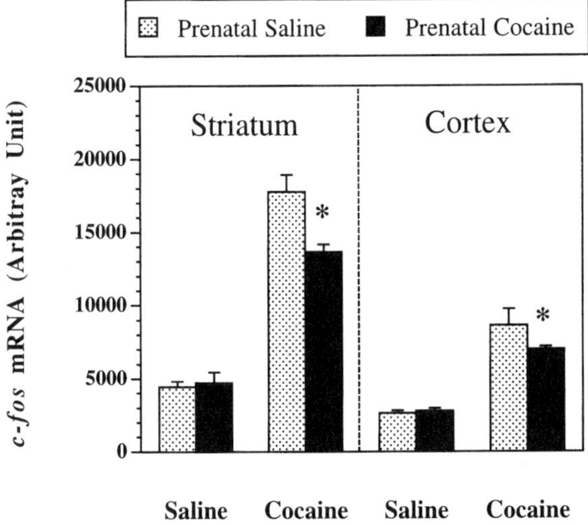

FIGURE 1. Cocaine-induced *c-fos* gene expression in prenatal saline-exposed or prenatal cocaine-exposed 20-day-old rabbits. Animals were sacrificed 60 minutes after an ip injection of saline solution or 40 mg/kg cocaine HCl. Striatum and frontal cortex were dissected out and total RNA was extracted. Ten micrograms of RNA from each tissue were used for assessing *c-fos* mRNA by Northern blots. Each bar represents the mean ± SEM of six individual measurements from six litter-matched animals. **p* <0.05 compared to prenatal saline-exposed animals.

exposed rabbits (FIG. 1). Pretreatment with the specific D_1 dopamine receptor antagonist SCH23390 (0.075 mg/kg, ip) almost abolished cocaine-induced *c-fos* gene expression. However, cocaine-induced *c-fos* gene expression was not affected by pretreatment with the specific D_2 dopamine receptor antagonist sulpiride (50 mg/kg, ip) (FIG. 2). These results confirm previous findings obtained in adult rats that cocaine-induced *c-fos* gene expression is mediated by D_1 but not by D_2 dopamine receptors.[5,6] Acute cocaine challenge increased the expression of *c-fos* mRNA by 301% in striatum and 229% in cortex of prenatal saline-exposed rabbits. However, in prenatal cocaine-exposed animals, cocaine-induced *c-fos* gene expression was reduced by 37.5% and 34.1% in striatum and cortex, respectively. Basal *c-fos* gene expression in the brain of both prenatal saline-exposed and prenatal cocaine-exposed rabbits was detected. This level of *c-fos* gene expression appears not to be induced by experimental stress, because levels of *c-fos* mRNA did not change over a period of 2 hours after injection of saline solution but rather may be due to active processes associated with this period of early postnatal rabbit brain development. These results suggest that prenatal cocaine exposure impairs D_1 dopamine receptor function, which may in part result from a deficit in D_1 dopamine receptor/Gs protein coupling which is produced by *in utero* cocaine exposure in rabbits.[7,8]

REFERENCES

1. ZUCKERMAN, B., D. A. FRANK, R. H. AMARO, S. M. LEVENSON & H. KAYNE. 1989. N. Engl. J. Med. **12:** 762–768.
2. CHASNOFF, I. J., C. FREIER & J. MURRAY. 1992. Pediatrics **89:** 284–289.

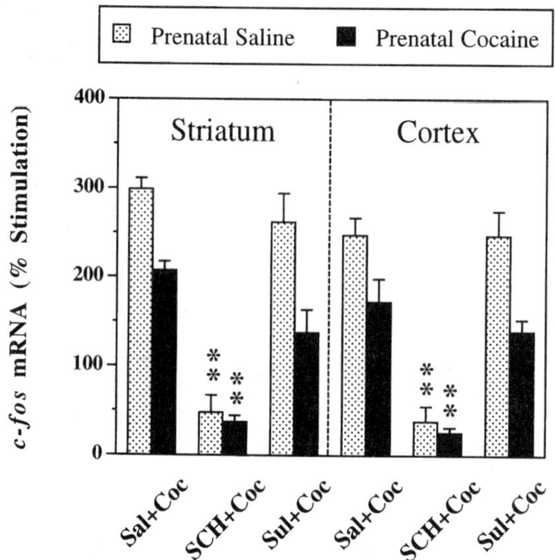

FIGURE 2. Antagonism of cocaine-induced *c-fos* gene expression in prenatal saline-exposed or prenatal cocaine-exposed 20-day-old rabbits. Animals were pretreated with ip injection of saline solution, 0.075 mg/kg SCH23390, or 50 mg/kg sulpiride 30 minutes before a challenge dose of 40 mg/kg cocaine HCl. Animals were sacrificed 60 minutes after injection of cocaine, and brain regions were dissected out for total RNA extraction. Ten micrograms of RNA from each tissue were used for detection of *c-fos* mRNA by Northern blots. Each bar represents the mean ± SEM of three individual measurements from three litter-matched animals. $^{**}p < 0.01$ compared to saline pretreated group in the respective prenatal saline-exposed or prenatal cocaine-exposed animal.

3. Graybiel, A. M., R. Moratalla & H. Robertson. 1990. Proc. Natl. Acad. Sci. USA **87:** 6912–6916.
4. Helton, T. E., J. B. Daunais & J. F. McGinty. 1993. Mol. Brain Res. **20:** 285–288.
5. Young, S. T., L. J. Porrino & M. J. Iadarola. 1991. Proc. Natl. Acad. Sci. USA **88:** 1291–1295.
6. Bhat, R. V. & J. M. Baraban. 1993. J. Pharmacol. Exp. Ther. **267:** 496–505.
7. Wang, H.-Y., S. Runyan, E. Yadin & E. Friedman. 1995. J. Pharmacol. Exp. Ther. **273:** 492–498.
8. Friedman, E., E. Yadin & H.-Y. Wang. 1996. Neuroscience **70:** 739–747.

Prenatal Cocaine Exposure Does Not Affect Selected $GABA_A$ Receptor Subunit mRNA Expression in Rabbit Visual Cortex[a]

JED S. SHUMSKY,[b,e] YUNXING WU,[c,f] E. HAZEL MURPHY,[b,e] JONATHAN NISSANOV,[d,g] AND DENNIS R. GRAYSON[b,c,f]

[b]*Department of Neurobiology and Anatomy, MCP ◆ Hahnemann University School of Medicine, Allegheny University of the Health Sciences, 3200 Henry Avenue, Philadelphia, Pennsylvania 19129, USA*

[c]*Department of Psychiatry, Allegheny University of the Health Sciences, 320 East North Avenue, Pittsburgh, Pennsylvania 15212, USA*

[d]*Imaging and Computer Vision Center, Drexel University, 32nd and Chestnut St., Philadelphia, Pennsylvania 19104, USA*

Our group previously showed[1] that in the dopamine-rich anterior cingulate cortex, significant increases in GABA immunoreactivity occur in the offspring of rabbits given intravenous injection of cocaine (3 mg/kg) twice daily during pregnancy. In contrast, such changes were not found in the dopamine-poor visual cortex. In ongoing studies we are investigating the effects of prenatal cocaine exposure on the developmental expression of specific $GABA_A$ receptor subunit mRNAs using *in situ* hybridization. We[2] previously reported laminar-specific alterations in selected $GABA_A$ receptor subunit mRNAs in anterior cingulate cortex at postnatal day 20 (P20). The aim of this study was to determine whether similar laminar-specific changes occurred in visual cortex at the same postnatal age.

METHODS

Dutch Belted rabbits (Myrtle's Rabbitry, Thompson Station, Tennessee) were bred in our animal facility according to our model,[3] and does were given cocaine (3 mg/kg, iv) twice a day from gestational day 8 to 29. Offspring were anesthetized with sodium pentobarbital and decapitated at P20. Brains were removed and frozen in isopentane cooled to −35°C with dry ice. Tissues were stored at −70°C until use. Coronal sections (14 μm) were cut on a cryostat and mounted onto silanated slides.

The α_1, β_2, or γ_2 subunit mRNA plasmids were constructed as previously described.[4] ^{35}S-labeled antisense cRNA probes were prepared by *in vitro* transcription of the linearized templates, and *in situ* hybridization was performed as previously de-

[a] This work was supported by P01DA06871 (E.H.M.), K04NS01647 (D.R.G.), and P41RR01638 (J.N.).

[e] Phone, 215/842-4641 or 4640; fax, 215/843-9082; e-mail: shumsky@auhs.edu or murphy@auhs.edu

[f] Phone, 412/359-4814; fax, 412/359-4364; e-mail: grayson@asri.edu or ywu@welchlink.welch.jhu.edu

[g] Phone, 215/895-1381; fax, 215/895-4987; e-mail: nissanoj@dunx1.ocs.drexel.edu

scribed.[2,5] *In situ* signals were visualized using slides and film. Four matched sections of visual cortex from four pairs of cocaine- and saline-treated P20 rabbit brains were quantitatively analyzed. Pairs of matched coronal sections were used for each of the α_1, β_2, and γ_2 $GABA_A$ receptor subunits to reduce within-subject variability. Nissl stained sections were used for the identification of specific laminae.

Histologically counterstained sections and their corresponding autoradiographic films were captured for image analysis using a Sony XC-77 camera mounted on a lightbox for macroautoradiographic analysis. Image capture and analysis relied on BRAIN 2.0 (Computer Vision Center for Vertebrate Brain Mapping, Drexel University, Philadelphia, Pennsylvania) and NIH Image 1.62 both running on a Macintosh. Histologic and autoradiographic images were aligned by the principal axis method.[6] Equivalent regions of interest for the six laminae of visual cortex were delineated on the histologic image, and their corresponding optical densities (OD) were measured on the autoradiographic image. We collected data from four sequential sections from four pairs of cocaine- or saline-exposed animals, with each pair matched for cortical level and processed together. Two-way (prenatal treatment × visual cortex layer) analysis of variance (ANOVA) was performed, with visual cortex layer taken as a repeated measure. Post-hoc analysis was performed using paired t tests.

RESULTS

As illustrated in FIGURE 1, the distribution of all three $GABA_A$ receptor subunit mRNAs was found to be laminar specific in visual cortex. ANOVA revealed a significant effect of visual cortex layer for all three $GABA_A$ receptor subunit mRNAs: α_1 [$F(5,30) = 25.9$, $p < 0.001$], β_2 [$F(5,30) = 67.4$, $p < 0.001$], and γ_2 [$F(5,30) = 147.9$, $p < 0.001$]. Levels of all three subunit mRNAs were found to be highest in visual cortex layer II. However, prenatal cocaine exposure produced no effect on the distribution of the three $GABA_A$ receptor subunit mRNAs across the visual cortex layers. Furthermore, post-hoc analysis using paired t tests revealed no significant differences between prenatal treatments in α_1, β_2, or γ_2 $GABA_A$ receptor subunit mRNA levels in any of the laminae of visual cortex and no differences for visual cortex layer II/III OD ratios (FIG. 2).

DISCUSSION

Prenatal cocaine exposure had no effect on levels of α_1, β_2, and γ_2 $GABA_A$ receptor subunit mRNAs in visual cortex. In contrast, prenatal cocaine exposure produced substantial alterations in the dopamine-rich anterior cingulate cortex,[7] including laminar-specific changes in $GABA_A$ receptor subunit mRNA levels at the same postnatal age,[2] long-term increases in GABA-immunoreactivity in anterior cingulate cortex neurons,[1] and long-term increases in parvalbumin-immunoreactivity in the dendrites of a subset of GABA neurons that stained positive for parvalbumin.[8] None of these changes was found in the dopamine-poor visual cortex. These findings cannot be explained by changes in cortical lamination, cell number, or soma size, because we found no differences in any of these parameters in either the anterior cingulate cortex or visual cortex.[1] Collectively, our data support the hypothesis that prenatal cocaine exposure alters the development of the GABAergic system only in areas of the brain that have substantial dopaminergic innervation.

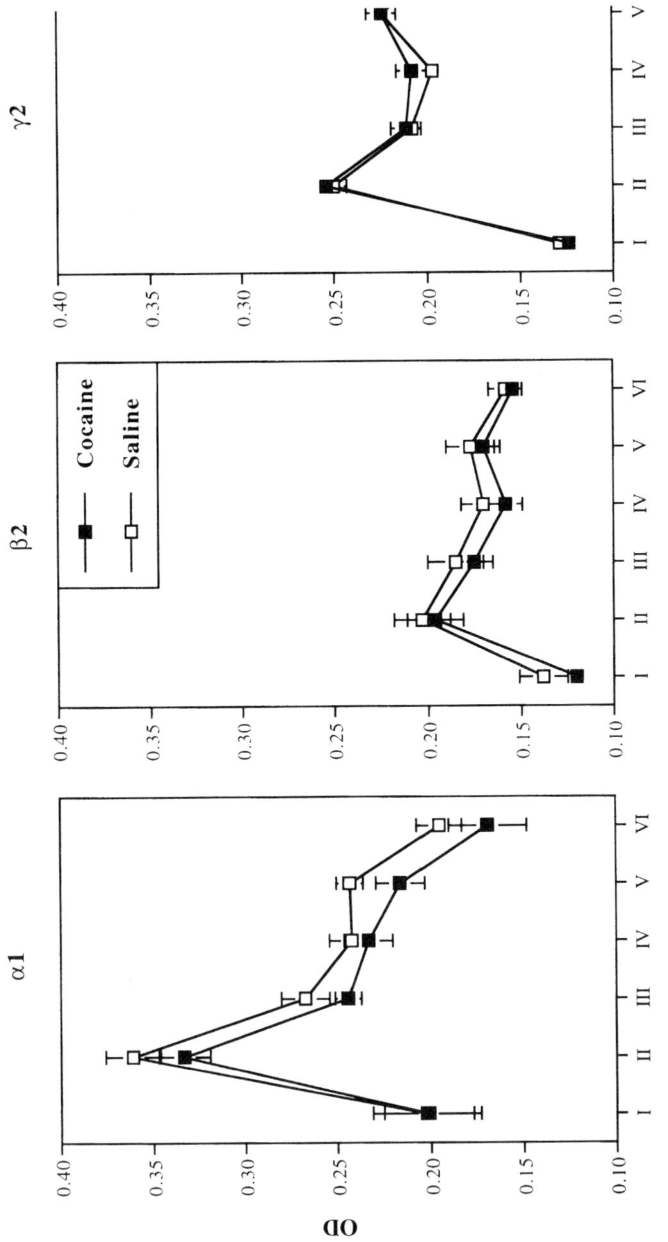

FIGURE 1. Effect of prenatal treatment with cocaine on α_1, β_2, and γ_2 $GABA_A$ receptor subunit mRNAs in visual cortex. Values represent mean OD intensity for animals prenatally exposed to cocaine ($n = 4$) or saline solution ($n = 4$) ± SEM.

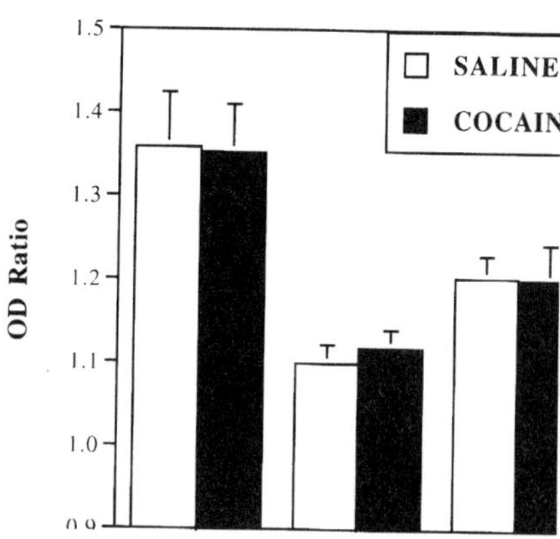

FIGURE 2. Effect of prenatal treatment with cocaine on the ratio between layers II and III for α_1, β_2, and γ_2 $GABA_A$ receptor subunit mRNAs in visual cortex. Values represent mean OD intensity ratios for animals prenatally exposed to cocaine ($n = 4$) or saline solution ($n = 4$) ± SEM.

REFERENCES

1. WANG, X.-H., P. LEVITT, D.R. GRAYSON & E.H. MURPHY. 1995. Intrauterine cocaine exposure of rabbits: Persistent elevation of GABA-immunoreactive neurons in anterior cingulate cortex but not visual cortex. Brain Res. **689:** 32–46.
2. WU, Y., J.S. SHUMSKY, E.H. MURPHY, J. NISSANOV, A. O'BRIEN-JENKINS & D.R. GRAYSON. 1997. Differential effects of prenatal cocaine exposure on selected subunit mRNAs of the $GABA_A$ receptor. Soc. Neurosci. Abstr. **23:** 103.
3. MURPHY, E.H., J.G. HAMMER, M.D. SCHUMANN, M.Y. GROCE, X.H. WANG & L. JONES. 1995. The rabbit as a model for studies of *in utero* cocaine exposure. Lab. Anim. Sci. **45:** 163–168.
4. WU, Y., J.S. SHUMSKY, E.H. MURPHY, J. NISSANOV, A. O'BRIEN-JENKINS, W. PALJUG & D.R. GRAYSON. 1998. The distribution of the α_1, β_2 and γ_2 $GABA_A$ receptor subunit mRNAs in the rabbit brain. Dev. Brain Res. Submitted.
5. MARLIER, L.N., T. ZHENG, J. TANG & D.R. GRAYSON. 1993. Regional distribution in the rat central nervous system of a mRNA encoding a portion of the cardiac sodium/calcium exchanger isolated from cerebellar granule neurons. Brain Res. **20:** 21–39.
6. NISSANOV, J. & D.L. MCEACHRON. 1991. Advances in image processing for autoradiography. J. Chem. Neuroanat. **4:** 329–342.
7. LEVITT, P., J.A. HARVEY, E. FRIEDMAN, K. SIMANSKY & E.H. MURPHY. 1997. New evidence for neurotransmitter influences on brain development. Trends Neurosci. **20:** 269–274.
8. WANG, X.-H., A. O'BRIEN-JENKINS, L. CHOI & E.H. MURPHY. 1996. Altered neuronal distribution of parvalbumin in limbic cortex of rabbits exposed *in utero* to cocaine. Exp. Brain Res. **112:** 359–371.

Prenatal Exposure to Cocaine Reduces Dopaminergic D_1-Mediated Motor Function but Spares the Enhancement of Learning by Amphetamine in Rabbits[a]

K. J. SIMANSKY,[b] G. BAKER, W. J. KACHELRIES, H. HOOD,
A. G. ROMANO, AND J. A. HARVEY

Department of Pharmacology, Allegheny University of the Health Sciences, Philadelphia, Pennsylvania 19129, USA

During recent years, several collaborating laboratories have used intravenous administration of low doses of cocaine (2–4 mg/kg, bid) during pregnancy in rabbits to model effects of prenatal exposure to this drug in humans.[1,2] Offspring exposed *in utero* to a maternal dose of either 3 or 4 mg/kg cocaine, bid, from day 8 through day 29 of gestation (G8-G29) had brains that were normal on gross examination. Finer analyses revealed structural and neurochemical aberrations in the CNS that included abnormal dendritic development in the anterior cingulate cortex[2,3] and impaired coupling of D_1-like receptors to their G-proteins.[2,4,5] The behavior of juvenile and adult offspring of mothers given cocaine appeared overtly normal. When challenged, however, the CNS abnormalities were associated with altered learning as assessed by associative (pavlovian) conditioning[6,7] and selectively diminished responsiveness to behavioral actions of the indirectly acting monoaminergic agonist D-amphetamine (D-AMPH).[8]

Previously, we reported that a moderately large dose of D-AMPH (5.0 mg/kg, sc) failed to elicit stereotyped head bobbing in juvenile (48–56 days old) Dutch rabbits that had been exposed prenatally to a maternal dose of cocaine of 4 mg/kg, bid, in the model just described. Locomotion and other motor actions of D-AMPH were normal in these rabbits. In 140-day-old rabbits, prenatal exposure to cocaine reduced head bobbing *and* other stereotypy. In 180-day-old rabbits, 6.0 mg/kg D-AMPH failed to elicit head bobbing, but smaller doses (0.3–3.3 mg/kg) produced identical effects on feeding and motor behavior in the cocaine progeny and their controls.[8]

A dose of 4 mg/kg cocaine, bid, produced a very low incidence of generalized tonic-clonic seizures (GTCS) in the pregnant does. A lower dose (3 mg/kg, bid), however, did not elicit GTCS in the does but still produced the fine structural and biochemical deficits just described in the offspring.[2] The present study, therefore, analyzed the effects of exposure during gestation to the lower dose of cocaine on behavioral responses. We tested the ability of acutely administered D-AMPH to stimulate head bobbing, which is mediated by D_1-like receptors.[8] Conversely, we determined the sensitivity of cocaine progeny to the cataleptic effect of blocking D_1 receptors with SCH23390. Finally, we

[a] This research was supported by United States Public Health Service Grant DA11164-01 from the National Institute on Drug Abuse.

[b] Address for correspondence: Kenny J. Simansky, Ph.D., Department of Pharmacology, MCP ◆Hahnemann School of Medicine, Allegheny University of the Health Sciences, 3200 Henry Avenue, Philadelphia, PA 19129-1137. Phone, 215/842-4675; 215/843-1515; e-mail: Simansky@AUHS.EDU

assessed whether D-AMPH would enhance the rate of acquisition of a classically conditioned (pavlovian) response in cocaine progeny as it does in normal rabbits.[9]

FIGURE 1 shows that fetal exposure to the smaller dose of cocaine essentially eliminated head bobbing normally elicited by D-AMPH. Analyses of the data based on litter ($n = 5$ litters per prenatal condition) as the unit (SAL, 77 ± 9 head bobs/10 min vs COC, 2 ± 1) or by gender (SAL male, $n = 6$, 81 ± 15 vs COC male, $n = 5$, 3 ± 3; SAL female, $n = 4$, 71 ± 12 vs COC female, $n = 5$, 1 ± 1) were consistent with the results shown in the figure. FIGURE 1 also demonstrates that cocaine progeny were more vulnerable to the cataleptic effect of blocking D_1 receptors. By contrast, a dose of D-AMPH that optimally enhanced associative learning in a dose-response study in normal rabbits (not shown) produced identical increases in the rate of acquisition of conditioned responses in cocaine progeny and their controls (FIG. 2). Note that the experimental parameters for conditioning were adjusted to equate baseline rates of acquisition (SAL-VEH and COC-VEH) in this study. In previous work using other parameters, prenatal

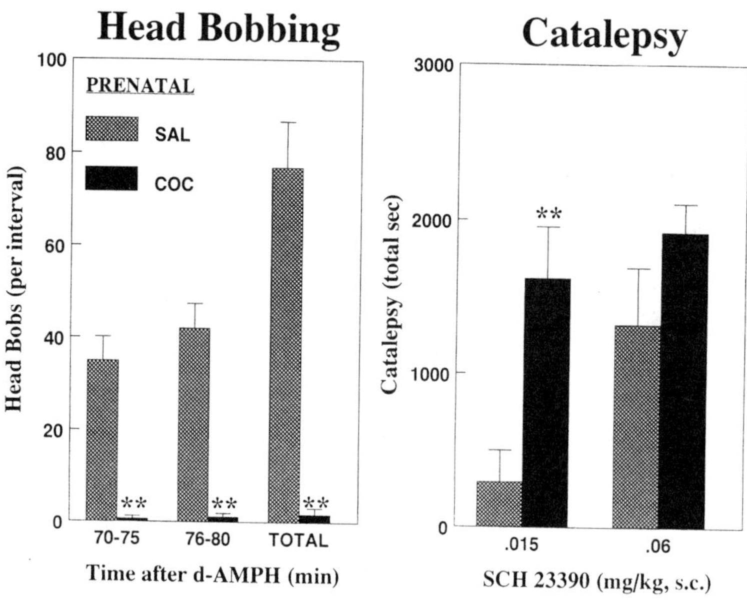

FIGURE 1. Prenatal exposure to cocaine reduces D_1-mediated motor function in rabbits. **(Left Panel)** Number of stereotyped vertical head movements (head bobs) elicited by 5 mg/kg sc of D-AMPH (sulfate salt) in 54–58-day-old rabbits exposed prenatally to cocaine (COC, $n = 10$) given iv to pregnant does (3 mg/kg, bid) or saline solution (SAL, $n = 10$). Rabbits were placed in an arena (76 cm^2 and 46 cm high), and the frequency of head bobbing was recorded by an observer for two successive 5-minute intervals at the time of peak responding.[8] $^{**}p < 0.01$ vs SAL; two-factor ANOVA (prenatal treatment vs time, TOTAL tested by significant main effect, intervals by Newman-Keuls tests). **(Right Panel)** Duration of catalepsy displayed by 10 cocaine progeny and 10 saline-exposed controls after administration of the D_1-like antagonist, R(+)-SCH 23390 HCl (5 pairs per dose), at 56–80 days of age. After an initial trial with saline solution (1 ml/kg, sc), rabbits were injected with SCH23390, placed with both forepaws on a bar suspended 18 cm above the surface of a table, and the latency to remove their paws from the bar (maximum 5 minutes) was measured every 15 minutes for 2 hours. $^{**}p < 0.01$, orthogonal t test.

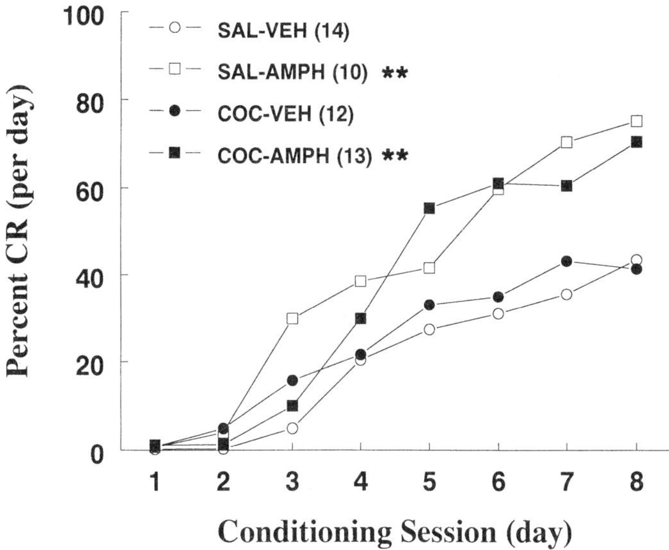

FIGURE 2. Prenatal exposure to cocaine does not prevent the enhancement by D-AMPH of associative conditioning of the nictitating membrane response (NMR) in rabbits. D-AMPH (1.8 mg/kg, sc) or vehicle injections were administered 20–30 minutes before the start of the training sessions, conducted on 8 successive days. Each session contained 60 paired stimulus presentations with a 90-db, 100-ms tone as a conditioned stimulus and a 100-ms corneal airpuff (unconditioned stimulus) presented 500 ms after conditioned stimulus onset. Percent CR was the percentage of the 60 trials in which the rabbits made a conditioned response. Cocaine and saline progeny (100–135 days old) were injected with either D-AMPH (e.g., COC-AMP, *n* in parentheses) or vehicle. $^{**}p < 0.01$ compared with rabbits injected with vehicle, ANOVA.

exposure to cocaine altered learning of a simple CS-US association and impaired learning of a complex discrimination.[6,7]

DISCUSSION

The current results demonstrated that fetal exposure to a smaller dose of cocaine than we tested previously[8] reproduced the deficit in responding stimulated by dopamine acting at D_1 receptors, probably in the striatum. This lower exposure did not produce GTCS in our model, but it did reduce D_1-G_S coupling in cocaine progeny.[2] Thus, this dopaminergic motor deficit is related to the dysfunction in cellular signaling. The data established for the first time that cocaine progeny are also more vulnerable to reduced motor function produced by blocking D_1-like receptors, probably also in the striatum. These dysfunctions appeared to be somewhat selective, because D-AMPH enhanced associative learning in cocaine progeny; however, the role of D_1 receptors in this behavior is unknown. Overall, the present evidence establishes the diminished capacity of D_1 dopaminergic mechanisms to support normal motor function. Cocaine-exposed offspring, however, may remain sensitive to therapeutic effects of D-AMPH or related agents in learning.

REFERENCES

1. LEVITT, P. *et al.* 1997. New evidence for neurotransmitter influences on brain development. Trends Neurosci. **20:** 269–274.
2. MURPHY, W. H. *et al.* 1997. Cocaine administration in pregnant rabbits alters cortical structure and function in their progeny in the absence of maternal seizures. Exp. Brain Res. **114:** 433–441.
3. JONES, L. *et al.* 1996. Nonuniform alteration of dendritic development in the cerebral cortex following prenatal cocaine exposure. Cereb. Cortex **6:** 431–445.
4. WANG, H.-Y. *et al.* 1995. Prenatal exposure to cocaine selectively reduces D1 dopamine receptor-mediated activation of striatal Gs proteins. J. Pharmacol. Exp. Ther. **273:** 492–498.
5. FRIEDMAN, E. *et al.* 1996. Effect of prenatal cocaine on dopamine receptor-G protein coupling in mesocortical regions of the rabbit brain. Neuroscience **70:** 739–747.
6. ROMANO, A. G. *et al.* 1995. Intrauterine exposure to cocaine produces a modality-specific acceleration of classical conditioning in adult rabbits. Pharmacol. Biochem. Behav. **52:** 415–420.
7. ROMANO, A. G. & J. A. HARVEY. 1996. Prenatal exposure to cocaine disrupts discrimination learning in adult rabbits. Pharmacol. Biochem. Behav. **53:** 617–621.
8. SIMANSKY, K. J. & W. J. KACHELRIES. 1996. Prenatal exposure to cocaine selectively disrupts motor responding to D-amphetamine in young and mature rabbits. Neuropharmacology **35:** 71–78.
9. HARVEY, J. A. *et al.* 1982. Effects of d-lysergic acid diethylamide, d-2-bromolysergic acid diethylamide, dl-2,5-dimethoxy-4-methylamphetamine and d-amphetamine on classical conditioning of the rabbit nictitating membrane response. J. Pharmacol. Exp. Ther. **221:** 289–294.

Neonatal Respiratory Control in the Rat after Prenatal Cocaine Exposure

A. N. DAVIES,[a,c] C. E. SULLIVAN,[a] AND P. D. C. BROWN-WOODMAN[b]

[a]*Department of Medicine, Faculty of Medicine (D06);* [b]*Department of Biomedical Sciences, Faculty of Health Sciences; The University of Sydney, NSW 2006, Australia*

Several clinical studies suggest that cocaine use by pregnant women increases the incidence of sudden infant death syndrome (SIDS) in their offspring.[1] It is linked to reproductive problems in humans including neurobehavioral abnormalities and congenital malformations such as loss of digits.[2] Many animal studies have given insight into possible mechanisms underlying these effects of cocaine. Webster and Brown-Woodman,[3] using rats, demonstrated that the digital defects were due to peripheral bleeding which was observed in fetuses soon after cocaine administration to the mother. Thus, as similar abnormalities are observed in the human and rat exposed to cocaine *in utero,* a study of respiratory control in this rat model may provide insight into physiologic mechanisms that could predispose some children to SIDS.

METHODS

In the current study, pregnant rats were given one intraperitoneal injection of cocaine (50 mg/kg) on day 16 of gestation and allowed to litter. Out of six litters exposed to cocaine *in utero,* only in one litter (617) were abnormalities observed (e.g., loss of digits). The results of tests of this litter were examined separately as well as pooled with other cocaine-treated litters. Ventilation was measured by a modification of the plethysmographic chamber method of Drorbaugh and Fenn.[4] Ventilation was measured in room air for 5 minutes; the response to the gas mixture was then measured for 10 minutes followed by measurement in room air for 5 minutes. The ventilatory response to hypoxia (8% O_2/N_2) and hypercapnia (10% CO_2/O_2) was measured in the pups exposed to cocaine and control pups in three age groups: days 5–8, 9–15, and 16–25 after birth.

RESULTS

In the 5–8-day-old animals, overall the cocaine-treated and control groups did not differ in response when exposed to hypoxia. However, litter 617 exhibited depression of resting ventilation ($p < 0.05$) and diminished initial response to hypoxia ($p < 0.001$) with respect to other cocaine-treated litters and control litters (FIG. 1). Resting ventilation in the 15–25-day age group was greater in cocaine-treated animals, especially litter 617 ($p < 0.05$) (FIG. 1). In the group of 9–14-day-old pups, the hypoxic response was similar overall in the cocaine-treated animals and in the control; however, ventilation of pups in litter 617 was depressed ($p < 0.001$) especially during rest before exposure to hypoxia. This may indicate sleep-onset hypoventilation. In the 16–25-day age group the response to hypoxia was similar in both treatment groups. The response to hypercap-

[c] Phone, 02/93512168; fax, 02/95503851; e-mail; and@mail.med.usyd.edu.au

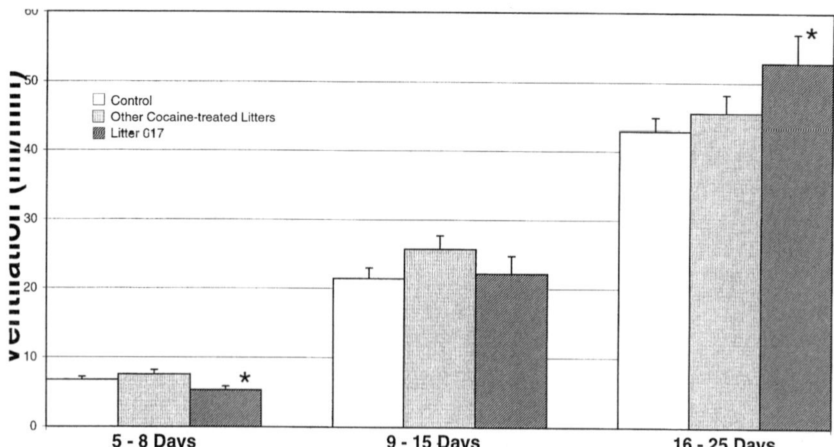

FIGURE 1. Resting ventilation in the three age groups studied: pups from control litters ($n = 80$), cocaine-treated litters excluding litter 617 ($n = 61$), and severely cocaine-affected litter 617 ($n = 9$). Cocaine exposure *in utero* initially depressed resting ventilation in the 5–8-day-old pups which later (16–25 days) developed enhanced resting ventilation. (*$p < 0.05$; error bars are standard error of the mean).

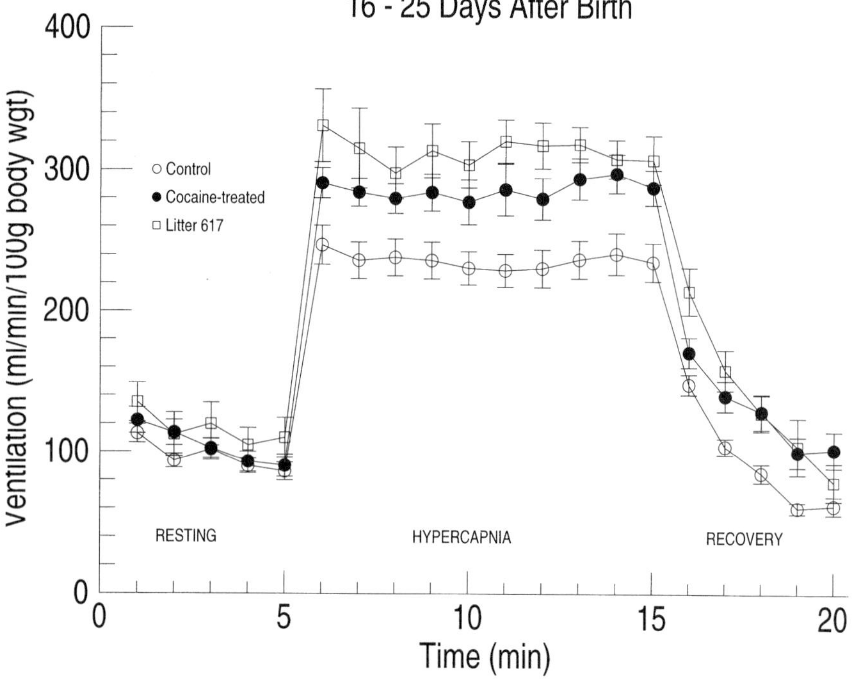

FIGURE 2. Response of 16–25-day-old pups to hypercapnia (10% CO_2/O_2). Ventilation is stimulated significantly more than that in control animals in all pups exposed to cocaine *in utero,* especially litter 617 ($p < 0.005$; control $n = 25$; cocaine-treated $n = 16$; litter 617 $n = 9$; error bars are standard error of the mean).

nia was similar for both the cocaine-treated and control animals in the younger age groups. However, in the 16–25 day age group exposed to hypercapnia, ventilation increased significantly more in cocaine-treated animals (p <0.005) (FIG. 2).

DISCUSSION

The results of this study suggest that cocaine exposure *in utero* depresses resting ventilation and response to hypoxia in neonatal rats. However, by the third week post partum, resting ventilation is greater in cocaine-exposed pups and they display a greater response to severe hypercapnia than do control animals. These results complement recent observations that prenatal cocaine exposure diminishes the hypoxic response in 5-day-old rat pups[5] and increases the ventilatory response to hypercapnia in neonatal guinea pigs.[6] The present study demonstrates that cocaine gives rise to these changes in respiratory function of the neonatal rat as a function of age. The early effects on respiratory control, by diminishing arousal, and the later effects, by increasing ventilatory effort, may increase the risk of SIDS in some infants, especially in a child with obstructive apnea during sleep.

REFERENCES

1. DURAND, D.J., A.M. ESPINOZA & B.G. NICKERSON. 1990. Association between prenatal cocaine exposure and sudden infant death syndrome. J. Pediatr. **117:** 909–911.
2. CHASNOFF, I.J., G.M. CHISUM & D. KAPLAN. 1988. Maternal cocaine use and genitourinary tract malformations. Teratology **37:** 201–204.
3. WEBSTER, W.S. & P.D.C. BROWN-WOODMAN. 1990. Cocaine as a cause of congenital malformations of vascular origin: Experimental evidence in the rat. Teratology **41:** 689–697.
4. DRORBAUGH, J.E. & W.O. FENN. 1955. A barometric method for measuring ventilation in newborn infants. Pediatrics **16:** 81–87.
5. LIPTON, J.W., T.L. DAVIDSON, P.M. CARVEY & D. WEESE-MAYER. 1996. Prenatal cocaine: Effect on hypoxic ventilatory responsiveness in neonatal rats. Resp. Physiol. **106:** 161–169.
6. OLSEN, G.D. & J.A. WEIL. 1992. *In utero* cocaine exposure: Effect on neonatal breathing in guinea pigs. J. Pharmacol. Exp. Ther. **261:** 420–428.

Ontogenic Cocaine Effects

Evidence for Multifactorial Mechanisms[a]

DIANA DOW-EDWARDS[b] AND YAMIT BUSIDAN

Laboratory of Cerebral Metabolism, Department of Pharmacology, State University of New York, Brooklyn, New York 11203, USA

Our model of embryonic exposure included cocaine administered at either 30 or 60 mg/kg/day by intragastric intubation during gestation day (G) 8-22 of the Sprague-Dawley rat (TABLE 1). We examined both behavioral and neurochemical parameters in the offspring. For example, 21-day-old pups exposed to cocaine at 60 mg/kg/day during G8-22 show decreased headgrooming following challenge with SKF38393, a dopamine D_1 agonist.[1] In addition, they show increased locomotor responses to challenge with quinpirole, the D_2-family agonist.[2] In adult males, prenatal cocaine reduces glucose utilization in multiple brain regions; this reduction may be related to both decreased functional activity within the forebrain dopamine circuits and hypoplasia of neuropil.[3] Direct evidence for hypoplasia of neuropil can be found in the brains of 21-day-old rats exposed to cocaine prenatally in that the branching of basal dendrites of cortical neurons is reduced in males compared to that in controls. (D.L. Dow-Edwards and M.W. Miller, unpublished data). Surprisingly, females show an increase in dendritic branching and no changes in glucose utilization. Therefore, prenatal cocaine exposure generally dampens functional activity and produces hypoplasia of neuropil in males and, at the same time, shifts the dopamine D_1:D_2 balance.

Human exposure during the fetal period, approximately 30–40 weeks' gestation, can be studied in the rat model by administering cocaine during postnatal days (PnD) 11–20. Postnatal exposure also alters functional activity and the D_1:D_2 balance, but the directions of the changes depend on the gender of the animal and the time of drug exposure (TABLE 1). For example, using the D_1 agonist SKF 82958 as a challenge drug, we found that pretreatment with cocaine dampened the responses of behaviors associated with the mesolimbic dopamine system in males and increased the behavioral responses associated with the nigrostriatal system in females.[4] PnD 11–20 cocaine at 50 mg/kg/day also suppressed sensitization of the locomotor response to 10 days of apomorphine (2 mg/kg/day) in adult males.[5] In addition, males did not exhibit normal inhibitory control over acoustic startle responses, suggesting impaired function in descending inhibitory pathways such as the mesolimbic dopamine circuit.[6] All of these behavioral changes can be attributed to altered function in a specific circuit involving the mesolimbic dopamine system and including the accumbens. The accumbens also showed reduced rates of glucose metabolism, and we have now found reduced levels of preprodynorphin (PPD) mRNA in the shell of the nucleus accumbens in adult males receiving cocaine during PnD 11–20.[7,9] Regulation of PPD neurons by the D_1 family of receptors has been established. Therefore, data from several studies indicate that PnD 11–20 cocaine produces accumbal PPD neurons expressing D_1 receptors that are in a reduced basal state and cannot respond to pharmacologic challenge in the normal manner.

[a] These studies were supported by National Institute on Drug Abuse Grant DA 04118.

[b] Phone, 718/270-3987; fax, 718/270-2241; e-mail, ddow-edw@netmail.hscbklyn.edu

TABLE 1. Cocaine Exposure during Human-Equivalent Gestational Periods

Human Embryonic (Prenatal rat G8–22)		Human Fetal (Postnatal Rat PnD 11–20)	
		Males	Females
1. Altered dopamine (DA) responses		1. ↓ Function in DA system	1. ↑ or no Δ in DA function
A. ↓ D_1 responses		A. ↓ D_1 locomotor response	A. ↑ D_1 sniffing
B. ↑ D_2 responses		B. No sensitization to apomorphine	B. No Δ sensitization
Males	*Females*	C. ↓ DAT mRNA vent mesencephalon	C. ND
2. ↓ Glucose utilization	no Δ	D. ↓ PPD mRNA in accumbens shell	D. ND
3. ↓ Intersections/basal dendrites	↑	E. ↓ Glucose utilization-accumbens	E. ↑ GU-striatum
		F. ↓ DA-mediated inhibition in acoustic startle	F. No Δ
		2. ↑ 5-HT activity	2. ↓ 5HT activity
		A. ↑ Quipazine response	A. ↓ Quipazine response
		B. ↑ 8-OH-DPAT response	B. No Δ DPAT response
		C. ↑ 5-HT transporter	C. No Δ 5HT transporter

NOTE: ↑ or ↓ indicates cocaine-induced differences compared to controls in the dependent measure indicated (ANOVA). No Δ indicates no change compared to controls. ND indicates not done (tissue not examined for that variable).

TABLE 2. Context-Dependent Effects on Glucose Utilization[a]

Brain Region	Condition	
	Standard[b]	Tented[c]
Motor	5/6↑	3/6↓
Sensory	3/9↑	2/9↓
Limbic	7/16↑	13/20↓

[a]Cocaine produces a condition which resembles that of a locus coeruleus lesion, Significant changes in metabolism are noted in PnD 11–20 cocaine-treated adult females.

[b]Experiment conducted with rats on open lab bench in plexiglas cages.

[c]Experiment conducted with rats habituated to small tents which reduce sensory stimulation and locomotor activity.

Perhaps due to this depressed state of the dopamine neurons, the 5-HT system shows increased responsivity in males (TABLE 1). For example, adult males that received cocaine (25 mg/kg PnD 11–20) showed increased sensitivity to the effects of low doses of quipazine[10] and an increased acoustic startle response following administration of the 5-HT_{1A} agonist 8-OH DPAT.[11] Neuroanatomic evidence of serotonergic hyperinnervation can be seen in the increased expression of 5-HT transporter mRNA in raphe of 21-day-old males treated with cocaine during PnD 11–21.[12]

We also produced evidence for an effect of cocaine on function of the noradrenergic system, the system that mediates attention and arousal (TABLE 2). Data on adult female rats that received cocaine at 50 mg/kg during PnD 11–20 indicate that cocaine dampens function in the ascending noradrenergic neurons arising in the locus coeruleus. Patterns of change in cerebral glucose utilization under standard lab-bench conditions or habituated and sensory/motor suppressed conditions resemble the differences produced by locus coeruleus-lesioned rats examined under varied noise conditions.[8,13]

Therefore, in addition to a depressed state of the D_1-regulated, PPD-expressing neurons within the mesolimbic system and hyperinnervation of the 5-HT neurons, cocaine appears to dampen function within the ascending noradrenergic neurons as well. Unfortunately, this noradrenergic hypothesis has only been proposed for females, and overall the data in females are quite different from those in males. The genders need to be studied under identical conditions to fully appreciate the differences in the responses to ontogenic cocaine exposure. Scientists should recognize the complex pharmacology of cocaine and the multiple ways in which the drug may affect developing neurons. We may never identify a specific clinical syndrome. However, it may be useful to use sensitive measures and consider how changes in attention and arousal may obscure the results from neuropsychological testing.

REFERENCES

1. GILDE, A.B. & D.L. DOW-EDWARDS. 1994. Prenatal cocaine exposure affects stereotypy following acute SKF-38393 injection in weanling rats. Am. Psychol. Assoc. Abstr.
2. GILDE, A.B., H.E. HUGHES & D.L. DOW-EDWARDS. 1993. Prenatal cocaine exposure affects motor activity following acute quinpirole injection in weanling rats. American Psychological Association's Abstr.
3. DOW-EDWARDS, D.L., L.A. FREED & T.A. FICO. 1990. Structural and functional effects of prenatal cocaine exposure in adult rat brain. Dev. Brain Res. **57:** 263–268.

4. Dow-Edwards, D.L. & Y. Busidan. 1998. Gender-specific responses to SKF 82958 in adult rats treated with cocaine or GBR 12909 during the postnatal period. Psychopharmacology. In revision.
5. Dow-Edwards, D.L., Y. Busidan & R. Yin. 1995. Behavioral sensitization to apomorphine in adult rats exposed to cocaine during the postnatal period. Soc. Neurosci. Abstr. **21:** 284.10.
6. Dow-Edwards, D.L. 1998. Impaired inhibitory processes in adult males exposed to cocaine or GBR 12909 during postnatal days 11–20. In preparation.
7. Dow-Edwards, D.L., L.A. Freed-Malen & H. E. Hughes. 1993. Long-term alterations in brain function following cocaine administration during the preweanling period. Dev. Brain Res. **72:** 309–313.
8. Dow-Edwards, D.L., G.S. Frick & R. Yin. 1996. Context-dependent effects of developmental cocaine exposure. Neurobehav. Teratol. Abstr.
9. Dow-Edwards, D. & Y. Hurd. 1997. Alterations in dynorphin mRNA in adult rats following postnatal cocaine exposure. CPDD Abstr. p. 82.
10. Dow-Edwards, D.L. 1998. Preweaning cocaine administration alters the adult response to quipazine: A comparison with fluoxetine. Neurotoxicol. Teratol. **20:** 133–142..
11. Dow-Edwards, D.L. 1996. Modification of acoustic startle reactivity by cocaine administration during the postnatal period: Comparison with a specific serotonin reuptake inhibitor. Neurotoxicol. Teratol. **18:** 289–296.
12. Dow-Edwards, D., Y Hurd & G. Frick. 1996. Alterations in serotonin transporter mRNA. Soc. Neurosci. Abstr. 361.8.
13. Justice, A., S.M. Feldman & L.L. Brown. 1989. The nucleus locus coeruleus modulates local cerebral glucose utilization during noise stress in rats. Brain Res. **490:** 73–84.

Prenatal Cocaine Exposure and Stimulus-Seeking Behaviors during the First Year of Life[a]

ROBERT L. FREEDLAND,[b] BERNARD Z. KARMEL,
JUDITH M. GARDNER, AND DAVID J. LEWKOWICZ

NYS Institute for Basic Research, Staten Island, New York 10314, USA

Our previous[1,2] and ongoing studies of neonates show that normal neonates modulate their attention to stimulation depending on their arousal level, preferring more stimulation when less aroused and less stimulation when more aroused, whereas neonates with CNS injury or prenatal cocaine exposure demonstrate poorer arousal modulation. The behaviors elicited for these two at-risk groups are diametrically opposite, with CNS-injured infants preferring less stimulation even when less aroused (i.e., stimulus avoiding) and cocaine-exposed (CE) infants preferring more stimulation, even when more aroused (i.e., stimulus seeking). We present the current results of arousal-modulated attention from newborn to 4 months as well as various methods that tap emerging perceptual and cognitive abilities in follow-up studies of older infants using visual recognition memory and habituation paradigms.

METHODS

Population. We report on data from 780 infants divided into four groups: one normal and three at-risk groups (two at-risk groups for the pattern complexity task). Demographic information is presented by Karmel *et al.* in this publication. CE status was obtained from maternal/infant urine toxicology, infant meconium toxicology, and maternal report. Any report of cocaine use during pregnancy was considered positive. Brain injury was obtained from worst case cranial ultrasound (US) and brainstem auditory-evoked response (BAER) findings. It should be noted that 18–20% of normal term CE infants have abnormal first BAERs versus 5–6% of the non-CE normal term population. These infants were excluded from analyses.

Arousal-Modulated Attention (newborn, 1 and 4 months). Infants viewed different random sequences of all possible pairs of three temporal frequencies for a total of six trials when in each of three different arousal conditions: (1) less aroused, after feeding; (2) more aroused (internal), before feeding; and (3) more aroused (external), after feeding with 8 Hz stimulation before each trial. Square-wave modulated frequencies were used across all three test ages, with a checkerboard pattern replacing a blank flash at 4 months to reduce fussiness.

Visual Recognition Memory (1 and 4 months). A one-trial paired comparison visual recognition memory task was administered after an infant-controlled familiarization

[a] This work was supported by National Institute of Child Health and Human Development Grant R01 HD21784 and National Institute on Drug Abuse Grants R01 DA06644 and K21 DA00236.

[b] Address for correspondence: Robert L. Freedland, NYS Institute for Basic Research in Developmental Disabilities, 1050 Forest Hill Road, Staten Island, NY 10314. Phone, 718/494-5278; fax, 718/494-3595; e-mail, FRESI@CUNYVM.CUNY.EDU

procedure (accumulated looking of 20 seconds and 10 seconds at 1 and 4 months) when infants were in two different aroused conditions (before/after feeding). Test trials were 20 seconds, with left-right position reversed after 10 seconds.

Fagan Infantest (7, 10, and 13 months). The standardized paired comparison visual recognition memory task was administered, using accumulated looking times and test trial durations.

Pattern Complexity (4 and 7 months). A paired comparison visual recognition memory task was administered. During familiarization, infants were presented with two patterns with identical orientations (vertical or horizontal [cardinals] or right/left obliques) until the infants reached an accumulated looking time of 10 and 8 seconds at 4 and 7 months. On subsequent paired-preference test trials, one of the two patterns was changed to a novel orientation, with the left-right position reversed after 10 and 5 seconds (at 4 and 7 months). Infants were presented with either the complex *herringbone* pattern, possessing a global orientation from the arrangement of local line segments oriented at right angles to each other, or *line gratings,* which do not possess the detail of local elements and multiple levels of orientations as does the herringbone.

RESULTS

Arousal-Modulated Attention. FIGURE 1 shows the proportion of looking to low, medium, and high temporal frequencies in each arousal condition of the visual preference procedure across the four risk categories at the three test ages. Similar to prior results, normal neonates (at 0 and 1 month) modulated their attention to stimulation depending on their arousal level, preferring more stimulation when less aroused and less stimulation when more aroused (note the X-pattern across conditions). CE infants showed a lack of arousal modulation (note the parallel lines across conditions), preferring more stimulation, even when more aroused. We refer to this robust and replicable result as *stimulus-seeking behavior.* CNS-injured infants also demonstrated poorer arousal modulation with increasing degrees of injury, but in a pattern opposite to that of the CE infants, with CNS-injured infants preferring less stimulation even when less aroused, a behavior we refer to as *stimulus-avoiding behavior.* By 4 months, there was only evidence of an arousal effect (stimulus-avoiding behavior) with CNS injury.

Visual Recognition Memory. The results indicated that 1-month-old infants shifted from familiarity preferences when more aroused to novelty preferences when less aroused, whereas 4-month-old infants had significant preferences for novelty in both conditions. CE infants preferred novelty in both conditions at both 1 and 4 months, suggesting poor arousal modulation and stimulus-seeking behavior.

Fagan Infantest. While the results showed significant novelty preferences across all groups, no differential pattern emerged across groups or ages.

Pattern Complexity. FIGURE 2 shows that normal infants more fully encoded the cardinal orientations, whereas CE infants encoded obliques as evidenced by their respective novelty responses. CE infants showed the strongest novelty preferences following familiarization to oblique herringbones, whereas normal infants showed the strongest novelty preferences after familiarization with the cardinal herringbones. Results from CNS-injured infants were equivocal, possibly suggesting their inability to differentiate orientational differences of the patterns. As the local elements within the oblique herringbones are oriented along the cardinal axes, CE infants may not be responding to the implied oblique orientation, but rather the orientation of the stimulation-rich local horizontal and vertical elements within the pattern. Such a response may be interpreted as a continuation of the "stimulation-seeking" behavior of CE neonates and was tested using line gratings, which do not possess the detail of local elements and multi-

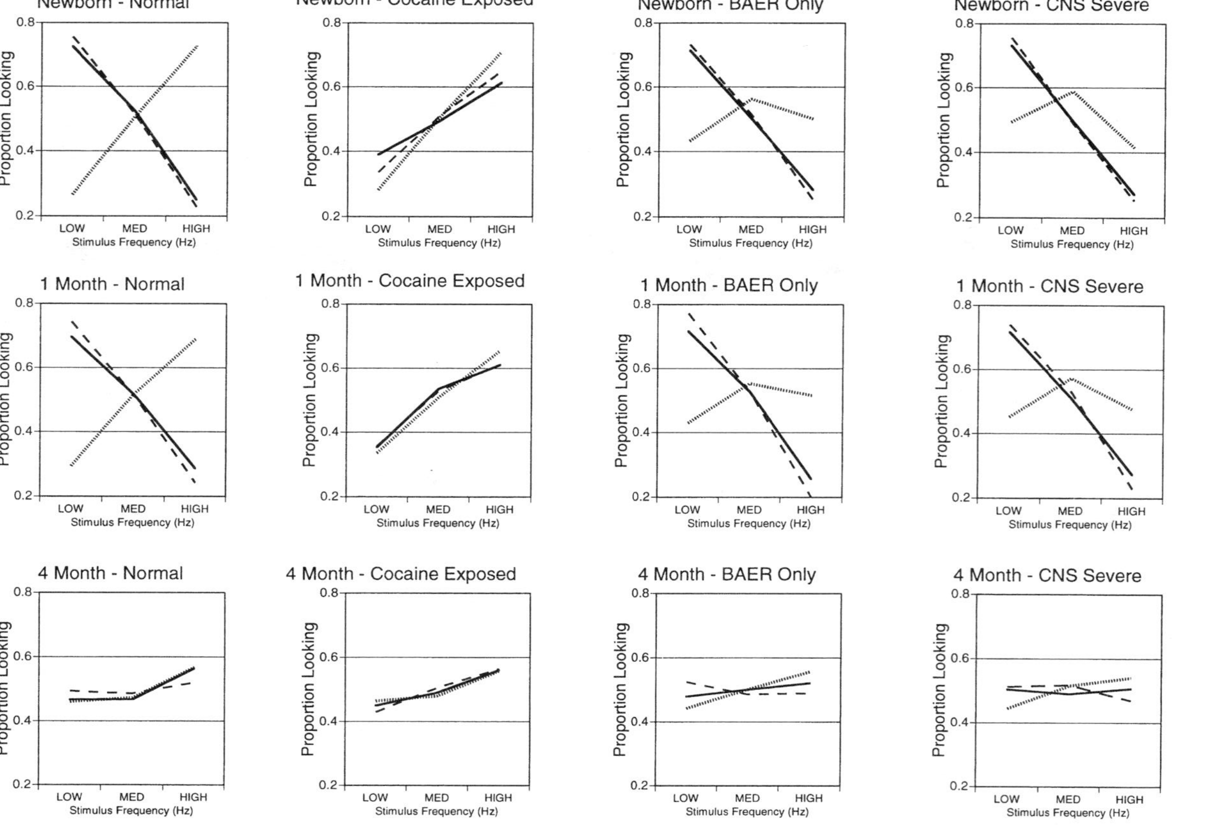

FIGURE 1. Amount of time infants looked at stimulus temporal frequencies when in more aroused and less aroused conditions as a function of co-

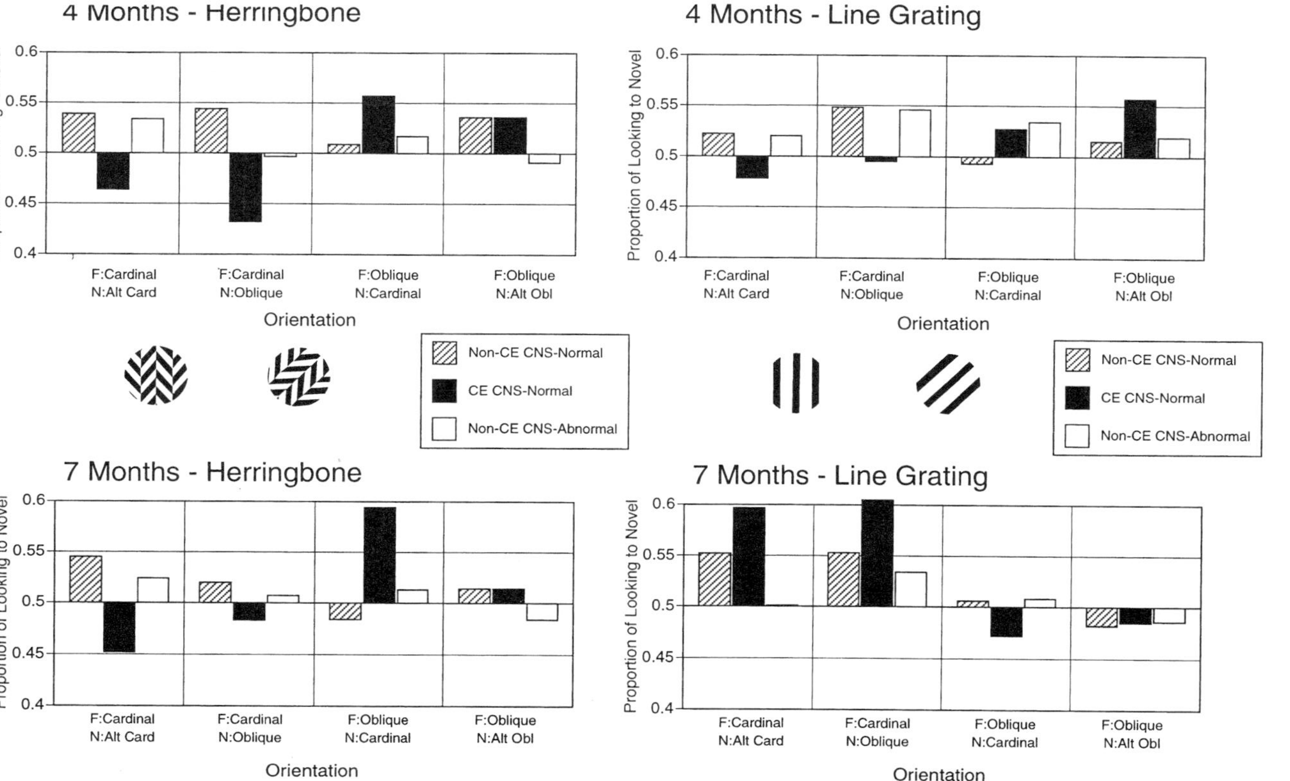

FIGURE 2. Proportion of looking at a novel orientation after familiarization with either a cardinal (horizontal or vertical) or oblique herringbone or line grating across three groups of infants at 4 and 7 months. Values below 0.50 indicate a preference for the familiar stimulus, whereas values above 0.50 indicate a preference for the novel stimulus. Examples of cardinal and oblique herringbone and line grating patterns are shown.

ple levels of orientations as the herringbone. However, as shown in FIGURE 2, the results from line gratings are not definitive, as CE infants at 4 months showed their strongest novelty preferences after familiarization with oblique line gratings, but at 7 months they showed their strongest novelty preferences after familiarization with the cardinal line gratings, a result most parsimonious with the "stimulus-seeking" hypothesis.

CONCLUSIONS

Similar to neonates, CE infants demonstrated behavioral responses uniquely different from those of both normal term and CNS-injured infants, in a manner that can be interpreted as *stimulus seeking.* CE infants remained differentiated as a group, *even past the neonatal period.* Differentiation past the neonatal period was accomplished by (1) targeting tasks that involve specific areas of neurofunction within the developing nervous system that are affected by cocaine (such as the dopaminergic system); and (2) specifying characteristics on US and BAER to better differentiate group membership.

REFERENCES

1. KARMEL, B.Z. & J.M. GARDNER. 1995. Prenatal cocaine exposure effects on arousal modulated attention during the neonatal period. Dev. Psychobiol. **29:** 463–480.
2. KARMEL, B.Z., J.M. GARDNER & R.L. FREEDLAND. 1996. Arousal-modulated attention at 4-months as a function of intrauterine cocaine exposure and CNS injury. J. Pediatr. Psychol. **21:** 821–832.

Neonatal Neurobehavioral Assessment and Bayley I and II Scores of CNS-Injured and Cocaine-Exposed Infants[a]

BERNARD Z. KARMEL,[b] JUDITH M. GARDNER, AND ROBERT L. FREEDLAND

NYS Institute for Basic Research, Staten Island, New York 10314, USA

Newborn neurobehavioral assessment procedures that are designed to evaluate early behavioral capabilities and dysfunctions as in sensory information processing, motor organization, attention, and arousal are frequently disrupted by injury or alterations of the CNS as from hypoxia or exposure to neurotoxic agents such as cocaine. Defining the consequences of CNS injury and drug exposure in newborns is important for both predicting recovery from acute problems and providing a basis for predicting long-term outcome. Our neurobehavioral procedure[1] is a categorical clinical evaluation of sensory and motor systems, appropriate for use with small, sick, high-risk neonates, with concurrent validity to brain insult as documented by cranial ultrasonography and brainstem auditory-evoked response (BAER) tests.[1–3] Six brain insult groups, defined by ultrasonography and BAER outcomes, were found to have different patterns of neurobehavioral abnormalities. We report here on neurobehavioral abnormalities in a subset of brain insult groups (from a longitudinal replication sample) and in a cocaine-exposed (CE) group at newborn and 1 month, and the relationship between these neonatal neurobehavioral abnormalities and later scores on the Bayley Scales of Infant Development (BSID).

METHODS

Participants. Neurobehavioral performance is reported from 780 infants divided into four groups: 1 normal and 3 at risk: Groups 1 (normal; $n = 263$) and 2 (CE; $n = 151$) were healthy term nursery infants having normal BAERs and ultrasonography (or assumed normal if not performed), with Group 1 non-CE while Group 2 was cocaine-exposed; Groups 3 (BAER-only; $n = 299$) and 4 (severe; $n = 67$) were NICU non-CE infants having abnormal BAERS, but where Group 3 had normal ultrasonography, Group 4 had severe brain injury with IVH Grade IV, hydrocephalus >10 mm, porencephaly, parenchymal hemorrhage or infarct, or seizures requiring medication. Demographic data for each group, respectively, are: birth weight (g) 3214, 2963, 2304, and 2476; gestational age (weeks) 39.1, 38.9, 34.9, and 35.1; intrauterine growth (z-score weight normalized for gestational age) 0.14, – 0.42, – 0.25, and 0.08; head circumfer-

[a] This work was supported by National Institute of Child Health and Human Development Grant R01 HD21784 and National Institute on Drug Abuse Grants R01 DA06644 and K21 DA00236.

[b] Address for correspondence: Bernard Z. Karmel, NYS Institute for Basic Research in Developmental Disabilities, 1050 Forest Hill Road, Staten Island, New York 10314. Phone, 718/494-5351; fax, 718/494-3595; e-mail, BZKSI@CON2.COM

ence (cm) 33.8, 33.1, 31.1, and 31.5; length (cm) 49.7, 48.4, 44.8, and 44.3; gender (% boys) 48, 48, 59, and 55. Note that healthy term CE infants still tended to have a lower birth weight even when corrected for gestational age. Cocaine exposure was obtained from maternal or infant urine or meconium toxicology or maternal report. Any report of use throughout pregnancy was considered positive. The worst case was used for ultrasonography and the first test was used for BAERs to determine brain insult. Of healthy term CE infants, 18–20% had abnormal first BAERs versus 5–6% of the non-CE healthy term population. These infants were excluded from this report.

Neurobehavioral Procedure. Neurobehavioral examinations were performed just prior to hospital discharge (at 38–40 weeks) and again approximately 1 month later (at 44–45 weeks). Each examination took about 10 minutes. Items were administered to enable decision-making as to any abnormalities on categories of behavior by a trained observer as follows. *Attention:* Visual: Inability to fixate checkerboard or bullseye paired with blank or to follow pattern smoothly across midline. Auditory: Inability to turn from midline to rattle or voice on right or left. *Sensory Symmetry:* Better visual or auditory orienting to right or left even if attention normal. *Head/Neck Control:* Extension/flexion (lag): Weak, little attempt to lift or pull head up. *Extremity Movements/Tone:* Hypo- or hypertonicity in arms or legs (or generalized); movement or tone differences between arms and legs. *Jitteriness:* Fine or gross tremors; spontaneous or elicited. *Motor Symmetry:* Better movement or tone on one side even if movements/tone normal. *State Control:* Peak excitement: Very low or high arousal; hyperresponsive; "all or none." Alertness: Eyes dull; unresponsive. *Feeding:* Weak or uncoordinated suck or swallow.

BSID Procedure. Infants return for follow-up every 3 months until 3 years of age. At each visit between 4 and 25 months, the BSID-II was administered with extra items filled in as necessary for the BSID-I. Thus, all infants were double-scored on both the BSID-I and the BSID-I.

RESULTS

Neurobehavioral. TABLE 1 provides the proportion of infants in each group with neurobehavioral abnormalities at newborn and 1 month. All neurobehavioral categories significantly differentiated risk groups from the normal group in some way. Four different patterns were apparent during the newborn period. Normal infants tended to have a lower incidence and severe infants tended to have a higher incidence of problems in most all categories (except in both cases for hypertonicity in the arms and legs). A greater proportion of CE infants were judged to have hypertonicity in both arms and legs with increased jitteriness, poorer state control (due to increased peak excitement and irritability), and increased deficits in visual attention. Infants in the BAER-only group tended to have a greater incidence of visual attention and visual asymmetry problems as well as poor head control, but less extremity problems. The visual attention and state control problems found for CE and brain insult infants may reflect arousal-modulated attention deficits (although in opposite directions) during this period.[4,5] Most neurobehavioral problems were transient and resolved by 1 month. The exception was jitteriness, which although decreased compared to that of newborn, was still a characteristic of the CE group. No other behavior distinguished infants at 1 month, although a general increased incidence of hypertonicity and visual asymmetry compared to newborn test results was observed across groups.

BSID. The Mental Development Index (MDI) and Psychomotor Development Index (PDI) for the BSID-I and II are shown in FIGURE 1. Of note is that even the normal group showed a decline across age on both versions. Inflation of BSID-I scores dur-

TABLE 1. Neurobehavioral Performance

	Newborn Infants				One-Month-Old Infants			
	Normal	Cocaine Exposed	BAER-Only	Severe	Normal	Cocaine Exposed	BAER-Only	Severe
n	(207)	(137)	(287)	(66)	(200)	(97)	(183)	(54)
Attention	.04	.13	.25	.30	.04	.03	.09	.15
Sensory asymmetry	.06	.09	.17	.29	.08	.11	.14	.31
Head extension	.12	.07	.34	.47	.05	.06	.11	.18
Head flexion	.16	.15	.34	.62	.15	.13	.16	.35
Hypotonia-arms	.06	.02	.19	.45	.10	.10	.14	.24
Hypertonia-arms	.32	.56	.11	.20	.19	.37	.32	.26
Hypertonia-legs	.24	.44	.25	.35	.09	.27	.14	.30
Motor asymmetry	.01	.01	.04	.12	.03	.09	.01	.15
Jitteriness	.14	.39	.09	.15	.03	.21	.08	.10
Feeding	.05	.04	.07	.15	.01	.00	.04	.07
State control	.02	.09	.03	.12	.02	.00	.04	.07

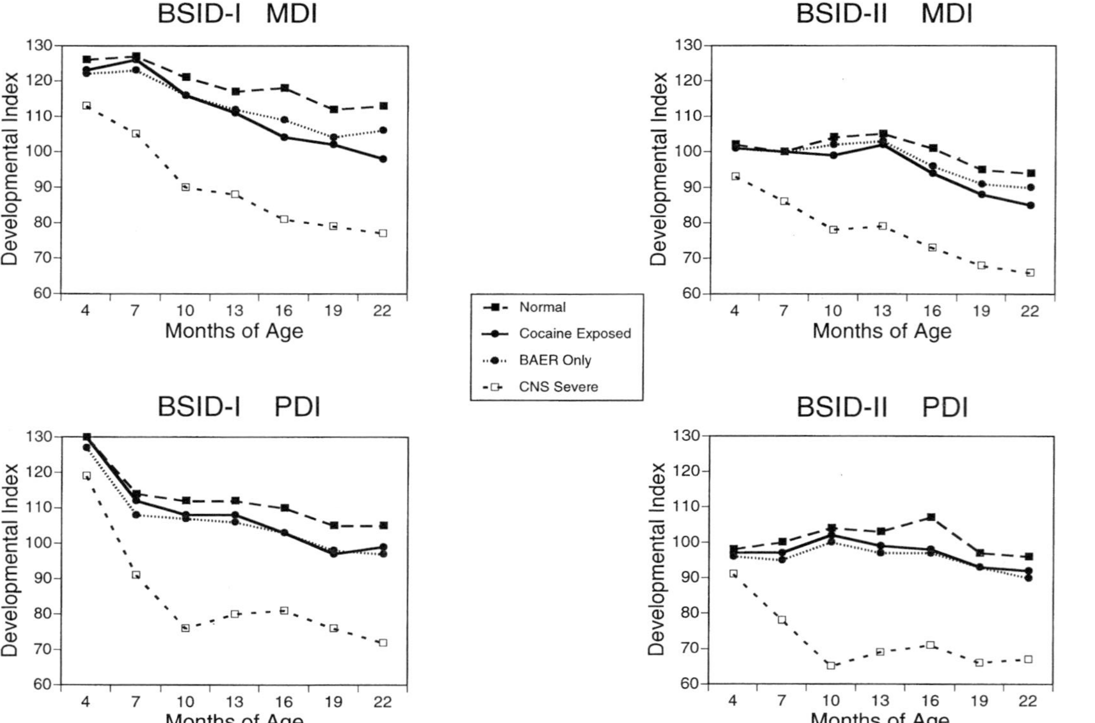

FIGURE 1. Mean Bayley Scale scores over age for four groups reflecting 2,463 tests from 536 infants. Group sample sizes: normal (984 tests; $n = 223$); CE (497 tests; $n = 105$); BAER-only (720 tests; $n = 149$); CNS severe (262 tests; $n = 59$). BSID-I = Original Bayley Scales of Infant Development; BSID-II = Revised Bayley Scales of Infant Development; MDI = Mental Development Index; PDI = Psychomotor Development Index.

ing the first few months was corrected by BSID-II; however, the normal group's BSID-II scores were lower than expected after the first year. Although the BAER-only and CE groups had scores within the normal range, they were lower (almost 1 SD; 10–15 points depending on the version) than those of the normal group, with the MDI decline starting towards the end of the first year. Lowered scores persisted even when confounds such as ethnicity, gender, inadequate prenatal care, and cigarette smoking were covaried. The severe group had lower scores on both indices of both versions from the earliest ages tested.

Relation between Neurobehavioral Assessment and the BSID. Logistic regression analysis provides a method for estimating the approximate weight each category in the neurobehavioral assessment carries in distinguishing each risk group from the normal group. From these weights, a composite brain insult-neurobehavioral score was calculated for each infant. The brain insult-neurobehavioral correlations with BSID-I and II MDI and PDI scores were significant at all ages. Although as neonates BAER-only infants tended to have more visual attention problems and CE infants tended to have more motor problems, BSID scores at older ages were similar.

CONCLUSION

From birth, different patterns of neurobehavioral functioning are detectable and differentially related to CNS pathology and neurotoxity due to prenatal cocaine exposure. These different patterns were all related to lower BSID scores later on, suggesting that several different atypical developmental trajectories may be identifiable. Because the CE group was composed of healthy term infants with no detectable brain insult on ultrasonography or BAERs and the decline in their scores was independent of environmental and social factors analyzed, we can only assume that prenatal exposure to cocaine had affected the developing nervous system in some way, despite the fact that their cognitive skills were within the normal range.

REFERENCES

1. Gardner, J.M., B.Z. Karmel, C.L. Magnano, K.I. Norton & E.G. Brown. 1990. Neurobehavioral indicators of early brain insult in high-risk neonates. Dev. Psychol. **26:** 563–575.
2. Gardner, J.M., B.Z. Karmel & C.L. Magnano. 1992. Arousal/visual preference interactions in high-risk neonates. Dev. Psychol. **28:** 821–830.
3. Karmel, B.Z., J.M. Gardner, R.A. Zappulla, C.L. Magnano & E.G. Brown. 1988. Brainstem auditory evoked responses as indicators of early brain insult. EEG Clin. Neurophysiol. **71:** 429–442.
4. Karmel, B.Z. & J.M. Gardner. 1995. Prenatal cocaine exposure effects on arousal modulated attention during the neonatal period. Dev. Psychobiol. **29:** 463–480.
5. Karmel, B.Z., J.M. Gardner & R.L. Freedland. 1996. Arousal-modulated attention at 4-months as a function of intrauterine cocaine exposure and CNS injury. J. Pediatr. Psychol. **21:** 821–832.

Perinatal Outcome after Cocaine ± Polydrug Exposure

O. GREENE,[a] A. VARGHESE, F. TUAMOKUMO, W.K. ASHE, AND P. TING
Howard University, Washington, DC 20001, USA

Cocaine abuse has increased dramatically in the United States. These disastrous upward trends in cocaine use have created epidemic numbers of prenatally exposed infants. Numerous reports have suggested that cocaine abuse during pregnancy is associated with increased perinatal morbidity and mortality.[1–3] Howard University Hospital serves a large number of underprivileged patients from the inner city, and a significant number of the patients are *in utero* cocaine-exposed infants. The specific aim of the current study is to examine the effects of *in utero* cocaine with or without polydrug (opioids and marijuana) exposure on neonatal morbidity, especially on the central nervous system.

A retrospective study was therefore conducted on 202 newborns exposed *in utero* to cocaine ± polydrugs (based on maternal history and/or urine toxicology screen, born at Howard University Hospital between January 1992 and 1996). The incidence of perinatal morbidity related to low birth weight (≤ 2,500 g), prematurity (<37 weeks), microcephaly (frontooccipital head circumference <10th percentile), *in utero* meconium passage, cerebral intraventricular hemorrhage, sexually transmitted diseases (HIV and congenital syphilis), and duration of hospital stay was studied. The data were compared with those of control newborns without *in utero* drug exposure or with all live births.

SPECIFIC AIMS

To examine perinatal adverse outcome associated with prenatal cocaine with or without opiates and marijuana (PDE) exposure on the developing brain, we analyzed the incidence of microcephaly and cerebral germinal matrix and intraventricular hemorrhage. Because cocaine is a potent vasoconstrictor, we examined the incidence of perinatal asphyxia by well established clinical markers including meconium-stained amniotic fluid, low birth weight, and Apgar score. We examined the economic impact on health care cost by focusing on the length of hospital stay of these babies after birth. Finally, other factors such as prenatal care and sexually transmitted diseases (syphilis and HIV) were also studied.

RESULTS

The incidence of low birth weight was 44%, but, it was 16% for all live births at Howard University Hospital (p <0.01). The prematurity (<37 weeks) rate was 35%, whereas, in non-cocaine-exposed infants it is 2–16%.[4] The incidence of microcephaly was 13% and was equally distributed between term and preterm infants. This was more than twice the figure of 6% in non-cocaine-exposed infants reported on elsewhere[4] (p

[a] Address for correspondence: Onaje Greene, 327 Elm Street, NW, Washington, DC 20001. Phone, 202/667-6260; fax, 202/672-9074; e-mail, ogreene@howard.edu

<0.01). Meconium-stained amniotic fluid was present in 22%, but, 4.5% occurred in preterm infants. The latter was significantly ($p < 0.01$) higher than 0.12% of all live births reported elsewhere.[5] Indeed, among cocaine-exposed preterm infants, 13% had meconium-stained amniotic fluid. Over 80% of mothers received poor (<7 prenatal visits) or no prenatal care. Average length of hospital stay was 19 days as compared to 8 days for all newborns at Howard University Hospital. Approximately 28% of the infants had drug withdrawal, and 8% required treatment. Surprisingly, none of the preterm infants in the study (including those with birth weight ≤1500 g) had interventricular hemorrhage but, the latter was reported to occur in 15 to 29% of all preterm infants.[6] An Apgar score of <7 at 1 and 5 minutes was noted, respectively, in 16% and 0.5% of the newborn. The incidence of HIV+ antibody was 3.5%, but newborns were not routinely screened. Serologic test for syphilis was routinely screened on all newborns at Howard University Hospital, and the test was positive in 8% of the drug-exposed infants (national average for all newborns was 11%).

DISCUSSION

The results corroborated the results of previous reports on increased incidence of low birth weight, premature infants, and microcephaly.[1–3] The complications associated with low birth weight and preterm infants can further compromise the developing brain to ischemic injury with subsequent psychomotor deficits. Because the incidence of microcephaly occurred with equal frequency in preterm infants and term newborns, we speculate that the toxic effect of cocaine on the developing brain occurs early in gestation and continues into the peak critical period of brain organization. Therefore, the long-term neuro-developmental outcome will be of special concern in these infants with microcephaly. Meconium-stained amniotic fluid occurred with a forty-fold increase in the incidence in preterm infants of cocaine ± polydrug exposure group when compared to preterm infants in all live births. The meconium aspiration syndrome can further compromise oxygenation/ventilation, thereby leading to hypoxic brain injury. The absence of interventricular hemorrhage in the cocaine-exposed group is a surprising finding, but a prospective study to examine the concurrent use of prenatal steroid and postnatal surfactant may clarify this issue. Both drugs reduce the incidence of interventricular hemorrhage significantly.[7]

Finally, the rising costs of health care and reshaping of medicine by HMOs makes the issues of prenatal care and hospital stay important factors. More preventive measures should be emphasized in dealing with drug-addicted pregnant mothers, and this

TABLE 1. Perinatal Morbidity Associated with Prenatal Cocaine ± Polydrug Exposure (PDE)

Factors of Morbidity	Cocaine ± PDE	No Cocaine ± PDE
Low birth weight (<2,500 g)	44%[a]	16%
Prematurity rate (<37 wk)	35%	2–16%
Microcephaly	13%[a]	6%
MSAF (preterm infants)	4.5%[a]	.12%[b]
Length of hospital stay (days)	19	8
Intraventricular hemorrhage	0%	15–29%[c]

[a] $p < 0.01$.
[b] All live births.
[c] All preterm infants.

may decrease the perinatal morbidity and subsequent health care cost. Finally, intensive efforts in public education, emphasizing the prenatal effects of drugs, the importance of adequate prenatal care, and the provision of much needed drug addiction and rehabilitation services may decrease morbidity and mortality of both mothers and babies.

CONCLUSION

The study revealed that *in utero* cocaine ± polydrug exposure is associated with significant increases in perinatal morbidity and length of hospital stay. The morbidity includes poor prenatal care, low birth weight, prematurity, microcephaly in both term and preterm infants, and meconium-stained amniotic fluid in preterm gestation (<37 weeks). However, there was no increase in the incidence of either interventricular hemorrhage or syphilis.

REFERENCES

1. Neerhof, M.G., S.N. MacGregor, S.S. Retzky & T.P. Sullivan. 1989. Cocaine abuse during pregnancy: Peripartum prevalence and perinatal outcome. Am. J. Obstet. Gynecol. **161:** 633–638.
2. Chasnoff, I.J. 1989. Cocaine, pregnancy, and the neonate. Women Health **15:** 23–35.
3. Chasnoff, I.J., K.A. Burns & W.J. Burns. 1987. Cocaine use in pregnancy: Perinatal morbidity and mortality. *Neurotoxicol. Teratol.* **9:** 291–293.
4. Handler, A., N. Kistin, F. Davis & C. Ferre. 1991. Cocaine use during pregnancy: Perinatal outcomes. Am. J. Epidemiol. **133:** 818–825.
5. Matthews, T.G. & J.B. Warshaw. 1979. Relevance of the gestational age distribution of meconium passage in utero. Pediatrics **64:** 30.
6. McLenan, D.A., O.A. Ajayi, R.J. Rydman & R.S. Pildes. 1994. Evaluation of the relationship between cocaine and intraventricular hemorrhage. J. Natl. Med. Assoc. **86:** 281–287.
7. Gunkel, J.H., B.R. Mitchell (Abbott Labs, Columbus, Ohio). 1995. Observational evidence for the efficacy of antenatal steroids from randomized studies of surfactant replacement. Am. J. Obstet. Gynecol. **173:** 281.

Chronic Cocaine Treatment Alters Social/Aggressive Behavior in Sprague-Dawley Rat Dams and in Their Prenatally Exposed Offspring[a]

J.M. JOHNS,[b,h] L.R. NOONAN, L.I. ZIMMERMAN,[d] B.A. McMILLEN,[e] L.W. MEANS,[f] C.H. WALKER,[b] D.A. LUBIN,[c] K.E. METER,[b] C.J. NELSON,[c] C.A. PEDERSEN,[b] G.A. MASON,[b] AND J.M. LAUDER[g]

Departments of [b]Psychiatry, [c]Psychology, and [g]Cell Biology and Anatomy, and [d]School of Social Work, University of North Carolina, Chapel Hill, North Carolina 27599–7096, USA

Departments of [e]Pharmacology and [f]Psychology, East Carolina University, Greenville, North Carolina 27858, USA

Maternal cocaine abuse during pregnancy has been correlated with a greater incidence of maternal neglect and problems with maternal-infant bonding.[1] Children of mothers who have abused cocaine during pregnancy have exhibited signs of increased irritability and altered state liability as newborns[2,3] and are aggressive, show poor social attachment, and display abnormal play behavior in unstructured environments as young children.[4] These data suggest cocaine-induced, abnormal development of socioemotional behavior, but it is difficult to determine if these deficits are a direct result of cocaine or are related to living in an unstable or abusive environment.

Animal research on the effects of prenatal cocaine exposure suggest that offspring exposed prenatally to cocaine exhibit signs of behavioral abnormalities including increased "emotionality" and neophobia[5,6] and aggression towards an intruder or other untreated conspecifics.[7–9] Long-term changes in specific neurotransmitter systems may be related to behavioral alterations.

On the basis of previous findings,[7–9] we focused our research on cocaine-induced alterations of both maternal and offspring social/aggressive behavior. The following data include a summary of results from several recent experiments.

METHODS

Treatment Groups. Dams received 15 mg/kg of cocaine-HCL (Sigma Chemical Co., St. Louis, Missouri) in a saline solution (CC) or an equal volume of (0.9%) normal saline (Sal) twice daily at approximately 9:00 AM and 4:00 PM from gestational days 1–20. An intermittent cocaine group received the same dose of cocaine on 2 consecu-

[a] These studies were supported in part by the National Institute on Drug Abuse Grant R29-DA08456-01 (to J.M.J.) and the UNC Neurosciences Center.

[h]Phone, 919/966-5961; fax, 919/966-5961; e-mail, jjohns@css.ujc.edu.

tive days every 4 days throughout gestation (days 2–3, 8–9, 14–15, and 19–20), and the amfonelic acid-treated (AFA, a selective dopamine uptake inhibitor) dams received 1.5 mg/kg of AFA dissolved in a pH 10 solution (Sterling Winthrop Labs, Rensselaer, New York) once daily (9:00 AM) on gestational days 1–20.

Procedure. Treatment dams were either yoke fed or fed ad libitum, were weighed daily, and had their daily food consumption measured. Dams were tested on postpartum days 6, 8, and 10 for aggression towards an intruder during a 10-minute period. On postpartum days 8 or 11, dams were killed and the ventral tegmental area, hippocampus, and amygdala were removed for oxytocin radioimmunoassay. Details of aggression testing procedures were published elsewhere.[10] Pups were placed with surrogates immediately after birth, weaned at 21 days of age, and separated into same sex groups of three for behavioral testing on postnatal days 30, 60, 90, and 180. Pups from three of the test periods (30, 60, and 180 days) were used for HPLC analyses of monoamines, and several pups were killed on postnatal days 1, 4, and 10 for assessment of 5-HT_{1A} receptor development using immunobinding assays (using a specific 5-HT_{1A} antipeptide antibody, which was a gift of John Raymond) and quantitative, competitive RT-PCR using internal standards. Frequency, duration, and latency of behaviors were recorded using a computer program (Behavior L.W.M.). Behaviors were usually videotaped and analyzed by two independent observers. Statistical analyses included factor analyses, Fisher's exact test, and analyses of variance.

RESULTS

Data on maternal indices, neonatal development, and other behavioral testing were previously reported.[11]

Maternal Aggression: Data for maternal aggression and oxytocin levels are summarized in FIGURE 1. Aggression towards an intruder was significantly increased in CC-treated dams on postpartum days 6, 8, and 10. Oxytocin was also reduced in the amygdala of the CC-treated dams relative to Sal- and AFA-treated dams, indicating more than a dopaminergic action of cocaine on aggression. (Intermittent cocaine-treated dams were not tested for maternal behavior.) Although dopamine-related behaviors (locomotor, rearing) were increased in the AFA-treated dams (relative to Sal- and CC-treated dams), they were not as aggressive as CC- or even Sal-treated dams, and they also had the highest levels of oxytocin in the amygdala of all groups.

Offspring Behavior. Abnormalities were age, sex, and task specific, as shown in TABLE 1. Cocaine-exposed pups show evidence of altered activity, social behavior, and aggression towards conspecifics which appears to occur in a developmental pattern with CC treatment having a stronger behavioral effect than intermittent cocaine. Serotonin and 5-HIAA levels were lower at postnatal day 60 in the striatum and hippocampus and in the striatum and amygdala at postnatal day 180.[12] Expression of 5-HT_{1A} receptors was increased in the brain overall at postnatal day 1, began to return to normal at postnatal day 4, and was significantly decreased in the brain overall at postnatal day 10 in male CC-exposed pups. Offspring prenatally exposed to the dopamine uptake inhibitor AFA were the most aggressive of all offspring followed by CC, intermittent cocaine, and Sal-treated rats, respectively. These data indicate a predominant dopaminergic effect on aggression in offspring. Aggression was decreased in all offspring groups by pretreatment with the anxiolytic gepirone, a 5-HT_{1A} partial agonist, although the AFA-treated pups were least affected by gepirone, and aggression was still evident in the CC-treated pups, even after gepirone treatment. These data

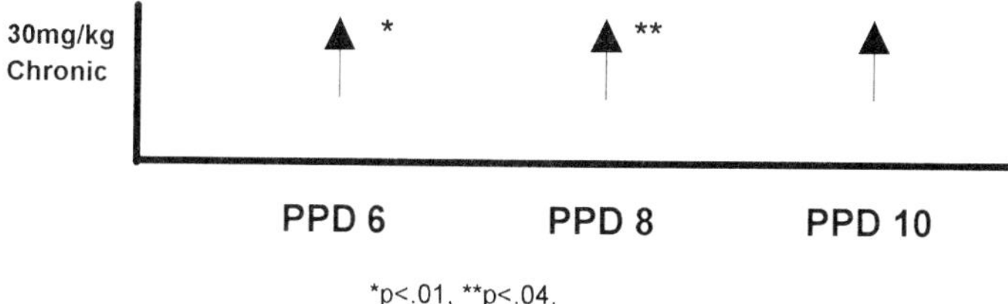

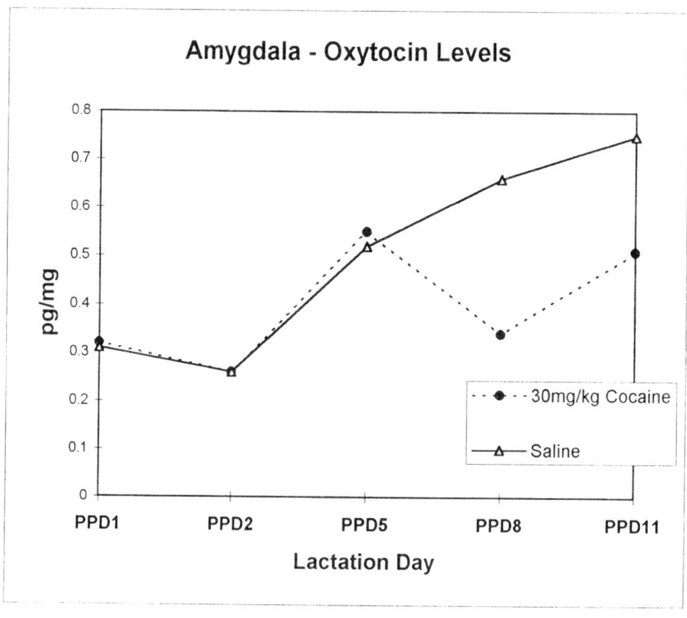

Note: PPD11 reflects a 25mg/kg dose.

FIGURE 1. Maternal aggression fight attacks relative to saline controls.

suggest that both dopaminergic and serotonergic systems as well as stress-related effects are probably involved in cocaine-induced aggression in prenatally exposed offspring.

Our results suggest that both maternal and offspring social/aggressive behavior are altered by CC treatment and that dopaminergic, serotonergic, and oxytocinergic (dams) systems probably mediate these effects. On the basis of these findings we hypothesized that changes in brain hormonal or neurochemical activity, as a result of chronic cocaine treatment (30 mg/kg) or prenatal exposure to chronic gestational cocaine treatment, alters the sensory or perceptual systems of both mothers and offspring so that, unlike untreated animals, they view stimuli as more threatening than they really are and react to a perceived threat in an abnormally aggressive manner.

TABLE 1. Behavioral Effects on Offspring after Prenatal Cocaine Exposure

	PND 30	PND 60	PND 90	PND 180
Chronic cocaine	Males: hypoactivity first 15 minutes of 6-hour activity test	Males: neophobic, did not enter open field in 1st 5 min. Female: spent more time rough grooming a conspecific, $p < 0.05$ and took longer to allow contact, ns	Males: took longer to reciprocate contact, $p < 0.02$. Males: spent more time rough grooming a conspecific, ns	Neophobic, males chased an intruder more often, $p < 0.01$, for a longer time, $p < 0.01$ & sooner, $p < 0.01$. Male intruders were threatened longer, $p < 0.05$. Females made more vocalizations, for a longer time in response to fewer airpuffs. Males took more trials to habituate responding to air puff (40% of baseline), $p < 0.05$. Following plus maze exposure, males decreased ACTH levels at 0 & 90 min, $p < 0.05$. Females decreased ACTH at 90 min, ns males decreased ACTH after exposure to an unfamiliar male, $p < 0.05$

Intermittent cocaine	Males-hypoactive during 3-hour dark phase of 6-hour activity test	Hyperactive in the open field, $p < 0.01$. Turned right on entrance, $p < 0.05$, spent more time in section 1 and less time in start box, $p < 0.05$. General decrease in activity, ns	N/A	
Amfonelic acid	ns	Hypoactive during dark cycle, $p < 0.05$. Spent more time in section 1 & less time in start box, $p < .05$.	N/A	Escaped an intruder faster, $p < 0.05$ Spent more time being aggressive towards an intruder (piloerection, aggressive posture, fight attack), following gepirone, $p < 0.01$.
Saline	ns	ns	ns	Took longer to escape intruder in Session 1 than Session 2. Females-required more air puffs to vocalize, vocalized less and for less time than males, $p < 0.05$.

ACKNOWLEDGMENT

Assistance with the assays was provided by the Mental Health Clinical Research Center of the Psychiatry Department #MH33127.

REFERENCES

1. Burns, K. A., W. J. Chethik, W. A. Burns & R. Clark. 1991. Dyadic disturbances in cocaine-abusing mothers and their infants. J. Clin. Psychol. **313:** 666–669.
2. Chasnoff, I. J., K. A. Burns & W. J. Burns. 1987. Cocaine use in pregnancy: Perinatal morbidity and mortality. Neurotoxicol. Teratol. **9:** 291–293.
3. Chasnoff, I. J., W. J. Burns, S. H. Schnoll & K. A. Burns. 1985. Cocaine use in pregnancy N. Engl. J. Med. **313:** 666–669.
4. Howard, J., L. Beckwith, C. Rodnig & V. Kropenske. 1989. The development of young children of substance-abusing parents: Insights from seven years of intervention and research. Zero to Three **9:** 8–12.
5. Church, M. W. & G. W. Overbeck. 1990. Prenatal cocaine exposure in the Long Evans rat. II. Dose-dependent effects on offspring behavior. Neurotoxicol. Teratol. **12:** 327–334.
6. Johns, J. M., M. J. Means, D. R. Anderson, E. W. Bass, L. W. Means & B. A. McMillen. 1992. Prenatal exposure to cocaine. II. Effects on open field activity and cognitive behavior in Sprague-Dawley rats. Neurotoxicol. Teratol. **14:** 343–349.
7. Johns, J. M., L. W. Means, E. W. Bass, M. J. Means, L. I. Zimmerman & B. A. McMillen. 1994. Prenatal exposure to cocaine: Effects on aggression in Sprague-Dawley rats. Dev. Psychobiol. **27:** 227–239.
8. Goodwin, G. A., C. J. Heyser, C. A. Moody, L. Rajachandran, V. A. Molina, H. M. Arnold, D. L. McKinzie, N. E. Spear & L. P. Spear. 1992. A fostering study of the effects of prenatal cocaine exposure. II. Offspring behavioral measures. Neurotoxicol. Teratol. **14:** 423–432.
9. Noonan, L. R. & J. M. Johns. 1995. Prenatal cocaine exposure affects social behavior in Sprague-Dawley rats. Neurotoxicol. Teratol. **17:** 569–576.
10. Johns, J. M., L. R. Noonan, L. I. Zimmerman, L. Li & C. A. Pedersen. 1994. Effects of chronic and acute cocaine treatment on the onset of maternal behavior and aggression in Sprague-Dawley rats. Behav. Neurosci. **108:** 1–7.
11. Johns, J. M., M. J. Means, L. W. Means & B. A. McMillen. 1992. Prenatal exposure to cocaine. I. Effects on gestation, development and activity in Sprague-Dawley rats. Neurotoxicol. Teratol. **14:** 337–342.
12. Henderson, M. G. & B. A. McMillen. 1993. Changes in dopamine, serotonin and their metabolites in discrete brain areas of rat offspring after in utero exposure to cocaine or related drugs. Teratology. **48:** 421–430.

Effects of *in Utero* Exposure to Cocaine and/or Opiates on Infants' Reaching Behavior

L.L. LAGASSE,[a] R.F. VAN VORST, S.M. BRUNNER, AND B.M. LESTER

Infant Development Center, Brown University School of Medicine, 79 Plain Street, Providence, Rhode Island 02905, USA

The importance of sensorimotor or exploratory activity to the acquisition or enrichment of knowledge has been suggested in different forms by several theorists.[1,2] By the second half of the first year, infants easily reach for stationary and moving objects, adjusting their grasp to accommodate the object they see.[3] Furthermore, infants can localize and reach for a stationary sound stimulus in the dark.[4,5] Recent evidence suggests that infants are capable of encoding and forming mental representations of objects in context with relatively brief experience.[6] Given these capacities, the present study explores infants' exploration of seen (light) and unseen (dark) events where only sound cues mark the activity and identity of an object previously represented.

Infants' exploratory behavior depends not only on cognitive and motor processes but also on motivational processes. During the last decade, cocaine or crack has become an increasingly common drug of abuse among young women, resulting in many infants who are exposed *in utero.* Cocaine is a central nervous system (CNS) stimulant that blocks the reuptake of monoaminergic transmitters (dopamine, norepinephrine, and serotonin) in the CNS, leading to more circulating catecholamines centrally and peripherally and increased neurophysiologic, autonomic, and behavioral arousal.[7,8] Cocaine easily crosses the placenta and the blood brain barrier. Based on its pharmacology, prenatal exposure to cocaine could lead to disturbances associated with limbic, hypothalamic, and extrapyramidal function that may compromise neuroregulatory mechanisms in the infant.[9]

Research to date supports concerns that *in utero* cocaine exposure may affect some of the processes that play a role in infants' exploration of the environment during the second half of the first year. First, cocaine-exposed infants show poorer gross and fine motor control than do nonexposed infants.[10,11] Second, while global cognitive deficits are unlikely, some findings suggest that *in utero* cocaine exposure affects encoding and recognition processes.[12] Third, exposed infants appear less motivated when they engage in interaction with objects and dyadic partners.[13] Poorer functioning in any of these domains may disrupt infants' exploration or understanding of events they experience. In this study, cocaine-exposed and nonexposed infants are presented with an interesting event in the light and dark to examine whether cocaine exposure is associated with exploration of the event.

METHODS

Subjects. Based on maternal history and meconium assay, 8 infants were identified as exposed *in utero* and 10 were nonexposed; all were full term, 7.5 to 8.5 months.

Procedure. Sixteen trials were presented to the infant in which four objects emitting

[a] Phone, 401/453-7640; fax, 401/453-7646; e-mail, linda__lagasse@brown.edu

sounds moved clockwise into the infant's reaching space at a fixed speed (5 cm/s) in the light and dark. Sessions were videotaped using infrared sensitive cameras for later coding of reaching, attention, affect, motivation, localization, and recognition by trained coders masked to the exposure status of the infant.

Data Reduction. Behavioral coding for reaching activity in the light and dark was completed by trained, reliable coders (Kappa >0.70; intraclass correlation >0.80). The dependent measures index related cognitive processes: *attention and motivation* (the rate of incomplete trials due to fussing and the rate of reaching); *auditory localization* (frequency of reaches and contacts with the object); *recognition* (frequency of object contacts with a closed grasp); *reaching efficiency* (trial duration and the distance of the object from the infant at first contact).

RESULTS AND DISCUSSION

Compared to the light condition, both groups reached and contacted the object less often, missed more often, and took longer to contact the object in the dark ($p < 0.01$ in all cases), reflecting the difficulty of the task in the dark. In both the light and dark, object contacts made with a closed grasp were faster than those involving open-handed touches ($p < 0.05$). No differences were noted between the groups in the number of trials terminated because of fussing. Although both groups reached for the object equally often in the light, cocaine-exposed infants reached less often than nonexposed infants in the dark ($p < 0.05$). When a reach was made, however, both groups missed the object equally often in the light and dark. Although the time to contact the object was similar in both groups in the light, cocaine-exposed infants were significantly slower to make contact with the object in the dark than were nonexposed infants ($p < 0.05$). Both groups used a closed grasp equally often in the light; however, exposed infants were more likely to use a closed grasp in the dark ($p < 0.05$).

In sum, the reaching behavior of cocaine-exposed infants did not differ from that of nonexposed infants in the light when both visual and auditory cues to the identity and localization of the object were available. But cocaine-exposed infants showed less engagement in sensorimotor activity when the task was more demanding and only auditory cues were available with which to recognize the object or its trajectory and guide their reaching. Given that cocaine-exposed infants as well as nonexposed infants localized objects when they tried, the decrement in reaching behavior may reflect attentional or motivational deficits that could affect the cognitive development of exposed infants.

REFERENCES

1. Piaget, J. 1952. The origins of intelligence in children. International Universities Press. New York, NY.
2. Gibson, A.J. 1988. Exploratory behavior in the development of perceiving acting and the acquiring of knowledge. Ann. Rev. Psychol. **39:** 1–41.
3. Von Hofsten, C. & L. Ronnqvist. 1988. Preparation for grasping an object: A developmental study. J. Exp. Psychol.: Hum. Percept. and Perform. **14:** 610–621.
4. Perris, E.E. & R.K. Clifton. 1988. Reaching in the dark toward sound as a measure of auditory localization in infants. Infant Behav. Dev. **11:** 473–491.
5. Clifton, R., E. Perris *et al.* 1991. Infants' perception of auditory space. Dev. Psychol. **27:** 187–197.
6. Clifton, R.K., P. Rochat *et al.* 1991. Object representation guides infants' reaching in the dark. J. Exp. Psychol.: Hum. Percep. Perform. **17:** 323–329.

7. Mayes, L.C. 1994. Neurobiology of prenatal cocaine exposure: Effect on developing monoamine systems. Infant Mental Health **15:** 134–145.
8. Volpe, J.J. 1992. Effect of cocaine use on the fetus. N. Engl. J. Med. **327:** 399–407.
9. Lester, B.M., L.L. LaGasse *et al.* 1996. Studies of cocaine-exposed human infants. *In* Behavior of Drug Exposed Offspring: Research Update. NIDA Monograph Series.: 175–210.
10. Fetters, L. & E. Z. Tronick. 1996. Neuromotor development of cocaine exposed and control infants from birth to 15 months: Poor and poorer performance. Pediatrics **98:** 938–943.
11. Schneider, J.W. & I.J. Chasnoff. 1987. Cocaine abuse during pregnancy: Its effects on infant motor development. A clinical perspective. Topics Acute Care Trauma Rehab. **2:** 59–69.
12. Alessandri, S.M., M.W. Sullivan *et al.* 1993. Learning and emotional responsivity in cocaine-exposed infants. Dev. Psychol. **29:** 989–997.
13. Tronick, E.Z., K.L. Olson *et al.* 1995. Mutual negative affect dominates the face-to-face interactions of 6-month-old infants who experienced in-utero cocaine exposure and their mothers. Presented at the Biennial Meeting of the Society for Research in Child Development, March–April, 1995.

Effects of Prenatal Cocaine Exposure on Responsiveness to Multimodal Information in Infants between 4 and 10 Months of Age[a]

DAVID J. LEWKOWICZ, BERNARD Z. KARMEL, AND JUDITH M. GARDNER

NYS Institute for Basic Research in Developmental Disabilities, 1050 Forest Hill Rd., Staten Island, New York 10314, USA

Our studies have shown that cocaine-exposed (CE) infants exhibit altered patterns of arousal that result in stimulus-seeking behavior. We previously suggested that initial, arousal-based behaviors transform themselves during development into higher-level, perceptual/cognitive modes of functioning and that the transition depends on the normal development of arousal-based modes of functioning. If arousal control mechanisms are altered in early development, the transition to the higher-level modes of functioning, such as intermodal integration, may be adversely affected. To test this possibility, we conducted studies to examine three aspects of CE infants' intermodal perception: (1) responsiveness to auditory-visual (A-V) synchrony relations; (2) preferences for multimodally represented exaggerated prosody information; and (3) responsiveness to the audible and visible components of the human face. Two groups of normal, healthy infants were tested: CE and non-CE. The CE infants had evidence of cocaine exposure based on maternal report and/or infant urine or meconium toxicology. Testing was carried out at 4, 7, and 10 months of age.

DETECTION OF AUDITORY-VISUAL ASYNCHRONY

An important basis for the perception of intermodal unity of diverse, multimodal sources of information is temporal intermodal synchrony. Normally developing infants can perceive A-V synchrony and can tell that the A and V components of a compound stimulus are asynchronous once they are separated by between 350 and 400 ms.[1] We asked whether prenatal exposure to cocaine might adversely affect the perception of A-V temporal synchrony. Using an infant-controlled habituation/test procedure, infants were first habituated to an object that bounced up and down and that made a sound each time it bounced. Following habituation, a series of test trials was given to each infant in which synchrony between the A and V bounce was disrupted by 300, 350, or 400 ms, and the amount of looking during each test trial was compared to that in a familiar test trial. The non-CE infants ($n = 116$, 105, and 85 at 4, 7, and 10 mo, respectively) discriminated an asynchrony of 400 ms at each of the 3 ages. By contrast, the CE infants ($n = 29$, 26, and 22 at 4, 7, and 10 months, respectively) failed to discriminate any of the asynchrony intervals. Power analysis of the CE data indicated that

[a] This work was supported by the National Institute on Drug Abuse Grant R01 DA06644.

[b] Address for correspondence: David J. Lewkowicz, NYS Institute for Basic Research in Developmental Disabilities, 1050 Forest Hill Rd., Staten Island, NY 10314. Phone, 718/494-5302; fax, 718/494-5395; e-mail, ddlsi@cunyvm.cuny.edu

the failure to obtain significant responsiveness was not due to insufficient power. Thus, it appears that prenatal cocaine exposure has a negative impact on the development of this basic sensory/perceptual task.

PREFERENCES FOR INFANT-DIRECTED TALK

Infants are highly responsive to infant-directed talk (IDT), a stylized type of speech that differs from adult-directed talk (ADT) in that it is higher in pitch, has a wider pitch range, has smooth and highly modulated pitch contours, is slower in tempo, is characterized by shorter utterances and greater prosodic repetition, and has longer pauses between utterances. Normally developing infants prefer to listen to IDT when given a choice between multimodally represented IDT and ADT, and this preference first appears at 4 months of age. The initial mechanism that mediates the facilitating effects of IDT is presumed to be an increase in arousal that typically is seen when infants are exposed to IDT. The increased arousal, in turn, is presumed to increase infants' attention to some of the key structural aspects of language that make it possible for them to "break" into the linguistic code and differentiate the basic structural aspects of their native language. To determine if prenatal cocaine exposure has a negative impact on a preference for IDT, each infant was allowed to view and listen to four 1-minute videotaped segments showing a woman speaking in IDT and in ADT in English and in Cantonese. Non-CE infants ($n = 49$, 52, and 30 at each age, respectively) looked and listened longer to IDT at each of the 3 ages ($p < 0.01$; see FIG. 1) regardless of language. The 4- and 7-month-old CE infants also preferred IDT ($n = 54$ and 41 at each of the ages, respectively; $p < 0.01$) regardless of language. By contrast, the 10-month-old CE infants ($n = 26$) did not exhibit a preference for IDT. This finding suggests that prenatal exposure to cocaine does not adversely affect the preference for IDT up to 6–7 months of age, but cocaine exposure does appear to have a deleterious effect later on. This decline in performance is similar to our findings indicating a decline in scores on the Bayley Mental Development Index starting at about this age.

RESPONSE TO THE COMPONENTS OF A FACE/VOICE COMPOUND STIMULUS

The human face is concurrently specified by various amodal and modality-specific attributes and is an important source of sensory, cognitive, linguistic, and social information for the infant. We used a multimodal component variation method, based on earlier work with normally developing infants,[2,3] to determine how CE infants respond to the various attributes of the face/voice compound stimulus. First, each infant was habituated to a video recording of a female reciting a prepared script in ADT and then was given four test trials: an auditory (A) test trial, where the same person was seen but a different person was heard singing; (2) a visual (V) test trial, where a new person was seen singing and the same person was heard speaking in ADT; (3) a combined auditory/visual (AV) test trial, where a new person was seen and heard singing; and (4) a familiar test trial where the same person that was seen talking in ADT during the habituation phase was seen and heard again. The non-CE infants ($n = 109$, 105, and 102 at 4, 7, and 10 months, respectively) discriminated the changes in all three types of test trials at all three ages (TABLE 1). By contrast, CE infants ($n = 33$, 25, and 32 at 4, 7, and 10 months, respectively) exhibited a delay in the emergence of responsiveness to the A attributes and a failure to respond to the visible change at older ages. The latter finding has never been observed in normally developing infants and may be due to the fact that the visible change from one person's face to another's is not as stimulating as is a change in voice from ADT to singing.

GENERAL CONCLUSIONS

Current studies showed that CE infants failed to discriminate A-V asynchrony at any of the ages tested, exhibited a decline in the preference for IDT, and produced a pattern of response to the components of a face/voice compound that is different from that found in normally developing infants. This overall pattern of findings appears to be consistent in a broad sense with the prediction that prenatal cocaine exposure leads to a disruption in arousal modulating mechanisms that, in turn, leads to a disruption in the developmental emergence of a variety of multimodal response mechanisms. Given that CE infants appear to seek stimulation, this set of findings may reflect the failure to make age-appropriate developmental transitions in arousal control mechanisms. This failure may, in turn, make it less possible for CE infants to perceive the stimulus differences that non-CE infants are able to discriminate because such differences may not have sufficiently differential arousal properties.

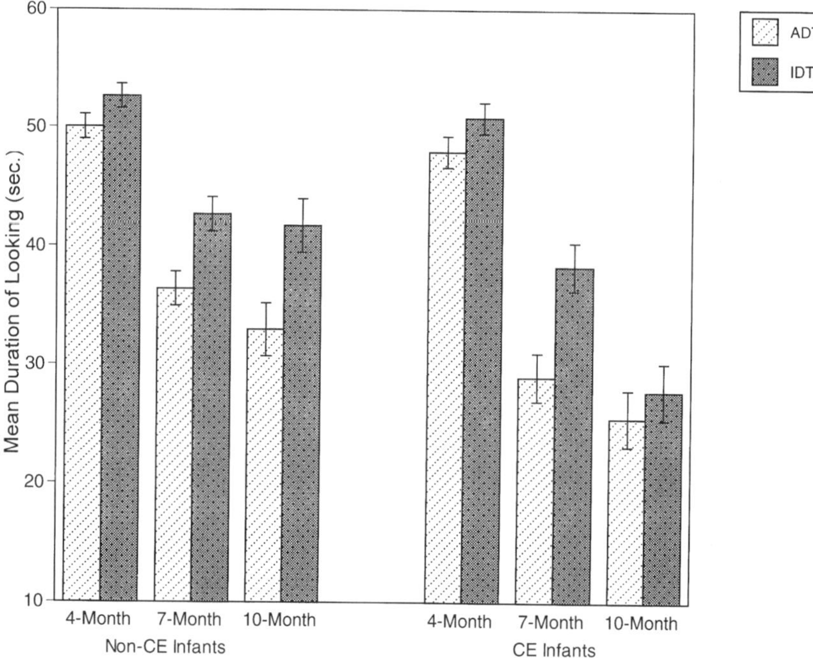

FIGURE 1. Mean duration of looking at multimodally specified infant-directed talk and adult-directed talk in cocaine-exposed (CE) and non-CE infants at each of three ages. Error bars indicate standard errors of the mean.

TABLE 1. Response to the Components of a Face/Voice Compound Stimulus in the Three Test Trials in Cocaine-Exposed and non-Cocaine-Exposed Infants

	Non-Cocaine-Exposed			Cocaine-Exposed		
	Auditory	Visual	Aud/Vis	Auditory	Visual	Aud/Vis
4 Mo.	*	*	*	ns	*	*
7 Mo.	*	*	*	m	ns	*
10 Mo.	*	*	*	*	ns	*

* = significant; m = marginal; ns = not significant.

REFERENCES

1. LEWKOWICZ, D. J. 1996. Perception of auditory-visual temporal synchrony in human infants. J. Exp. Psychol.: Hum. Percept. Perform. **22:** 1094–1106.
2. LEWKOWICZ, D. J. 1996. Infants' response to the audible and visible properties of the human face. I. Role of lexical/syntactic content, temporal synchrony, gender, and manner of speech. Dev. Psychol. **32:** 347–366.
3. LEWKOWICZ, D. J. 1998. Infants' response to the audible and visible properties of the human face. II. Effects of singing. Dev. Psychobiol. In press.

Effects of Prenatal Cocaine Exposure on Serotonin and Norepinephrine Transporter Density in the Rat Brain[a]

ALISON M. MCREYNOLDS[b] AND JERROLD S. MEYER

Department of Psychology, Neuroscience and Behavior Program, Tobin Hall, University of Massachusetts, Amherst, Massachusetts 01003, USA

A variety of both neurochemical and behavioral abnormalities have been observed following prenatal cocaine exposure.[1] Cocaine's acute action in the central nervous system is to block the dopamine (DA), norepinephrine (NE), and serotonin (5-HT) reuptake transporters, which are known to have similar properties in the adult and fetal brain.[2] Numerous reports suggest that exposure to cocaine during early development may alter the postnatal organization of the serotonergic[3] and noradrenergic[4] systems. To help characterize the nature of these changes, we used quantitative *in vitro* autoradiography to determine the effects of prenatal cocaine treatment on the expression of the 5-HT and NE reuptake transporters at three postnatal time points.

METHODS

Pregnant Sprague-Dawley rats (Charles River CD strain) were given subcutaneous injections of 40 mg/kg cocaine-HCl or an equivalent volume of saline solution once daily from gestational days 8 through 20. Saline-treated controls were pair-fed to the cocaine-treated dams. Litters were culled to four males and four females on postnatal day (PD 1), fostered to untreated surrogate dams, and weaned at PD 21. At PD 1, 10, 25, and 60, one male from each litter was sacrificed by decapitation, and the brain was quickly removed and frozen on dry ice. Brains were sectioned at 10 µm (PD 10) or 20 µm (PD 25 and 60) (PD 1 tissue samples have not yet been studied). Different sections from the same animal were incubated with either 1 nM [^{3}H]paroxetine to label the 5-HT transporter (SERT) or 3 nM [^{3}H]nisoxetine to label the NE transporter (NET). Nonspecific binding was determined in the presence of fluoxetine or mazindol, respectively. Following exposure of sections and plastic standards for appropriate time periods, films were developed and densitometry was performed using NIH Image software.

RESULTS AND CONCLUSIONS

The treatment paradigm used in this study had no effect on litter size or pup weight (data not shown), indicating that this regimen was not grossly teratogenic to the offspring. Analyses of the autoradiograms from PD 10 indicate that prenatal cocaine exposure did not alter SERT or NET density in any region examined at this time point

[a] This research was supported by National Institute on Drug Abuse Grant DA-06495.

[b] Phone, 413/545-2709; fax, 413/545-0996; e-mail, amcreynolds@nsm.umass.edu

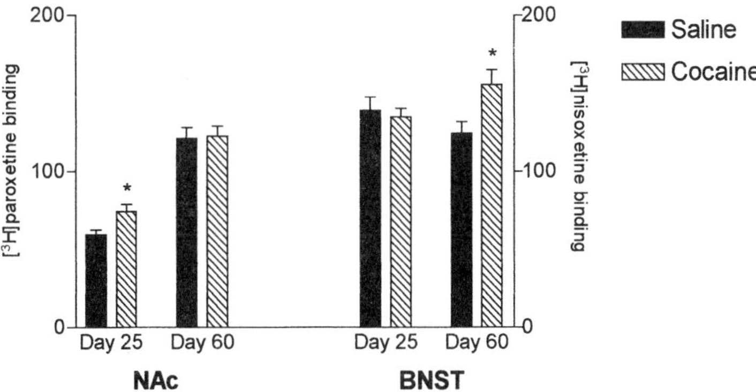

FIGURE 1. Characterization of [^{3}H]paroxetine and [^{3}H]nisoxetine binding to serotonin and norepinephrine transporters in postnatal day 25 and 60 male rats treated from gestational day 8–20 with cocaine-HCl versus saline solution. Values shown represent the mean ± SEM of fmol/mg tissue.

(data not shown). Similarly, no changes in NET binding were observed at PD 25; however, analysis of [^{3}H]paroxetine binding revealed a significant 25% increase in SERT density in the nucleus accumbens at this age (FIG. 1 and TABLE 1). At PD 60, the group difference in [^{3}H]paroxetine binding was no longer evident, whereas [^{3}H]nisoxetine binding to NET in the bed nucleus of the stria terminalis was increased in cocaine-exposed animals compared with saline-treated controls. Changes in SERT and NET binding were not observed in any other brain region examined at PD 25 and 60. (See Table 1 for selected examples.)

TABLE 1. Effects of Prenatal Cocaine Exposure on Serotonin and Norepinephrine Transporter Binding[a]

		Region *(n)*	Saline (± SEM)	Cocaine (± SEM)
[^{3}H]Paroxetine	PD 25	Nucleus accumbens (6)	59.5 ± 3.0	74.3 ± 4.4*
		Striatum (5)	154.0 ± 13.1	160.1 ± 11.2
		Hippocampus CA3 (5)	153.9 ± 18.0	153.8 ± 9.3
	PD 60	Nucleus accumbens (7)	120.0 ± 7.1	122.6 ± 6.2
		Striatum (7)	148.9 ± 9.8	141.2 ± 10.7
		Hippocampus (7)	106.9 ± 3.0	107.5 ± 5.2
[^{3}H]Nisoxetine	PD 25	Bed nucleus of the stria terminalis (4)	138.9 ± 8.7	134.8 ± 5.4
		Anteroventral thalamic nucleus (4)	101.2 ± 6.2	87.9 ± 6.1
		Hippocampus CA3 (5)	77.9 ± 12.6	68.8 ± 3.7
	PD 60	Bed nucleus of the stria terminalis (7)	124.4 ± 7.3	155.7 ± 9.4*
		Anteroventral thalamic nucleus (7)	95.8 ± 3.7	105.6 ± 5.5
		Hippocampus (7)	37.3 ± 3.7	39.4 ± 5.0

[a]Values represent fmol/mg tissue (mean ± SEM) of [^{3}H]paroxetine and [^{3}H]nisoxetine binding for each treatment group.

*$p < 0.05$.

The data presented here provide further evidence for alterations in serotonergic and noradrenergic development following prenatal cocaine exposure and indicate that these changes can be region specific. However, it remains unclear whether the observed changes in NET binding are persistent or transient, like those observed with SERT binding, and whether the increased transporter density seen here represents an upregulation of the transporter per terminal or an altered innervation pattern. Given the widespread modulatory role of 5-HT and NE in the central nervous system, cocaine-induced alterations in the development of these systems are of particular interest. Such neurochemical alterations may contribute to the observed behavioral abnormalities following cocaine exposure *in utero.*

REFERENCES

1. FRANK, D.A., K. BRESNAHAN & B.S. ZUCKERMAN. 1993. Maternal cocaine use: Impact on child health and development. Adv. Pediatr. **40:** 65–99.
2. MEYER, J.S., L.P. SHEARMAN & L.M. COLLINS. 1996. Monoamine transporters and the neurobehavioral teratology of cocaine. Pharmacol. Biochem. Behav. **55:** 585–593.
3. AKBARI, H.M. *et al.* 1992. Prenatal cocaine exposure disrupts the development of the serotonergic system. Brain Res. **572:** 57–63.
4. WALLACE, D.R., C.F. MACTUTUS & R.M. BOOZE. 1995. Prenatal intravenous cocaine: Persistent regional alterations in α_2-adrenergic receptor density [abstr.]. Neurotoxicol. Teratol. **17:** 385.

Sources of Heart Rate Variation during Sleep in Cocaine-Exposed Neonates[a]

MICHAEL G. REGALADO,[b,f,g] VICKI L. SCHECHTMAN,[c,h] MICHAEL C.K. KHOO,[d,i] JOHN SHIN,[d,i] AND XYLINA D. BEAN[e,j]

[b]*Department of Pediatrics, University of Southern California School of Medicine, Childrens Hospital Los Angeles, 4650 Sunset Boulevard, MS # 76, Los Angeles, California 90027, USA*

[c]*Brain Research Institute, UCLA School of Medicine, Los Angeles, California 90095–1761, USA*

[d]*Department of Biomedical Engineering, University of Southern California, Los Angeles, California 90089–1451, USA*

[e]*Department of Pediatrics, Charles R. Drew University of Medicine, 12021 S. Wilmington Avenue, Los Angeles, California 90059, USA*

A few reports have examined various aspects of the effects of chronic *in utero* cocaine exposure on autonomic control of heart rate in the neonate, and these have been inconclusive.[1–4] We previously reported a trend toward slower heart rates, significantly greater changes in heart rate between sleep states, and significantly greater overall heart rate variability across sleep states in cocaine-exposed neonates compared to controls.[4] In this paper we report the results of spectral analysis of heart rate variation in that sample of cocaine-exposed neonates. The purpose of the analyses is to determine what types of heart rate variation account for the increased heart rate variability (respiratory sinus arrhythmia vs low frequency heart rate variation) in neonates with chronic cocaine exposure *in utero.*

METHODS

The subjects were 11 full-term cocaine-exposed infants and 11 full-term control infants. All were healthy infants 2-weeks postnatal age at the time of the study with birth weights greater than 2,500 g and Apgar scores at 5 minutes greater than 7. Cocaine exposure was determined initially by maternal self-report or neonatal toxicological urinalysis (EMIT procedure). Radioimmunoassay of mothers' hair[5] was used to verify cocaine exposure and lack thereof in the cocaine group and the control group, respectively. The infants with cocaine exposure had significantly greater exposure to tobacco and alcohol.[4] Infants with identified exposure to substances other than cocaine, alcohol, and tobacco were excluded.

Four-hour daytime recordings of the electrocardiogram (ECG) were obtained from the infants during spontaneous sleep and wakefulness. Each 1-minute epoch was clas-

[a] This research was supported by March of Dimes Birth Defects Foundation Grant No. 12-FY92-0833, Biomedical Research Support Grant No. 2S07-RR05780-15, and UCLA Academic Senate awards to Michael Regalado and National Institutes of Health Grant RR-01861 to Michael Khoo.

[f] Corresponding author.

[g] Phone, 213/669–2110; fax, 213/663-6707; e-mail, regalado@hsc.usc.edu

[h] Phone, 310/206-1679; fax, 310/206-5855; e-mail:vicki@aunix.loni.ucla.edu

[i] Phone, 213/740–0347; fax, 213/740–0343; e-mail:khoo@bmsrs.usc.edu

[j] Phone, 310/668–3150; fax, 310/763–2638

sified as quiet sleep, active sleep, or waking based on behavioral criteria. The intervals between successive R waves of the ECG (R-R intervals) were determined, and a linear interpolation algorithm was used to convert the R-R intervals to equally-spaced measures of heart rate. For each 1-minute epoch, the power spectrum of the interpolated heart rate signal was computed using a prewhitened autoregressive method (6). The power spectrum was integrated from 0 to 8 Hz to obtain the total power. Spectral power was then determined for a high-frequency band (0.3 to 2 Hz), primarily respiratory sinus arrhythmia, which is predominantly under vagal control, and for mid-frequency (0.1 to 0.2 Hz) and low-frequency bands (0.03 to 0.1 Hz), both arising from sympathetic and parasympathetic mechanisms. Median values for spectral power in each band were determined for quiet and active sleep. Differences between groups were examined using a 2-tailed Mann-Whitney rank sum test.

RESULTS

Total power was enhanced in cocaine-exposed infants relative to control infants in both quiet and active sleep ($p < 0.05$ in both cases). In quiet sleep, both mid- and low-frequency heart rate variation were increased in infants of cocaine-abusing mothers compared to controls ($p < 0.05$ for low-frequency; $p < 0.02$ for mid-frequency; FIG. 1). In active sleep, only low-frequency variation was significantly increased in cocaine-exposed infants compared to controls ($p < 0.05$, FIG. 2). Power of respiratory sinus arrhythmia did not differ between the two groups in either sleep state.

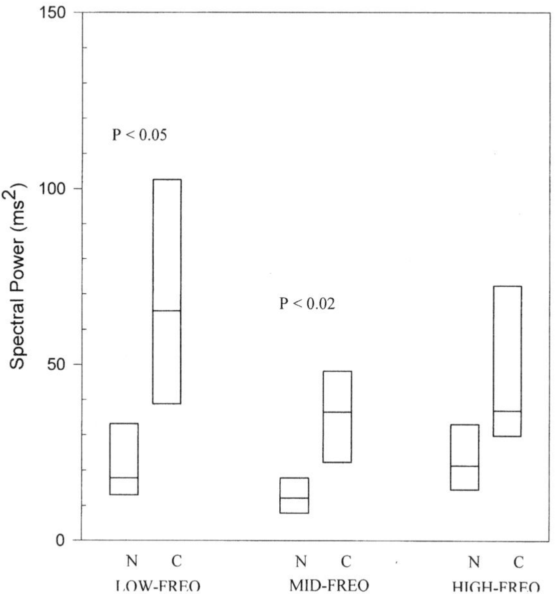

FIGURE 1. Spectral composition of heart rate variability in normal controls (N) versus cocaine-exposed (C) infants in quiet sleep. Low-frequency power and mid-frequency power were significantly higher in cocaine-exposed infants. (*Box plots* represent medians and interquartile ranges.)

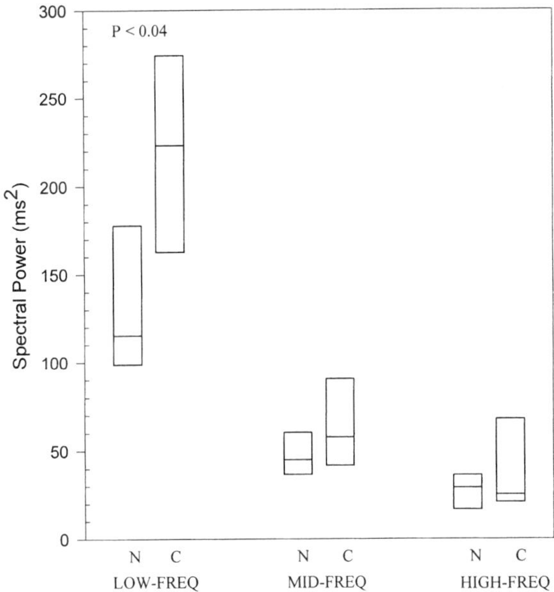

FIGURE 2. Spectral composition of heart rate variability in normal controls (N) versus cocaine-exposed (C) infants in active sleep. Low-frequency power was significantly higher in cocaine-exposed infants.

CONCLUSION

These results suggest differences at 2 weeks of age in sympathetic control of heart rate in cocaine-exposed infants compared to infants without cocaine exposure. Although it is possible that behavioral factors, such as a higher incidence of periodic breathing in cocaine-exposed infants, may contribute to these findings, increases in mid- and low-frequency heart rate variation without changes in respiratory sinus arrhythmia are suggestive of specific effects of prenatal cocaine exposure on catecholamine sensitivity and/or metabolism. Findings of increased sympathetic tone in the neonatal period may have significance for concurrent neurobehavioral phenomena described in cocaine-exposed infants.[7]

REFERENCES

1. DiPietro, J.A. *et al.* 1995. Reactivity and regulation in cocaine-exposed neonates. Infant Behav. Dev. **18:** 407–414.
2. Mehta, S.K. *et al.* 1993. Transient myocardial ischemia in infants prenatally exposed to cocaine. J. Pediatr. **122:** 945–999.
3. Oriol, N.E. *et al.* 1993. Cocaine effects on neonatal heart rate dynamics: Preliminary findings and methodological problems. Yale J. Biol. Med. **66:** 75–84.
4. Regalado, M. *et al.* 1996. Cardiac and respiratory patterns during sleep in cocaine-exposed neonates. Early Hum. Dev. **44:** 187–200.

5. BAUMGARTNER, W. *et al.* 1989. Hair analysis for drug abuse. J. Forensic Sci. **34:** 1433–1453.
6. BIRCH, G.E. *et al.* 1988. Application of prewhitening to AR spectral estimation of EEG. IEEE Trans. Biomed. Eng. **35:** 640–645.
7. MIROCHNICK, M. *et al.* 1997. Elevated plasma norepinephrine after in utero exposure to cocaine and marijuana. Pediatrics **99:** 555–559.

Prenatal Cocaine Exposure Increases Susceptibility to Drug-Induced Seizures

c-fos Induction and Brain Cocaine Levels[a]

ABIGAIL SNYDER-KELLER[b,d] AND RICHARD W. KELLER, JR.[c]

[b]*Wadsworth Center for Laboratories and Research, New York State Department of Health, and* [c]*Department of Pharmacology and Neuroscience, Albany Medical College, Albany, New York* [b]*12201 or* [c]*12208*

Infants exposed to cocaine *in utero* display a higher incidence of neonatal seizures.[1] Although these infants appear to recover from this period of heightened epileptogenicity, the degree to which underlying brain abnormalities might lead to seizures under conditions of stress or pharmacologic challenge later in life remains to be determined. We previously reported that prenatally cocaine-treated rats are more susceptible to cocaine-induced seizures (both acute and kindled) as adults.[2] We now extend these findings and examine the basis for this differential susceptibility.

Sprague-Dawley rats derived from the Griffin Lab strain (New York State Department of Health) were time mated (day sperm seen was considered embryonic day [E] 0) and injected with cocaine (40 mg/kg, sc) from E10–E20. Controls consisted of pups born to females injected with saline solution during the same period. All procedures were approved by the Institutional Animal Care and Use Committees.

SEIZURE TESTS

At 2–3 months of age, rats were tested for their sensitivity to acute drug-induced seizures. Each animal was administered a single dose of cocaine ip (males received 50, 55, or 60 mg/kg; females 45, 50, or 55 mg/kg) or 30 mg/kg pentylenetetrazol (PTZ). As seen in TABLE 1, a greater percentage of prenatally cocaine-treated females seized in comparison to prenatally saline-treated females in response to 50 mg/kg cocaine; prenatally cocaine-treated males were not different from controls. Both male and female prenatally cocaine-treated rats were more susceptible to PTZ-induced seizures; however, the *severity* of the seizures was greater only in prenatally cocaine-treated females relative to controls. The increased susceptibility of prenatally cocaine-treated rats to PTZ-induced as well as cocaine-induced seizures argues against a specific increase in sensitivity to cocaine and suggests that the balance between excitatory and inhibitory mechanisms may be upset in the brains of prenatally cocaine-treated rats.

FOS IMMUNOCYTOCHEMISTRY

As a means of determining the degree of neuronal excitation produced by these drugs (or drug-induced seizures),[3] we examined the distribution and density of Fos-

[a] This work was supported by National Institutes of Health Grants DA08694 (to A.S.-K.) and DA06199 (to R.W.K.).

[d] Address for correspondence: Abigail Snyder-Keller, Wadsworth Center for Laboratories and Research, New York State Department of Health, P.O. Box 509, Empire State Plaza, Albany, NY 12201. Phone, 518/486-2590; fax; 518/474-5049; e-mail; snykell@wadsworth.org

TABLE 1. Percentage of Animals Seizing in Response to Acute Injections of Cocaine or Pentylenetetrazol as Adults as a Function of Prenatal Treatment and Sex

	COC45	COC50	COC55	COC60	PTZ30
Prenatal saline					
Males	—	0	36	44	46 (1.7)
Females	0	14	31	—	13 (1.0)
Prenatal cocaine					
Males	—	11	33	44	76* (1.9)
Females	0	50*	67	—	50* (1.9*)

Numbers indicate percentage of animals seizing in response to an acute injection of cocaine (COC) at one of the doses indicated (45–60 mg/kg; 9–12 rats/group) or pentylenetetrazol (PTZ) at 30 mg/kg (15–24 rats/group). No more than two rats of each sex from each litter were used for the same behavioral test, and each rat was tested only once. Numbers in parentheses indicate the mean severity of PTZ-induced seizures (of those having seizures) when scored according to the following rating scale: **0** = no seizure; **1** = head clonus or "jerks"; **2** = head torsion; **3** = wild running/bouncing; **4** = tonic extension of the limbs.

*Significantly different from control group of the same sex ($p < 0.05$).

immunoreactive cells in striatum, nucleus accumbens, area tempestas[4] (anterior piriform cortex), piriform cortex (posterior), and basolateral and medial amygdala. We reasoned that differences in the number of Fos-immunoreactive cells may indicate the locus of differential sensitivity to cocaine or PTZ or differences in threshold for cocaine- or PTZ-induced seizures, particularly in limbic system regions known to be involved in cocaine-induced seizures.[5]

Animals were perfused (4% paraformaldehyde) 2 hours after cocaine- or PTZ-induced seizures. Sections were immunostained for Fos (sheep polyclonal antibodies from Cambridge Research Biochemicals [now Genosys]; 1:6000) using standard avidin-biotin-peroxidase procedures. Fos-immunoreactive nuclei were counted in a 600 × 800 μm box (using a 20× objective) placed in each of six brain regions, using the NIH Image program. For each region, each animal's count consisted of the average of the left and right side. Means were calculated from five to six females/condition for cocaine, and three to five males/group for PTZ. At threshold doses of cocaine (50–55 mg/kg), nonseizing female rats that were prenatally cocaine treated exhibited lower numbers of Fos-immunoreactive cells in piriform cortex and medial amygdala (FIG. 1). This may reflect a lower threshold in prenatally cocaine-treated rats, so that a lower level of excitation (i.e., fewer Fos-immunoreactive cells) is necessary to generate a seizure in these rats. Once a seizure was elicited, a dramatic increase occurred in the number of Fos-immunoreactive cells in piriform cortex and amygdala, although there were no differences as a function of prenatal treatment (FIG. 1). The percentage increase above nonseizing levels was much greater in prenatally cocaine-treated rats because the number of Fos-immunoreactive cells in the nonseizing condition was lower. Pretreatment with the noncompetitive NMDA antagonist MK-801 (0.5–1.0 mg/kg, ip 30 minutes prior) blocked cocaine-induced seizures and increases in Fos immunoreactivity in striatum, piriform cortex, and both regions of amygdala. The dopamine D_1 antagonist SCH23390 (0.5 mg/kg, ip, 30 minutes prior) blocked cocaine-induced seizures and increases in Fos immunoreactivity in all regions.

Similarly, stage 1 PTZ seizures were induced with a lower level of neural activation (lower numbers of Fos-immunoreactive cells) in prenatally cocaine-treated rats, in area tempestas and medial amygdala. Stage 2 PTZ seizures were induced with a lower level

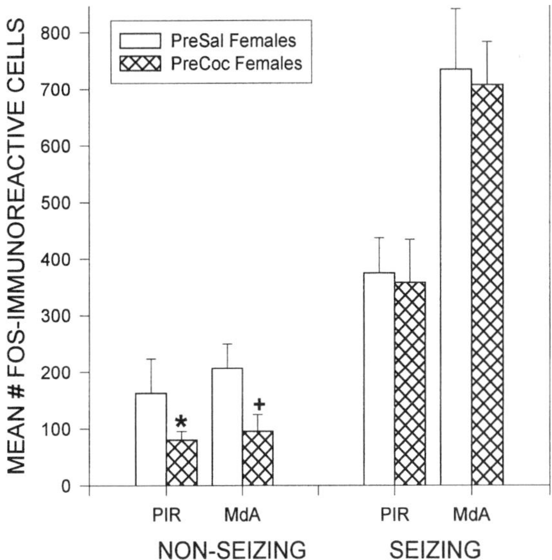

FIGURE 1. Mean number of Fos-immunoreactive cells in non-seizing and seizing rats 2 hours after 50–55 mg/kg cocaine ip. Counts were obtained from piriform cortex (PIR) and medial amygdala (MdA) of five prenatally saline-treated females *(open bars)* and five prenatally cocaine-treated females *(cross-hatched bars)*. *Significant difference from corresponding prenatally saline-treated group (*t* test; $p < 0.05$). $^{+}(p = 0.067)$.

of neural activation in prenatally cocaine-treated rats, in area tempestas. MK-801 (0.5–1.0 mg/kg, ip), but not SCH23390 (0.5 mg/kg, ip), pretreatment blocked PTZ seizures and increases in Fos immunoreactivity in area tempestas, amygdala, and piriform cortex. Thus, comparisons of the numbers of Fos-immunoreactive cells in prenatally cocaine-treated versus prenatally saline-treated rats, as well as the ability of drugs that block the drug-induced seizures to block accompanying c-fos induction, implicate the piriform cortex and amygdala as regions that may be altered after prenatal cocaine exposure, in such a way as to confer increased seizure susceptibility in response to drugs that alter the balance between excitatory and inhibitory mechanisms in the brain.

COCAINE LEVELS

We also tested the hypothesis that prenatal cocaine treatment might alter the delivery of cocaine to the brain by measuring the amount of cocaine in brain tissue samples after these rats were challenged with cocaine as adults. Tissue samples were dissected from frontal cortex, nucleus accumbens, striatum, amygdala, and hippocampus 20 minutes after ip injection of 40 mg/kg cocaine; sonicated in 0.1N perchloric acid; and analyzed by HPLC with UV-detection using lidocaine as internal standard. The samples were separated on a 3-µm reverse-phase column (Rainin Microsorb MV Column C18; 4.6 × 10 cm) using a mobile phase of 0.1 M KH_2PO_4 containing 5 mM triethylamine and adjusted to pH 3.0 with phosphoric acid, 1.88 g/l heptane sulfonic acid, and

25% acetonitrile at a flow rate of 1.2 ml/min. Cocaine had a retention time of about 6 minutes and was detected at 235 nm. No differences were found in the amount of cocaine measured in the tissue homogenates obtained from prenatally cocaine-treated versus prenatally saline-treated rats. Similarly, no increase was noted in the amount of cocaine detected in striatal dialysates obtained after cocaine challenge in adult Long-Evans rats prenatally treated with 20 mg/kg cocaine, despite the fact that cocaine challenge during the first month after birth did result in elevated cocaine in the striatum of prenatally cocaine-treated rats.[6] These findings suggest that the increased seizure susceptibility of prenatally cocaine-treated rats, when tested as adults, is not due to the increased delivery of cocaine to the brains of these animals.

REFERENCES

1. Chasnoff, I.J. & D.R. Griffith. 1989. Cocaine: Clinical studies of pregnancy and the newborn. Ann. N.Y. Acad. Sci. **562:** 260–266.
2. Snyder-Keller, A.M. & R.W. Keller, Jr. 1995. Prenatal cocaine alters later sensitivity to cocaine-induced seizures. Neurosci. Lett. **191:** 149–152.
3. Sagar, S.M., F.R. Sharp & T. Curran. 1988. Expression of c-fos protein: Metabolic mapping at the cellular level. Science **240:** 1328–1331.
4. Maggio, R. & K. Gale. 1989. Seizures evoked from area tempestas are subject to control by GABA and glutamate receptors in substantia nigra. Exp. Neurol. **105:** 184–188.
5. Clark, M., R.M. Post, S.R.B. Weiss & T. Nakajima. 1992. Expression of c-fos mRNA in acute and kindled cocaine seizures in rats. Brain Res. **582:** 101–106.
6. Keller, R.W., Jr., M.T. Chen, A. Snyder-Keller, J.N. Carlson & S.D. Glick. 1997. Prenatal cocaine exposure alters subsequent cocaine entry into the brain in young rats as monitored by *in vivo* microdialysis. Soc. Neurosci. Abstr. **23:** 262.

Mortality in Neonatal Rats Is Increased by Moderate Prenatal Exposure to Some Monoamine Reuptake Inhibitors

A Brief Review

STEVEN SPARENBORG[a]

Pharmacology & Toxicology Branch, Medications Development Division, National Institute on Drug Abuse, National Institutes of Health, Rockville, Maryland 20857, USA

Many developmental effects of cocaine exposure *in utero* have been reported, including those in this volume. These neurochemical, anatomical, and behavioral effects were studied in the postnatal animal and were produced by moderate doses of cocaine that were not fatal to either mother or offspring. Other reports have focused on the fatal effects of greater *in utero* exposure. Increases in pup mortality when cocaine was given during pregnancy were accompanied by increases in maternal mortality at the same dose levels.[1,2] The mechanism of the fatal effects is unknown. Cocaine is known to block the uptake of the monoamines dopamine, serotonin (5-HT), and norepinephrine (NE) in an equal manner. Mazindol also blocked the uptake of these neurotransmitters equally and caused postnatal rat pup death and pre- and postnatal rat dam death at doses that produced no toxicity in males or non-gravid females[3] (TABLE 1). Transporters for these monoamine neurotransmitters are functional in fetal rat brain as early as gestational day 15.[4] 5-HT and NE transporters are found in the placenta on gestational day 20, but none for dopamine are apparent.

As with cocaine, many developmental effects induced by the selective serotonin reuptake inhibitor fluoxetine have been noted and are anatomical, neurochemical, and behavioral. However, fluoxetine and other drugs that inhibit the reuptake of 5-HT selectively or 5-HT and NE but not dopamine, also increase the mortality of rat pups (TABLES 1 and 2). This effect occurred when dams were given daily oral doses of fluoxetine,[5] fluvoxamine,[6] sertraline,[7] paroxetine,[8] venlafaxine[9] or nefazodone[10] from gestational day 15 through postnatal day 21. Pup death typically occurred within the first few days after birth and not at later times. An increased stillbirth rate and low birth weight were also associated with the increased mortality rate. There were no other indications of fetotoxicity, and all surviving pups reached developmental milestones at normal rates and appeared normal under external examination.

The doses that resulted in these effects were not toxic to the dams, except that they mildly reduced food consumption and weight gain. It is unlikely that reduced weight gains of 5–15% affected mortality of pups. Voorhees and colleagues[11] reported that although prenatal treatment with fluoxetine (12 mg/kg po) increased pup mortality and decreased birth weight, pair-feeding a group of pregnant rats to the level of food con-

The views and opinions expressed herein are those of the author and do not necessarily reflect those of the National Institute on Drug Abuse.

[a] Address for correspondence: Room 11A-55, 5600 Fishers Lane, Rockville, MD 20857. E-mail, ss292q@nih.gov

TABLE 1. Toxic Findings in Rat Pups Born to Dams Dosed with Monoamine Reuptake Inhibitors during Gestation[a]

Drug Name	Control	Low Dose	Middle Dose	High Dose
Nonselective				
Mazindol				
Dose	0	5	10	20
Survival	94	84	57	22
Stillborn	ne	ne	ne	ne
Birth weight	—	d	d	d
Dopamine and NE only				
Bupropion				
Dose	0	100	200	300
Survival	—	ne	ne	ne
Stillborn	nr	nr	nr	nr
Birth weight	—	ne	ne	ne
5-HT and NE only				
Venlafaxine				
Dose	0	10	30	80
Survival	86	80	76	41
Stillborn	4	5	10	22
Birth weight	—	nr	92	88
Nefazodone				
Dose	0	75	150	300
Survival	99	nr	96	65
Stillborn	ne	ne	ne	ne
Birth weight	—	nr	95	86

[a]These data were taken from reviews of reproductive toxicity studies submitted to the FDA by sponsors of the drugs. These drugs were given by oral gavage to pregnant Long-Evans (bupropion only) or Sprague-Dawley rats on day 15 of gestation through weaning, except for mazindol which was given only through day 20 of gestation and bupropion in which dams were dosed beginning 15 days prior to mating and continued through weaning.

Dose is expressed as mg/kg body weight of the dam.

Survival numbers are percentages of live births.

Stillborn numbers are percentages of all births.

Birth weights are percentages of controls.

Abbreviation: nr = not mentioned in the FDA review. The following letters are used here when the FDA review did not include actual values. si = slight increase over control group levels; ne = no effect; d = decreased compared to control group.

sumption in the fluoxetine-treated group did not affect pup mortality or birth weight. Some dams dosed with sertraline at either 20 or 80 mg/kg were observed to be hyperactive and aggressive during the first few days of dosing. Neither pre- nor postnatal sertraline dosing affected the quality of care given by dams to their pups. In a cross-fostering study, only 40% of pups born to dams dosed with sertraline (80 mg/kg) survived, whether they were raised by their birth mother or a saline-treated foster mother. Survival of the offspring of saline-treated dams was not adversely affected by cross-fostering to drug-treated dams. Cross-fostering studies were not done with the other selective uptake inhibitors. Venlafaxine reduced pup retrieval by dams, but this effect might be attributable to dysfunctional pups.

There appears to be a critical period during which dosing pregnant rats with these drugs increases pup mortality. Sertraline did not affect pup survival when given at 80 mg/kg during gestation days 0–15, but only half the pups survived when dams were

TABLE 2. Toxic Findings in Rat Pups Born to Dams Dosed with Selective Serotonin Reuptake Inhibitors during Gestation[a]

Drug Name	Control	Low Dose	Middle Dose	High Dose
Fluoxetine				
Dose	0	2	5	12.5
Survival	92	nr	87	61
Stillborn	7	nr	nr	14
Birth weight	—	100	100	83
Fluvoxamine				
Dose	0	5	20	80
Survival	96	83	83	75
Stillborn	nr	nr	nr	si
Birth weight	—	nr	nr	nr
Sertraline				
Dose	0	10	20	80
Survival	99	93	75	47
Stillborn	0	3	8	16
Birth weight	—	98	89	83
Paroxetine				
Dose	0	1	4	15
Survival	90	78	65	28
Stillborn	nr	nr	nr	nr
Birth weight	—	98	nr	nr

[a]These data were taken from reviews of reproductive toxicity studies submitted to the FDA by sponsors of the drugs. These drugs were given by oral gavage to pregnant Sprague-Dawley or Wistar-derived rats on day 15 of gestation through weaning, except for fluoxetine in which dosing began pre-mating and for paroxetine middle and high doses which were given only on the last 4 days of gestation and the first 4 postnatal days. Other notations as in TABLE 1.

Abbreviation: nr = not mentioned in the FDA review.

given the drug from day 0 through parturition. Paroxetine did not reduce pup survival when given to dams at 10 mg/kg starting on postnatal day 5.

The actual mechanism by which the deaths occurred is unclear. In some cases, entire litters were lost, but most frequently, most litters were affected by the loss of some pups. Most dead pups in the sertraline study did not have milk in their stomachs. The pattern of increased pup mortality, stillbirth rate, and lower birth weight in rat reproduction studies is unique to drugs that inhibit the reuptake of 5-HT. An electronic search of the "Physicians Desk Reference"[12] found information about reproductive toxicity with this pattern of effects only for those drugs that inhibit serotonin uptake. As noted earlier, drugs that inhibit the uptake of both 5-HT and dopamine (i.e., cocaine and mazindol) cause this pattern, but maternal fatalities also occur at doses that produce the pattern. The differing structures of the 5-HT uptake inhibitors suggest that a common toxic effect would be due to an exaggerated pharmacologic effect rather than to common interaction at a nonserotonergic locus. Prenatal exposure to fluoxetine is known to disrupt normal serotonergic neurotransmission.[13] Death may have resulted from undernutrition secondary to abnormal pup behavior, but this does not explain stillbirths. Disrupted nervous system development could alter cardiovascular and respiratory impulses, causing both stillbirths and early postnatal death. Abnormally high 5-HT levels can fatally disrupt breathing patterns in 4-day-old rat pups.[14] Victims of sudden infant death syndrome have elevated levels of 5-HT and dopamine metabolites in their cerebrospinal fluid.[15]

Increased pup mortality, stillbirths, and lower birth weights seem to be related to blockade of 5-HT transporters during development. Simultaneous blockade of the 5-HT and dopamine transporters, in the cases of cocaine and mazindol, increased the toxicity of 5-HT transporter blockade by also producing maternal death. NE transporter blockade probably does not contribute to pup or dam deaths. Bupropion, a dopamine uptake blocker and mild NE uptake blocker, was not toxic to either pups or dams at high doses.[16] Further study of this issue may reveal interesting interactions of the monoamines in their influence on development.

ACKNOWLEDGMENT

Kimberly Woodard is greatly appreciated for conducting the search of the "Physicians Desk Reference."

REFERENCES

1. Church, M. *et al.* 1990. Prenatal cocaine exposure in the Long-Evans rat. I. Dose-dependent effects on gestation, mortality, and postnatal maturation Neurotoxicol. Teratol. **12:** 327–334.
2. Wiggins, R & B. Ruiz 1990. Development under the influence of cocaine. I. A comparison of the effects of daily cocaine treatment and resultant undernutrition on pregnancy and early growth in a large population of rats Metab. Brain Dis. **5:** 85–99.
3. Pharmacologist Review of NDA 17–297, FOI Office, FDA, Rockville, MD 20857.
4. Meyer, J.S., L.P. Shearman & L.M. Collins. 1996. Monoamine transporters and the neurobehavioral teratology of cocaine. Pharmacol. Biochem. Behav. **55:** 585–593.
5. Pharmacologist Review of NDA 18-936, FOI Office, FDA, Rockville, MD 20857.
6. Pharmacologist Review of NDA 20-350, FOI Office, FDA, Rockville, MD 20857.
7. Pharmacologist Review of NDA 19-839, FOI Office, FDA, Rockville, MD 20857.
8. Pharmacologist Review of NDA 20-031, FOI Office, FDA, Rockville, MD 20857.
9. Pharmacologist Review of NDA 20-151, FOI Office, FDA, Rockville, MD 20857.
10. Pharmacologist Review of NDA 20-152, FOI Office, FDA, Rockville, MD 20857.
11. Vorhees, C.V. *et al.* 1994. A developmental neurotoxicity evaluation of the effects of prenatal exposure to fluoxetine in rats. Fund. App. Tox. **23:** 194–205.
12. PDR Electronic Library. 1997. Medical Economics Company, Montvale, NJ.
13. Cabrera, T.M. & G. Battaglia. Delayed decreases in brain 5-hydroxytryptamine$_{2A/2C}$ receptor density and function in male rat progeny following prenatal fluoxetine. J. Pharmacol. Exp. Ther. **269:** 637–645.
14. Hilaire, G., D. Morin, A.-M. Lajard & R. Monteau. 1993. Changes in serotonin metabolism may elicit obstructive apnoea in the newborn rat J. Physiol. **466:** 367–382.
15. Caroff, J., E. Girin, D. Alix, C. Cann-Moisan *et al.* 1992. Neurotransmission and sudden infant death syndrome. Study of cerebrospinal fluid. C. R. Acad. Sci. Paris **t. 314, Serie III:** 451–454.
16. Pharmacologist Review of NDA 18-644, FOI Office, FDA, Rockville, MD 20857.

Cocaine-Inhibited Neuronal Differentiation in NGF-Induced PC12 Cells and Altered C-fos Expression Are Reversed by C-fos Antisense Oligonucleotide[a]

DITZA A. ZACHOR,[b] JOHN F. MOORE, ANNE B. THEIBERT, AND ALAN K. PERCY

Department of Pediatrics and Neurobiology, University of Alabama at Birmingham, Birmingham, Alabama 35294-0017, USA

Cocaine is a major drug of abuse and involves 10–20% of urban pregnancies.[1] In previous studies we examined the effects of cocaine on PC12 cells, a well-characterized neuronal model.[2] Application of nerve growth factor (NGF) to PC12 cells induces morphologic and biochemical changes, resulting in differentiation to a sympathetic neuron-like phenotype. Cells stop dividing, extend neurites, and express neuronal genes.[3] Using this cellular model, we demonstrated that cocaine has direct dose-dependent inhibitory effects on NGF-induced neuronal differentiation without being toxic to the cells. Neurite outgrowth was significantly reduced upon exposure to cocaine levels commonly found in the blood of known drug users.[4] Partial recovery was noted in cells that were reexposed to NGF without cocaine.[5] NGF exerts its action through interaction with its high affinity surface receptor which leads to activation of its intrinsic tyrosine kinase and thereafter a cascade of intracellular signaling proteins. The latter eventually induce the transcriptional activation of specific immediate early genes (IEGs). Finally, activation of late genes occurs, and their protein products are responsible for the differentiated neuronal phenotype.[6] We concentrated on the stage of immediate early gene expression, as IEGs play a major role in regulating cell cycle and differentiation. Our hypothesis was that cocaine alters the expression of c-fos and therefore blocks NGF-mediated neurite extension.

METHODS

PC12 cells were grown in serum-free media to eliminate cocaine breakdown by serum enzymes. Cells were treated with NGF 20 ng/ml, a dose yielding 50% of the maximal response.[4] We determined the time course of c-fos expression in PC12 cells treated with NGF at the ED_{50} and cocaine 10 μg/ml, a moderately toxic dose. C-fos expression was measured at 0.5, 6, 24, 48, and 72 hours after exposure to NGF with and without cocaine by RT-PCR analysis. RNA was isolated from PC12 cells.[7] Total RNA was reverse transcribed using gene-specific primers to generate first-strand cDNA. The cDNA

[a] This work was supported by The Research Institute at The Children Hospital of Alabama Research Foundation Grant.

[b] Address for correspondence: Ditza A Zachor, The University of Alabama at Birmingham, 331C Sparks Building, 1720 Seventh Avenue, South, Birmingham, AL 35294-0017. Phone, 205/975-5508; fax, 205/975-2380; e-mail, dzachor@civmail.circ.uab.edu

was then amplified using multiplex PCR with the same gene-specific primers. The PCR products were separated out in an agarose gel and photographed, and relative band densities were determined. The densities of the amplified genes were proportional to their initial concentration in the cell system. C-fos was reported relative to cyclophilin mRNA to minimize any sample-to-sample variation.[8]

RESULTS

C-fos and cyclophilin expression pattern of PC12 cells treated with NGF differed from that of cells treated with NGF and cocaine over the exposure time (FIG. 1). During the first 6 hours, c-fos expression followed the same pattern in both groups. However, from 24–72 hours, c-fos expression in cocaine-treated cells exceeded that of control cells by 2–6 times. In NGF-treated control cells, c-fos expression declined after a rapid initial rise and returned to baseline levels after 24 hours. By contrast, c-fos expression in the cocaine-treated cells remained above the baseline expression during the entire treatment period.

To further explore the significance of the prolonged cocaine-induced c-fos expression, we treated PC12 cells with NGF, cocaine, and c-fos antisense in doses ranging from 0.2–10 μM to inactivate the gene.[9] Adding c-fos antisense to the media of cocaine-treated cells resulted in improved neuronal differentiation (FIG. 2). However, the c-fos antisense effect was only significant over a narrow concentration range.

DISCUSSION

The foregoing observations suggest that cocaine has striking effects on the temporal expression of c-fos in NGF-stimulated PC12 cells. Previous *in vivo* studies noted that cocaine also induced c-fos in rat striatal neurons after acute and chronic administration.[10] In PC12 cells, NGF induces only transient c-fos expression, whereas constitutive expression of c-fos and other immediate early genes blocks the NGF-mediated exit from the cell cycle and interferes with expression of late genes, resulting in impaired neurite extension.[11] C-fos antisense treatment significantly reduced the inhibitory effect of cocaine on neurite outgrowth. Therefore, cocaine inhibitory effects on NGF-induced neuronal differentiation may be attributed to cocaine's striking effects on the temporal

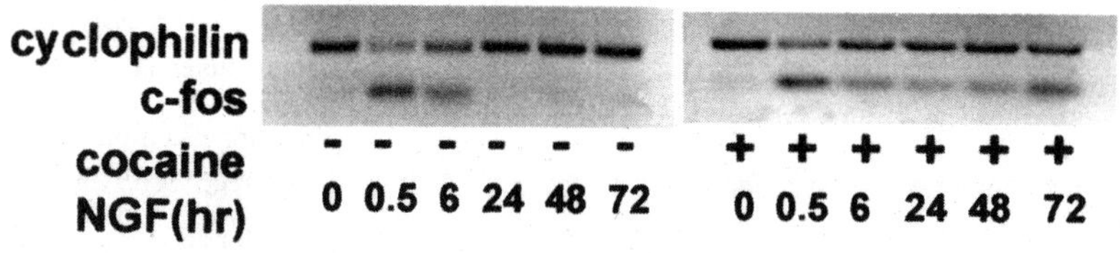

FIGURE 1. RT-PCR products of c-fos and cyclophilin are shown on agarose gel from control PC12 cells treated with nerve growth factor (NGF) and cells treated with cocaine and NGF. In both control and cocaine-treated cells, c-fos expression peaks after 0.5 hours. In control cells, c-fos expression declined rapidly and returned to baseline expression after 24 hours. By contrast, c-fos expression in cocaine-treated cells remained above baseline expression during the entire exposure time of 72 hours.

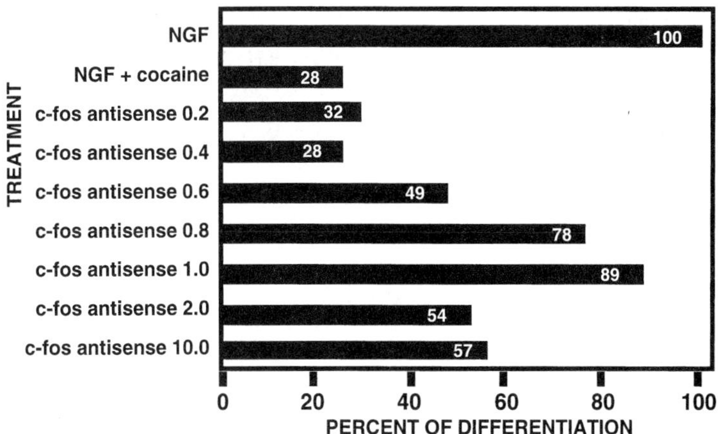

FIGURE 2. Effects of three types of treatments on NGF-induced neuronal differentiation in PC12 cells: a control group treated with NGF alone, a group treated with NGF and cocaine, and a third group treated with NGF, cocaine, and c-fos antisense (to inactivate c-fos expression). Cocaine inhibited neuronal differentiation, measured morphologically as cells bearing neurites longer than 1 cell diameter, to as low as 20% of the control cells. In the group treated with c-fos antisense, neuronal differentiation increased significantly to 89% of the control group only in a narrow concentration range between 0.6 and 2 μM.

expression of c-fos. Further studies will be required to explore the effects of cocaine on other immediate early genes and on other components of NGF signal transduction.

REFERENCES

1. Frank D.A., B.S. Zuckerman & H. Amaro. 1988. Cocaine use during pregnancy: Prevalence and correlates. Pediatrics **82:** 888–895.
2. Green, L.A. & A.S. Tischler. 1976. Establishment of a noradrenergic clonal line of rat adrenal pheochromocytoma cells which respond to nerve growth factor. Proc. Natl. Acad. Sci. USA **73:** 2424–2428.
3. Greenberg, E., L. A. Greene & E.B. Ziff. 1985. Nerve growth factor and epidermal growth factor changes in protooncogene transcription in PC12. J. Biol. Chem. **260:** 14101–14110.
4. Zachor, D. A., J. K Cherkes, C.T. Fay & I Ocrant. 1994. Cocaine differentially inhibits neuronal differentiation and proliferation in vitro. J. Clin. Invest. **93:** 1179–1185.
5. Zachor A.D., J.F. Moore, T.M. Smoot & A.K. Percy. 1996. Inhibitory effects of cocaine on NGF-induced neuronal differentiation: Incomplete reversibity after a critical time period. Brain Res. **729:** 270–272.
6. D'Arcangelo, G & S. Halegoua. 1993. A branched signaling pathway for nerve growth factor is revealed by Src-, Ras, and Raf-mediated gene induction. Mol. Cell. Biol. **13:** 3146–3155.
7. Chomczynski, P. & N. Sacchi. 1987. Single-step method of RNA isolation by acid guanidinium thiocyanate-phenol-chloroform extraction. Anal. Biochem. **162:** 156–159.
8. Ausubel, F. M. *et al.* Eds. 1995. Current Protocols in Molecular Biology. **2:** Unit 15.4 15.4.1–15.4.6. John Wiley & Sons, Inc. New York.
9. Majocha, R.E., S. Agrawal & J.Y. Tang. 1994. Modulation of PC12 cells response to

NGF by antisense oligonucleotide to amyloid precursor protein. Cell. & Mol. Neurobiol. **14:** 425–437.

10. MORATALLA, R., E.A. VICKERS, H.A. ROBERTSON, B.H. COCHRAN & A.M. GRAYBIE. 1993. Coordinated expression of c-fos and jun-B is induced in the rat striatum by cocaine. J. Neurosci. **13:** 423–433.
11. BRASELMANN, S., G. GERGERS, C. WRIGHTON, P. GRANINGER, G. SUPERTI-FURGA & M. BUSSLINGER. 1992. Identification of Fos target genes by the use of selective induction systems. J. Cell Sci. **16:** 97–109.

Central and Autonomic Nervous Systems' Signs Associated with *in Utero* Exposure to Cocaine/Opiates

HENRIETTA S. BADA,[a,j] CHARLES R. BAUER,[b] SEETHA SHANKARAN,[c] BARRY LESTER,[d] LINDA L. WRIGHT,[e] JOEL VERTER,[f] VINCENT L. SMERIGLIO,[g] LORETTA P. FINNEGAN,[h] AND PENELOPE L. MAZA[i]

[a]*The University of Tennessee, Memphis, Memphis, Tennessee 38163*
[b]*University of Miami, Miami, Florida*
[c]*Wayne State University, Detroit, Michigan*
[d]*Brown University, Providence, Rhode Island*
[e]*National Institute of Child Health and Human Development*
[f]*George Washington University, Washington, DC*
[g]*National Institute on Drug Abuse*
[h]*Center for Substance Abuse Treatment*
[i]*Administration of Children, Youth and Families*

Central nervous system (CNS) and autonomic nervous system (ANS) manifestations are reported in neonates born to mothers addicted during pregnancy to opiates, such as heroin and methadone.[1,2] These CNS and ANS signs comprise the manifestations reported with neonatal "abstinence syndrome".[3] However, variation in the reported prevalence of these manifestations is evident when *in utero* neonatal exposure primarily involves cocaine.[4,5]

METHODS

The objectives of this study were: (1) to determine the prevalence of CNS/ANS signs in neonates born to mothers who abused cocaine and/or opiates during pregnancy, and (2) to determine the prevalence of these signs with *in utero* exposure involving cocaine use only.

The study involved a multisite evaluation of the effects of maternal lifestyles on their infants' acute and long-term outcomes in 4 of the 12 participating centers of the National Institute of Child Health and Development Neonatal Research Network. The participating sites included Brown University (Providence, Rhode Island), University of Miami (Miami, Florida), The University of Tennessee, Memphis (Memphis, Tennessee), and Wayne State University (Detroit, Michigan). The Biostatistics Coordinating Center of George Washington University, Washington, DC, provided data management, research coordination, and statistical consultation/support.

The enrollment period was between May 1993 and May 1995. Eligibility for enrollment into the study included (1) birth weight greater than 500 g, (2) best obstetrical estimate of gestational age less than 43 weeks, (3) likelihood to survive, and (4) birth

[j]Address for correspondence: Henrietta S. Bada, MD, Newborn Center, 853 Jefferson Avenue, Room 201, Memphis, TN 38163. Phone, 901/448–5950; fax, 901/448–1691

within the stipulated time frame specific to each clinical site as determined by each site's number of live births and prevalence of drug use among pregnant women. Mothers were approached in the hospital for informed consent, and a brief interview was conducted to obtain a drug history during pregnancy and within a year prior to delivery.

After consent was obtained, meconium collection was begun, and the infant was assessed by a certified research nurse masked to the infant's drug exposure status. Infant assessment included determination of vital signs, growth measurements, and gestational age by the New Ballard examination, physical examination, and evaluation for the presence of CNS/ANS signs.

After discharge, both mother and infant's medical records were reviewed to obtain a summary of medical treatment, procedures, symptoms, and diagnoses. Meconium specimens were sent to a reference laboratory (El Sohly Laboratories, Oxford, Mississippi) for radioimmune assay, with subsequent confirmation of positive samples using gas chromatography/mass spectroscopy (GC/MS).

Infants were considered nonexposed (NON) when their mothers denied cocaine and opiate use during pregnancy and absence was confirmed by meconium analysis. Exposed infants (EXP) were those born to mothers who admitted to cocaine and/or opiate use during pregnancy or who denied cocaine and/or opiate use but meconium tested positive for metabolites of cocaine and/or opiates. For this report, exposure to cocaine only (C) indicated that mothers admitted to the use of cocaine only without opiates and confirmed by meconium analysis or a negative history, but meconium analysis confirmed the presence of only cocaine metabolites. Opiate exposure (OC) was defined as a maternal admission of opiate use with or without cocaine or a negative maternal history for drug use, but meconium analysis yielded positive results for opiates and its metabolites with or without the presence of cocaine metabolites.

Statistical methods included determination of prevalence of each of the CNS/ANS signs in the NON, EXP, C, and OC groups. The EXP, C, and OC groups were each compared against the nonexposed group by determination of odds ratios for each of the CNS/ANS signs and 95% confidence intervals. Multivariable analysis was carried

TABLE 1. Maternal and Infant Characteristics (%)

	NON (n = 7,442)	EXP (n = 1,185)	C (n = 977)	OC (n = 208)
Maternal Characteristics				
Black	48	76*	81*	53
Married	39	13*	11*	22*
Medicaid recipient	62	87*	89*	79*
Education ≤12 yr	71	84*	85*	77
Alcohol use (pregnancy)	31	69*	74*	46*
Smoker (pregnancy)	20	80*	82*	72*
Marijuana use (pregnancy)	5.0	37*	40*	22*
Infant characteristics				
Male	52	52	52	52
Gestational age 25–32 wk	9	16*	16*	15*
33–36 wk	14	26	27	23
37–42 wk	77	58	57	63
Birth weight 501–1,500 g	6	10*	10*	13*
1,501–2,500 g	16	33	33	28
>2,500 g	78	57	57	59

*p <0.01 compared to NON.

TABLE 2. Prevalence (%) of CNS/ANS Signs and Odds Ratios in the NON, EXP, C, and OC Groups

CNS/ANS	NON (n = 7,442)	EXP (n = 1,185)	C (n = 977)	OC (n = 208)	EXP/NON	C/NON	OC/NON
Signs	%	%	%	%	Odds Ratio (95% Confidence Interval)		
Hypertonia	0.8	3.2	2.0	9.6	4.27 (2.9–6.3)	2.5 (1.5–4.2)	13.8 (9.1–21.0)
Jittery, tremors	5.9	16.6	13.0	33.8	3.15 (2.6–3.8)	2.4 (1.9–2.9)	8.1 (6.2–10.6)
High-pitched cry	1.5	4.0	2.4	12.0	2.79 (2.0–4.0)	1.6 (1.04–2.6)	9.2 (6.2–13.6)
Difficult to console	1.0	2.9	1.8	8.6	3.10 (2.1–4.6)	1.9 (1.1–3.1)	9.7 (6.2–15.2)
Difficult to arouse	0.4	1.0	1.1	0.5	2.72 (1.4–5.2)	3.0 (1.5–5.9)	1.3 (0.2–9.8)
Irritability	5.8	14.9	11.3	32.3	2.86 (2.4–3.4)	2.1 (1.7–2.6)	7.8 (6.0–10.3)
Sneezing	3.1	4.2	3.0	8.2	1.36 (1.0–1.9)	1.1 (0.7–1.6)	2.8 (1.7–4.6)
Excessive suck	0.7	3.4	2.2	10.5	5.30 (3.6–7.8)	3.0 (1.8–5.0)	17.4 (11.7–25.8)
Nasal stuffiness	1.7	3.0	2.6	4.9	1.77 (1.2–2.6)	1.5 (1.0–2.4)	2.9 (1.6–5.6)
Hyperalertness	0.1	1.3	0.7	3.9	13.10 (6.6–26.3)	7.4 (3.0–18.0)	41.3 (22.3–76.3)

out using logistic regression models. Covariates chosen were the factors significantly different between exposed and nonexposed such as gestational age, race, birth weight, maternal marital status, prenatal care, marijuana use, alcohol use during pregnancy, abruptio placentae, smoking during pregnancy, known sexually transmitted diseases, education (highest grade completed), clinical site, and infant's postnatal age at examination. Odds ratios (EXP/NON, C/NON, OC/NON) for each of the CNS/ANS signs were derived from multivariable estimates.

There were 19,079 mother/infant dyads screened for recruitment into this study; 16,988 met eligibility criteria, and 11,811 consented to study participation. A total of 10,626 infants were born to mothers who denied use of cocaine and/or opiates during pregnancy. Of these infants, it was possible to collect adequate meconium in 7,442 infants to allow confirmation of a negative exposure history; these infants were therefore considered in the NON group. The remaining infants ($n = 3,184$) who had no meconium collected or inadequate meconium were excluded from the NON group. There were 1,185 infants who were born to mothers who admitted to abusing cocaine and/or opiates (EXP group). Exposure in 977 involved cocaine only (C group) and in 208 exposure involved opiates with or without cocaine (OC group). TABLE 2 shows the prevalence rates of CNS/ANS signs in the NON, EXP, C, and OC groups, odds ratios, and 95% confidence intervals. After multivariable analysis, the odds ratios changed little in magnitude.

SUMMARY

In summary, we found that the prevalence of CNS/ANS signs was significantly higher in the infants exposed to cocaine and/or opiates than in nonexposed infants. However, the prevalence of a large number of these signs was less than 5%. The prevalence rates of these signs are lower when exposure involved cocaine only; thus, their assessment has limited clinical utility.

REFERENCES

1. ROTHSTEIN, T. J. & J. B. GOULD. 1974. Born with a habit: Infants of drug addicted mothers. Pediatr. Clin. North Am. **21:** 307–321.
2. ROBERTS, R. J. 1984. Fetal and infant intoxication. *In* Drug Therapy in Infants: Pharmacologic Principles and Clinical Experience.: 322–383. W. B. Saunders. Philadelphia, PA.
3. FINNEGAN, L. P. 1985. Neonatal abstinence. *In* Current Therapy in Neonatal Perinatal Medicine. N. M. Nelson, Ed.: 262–270. B. C. Decker. Toronto, Canada; Philadelphia, PA.
4. NEUSPIEL, D. R. & S. C. HAMEL. 1991. Cocaine and infant behavior. Dev. Behav. Pediatr. **12:** 55–64.
5. YOUNG, S. L., H. J. VOSPER & S. A. PHILLIPS. 1992. Cocaine: Its effects on maternal and child health. Pharmacotherapy **12:** 2–17.

Index of Contributors